SECOND EDITION

AVIAN MEDICINE

For Elsevier:

Commissioning Editor: Joyce Rodenhuis
Development Editor: Rita Demetriou-Swanwick, Louisa Welch
Project Manager: Andrew Palfreyman
Designer: Sarah Russell
Illustrations Manager: Bruce Hogarth
Illustrator: Samantha Elmurst

SECOND EDITION

AVIAN MEDICINE

Edited by

Jaime Samour MVZ, PhD, Dip ECAMS

Director,
Wildlife Division,
Wrsan,
Abu Dhabi,
United Arab Emirates

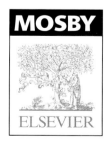

EDINBURGH   LONDON   NEW YORK   OXFORD   PHILADELPHIA   ST LOUIS   SYDNEY   TORONTO   2008

MOSBY
ELSEVIER

An imprint of Elsevier Limited

First published 2000
Reprinted 2003, 2004
Second edition 2008

ISBN 978 0 7234 3401 6

1005 364217

British Library Cataloguing in Publication Data
A catalogue record for this book is available from the British Library

Library of Congress Cataloging in Publication Data
A catalog record for this book is available from the Library of Congress

ELSEVIER your source for books,
journals and multimedia
in the health sciences

www.elsevierhealth.com

Working together to grow
libraries in developing countries

www.elsevier.com | www.bookaid.org | www.sabre.org

ELSEVIER   BOOK AID International   Sabre Foundation

The
Publisher's
policy is to use
**paper manufactured
from sustainable forests**

Printed in Spain

Contents

Contributors

M.M. APO, BSc, ACS
Wildlife Division, Wrsan,
Abu Dhabi, United Arab Emirates

T.A. Bailey, BSc, BVSc, MRCVS, Cert Zoo Med, Dip ECAMS,
MSc (Wild Animal Health), PhD
Dubai Falcon Hospital,
Dubai, United Arab Emirates

F. Cavalli, MD, Gen Rad
Radiodiagnostic Unit,
Department of Diagnostic Imaging,
Maggiore Hospital, Trieste,
Italy

M.E. Cooper, LLB, FLS
The University of the West Indies,
School of Veterinary Medicine,
St. Augustine,
Trinidad and Tobago

Professor J.E. Cooper, DTVM, FRCPath, FIBiol, FRCVS
Diplomate, European College of Veterinary
Pathologists,
Professor of Veterinary Pathology,
The University of the West Indies,
St. Augustine,
Trinidad and Tobago

L. Cruz-Martinez, DVM
Veterinary Resident,
The Raptor Center,
College of Veterinary Medicine,
University of Minnesota,
St. Paul, Minnesota,
USA

F.J. Dein, VMD, MS
USGS, National Wildlife Health Center

School of Veterinary Medicine,
University of Wisconsin–Madison,
Madison, Wisconsin,
USA

M. Delogu, DVM, PhD
Department of Public Veterinary Health and
Animal Pathology
Faculty of Veterinary Medicine, University of Bologna,
Italy

A. Di Somma, Dr Vet Med
Specialist in Small Animal Medicine
Dubai Falcon Hospital,
Dubai, United Arab Emirates

N.A. Forbes, BVetMed, CBiol MIBiol, Dip ECAMS,
FRCVS, RCVS
Specialist Zoo Animals and Wildlife Medicine (Avian),
Great Western Referrals, Swindon,
UK

N.H. Harcourt-Brown, BVSc, Dip ECAMS, FRCVS
Harrogate, Yorkshire,
UK

J.C. Howlett, RVN, BSc (Hons), Dip Nat Sci
National Avian Research Center,
Environment Agency,
Abu Dhabi, United Arab Emirates

P.J. Hudson, BSc, DPhil
Department of Biological and Molecular Sciences,
Institute of Biological Sciences,
University of Stirling, Stirling,
UK

S.J. Kellner Dr med vet, MRCVS, Cert VOphthal
Animal Eye Clinic, Frauenfeld,
Switzerland

I.F. Keymer, PhD, FRCVS, FRCPath, CBiol, DLSHTM
Edgefield
Melton Constable,
UK

Professor J.K. Kirkwood,
BVSc, PhD, MRCVS, C Biol FIBiol
Scientific Director, Universities Federation for Animal
Welfare,
Wheathampstead,
UK

Professor M.E. Krautwald Junghanns,
Dr med vet, Dr med habil, Dip ECAMS
Clinic for Birds and Reptiles,
University of Leipzig,
Germany

M.P.C. Lawton, B Vet Med, Cert VOphthal, Cert LAS, D Zoo
Med, CBiol MIBiol, FRCVS,
Specialist in Exotic Animal Medicine,
Exotic Animal Centre, Harold Wood,
UK

P.A. McKinney, MVB, Cert Zoo Med, MRCVS
Wildlife Protection Office,
Dubai, United Arab Emirates

C.G. Martinez, Lic Vet, MRCVS, MSc
Cheltenham,
UK

J.L. Naldo, DVM
Wildlife Division, Wrsan,
Abu Dhabi, United Arab Emirates

M.A. Peirce, PhD, CBiol FIBiol, FZS
MP International Consultancy, Bexhill-on-Sea
UK

M. Pees, Dr med vet, Dip ECAMS
Clinic for Birds and Reptiles,
University of Leipzig,
Germany

Professor P.T. Redig, DVM, PhD
Director, The Raptor Center, College of Veterinary
Medicine,
University of Minnesota,
St. Paul, Minnesota,
USA

J. Samour, MVZ, PhD, Dip ECAMS
Director, Wildlife Division, Wrsan,
Abu Dhabi, United Arab Emirates

C. Silvanose, BSc, DMLT, DCPath
Dubai Falcon Hospital,
Dubai, United Arab Emirates

P. Thorsen, DVM
Laboratory Animal Resource Center,
University of California San Francisco, San Francisco,
California,
USA

Professor U. Wernery, Priv Doz Dr Dr habil
Scientific Director, Central Veterinary Research
Laboratory,
Dubai, United Arab Emirates

P. Zucca, DVM, PhD
Department of Comparative Biomedical Sciences,
Faculty of Veterinary Medicine, University of Teramo,
Teramo,
Italy

Professor Emeritus P. Zwart, DVM, PhD
Professor in Diseases of Exotic Animals, Department
of Veterinary Pathology,
Utrecht University,
The Netherlands

Foreword

The production of a second edition of Avian Medicine is testimony to the success of the book and the quality of its contents. First published in 2000, it brought a new look to disseminating information about birds and their health. Beautifully illustrated, with much of the emphasis on species and situations that were different from more conventional North American and European volumes, Avian Medicine not only quickly caught the eye of veterinarians and biologists but rapidly became recognised as both a scientifically sound and a practically orientated authoritative text.

The Editor, Dr. Jaime Samour, has had a life-long interest in birds and other wildlife. Following university and post-graduate studies, he started in earnest to apply his veterinary training, practical skills and empathy with animals to promote the health, welfare and conservation of diverse creatures. Most of these species had previously attracted relatively little attention from the veterinary profession and therefore much needed to be done. In a career that has included spells as a lecturer, museum assistant, taxidermist, film consultant, expedition leader and park manager, as well as more conventional veterinary appointments, Jaime has managed to contribute much to our knowledge of the biology and care of a wide range of animals.

Jaime has an international background, having been born in El Salvador and then educated in Mexico and England. This has been strengthened through his many years of working as a veterinarian in the Middle East - Bahrain, Saudi Arabia and the United Arab Emirates. He has friends and colleagues all over the world which, coupled with his communication and language skills, means that he reads and refers to a wide array of literature. This is also reflected in his numerous publications, scientific papers, conference proceedings, articles, reports and several books.

For thousands of years birds have fascinated the human race. The Class Aves has served us well in many different ways, including the provision of companionship and assistance as well as being the source of eggs, meat and feathers. They have been both revered and feared in various cultures. The requirement to treat them humanely is stressed in both Christian and Muslim writings and in the teaching of the other great religions.

The need for this book has never been greater. Many of the world's 9000 species of bird are threatened in the wild by such factors as habitat destruction, unsustainable hunting, persecution, poisoning and infectious diseases. In captivity the maintenance of the health of birds is crucial and there is increasing international pressure, from the public and scientists alike, that their welfare should be paramount. Avian Medicine is a rich source of information for all those who work with birds, whether in the wild or in captivity, and I therefore warmly welcome this revised edition.

John E. Cooper DTVM, FRCPath, FIBiol, FRCVS
Diplomate, European College of Veterinary Pathologists
Professor of Veterinary Pathology,
The University of the West Indies,
St. Augustine,
Trinidad and Tobago

Acknowledgments

I should like to thank Professor J.E. Cooper, one of the founders of avian medicine, for his professional support throughout the years and for his encouragement to produce this book. His contagious enthusiasm and dedication to veterinary sciences have always been a source of inspiration in my career. I am grateful to Amado Azur, Tom Bailey, Judith Howlett, Nafeez Mohammed Jainudeen, Jesus Naldo and Christudas Silvanose, my colleagues and personal friends: without their understanding and support the production of this book would not have been possible. Thanks also to Dr. Ali Ridah, Dr. Ulrich Wernery, Mrs. Renate Wernery and all the technical staff at the Central Veterinary Research Laboratory, Dubai, United Arab Emirates for their friendship and technical collaboration throughout the years. I should also like to express my deep and most sincere gratitude to HE Mohammed Al-Bowardi, Managing Director of the Environment Agency (formerly Environmental Research and Wildlife Development Agency), Abu Dhabi, United Arab Emirates for his personal friendship and for his support for the clinical and research work of the Veterinary Science Department; to Mr. Abdullah Ghanem Al-Ghanem, Dr. Fahad Mohammed Al-Nafjan and Mr. Basil Al Abbasi for all their help and support during the establishment of the Fahad bin Sultan Falcon Center; to H. H. Sheikh Sultan bin Zayed Al Nahyan for his interest and dedication to the preservation of flora and fauna in Abu Dhabi; to Linda Duncan, Teri Merchant and the staff at Mosby Year Book Inc., St. Louis, USA and to Deborah Russell, Mark Sanderson, Philip Dauncey, Hilary Hewitt and all the editorial and production staff at Harcourt Publishers Ltd., London, UK, for their patience, dedication and understanding throughout the inception, preparation and completion of the first edition of this book; I am thankful to all contributors to the first edition for agreeing to update their sections with new material and for their continuing support for *Avian Medicine*; I am deeply indebted to Joyce Rodenhuis, Zoë A. Youd, Rita Demetriou-Swanwick and all the editorial and production staff at Elsevier Ltd., UK for their encouragement, assistance and incredible patience during the preparation of this second edition; finally I would like to acknowledge the invaluable assistance provided by Generoso Quiambao in producing a large part of the photographic material used in the second edition of this book.

x

Dedications

This book is dedicated to Mr. David M. Jones and Dr. Christine M. Hawkey, my mentors and friends in times when a helping hand and guidance in my professional career was needed. Your kindness, wisdom and professionalism are still a shining light on the path of my life. My heartfelt gratitude for your unstinting support, your deep understanding and for believing in me. Thank you for being who you are.

I also would like to dedicate this book to the memory of my father Oscar and mother Clarita, who devoted their entire lives to giving us a better future; to my sister Jeannette and brothers Oscar and wife Gilda, Eduardo and wife Charito, Carlos Roberto and wife Anita and to Hayde for sharing throughout the years all those precious moments with me. Finally, to my wife Merle, my sons Omar Ricardo and Adam and my daughters Miriam and Yasmeen with all the love a husband and a father can give… and to all of those who in one way or another believed in me and have made easier my voyage through life.

Jaime Samour
Abu Dhabi, United Arab Emirates, 2008

Preface to the second edition

One day a man walked by a large construction site where there was a flurry of activity around the building of a new church for the city. The man saw a laborer carrying bricks in a wheelbarrow and asked him, 'What are you doing?' The laborer looked at him, startled, and answered swiftly, 'I am carrying bricks.' The man continued walking and saw another laborer doing the same task and asked him the same question, 'What are you doing?' and the laborer, with a smile on his face, said 'I am earning bread for my family.' The man continued walking and saw another laborer, who was also carrying a large number of bricks in a wheelbarrow, and asked him, 'What are you doing?' and he answered proudly, 'I am building a cathedral.'

In the course of our professional lives we have to reflect and ask ourselves a similar question, 'What are we doing?' Are we working for the sake of working? Are we working in order to sustain our families? …or are we also working with more profound objectives in mind? As professionals we work with birds because we like and enjoy working with them and, indeed, this allows us to provide for our families …but as professionals we also have the responsibility to continue learning, as professionals we have the responsibility to improve our skills, as professionals we have the responsibility to strive for excellence in order to give others the best of us, and this is what we are intending to do with the second edition of *Avian Medicine* – to provide you with a new building block to help you develop your career.

I am deeply indebted and honored to have the participation of some of the most important figures of the avian medicine world as new contributors to the second edition of *Avian Medicine*. I am referring to the distinguished educator and prominent pathologist Professor John E. Cooper, together with Christudas Silvanose for the new section on Cytology, to my long-time friend and top avian specialist Neil Forbes for his outstanding contribution on Soft tissue surgery and to the world-renowned Professor Maria-Elisabeth Krautwald-Junghanns, together with newcomer Michael Pees, for the section on Ultrasonography. I am also deeply grateful to my dear friends Paolo Zucca, with newcomers Mauro Delogu and Fabio Cavalli, for their excellent contribution on Advanced anatomical imaging, and to Thomas A. Bailey and newcomers Antonio Di Somma and Celia Garcia Martinez for preparing the exceptional section on Image-intensified fluoroscopy. I also would like to thank Thomas A. Bailey for preparing the much-needed section on Biochemistry and Nigel Harcourt-Brown for contributing the interesting new section on Behavioral osteodystrophy.

I would like to acknowledge, in particular, the generous and unselfish assistance of my dear friend Tom Bailey for providing me with new ideas for the production of this edition, but above all, for his friendship and unwavering support throughout the years – thank you.

Jaime Samour
Abu Dhabi, United Arab Emirates, 2008

Preface to the first edition

For the past 25 years, clinicians and veterinary scientists from all over the world have contributed substantially to establish avian medicine as a rightful specialty of veterinary science. In this respect, significant advances have been made in the disciplines of therapeutics, anesthesia, surgery and diagnosis in birds and there appears to be no end to the vast number of publications portraying such achievements. From the humble beginnings with text books such as those from Arnall and Keymer (1975) and Cooper (1978), followed a few years later by those from Cooper and Greenwood (1981), Heidenreich (1982), Coles (1985), Harrison and Harrison (1986) and Burr (1987), to the most recent master pieces such as those by Redig *et al.*, (1993), Ritchie *et al.*, (1994), Beynon *et al.*, (1995), Ritchie (1995), Beynon *et al.*, (1996), Rosskopf and Woerpel (1996), Tully and Shane (1996), Altman *et al.*, (1997), Heidenreich (1997), Rupley (1997), Altman and Forbes (1998), Coles and Krautwald-Junghanns (1998), Olsen and Orosz (2000), Lumeij *et al.*, (2000), Tully *et al.*, (2000), Cooper (2002), Wernery *et al.*, (2004) and Harrison and Lightfoot (2006) all remarkable examples reflecting the current status of avian medicine.

Avian Medicine was conceived as a hybrid publication combining the formality of a textbook, the pictorial guide of an atlas and the practicality of a manual. While striving to provide the most up-to-date information available, we tried to keep heavy and continuous text to a minimum. Unfortunately, it was not possible to achieve this in all chapters, as some subjects are difficult to depict in a condensed manner or even to illustrate. However, throughout the book, the text is liberally sprinkled with information in the form of bullet points and tables in order to ease comprehension at a glance. Moreover, some sections include practical guidelines on the medical management of the single patient or flock, useful tips on clinical-laboratory diagnosis and suggested treatments. The Appendix section brings together data from a wide variety of species on hematology and blood chemistry reference values, sex-linked bodyweights,

incubation periods, commonly used pharmaceutics and other information relevant to avian practitioners. Some of the data contained in this section is unique and has never been published before.

The photographic material of *Avian Medicine* illustrates a wide diversity of clinic and pathologic cases from *A*(mazon parrot) to *Z*(ebra finch) in the avian world. Some of the photographs may be candidates to win competition prices, since they were obtained under 'studio' conditions, while others were taken by clinicians going about doing their job. Moreover, the photographs were procured from individuals engaged in clinical work in zoological parks, as well as from individuals involved in private practice and clinical research. The reader will also notice that many of the photographs are from the cultural characteristics and morphological appearance of the pathogens themselves rather than the pathological lesions caused by them. Diversity, I think, is the right word to describe the photographic material presented, being perhaps the best asset of *Avian Medicine*.

During the preparation of each individual section of *Avian Medicine* we tried to compile a set of bibliographical references as comprehensive as possible. In addition, some sections were also provided with a suggested list of additional papers or books to which the reader may refer to if needed. While attempting to provide an up-to-date reference list, we also intended to include references originated from both sides of the Atlantic, an important detail that we tried hard not to overlook. If we have failed in this respect and have omitted any important reference, we can assure you that this was not intentional and most sincerely beg your pardon.

Many of the early publications on avian medicine had a resolute tendency to focus almost exclusively on medical aspects and management of psittacine species. To many, avian medicine was synonymous to psittacine medicine. This may have been due to the fact that many of the early pioneers of avian medicine developed their expertise working with psittacines. In this respect, I would like to pay tribute to all those who through **xiii** hard work and vision created a true specialty. Their skills acquired and refined throughout the years and their dedication to psittacine medicine has been a source of inspiration to us all. However, times have changed and we have to change with it. There are now numerous colleagues, not only on both sides of the Atlantic, but also elsewhere in the world, working to promote avian medicine as a specialty on a wide variety of avian species. Thus, it is so refreshing to see recent publications devoted to pigeon, raptor, ratite and waterfowl medicine, as well as psittacine medicine.

Avian Medicine portrays general medical aspects in a wide variety of bird groups, but particular emphasis is made on some which are very seldom mentioned in the literature such as bustards. There is also a strong emphasis on falcons, since many of the contributors have been fortunate enough to have been exposed to raptor medicine while working in the Middle East and in many other parts of the world. In addition, *Avian Medicine* includes some topics rarely described in conventional text books such as neck dislocation and fracture and paresia and, unique subjects such as the use of TOBEC in the assessment of bodily condition in avian species or the novel orthopedic techniques described by Professor Patrick Redig. Some sections are just simply celebrations to the long years of service and extensive experience of the contributor, such as the Chapter on necropsy by Dr. Ian F. Keymer and the section on bacterial diseases by Professor Peernel Zwart. Other sections have offered the opportunity for many new comers, to express and share our experience with other members of the veterinary profession.

Avian Medicine was brought into existence as a pictorial and illustrated guide to some of the most important aspects of avian medicine. Our intent was to target veterinary medicine students by opening their eyes to the numerous facets of medicine in birds, but it was also intended for the busy veterinarian in mind. If, after going through the text and illustrations of this book, we were able to influence one single member of the veterinary profession to embrace avian medicine as specialty, our intention of producing this book would have been amply rewarded.

Jaime Samour   Riyadh, Kingdom of Saudi Arabia, 1998

Capture and handling

Capture

Thomas A. Bailey

Physical capture

In order to handle the avian patient for a physical examination it must first be captured (Figs. 1.1–1.5). The method of capture depends on the species, the age, the level of tameness, the size of the cage/enclosure and the environment.

Many patients are presented in small cages and before capture is attempted all perches, and food and water bowls should be removed. Small cage doors do not allow easy access and it may be more practical to remove the entire top of the cage in a darkened room. A paper towel or cloth may be used to serve as a visual barrier to enable the capture of many birds. Many tame cage-birds may have been trained to hop on to your finger or wrist, after which they can be grasped from behind. Trained raptors are best hooded before they are captured. Army night vision goggles (Fig. 1.5) can be used to capture birds by hand in darkened rooms or aviaries at night.

Birds housed in larger aviaries are often able to escape by flying or running and they may be captured using nets or corrals. A single bird in a small aviary can be captured by hand by one person if the bird is tame or by using a net by one or more people if the bird is of a nervous temperament. Nets may be used either with or without a handle. The decision regarding whether to use a handle will depend on the available space within the aviary. The catcher should push the bird into a corner before closing in and netting the bird. If the bird attempts to run or fly past the catcher the net should be placed in front of it, so that the bird runs or flies into it. Care should be taken when netting flying birds so as not to cause any injuries. In all cases, if there is any doubt the catcher should allow the bird to pass by. Once netted the bird should be carefully removed and either held in the hands or placed in a box or carrier. While removing the bird from the net, special attention should be paid to the feet, head and carpometacarpal joints to ensure that they are not entangled in the netting as the bird is pulled out.

In larger aviaries, flocks of birds may be caught by making a corral from shade cloth. This should be hung or fastened to extensible metal poles and shaped into a blind-ended funnel with a wide mouth and a small circular catching area at the blind end. Some larger species, such as kori bustards (*Ardeotis kori*), may best be captured by cornering and grabbing them by hand. However, even with such large birds a net placed over their head and upper body makes capture easier and therefore less stressful for the bird. Specialized texts should be referred to for the capture of ratites.

Examples of devices for the capture of free-living birds include the following:

- Walk or swim-in traps (wildfowl)
- Cannon or rocket nets (wildfowl, gamebirds and ostriches)
- Balchatri (raptors)
- Boma (ratites)
- Pop-up corral (ostriches)
- Doghaza (raptors).

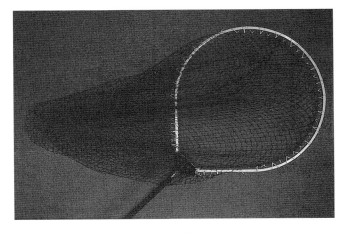

Fig. 1.1 A net for capturing medium-sized birds.

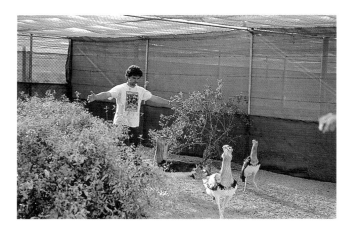

Fig. 1.2 Larger species of bird can be pushed towards a corner where they can be captured.

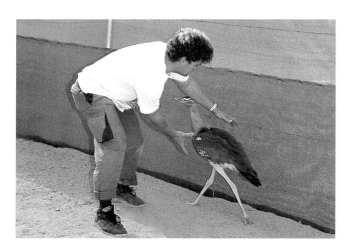

Fig. 1.3 Kori bustards (*Ardeotis kori*) may be captured when they pass between the handler and the side of an enclosure.

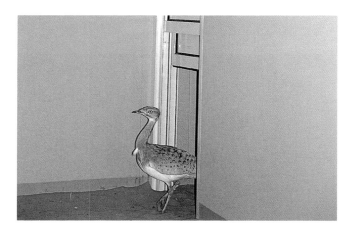

Fig. 1.4 The use of sliding gates facilitates moving birds, such as houbara bustards (*Chlamydotis undulata*), from one quarter to another. Using this system, a bird can be singled out from a larger group to ease physical capture.

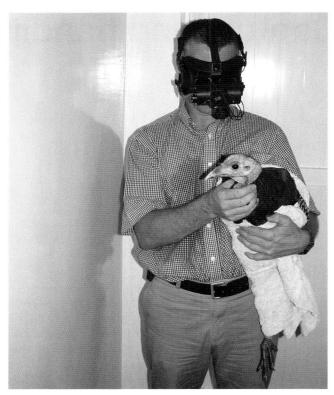

Fig. 1.5 Army night vision goggles can be used to capture birds, such as this wild turkey (*Meleagris gallopavo*), by hand in darkened rooms or aviaries at night.

Trapping-related injuries are not uncommon and before attempting to trap free-living birds, veterinarians should be familiar with local wildlife regulations and should ensure familiarity with the particular trapping method that is to be used.

FURTHER READING

Austin DH, Peoples TE, Williams LE (1972) Procedures for capturing and handling live wild turkeys. *Southeastern Association of Game and Fish Commissioners* **26**: 222–236.

Cooper JE (1991) Caged and wild birds. In: Anderson RS, Edney AT (eds) *Practical Animal Handling*, pp. 147–155. Pergamon Press, Oxford.

Forbes NA (1996) Examination, basic investigations and handling. In: Beynon PH, Forbes NA, Harcourt-Brown NH (eds) *Manual of Raptors, Pigeons and Waterfowl*, pp. 17–29. British Small Animal Veterinary Association Ltd, Cheltenham.

Fowler ME (1995) *Restraint and Handling of Wild and Domestic Animals*. Iowa State University Press, Ames, IO.

Sleigh I, Samour JH (1996) *The National Avian Research Centre Birdcare Manual – management techniques for a collection of bustards* (Otididae). Internal Report, National Avian Research Centre, Abu Dhabi.

Sonsthagen TF (1991) *Restraint of Domestic Animals*, pp. 131–137. American Veterinary Publications, Goleta, CA.

White J (1990) Raptor restraint. *Journal of the Association of Avian Veterinarians* **4**: 91–92.

Chemical capture

Drugged baits were first used by J.L. Daude in 1942 to capture pest birds in France and are considered to be the most effective method for capturing free-living birds, particularly gamebirds and waterfowl (Jessup, 1982). Larger birds such as ratites may be chemically immobilized, under both captive and field conditions, using blow guns or pole syringes to deliver intramuscular drugs.

Avian veterinarians may be involved in the capture of free-living birds for the following reasons:

- Biomedical studies
- Disease control
- Game management
- Nuisance animal control
- Population control
- Ringing and biological studies
- Translocation.

Baited food items include corn, eggs and meat for the capture of granivorous; gruiformes and waterfowl; and corvids and raptors, respectively (Jessup, 1982; Garner, 1988; Stouffer and Caccamise, 1991; Belant and Seamans, 1997; Hayes *et al.*, 2003). Their use has been reported in the following species:

- American crows (*Corvus brachyrhynchos*)
- Canada geese (*Branta canadensis*)
- Doves (*Zenaidura macroura*)
- Ducks (*Anas platyrhynchos*)
- Harris hawk (*Parabuteo uncinatus*)
- Pheasants (*Phasianus colchicus*)
- Red-winged blackbirds (*Agelaius phoeniceus*)
- Sandhill cranes (*Grus canadensis*)
- Wild turkey (*Meleagris gallopavo*)
- Wood pigeons (*Columba palumbus*).

Dose rates for some oral drugs are presented in Table 1.1. Combinations of drugs have also been used (Jessup, 1982; Cyr and Brunet, 1992), for example diazepam and alpha-chloralose in waterfowl (0.3–0.4 g and 0.1–0.12 g per cup of bait, respectively), and alpha-chloralose and secobarbital in red-winged blackbirds (*Agelaius phoeniceus*) (0.02–0.025 mg and 0.025–0.03 mg, respectively). Although oral ketamine has been used to successfully sedate an escaped raptor (Garner, 1988), it was not found to be effective for capturing turkeys (Clutton, 1988). The use of 1–2 grains of pentobarbital mixed with bread has also been reported to immobilize free-living ducks sufficiently for capture within 15–20 min (Harrison, 1986).

When drugged baits are used it is difficult to control the dose and rate of absorption of drugs that have been ingested, because of range of sizes and species, health status, the weather and other environmental conditions. Complications can also occur in sedated individuals that are not captured, including:

- Hypothermia
- Hyperthermia
- Overdose
- Suffocation
- Aspiration pneumonia
- Drowning
- Predation
- Peer-inflicted trauma.

Once the sedated birds have been caught they may have to be confined to a recovery pen until the effects of the drug have worn off. If birds are overdosed they can often be saved if an incision is made in the crop, the drugged

TABLE 1.1 Drugs given as oral baits that have been used to capture free-living birds			
Agent	**Species**	**Dose**	**Reference**
Alpha-chloralose	Wild turkey	2.0 g pcb	Williams *et al.*, 1973; Austin *et al.*, 1972
	Sandhill cranes	0.45–0.5 g pcb	Williams and Phillips, 1973
	Canada geese	0.25 g pcb	Jessup, 1982
	American crows	0.035 g per egg	Stouffer and Caccamise, 1991
Ketamine	Harris hawk	100 mg/kg meat	Garner, 1988
Methoxymol	Wild turkey	4.0 g pcb	Jessup, 1982
	Doves	1.5–2.0 g pcb	
Methohexital	Doves	1.25 g pcb	Jessup, 1982
Sodium amobarbital	Mallards	900 mg	Gordon, 1977
Sodium secobarbital	Doves	1.25 g pcb	Jessup, 1982
Tribromoethanol	Wild turkey	10–11 g	Williams *et al.*, 1973
	Pheasant	40 g/kg corn	Fredrickson and Trautman, 1978

pcb = per cup of bait (usually corn).

bait is removed and the crop is washed out (Jessup, 1982). Although it is impossible to control the amount of bait that is consumed, drugged baits are considered to cause less than 10% mortality when properly applied (Jessup, 1982). Before attempting oral baiting, veterinarians should be familiar with local wildlife regulations and the relevant literature.

Intramuscular ketamine has even been given by remote-controlled injector placed in the nest of breeding seabirds (Wilson and Wilson, 1989). African penguins (*Spheniscus demersus*), cape gannets (*Morus capensis*), bank cormorants (*Phalacrocorax neglectus*) and crowned cormorants (*Phalacrocorax coronatus*) anesthetized in this way were easily captured for biological studies.

Combinations of etorphine hydrochloride, acepromazine maleate, ketamine, medetomidate hydrochloride and xylazine hydrochloride delivered intramuscularly by blow guns or pole syringes have been used to immobilize ostriches (*Struthio camelus*) and double wattled cassowary (*Casuarius casuarius*) (Robinson and Fairfield, 1974; Stoskopf *et al.*, 1982; Samour *et al.*, 1990; Ostrowski and Ancrenaz, 1995). Grobler and Begg (1997) reported the capture of three free-living kori bustards in the Kruger National Park using a dart gun and 1 mg etorphine hydrochloride and 100 mg ketamine/5 mg xylazine to catch two birds (reversed with antidotes to etorphine and xylazine) and 30 mg/kg zolazepam/tiletamine (Zoletil) for one bird. Birds captured with Zoletil need to be kept in a quiet, dark, undisturbed environment for at least 12 h and based on their experience Grobler and Begg (1997) recommended using 20–25 mg/kg. Complications of chemical immobilization include hyperthermia, regurgitation, inhalation pneumonia and myopathy. Dosages of chemical agents used to anesthetize ratites are dealt with in depth by Keffen (1993) and Tully and Shane (1996).

REFERENCES

Austin DH, Peoples TE, Williams LE (1972) Procedures for capturing and handling live wild turkeys. *Southeastern Association of Game and Fish Commissioners* **26**: 222–236.

Belant JL, Seamans TW (1997) Comparison of three formulations of alpha-chloralose for immobilization of Canada geese. *Journal of Wildlife Diseases* **33**: 606–610.

Clutton RE (1988) Inefficacy of oral ketamine for chemical restraint in turkeys. *Journal of Wildlife Diseases* **24**: 380–381.

Cyr A, Brunet J (1992) Anesthetization of captive red-winged black-birds with mixtures of alpha-chloralose and secobarbital. *Journal of Zoo and Wildlife Medicine* **24**: 80–82.

Garner MM (1988) Use of an oral immobilizing agent to capture a Harris hawk (*Parabuteo uncinatus*). *Journal of Raptor Research* **22**: 70–71.

Grobler DG, Begg S (1997) Chemical capture of kori bustard (*Ardeotis kori*). *Newsletter of the World Association of Wildlife Veterinarians.*

Harrison GJ (1986) Anesthesiology. In: Harrison GJ, Harrison LR (eds) *Clinical Avian Medicine and Surgery*, pp. 549–559. WB Saunders, Philadelphia.

Hayes MA, Hartup BK, Pittman JM, Barzen JA (2003) Capture of sandhill cranes using alpha-chloralose. *Journal of Wildlife Diseases* **39**: 859–868.

Jessup DA (1982) Chemical capture of upland game birds and waterfowl: oral anesthetics. In: Nielsen L, Haigh JC, Fowler ME (eds) *Chemical Immobilization of North America Wildlife*, pp. 214–226. Wisconsin Humane Society, Milwaukee, WI.

Keffen RH (1993) The ostrich *Struthio camelus*: capture, care, accommodation, and transportation. In: McKenzie AA (ed.) *The Capture and Care Manual*, pp. 634–652. Wildlife Decision Support Services, Pretoria, South Africa.

Ostrowski S, Ancrenaz M (1995) Chemical immobilisation of rednecked ostriches (*Struthio camelus*) under field conditions. *Veterinary Record* **136**: 145–147.

Robinson PT, Fairfield J (1974) Immobilization of an ostrich with ketamine HCl. *Journal of Zoo and Wild Animal Medicine* **5**: 11.

Samour JH, Irwin-Davies J, Faraj E (1990) Chemical immobilisation in ostriches (*Struthio camelus*) using etorphine hydrochloride. *Veterinary Record* **127**: 575–576.

Stoskopf MJ, Beall FB, Ensley PK, Neely E (1982) Immobilization of large ratites: blue necked ostrich (*Struthio camelus australis*) and double wattled cassowary (*Casuarius casuarius*), with hematologic and serum chemistry data. *Journal of Zoo and Wild Animal Medicine* **13**: 160–168.

Stouffer PC, Caccamise DF (1991) Capturing American crows using alpha-chloralose. *Journal of Field Ornithology* **62**: 450–453.

Tully TN, Shane SM (1996) *Ratite Management, Medicine and Surgery*, pp. 79–94. Krieger Publishing, Malabar, FL.

Williams LE, Phillips RW (1973) Capturing sandhill cranes with alpha-chloralose. *Journal of Wildlife Management* **37**: 94–97.

Williams LE, Austin DH, Peoples TE, Phillips RW (1973) Capturing turkeys with oral drugs. *National Wild Turkey Symposium.*

Wilson RP, Wilson M-PTJ (1989) A minimal-stress bird-capture technique. *Journal of Wildlife Management* **53**: 77–80.

FURTHER READING

Fredrickson LF, Trautman CG (1978) Use of drugs for capturing and handling pheasants. *Journal of Wildlife Management* **42**: 690–693.

Gordon B (1977) The use of sodium amobarbital for waterfowl capture. *Journal of Zoo and Wild Animal Medicine* **8**: 34–35.

Loibl MF, Clutton RE, Marx BD, McGrath CJ (1988) Alpha-chloralose as a capture and restraint agent of birds: therapeutic index determination in the chicken. *Journal of Wildlife Diseases* **24**: 684–687.

Handling

Thomas A. Bailey

Immobilization

The main aims when restraining birds are to immobilize the wings, and to control the legs and heads of species with powerful feet and beaks (Figs 1.6–1.34). Time spent practicing techniques, along with a dose of patience, are essential prerequisites to minimize the possibility of injury and stress to both the bird and handler. Items

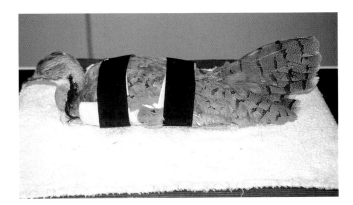

Fig. 1.6 Restraining a houbara bustard (*Chlamydotis undulata*) using a body harness. These are manufactured from a medium-weight canvas cloth and Velcro® bands. These devices are commonly used to restrain large waterfowl, such as swans, and some birds of prey.

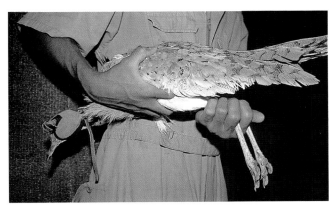

Fig. 1.7 Restraint technique for a medium-sized houbara bustard with a falconry hood in place.

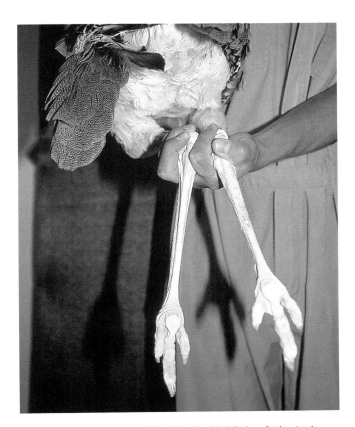

Fig. 1.8 Correct procedure for holding the hind limbs of a bustard, by placing one or two fingers between them.

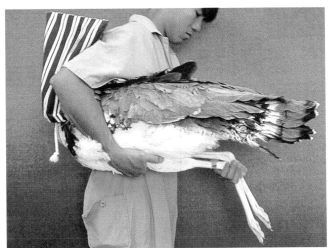

Fig. 1.9 Restraint technique for a large kori bustard (*Ardeotis kori*) with a cloth hood in place.

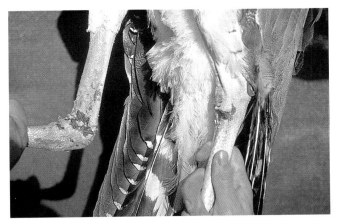

Fig. 1.10 Superficial pressure damage to the skin on the medial aspect of the hocks of a kori bustard after incorrect handling.

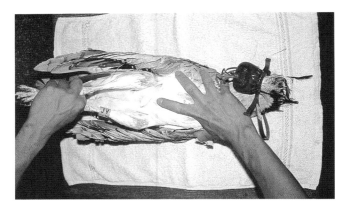

Fig. 1.11 Restraining a houbara bustard in dorsal recumbency on a padded cushion to enable venepuncture.

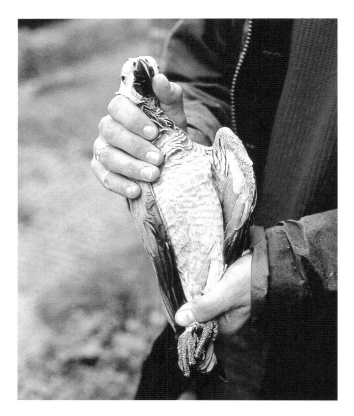

Fig. 1.12 Correct method of restraint of an African gray parrot (*Psittacus erithacus*). (Courtesy of Mr. A. Jones).

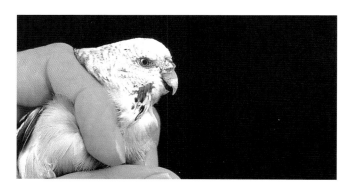

Fig. 1.13 Correct method of restraint for examination of a budgerigar (*Melopsittacus undulatus*). (Courtesy of Mr. A. Jones).

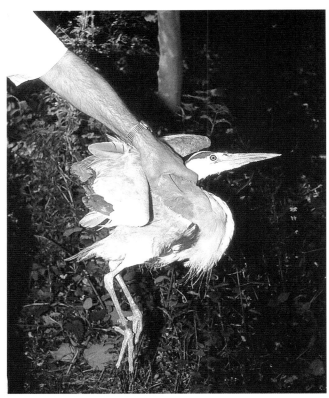

Fig. 1.14 Heron (*Ardea cinerea*) restrained in one hand controlling wings, neck and beak, leaving the other hand free to examine the bird or treat. (Courtesy of Mr. A. Jones).

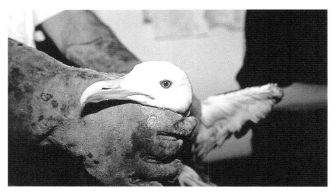

Fig. 1.15 Gulls will often attempt to stab with their beaks, and it may be necessary to place an elastic band on the beak. (Courtesy of Mr. A. Jones).

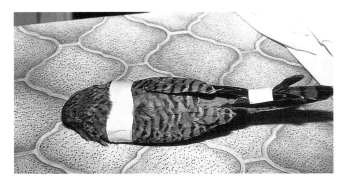

Fig. 1.16 Masking tape has been used to help immobilize a common kestrel (*Falco tinnunculus*) as a first aid remedy to secure the wings temporarily following wing fracture, until such time as a more precise fracture fixation could be performed. (Courtesy of Mr. A. Jones).

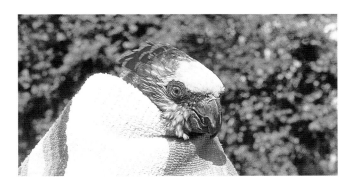

Fig. 1.17 Hawkhead parrot (*Deroptyus accipitrinus*) restrained in a towel. (Courtesy of Mr. A. Jones).

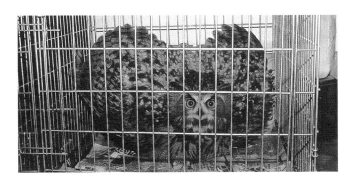

Fig. 1.18 European eagle owl (*Bubo bubo*) threat display. The approach to handling a bird will vary according to the species and the temperament of the bird!. (Courtesy of Mr. A. Jones).

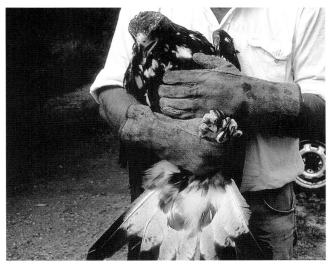

Fig. 1.19 Potentially dangerous birds such as this golden eagle (*Aquila chrysaetos*) should be restrained with gloves. (Courtesy of Mr. A. Jones). In addition, female handlers should also wear a leather apron whenever handling large raptors.

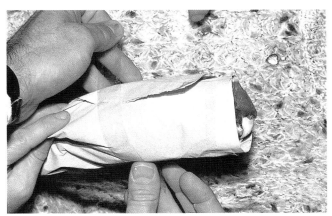

Fig. 1.20 Wrapping a psittacine in a paper towel while recovering from anesthesia. (Courtesy of Mr. A. Jones).

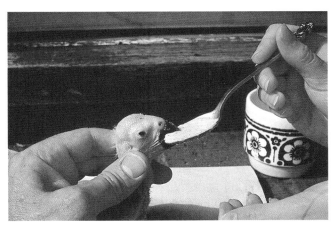

Fig. 1.21 Restraint of a neonatal parrot for hand-feeding. (Courtesy of Mr. A. Jones).

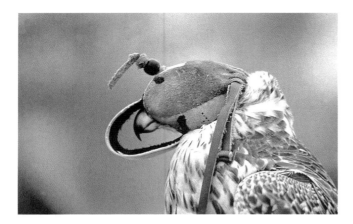

Fig. 1.22 Saker falcon (*Falco cherrug*) with an adapted hood to prevent self-inflicted injuries. (Courtesy of Dr. J. Samour).

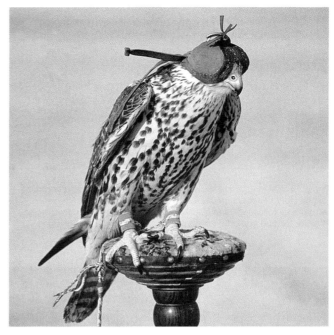

Fig. 1.23 Saker falcon with a hood on a Middle Eastern style block. (Courtesy of Dr. J. Samour).

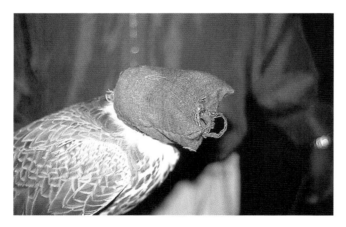

Fig. 1.24 In an emergency, a hood may need to be improvised. (Courtesy of Dr. J. Samour).

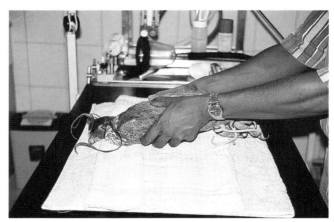

Fig. 1.25 Correct way of 'casting' a falcon. The operator grabs the hooded bird from the sides holding the wings firmly and placing the thumbs at the back of the falcon. The falcon has been cast on a soft towel. Note the 'tea towel' already in place to wrap the body. (Courtesy of Dr. J. Samour).

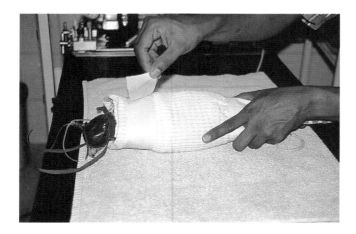

Fig. 1.26 Correct way of wrapping a falcon using a 'tea towel' and masking tape. Care should be exercised with the talons at all times. (Courtesy of Dr. J. Samour).

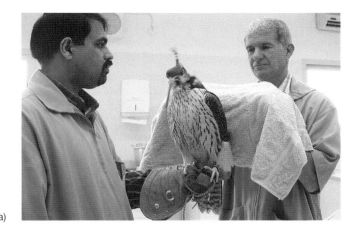

(a)

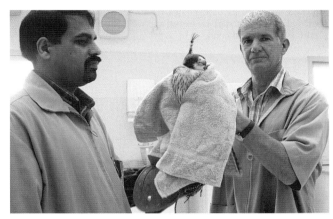

(b)

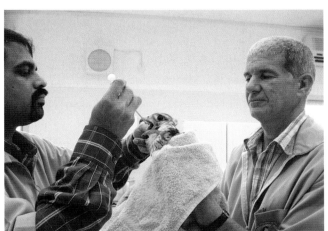

(c)

Fig. 1.27 Restraining a hooded falcon using a towel. (a) The assistant is holding the hooded falcon on his gloved hand. The operator holds a soft towel ready to place it around the body of the bird. (b) The operator wraps the towel around the body of the bird and holds the falcon firmly. (c) The assistant has removed the glove from his hand and can now proceed with administering oral medication to the falcon.

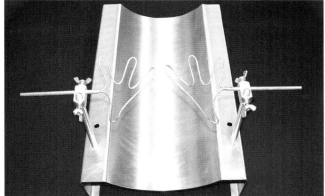

(a)

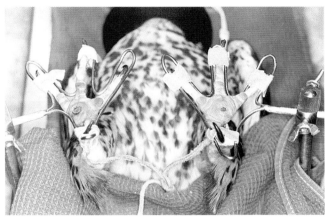

(b)

Fig. 1.28 (a) Customized restraint device for surgery on the avian foot. (b) The device used to immobilize the feet of a falcon prior to bumblefoot surgery. (Courtesy of Dr. J. Samour).

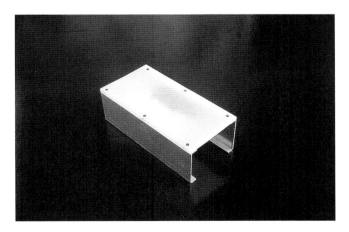

Fig. 1.29 Operating table (20 × 15 × 10 cm) used for surgical procedures in small birds (< 50 g). Note that the sides are made of aluminum and the top is made of Perspex molded to accommodate the shape of the body. The table can be placed over a heating pad to maintain a suitable temperature during surgery. (Courtesy of Dr. J. Samour).

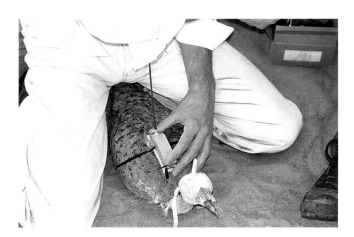

Fig. 1.30 Free-living birds, such as this houbara bustard, may need to be restrained to assist with placing satellite transmitters for field biologists. (Courtesy of Dr. J. Samour).

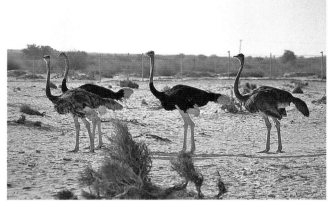

Fig. 1.33 Ostriches (*Struthio camelus*) are very dangerous birds and should always be handled by expert and well trained personnel. (Courtesy of Dr. J. Samour).

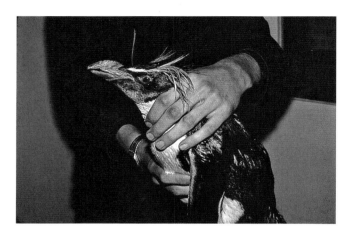

Fig. 1.31 Restraining a rockhopper penguin (*Eudyptes chrysocome*). (Courtesy of Dr. J. Samour).

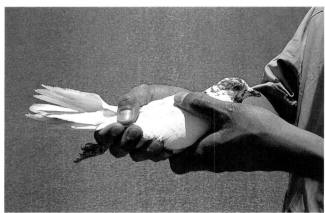

Fig. 1.34 Correct method of restraint of a domestic pigeon (*Columba livia*).

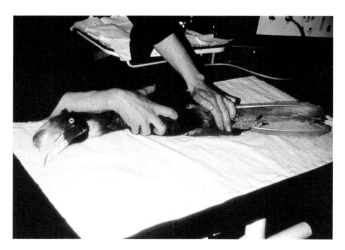

Fig. 1.32 Restraining a hornbill. (Courtesy of Dr. J. Samour).

of equipment that are used to assist in the restraint of birds for physical examination are listed in Table 1.2.

The strategies for resisting human handling vary between bird species. Hawks generally tend to use their feet to resist the handler while falcons, imprinted birds of prey, vultures, some eagles and some owls are likely to bite as well as 'foot' the handler. Larger birds, such as swans, can cause injuries with their wings, while ratites have a dangerous kick. Knowing what the strategy of the animal is likely to be may assist the handler in making split-second decisions that are necessary to restrain a bird safely. Recommended techniques for the handling and restraint of different groups of birds are given in Table 1.3. Further specialized information on handling techniques for different species of birds may be gleaned from the texts listed in the bibliography.

TABLE 1.2 Equipment that may facilitate the handling and restraint of birds

Equipment	Purpose	Comments
Cardboard tubing	In which to place bird so as to minimize struggling and to facilitate weighing and other procedures	Often used by field biologists. The bird appears quieter and less easily stressed
Cloth bag, sack, stocking or pillow case	As above	Care must be taken not to asphyxiate or damage the bird. If cloth material is used it should be washed and autoclaved between each bird to prevent transmission of infections
Cork or rubber tubing	Can be placed over bills that have a sharp tip to reduce potential damage to handler's face	
Ear protectors	To prevent hearing loss that can occur from repeated exposure to screaming patients	
Elastic bands and sticky tape	To seal beak and protect the handler	Remember that the bird can still stab, and to remove the band or tape before release
Foot-wraps	To immobilize the feet of birds of prey	Place a roll of cotton or gauze on the footpad and wrap the feet with a non-adhesive wrap to immobilize the talons
Forked stick or handlebars	To fend off large ostriches or other ratites	
Gloves	Reduction of damage to handler	Avoid unless essential. Should not be used to restrain psittacines or passerines. Use thin gloves wherever possible. Elbow length gloves can be useful for large, aggressive birds
Harness and other devices	To restrain birds so as to minimize struggling and facilitate procedures	The 'Guba' is a design used to restrain falconers' birds, while 'swan jackets' have been designed for restraining large waterfowl
Hoods	To cover the head of a diurnal bird in order to minimize struggling and facilitate procedures	A standard method of quieting and restraining falconers' birds and can be used to advantage in many other species. A loose cloth bag or sock can be used if a well-fitted hood is not available. Falconry hoods must fit the bird well
Padded examination table	Birds should be examined on a soft surface in order to prevent trauma as the bird struggles	Blankets, towels, covered cushions or foam may be used
Padded sheets of plywood or Plexiglas	Such shields are used to allow handlers to move large, fractious ratites	Handlers should be prepared to withstand solid blows to the board
Paper or cloth towels	To wrap around bird in order to facilitate handling and permit restraint	Paper towels are better because they can be discarded after use. Material should be washed and autoclaved between each bird, as above
Safety glasses	To protect the face and eyes of the handler	May be considered when dealing with aggressive birds such as storks or herons
Stanchions or 'plucking boxes'	Used to restrain ostriches for feather harvesting	

Source: modified from: Cooper JE (1991) Caged and wild birds. In: Anderson RS, Edney AT (eds). *Practical Animal Handling*, pp. 147–155. Pergamon Press, Oxford.

Restraining devices made up of medium-weight canvas and Velcro® straps have been designed and successfully used in bustards (Fig. 1.6) and other species such as swans and large birds of prey (Harris and Brown, 2003). These devices protect the birds from trauma within transport boxes or crates and protect the integrity of the feathers.

Birds are highly sensitive to stress, and incorrect handling can cause:

- Temporary or permanent limb paresia or paralysis
- Hyperthermia
- Fractures of legs or wings
- Skin lacerations, bruising and feather loss
- Luxation of the tibiotarsal bones
- Dislocation of the cervical vertebrae
- Compression of the flexible trachea and internal organs
- Progression of a disease process and even death.

Before attempting to catch and handle small and obviously sick birds, it is wise to warn the owner that there is a risk that the bird may suddenly die of heart failure. Birds that are brought in from the wild are unaccustomed to humans and because of this handlers must consider the effects of stress and minimize restraint time.

TABLE 1.3 Methods of handling and restraint of various groups of birds

Bird group	Handling technique	Additional comments
Small passerines	Place the head between two fingers so that the body rests in the palm of the hand, or it can be restrained by holding the head gently between the thumb and first finger	May stab or bite with beak; thin gloves will help to minimize effect. Elastic band or sticky tape may be used to seal beak
Large passerines	Hold with two hands, round wings	
Small psittacines	As for small passerines	
Large psittacines	As for large passerines	
Small and medium-sized birds of prey	As for large passerines. Falconry hoods are very helpful in blocking visual stimuli and have a calming effect	Raptors will often grasp air with their feet when restrained and it is important not to allow them to puncture themselves with their talons (use foot-wraps)
Large birds of prey	As for small and medium birds of prey. Can use a cloth towel to grasp round wings. Alternatively catch while perching by seizing legs and quickly turning the bird upside down: the wings will usually be extended but can be readily folded into the body	Use heavy gloves and wear appropriate falconers' equipment. Vultures may regurgitate food from their crop when handled
Pigeons and doves	As for small and large passerines. Pigeon fanciers prefer to hold birds with one hand around the base of the tail	Rarely bite or scratch. Inclined to defecate during handling. Feathers easily lost
Small waterfowl	Can be restrained by their wings or by grasping the back and wings and using the thumb and fingers to restrain the feet	Heavy-bodied species should not be carried by using the wings or feet alone
Large waterfowl	The base of both wings should be grasped with one hand while the other hand and arm supports the body. These birds may be carried under one arm, with their head facing to the back. The arm is wrapped around the wings and a hand is used to support the body and control the legs	Some geese have sharp claws and powerful legs and cause scratches. Swans and geese may flap wings which may deliver painful blows, and prove difficult to restrain. These species should not be carried by the wings alone, since temporary or permanent brachial paralysis may ensue
Gamebirds	In the larger species the base of the wing is fixed with one hand and the legs are controlled with the other hand. The abdomen should be supported from below	Never restrain gamebirds by the feathers alone – the whole body must be secured to prevent a shock molt. Cocks with spurs can injure handlers and the beak also serve as a weapon
Waders, herons, storks, flamingoes, cranes	As above depending on size. Grasp neck of herons, storks and cranes first in order to restrain head. When the bird is picked up the legs should be extended parallel to the ground. It is important to place one or two fingers or a rolled towel between the hocks to prevent injuries	May stab with beak: protect eyes and exposed skin. Handle with care as long legs and wings are prone to damage. Storks and cranes have strong legs and will kick. The margins of the blunt bill of the flamingo are serrated and can lacerate fingers or arms. Storks may regurgitate food when handled
Bustards	As above depending on size	Rarely bite or scratch. Inclined to defecate during handling. Feathers easily lost. Handle with care as long legs are prone to damage, including fractures. Some species have strong legs and will kick
Gulls, terns, petrels, shearwaters	As above depending on size	Gulls very likely to stab with beak: always use an elastic band. All this group inclined to vomit during handling and fulmars may regurgitate oil
Ratites	Small or immature ratites can be caught by grasping the legs firmly and picking the bird off the ground. Large ratites are handled by catching the head and pulling it forward and down until the vision of the animal is blocked. Additional handlers grasp the wings from the sides and place pressure in a downward direction to prevent the bird from jumping. More steady pressure will cause the bird to sit down	Darkness (hooding or subdued lighting) is one of the best restraint techniques, which may be used in ratites of all sizes. Manual restraint of ratites is potentially dangerous to both the handler and the animal. Ratites can react rapidly when frightened and can jump and flail with their legs. Male ostriches can be more dangerous during the breeding season
Hummingbirds	Most easily restrained and transported wrapped in cloth jackets with their heads protruding so that they can be fed	
Penguins	*Spheniscus* penguins and most crested penguins should be restrained by grasping them suddenly by the neck and hoisting them into the air at the length of the arm. The feet can be controlled with the other hand. From this position the bird can be supported on the lap of the handlers and examined thoroughly	These birds can pummel an aggressor with their powerful flippers, which can be painful

Source: modified from: Cooper JE (1991) Caged and wild birds. In: Anderson RS, Edney AT (eds) *Practical Animal Handling*, pp. 147–155. Pergamon Press, Oxford.

Transport

Birds should be transported in a secure, darkened and well ventilated container (Figs 1.35–1.38). Containers should have ventilation holes low on their sides (to minimize light at eye level) and have a new piece of carpet, rubber matting (which has the advantage that it can be disinfected and reused), or similar material on the floor to allow the bird adequate grip. Straw, peat or hay should be avoided as bedding because of the risk of contamination with spores of *Aspergillus* sp. The container must be free of sharp edges or protrusions that could

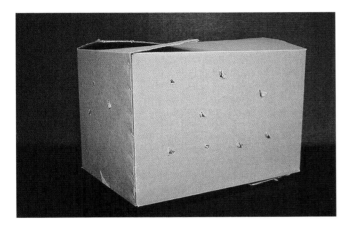

Fig. 1.35 Cardboard box for transporting medium-sized birds. One of the main advantages of cardboard (or similar material) boxes is that they are relatively cheap and can be incinerated after use.

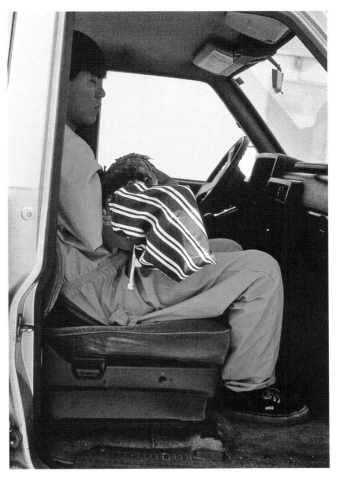

Fig. 1.36 For short journeys, large birds may be manually restrained and transported by car.

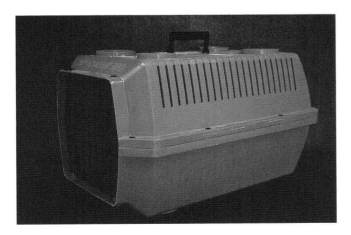

Fig. 1.37 Commercial pet carriers may be used to transport medium-sized birds, such as houbara bustards (*Chlamydotis undulata*). To reduce the risk of birds slipping while in the carrier, a piece of rubber matting is attached to the base. A piece of hessian sacking may be used to cover the front grid to reduce disturbance to the bird and effectively darken the carrier.

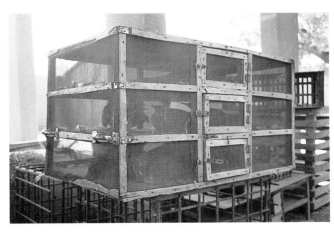

Fig. 1.38 Three-tiered crates are often used to transport poultry, houbara bustards, ducks, partridge and many other avian species in the Middle East. The birds are transported long distances in such cramped, overcrowded conditions and may arrive in a weakened state.

cause injury. Padding the ceiling and sides of a container can reduce injuries. The bird should be maintained at an ambient temperature of 21.1–26.6°C (70–80°F) and should never be left unattended. The size of the container should not permit wing flapping but must allow the bird room to stand up in a natural position and turn around.

The transport requirements of birds vary greatly between different groups. Pigeons and smaller waterfowl can be carried in small disposable cardboard boxes. Long-legged birds such as flamingoes must not only be able to stand up in transit but also have their bodies supported ventrally, for example by a sling, in order to prevent collapse. Swans and large geese may be restrained in purpose-made restraints. Free-living raptors can be transported in small, strong cardboard boxes. Falconers' birds can be transported hooded on cadges or on the fist of the falconer. Passerines and psittacine birds can be transported in their cages but should have the water dish emptied. Toys and all but one perch should be removed, and a blanket can be placed over the cage to provide darkness. Crates for transporting wildfowl need to have good ventilation and a receptacle for water (if the trip is for more than a few hours). Adult ratites can be transported in a shipping crate or an enclosed horse trailer, while young ratites can be transported in pet carriers. Transporting at night is recommended for birds such as ratites, as they are calmer and subject to less thermal stress. Further specialized information on handling different species of birds may be gleaned from the texts listed in the bibliography.

Containers that have been previously used to transport birds must be cleaned and disinfected before re-use. Wooden crates are not ideal for transporting birds as they are difficult to disinfect. Carrier specifications for international air transportation of birds are set by the International Air Transport Association (IATA 1998).

REFERENCES

Cooper JE (1991) Caged and wild birds. In: Anderson RS, Edney AT (eds). *Practical Animal Handling*, pp. 147–155. Pergamon Press, Oxford.

Harris JM, Brown B (2003) A restraint and transportation device for raptors. *Proceedings of the Association of Avian Veterinarians*, Pittsburgh, pp. 91–93.

IATA (1998) *Live Animal Regulations*, 25th edn. International Air Transport Association, Geneva. Webpage: http://www.iata.org/index.asp

FURTHER READING

Cooper JE, Hutchinson MF (1985) *Manual of Exotic Pets*. British Small Animal Veterinary Association, Cheltenham.

Forbes NA (1996) Examination, basic investigations and handling. In: Beynon PH, Forbes NA, Harcourt-Brown NH (eds) *Manual of Raptors, Pigeons and Waterfowl*, pp. 17–29. British Small Animal Veterinary Association, Cheltenham.

Fowler ME (1986) *Zoo and Wild Animal Medicine*, 2nd edn. WB Saunders, Philadelphia.

Jensen JM (1993) Ratite handling and restraint. In: Fowler ME (ed.) *Zoo and Wild Animal Medicine, Current Therapy 3*, pp. 198–200. WB Saunders, Philadelphia.

Mouser M (1996) Restraint and handling of the emu. In: Tully TN, Shane SM (eds) *Ratite Management, Medicine and Surgery*, pp. 41–45. Krieger Publishing, Malabar, FL.

Ritchie BW, Harrison GJ, Harrison LR (1994) *Avian Medicine: Principles and Application*. Wingers Publishing, Lake Worth, FL.

Sleigh I, Samour JH (1996) *The National Avian Research Centre Birdcare Manual – management techniques for a collection of bustards* (Otididae). National Avian Research Centre Internal Report, Abu Dhabi.

Sonsthagen TF (1991) *Restraint of Domestic Animals*, pp. 131–137. American Veterinary Publications, Goleta, CA.

Wade JR (1996) Restraint and handling of the ostrich. In: Tully TN, Shane SM (eds) *Ratite Management, Medicine and Surgery*, pp. 37–40. Krieger Publishing, Malabar, FL.

White J (1990) Raptor restraint. *Journal of the Association of Avian Veterinarians* 4: 91–92.

Clinical examination

2

General considerations

Jaime Samour

Clinical examination is a key part of the diagnosis of diseases of birds. It implies handling and restraint of the bird in order to carry out the necessary investigations.

Even before a bird is handled for examination, there are important prerequisites. The first of these is to ensure that one has as full a case history as possible. This should include information not only about the bird(s) itself but also about the environment in which the bird lives and the management to which it is subjected. It may be advisable for the clinician to visit the premises or, at the very least, see the cage and accessories before an attempt is made at clinical examination. Supporting tests such as examination of feces or of food remains in the cage, or analysis of possible toxic material may usefully precede clinical examination and give some guidance as to further investigations that may be necessary. Following collation and analysis of history and records, the bird(s) should be observed. Observation implies that the bird is not handled or restrained but is carefully watched (Figs 2.1–2.7). There are many ways of observing a bird and the method chosen will depend upon the circumstances, the facilities, the purpose of the procedure, etc. In general terms, observation can be divided into two types: 1) with the bird aware of the observer's presence and 2) with the bird unaware of the observer's presence. Ideally, a bird should be subjected to both, since neither one will necessarily provide all the relevant information. Thus, certain behavioral traits may be exhibited by a bird when it is alone and the observer is not apparently in the vicinity but may not be shown when the same observer is in view, when the behavioral traits may be suppressed. Conversely, some traits are exhibited when a person is present, especially those that are psychological and that can be triggered by human presence or other stimuli. Therefore, whenever possible, the patient should be observed first without being aware and then subsequently when it is aware of the observer's presence. The first of these is best carried out using a peephole observation panel through which the bird can be watched, preferably in its own environment. An alternative method is to film the behavior of the bird using a video camera or closed-circuit television. However, caution must still be exercised, since a bird that is not accustomed to a video camera or similar equipment may exhibit atypical behavior in response.

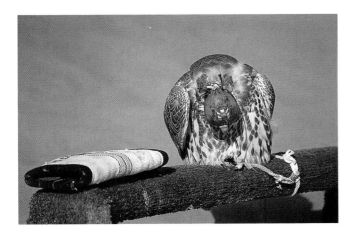

Fig. 2.1 The avian clinician has to be familiar with the basic biology of the different species. In the photograph, this gyrfalcon (*Falco rusticolus*) may appear, to the untrained eye, to be in mortal agony and about to drop dead. The answer is very simple, the bird is sleeping! Gyrfalcons, unlike other falcons, have a tendency to bend the body and tuck the head very low in the early hours of the day if they are still sleepy.

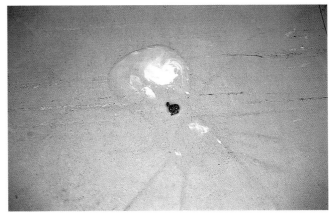

Fig. 2.2 Normal mutes of a falcon. Note the normal abundant watery/urate part and the solid dark-brown/black part. Differences in the consistency and appearance may reflect general disease.

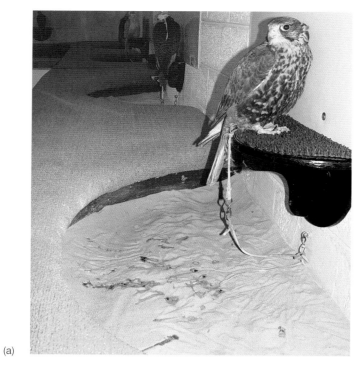

(a)

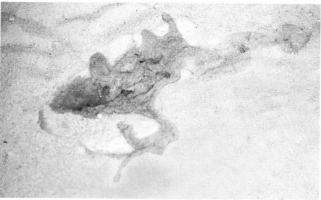

(b)

Fig. 2.3 The falcon shown in (a) was admitted with a complaint of passing of metallic green-colored urates. On radiological examination the liver was found to be severely enlarged. Subsequent liver biopsy and histopathology analysis confirmed the diagnosis of severe hepatic amyloidosis. This medical disorder is characterized by gradual weight loss and biliverdinuria. The photographs show the mutes passed overnight. (b) Close-up photograph of the mute of the falcon in (a). Note the metallic green color of the urates.

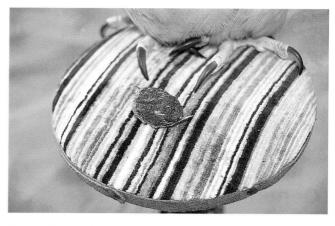

Fig. 2.4 Casting of pellets is a normal physiological aspect of the digestive system of birds of prey. The regurgitated pellets of birds of prey are formed in the gizzard and contain indigestible elements of the diet such as bone fragments, feathers and fur.

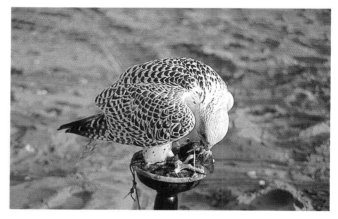

Fig. 2.5 A clinically normal falcon will show immediate interest in its food and will normally eat fast and actively.

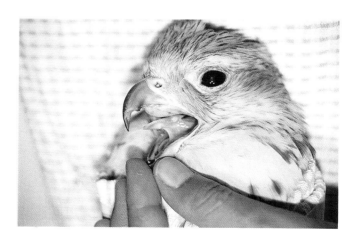

Fig. 2.6 While eating, a falcon with clinical trichomoniasis will very often shred pieces of meat and toss them away. Note the large trichomoniasis caseous growth located in the nasal cavity and protruding through the hard palate.

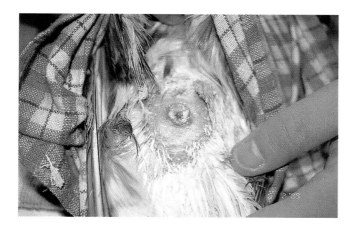

Fig. 2.7 An unusual clinical case in a saker falcon (*Falco cherrug*) showing an abdominal hernia. The only sign shown by the bird was the inability to expel the mutes without soiling the feathers.

Observation with the patient aware is far easier to carry out but even so must be performed in a systematic and logical way. The bird should be observed from a distance initially and only subsequently approached. The response of the bird to the presence of a person or to stimuli such as sound should be noted, but the general attitude or composure of the bird should also be recorded. It is most important that observation is carried out of the bird as a whole – which means, for example, that both eyes should be observed, both nostrils, the right side of the bird, the left side of the bird, back view, front view, etc. (Fig. 2.5). If this approach is not followed, mistakes can ensue. A bird may even attempt to disguise clinical signs by, for example, only turning one side of its head (one eye) to the observer, thus protecting and concealing the other eye, which may be partly closed, or discharging, or have a corneal ulcer. During observation other parameters may also be measured, for instance respiration rate. The breathing movements, often indicated by a bobbing of the tail, will be more easily and accurately recorded at this stage before the bird is handled. Indeed, there is merit in recording the respiration rate during initial observation (patient unaware), during subsequent observation (patient aware) and finally when the patient is handled for clinical examination. Such a comparison can often yield important information.

Generally speaking, observation should be carried out by the veterinary surgeon alone, without others present. The influence of proximity to humans is thus lessened and the clinician is able to concentrate on the task in hand. There are occasions, however, when observation with the owner can be beneficial. Examples are when there is a psychological disorder and the veterinarian believes that this may be triggered by the presence or actions of the owner or when a particular behavioral trait can only be demonstrated with the assistance of the owner. For instance, a parrot may come out of its cage and show a particular trait when encouraged to do so by the owner, but not otherwise.

The advantage of videotaping the behavior of the bird, both before and after it is aware of the observer's presence, is that the recording can be reviewed time and time again. It can also be used at a later date to monitor the progress of the bird or for educational purposes for clients or students.

Clinical history

Jaime Samour

In avian practice, veterinary surgeons are normally confronted with the individual pet bird in their surgery, but a visit to inspect a single bird or a flock where it is kept is often necessary. In both cases, a comprehensive and well detailed clinical history, gathered from the owner or keeping staff, is essential for the establishment of an accurate diagnosis. However, the inquiry has to be conducted in a methodical and systematic way. This is of paramount importance, since a well organized data collection exercise creates a good impression and achieves its objectives in a relatively short time. Very often, diagnostic mistakes are made by omitting a basic question or by overlooking one aspect in the management of a bird or a flock.

The collection of a clinical history in avian practice is very similar to and has many aspects in common with the gathering of information in general veterinary practice (Figs 2.8–2.10). However, clinical signs in mammals are more conspicuous to owners or keeping staff than those in birds. Therefore, careful, methodical and logical questioning is essential when dealing with birds.

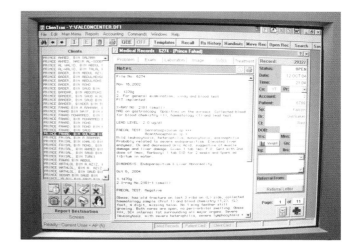

Fig. 2.8 Sophisticated medical databases are very popular nowadays for record keeping in busy clinical practices. This commercially available program (Clientrax®a) is a comprehensive database able to handle the medical and financial records of patients and owners. Conversely, tailor-made databases can be made to suit the particular need to the practice, breeding or research facility.

Fahad bin Sultan Falcon Center

Clinical Record Form

Record No [_____]

Patient data (please fill/tick✓)

Name: [_____] Species:[_____] Sex: M (   ) F (   )

Age: Juvenile (   ) Adult (   )   Colour:[_____] Origin: Wild-caught (   ) Captive bred (   )

PIT No [_____] Ring No: [_____]

Owner data (please fill/tick✓)

Owner [_____]

Falconer [_____]

Contact numbers: Office/home [_____] Mobile[_____]

Owner account No [_____] City [_____] Country [_____]

Clinical history

Date	Weight	Medical history/treatment

Fig. 2.9 A simple and compact clinical form used at the Fahad bin Sultan Falcon Center. This form can be adapted for routine clinical work in other avian species.

Fahad bin Sultan Falcon Center

Clinical Pathology Form - Hematology

Record No [_____]

Submission information (please fill/tick✓)

Collection date [_____] Time of collection [_____] Health status: Normal ( ) Abnormal ( )

Specimen: Blood - EDTA ( ) Blood - Heparin ( ) Blood - smear ( ) Restraint: Manual ( ) Chemical ( ) Type [_____]

Fasting time: <3 hrs ( ) 3–6 hrs ( ) 6–12 hrs ( ) 12–24 hrs ( ) 24–48 hrs ( ) >48 hrs ( ) Unknown ( )

Submission reason: Clinical ( ) Quarantine ( ) Health screen ( ) PME ( ) Others [_____]

Clinical summary [_____]

Tests required: Profile No 1 ( ), Profile No 2 ( ), Profile No 3 ( ), Profile No 4 ( ). Please specify individual tests on table

Laboratory use only

Analysis information (please fill/tick✓)

Date examined [_____/_____/_____] Time examined [_____] Lab sample ID [_____]

Storage condition: Fresh 0–3 hrs ( ) Refrigerated <24 hrs ( ) Refrigerated >24 hrs ( )

Specimen appearance: Normal ( ) Abnormal: Hemolytic ( ) Icteric ( ) Lipemic ( )

Analysis results (please select individual test required)			Normal range (Absolute value)			
Analysis	Results (Absolute)	Results (%)	Saker	Peregrine	Gyr	Lanner
RBC (x10^{12}/1)			2.54–3.96	2.95–3.94	3.1–5.1	2.6–3.9
Hb (g/dl)			11.5–16.5	11.8–18.8	16.0–21.2	12.2–17.1
PCV (%)			38–49	37–53	44–59	37–53
MCV (fl)			124–147	118–146	106.1–162.3	127–150
MCH (pg)			41.4–45.4	40–48.4	39.2–59.6	42.3–48.8
MCHC (g/dl)			30.4–34.9	31.9–35.2	35.5–37.8	31.7–35.3
WBC (x10^9/1)			3.8–11.5	3.3–11	4.2–10.8	3.5–11
Heterophils (x10^9/1)			2.6–5.85	1.4–8.55	2.3–8.8	1.65–8.8
Lymphocytes (x10^9/1)			0.8–4.25	1.1–3.3	0.5–2.4	1.1–5.13
Monocytes (x10^9/1)			0–0.8	0.1–0.86	0.03–0.9	0–0.9
Eosinophils (x10^9/1)			0–0.02	0–0.3	0.0–0.6	0–0.2
Basophils (x10^9/1)			0–0.45	0–0.64	0.0–0.3	0–0.45
Thrombocytes (x10^9/1)			12–25	6–46	12.7–29.9	5–40
Fibrinogen (gl)			1.78–4.7	<4.2	1.7–5.6	<4

Film findings

Note:
- Profile No 1. - WBC count, aemoglobin estimation, film examination for differential and blood cell morphology.
- Profile No 2. - WBC count, RBC count, PCV, hemoglobin estimation, film examination for differential, blood cell morphology and haemoparasites.
- Profile No 3. - WBC count, RBC count, PCV, hemoglobin estimation, MCV, MCH, MCHC, film examination for differential, blood cell morphology and hemoparasites and fibrinogen..
- Profile No 4. - Individual hematology tests.

Fig. 2.10 A more complex and sophisticated clinical laboratory diagnostic form used at the laboratory of the Fahad bin Sultan Falcon Center. The filling up of such complex forms is made easier by including 'fill up spaces' and 'tick boxes'. Established normal values are also included to ease the interpretation of results.

Initially, it is important to collect basic information related to the owner and the patient as follows:

Owner data

- Name
- Address
- Contact numbers (house/office/mobile telephone, fax)
- E-mail.

Patient data

- Species
- Sex
- Age
- Identification (name, passive induced transponder [PIT], ring, tattoo)
- Origin/source
- Duration of ownership.

The first step in obtaining a clinical history is to inquire about the purpose of the visit. The patient may be presented, or the inspection of the flock may be requested, for a routine health assessment or because of a medical condition. This question has to be asked in a courteous manner, since it is essential to create a suitable impression and provide confidence for further questioning.

The second step is to gather clinical information relevant to the medical condition. It is always advisable to begin with general questions, proceeding to more particular or specific ones. It is also highly recommended for veterinary surgeons interested in avian practice to be familiar with the biology of the most common avian species. This would certainly help to address all questions correctly and to avoid making important mistakes. For instance, the practitioner should know whether the species exhibits sexual dimorphism, its normal feeding habits and its breeding season before beginning to ask relevant questions. A reassuring smile will encourage owners or keeping staff to talk. Allow them to talk while listening attentively and do not interrupt abruptly to ask further questions. Patience and politeness are key psychological factors in clinical history collection. Important aspects to consider during the gathering of the clinical history include general clinical details, housing and feeding.

General clinical details

- Clinical signs (symptoms)
- Duration of ailment/disease
- Attitude of bird
- Performance (flight)
- Food passage from crop to stomach (Falconiformes)
- Regurgitation/vomition

- Casting (Falconiformes)
- Consistency of feces and appearance
- Changes in plumage/molting
- Bodyweight
- Reproductive status
- Medication/treatments.

Housing

- Type of cage/enclosure/aviary
- Size (height, length and width)
- Structural materials (poles, netting)
- Vegetation (trees, shrubs, ground cover plants, edible plants)
- Location of cage/aviary in relation to other buildings/disturbance
- Cage furniture/appliances (perches/ledges/nesting boxes)
- Floor of aviary (substrate/contours of floor)
- Feeding utensils (feeding/watering)
- Companions (number/sex)
- Contact with feral or free-living birds.

Feeding

- Type of diet
- Changes in the diet
- Food source and storage
- Appetite
- Water consumption.

Obviously, not all these questions are relevant to all situations. The veterinary surgeon should, therefore, conduct the inquiry according to the species, the clinical condition and the general circumstances of the case.

FURTHER READING

Brown SA (1996) Taking an accurate patient history. In: Rosskopf WJ Jr, Woerpel RW (eds) *Diseases of Cage and Aviary Birds*, 3rd edn, pp. 242–244. Williams & Wilkins, Baltimore.

Forbes NA (1996) Examination, basic investigations and handling. In: Beynon PH, Forbes NA, Harcourt-Brown NH (eds) *Manual of Raptors, Pigeons and Waterfowl*, pp. 17–29. British Small Animal Veterinary Association, Cheltenham.

Harrison GJ, Ritchie BW (1994) Making distinctions in the physical examination. In: Ritchie BW, Harrison GJ, Harrison LR (eds) *Avian Medicine: Principles and Application*, pp. 144–175. Wingers Publishing, Lake Worth, FL.

Physical examination

Jaime Samour

Physical examination implies that the bird is handled or restrained. These, in turn, can be distinguished. Handling means that the bird is touched but is not necessarily physically restrained so that its movements and activity are curtailed. Thus, a pet budgerigar may be handled in the sense that it climbs or stands on the hand, or a trained hawk (falcon) may be handled in the sense that it sits on the fist of its owner.

In both cases, a certain amount of examination can be carried out and it may even be possible to take samples. In many other cases, however, physical restraint is necessary, ranging from grasping a small cage-bird in the hand by use of a net or strong gloves or wrapping a bird in a towel or similar material. By definition, the more a bird is restrained the less 'normal' it is likely to be and this can complicate examination and interpretation of findings. However, the bird that is wrapped in a towel for examination may well be attempting to bite the handler, may have an accelerated respiration and heart rate and may not respond normally to visual or other stimuli. Therefore, the extent to which forceful restraint is carried out should be limited, certainly at the beginning of the examination, so that relatively reliable data can be obtained. The impact of handling and restraint can be reduced in a number of ways, for example by use of subdued light or by applying a hood or cloth bag to the head of the bird. In some cases, it may prove necessary or desirable to anesthetize (sedate) a bird lightly to facilitate clinical examination. This has much to commend it, particularly if otherwise the bird is adversely affected by handling and restraint, but the effect of chemical restraint has to be borne in mind, particularly in so far as it can affect parameters such as heart rate, hematological values and response to stimuli.

Weighing and morphometrics

A bird should be weighed whenever it is handled or restrained (Figs 2.11–2.13). Weighing provides important data (particularly when combined with morphometrics such as wing or leg measurements; Fig. 2.14) that can be used in assessment of health, in monitoring response to treatment and for other purposes such as sex determination, taxonomy or providing information for subsequent legal cases.

Sometimes it is possible for a bird to be weighed voluntarily, for example a hooded hawk can be placed on scales and weighed without difficulty. A hand-tame psittacine bird will usually permit the owner to place it on to a balance or it may grasp a cloth bag suspended from a spring balance. In many cases, however, weighing has to be carried out during physical restraint. In this case, the bird is either placed in a small cloth bag or wrapped in a towel or placed in a holding device and then weighed on scales or a balance. Electronic scales, which can be zeroed to take account of the bag or the towel, are usually ideal for the purpose. However, spring balances specially designed for use by bird ringers have

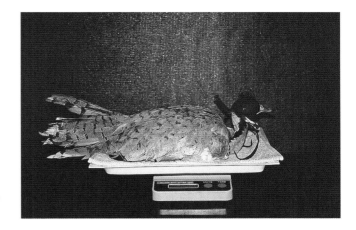

Fig. 2.11 Accurate weight determination is essential for administering anesthetics or medications. Weighing a houbara bustard (*Chlamydotis undulata*) is straightforward once the bird is hooded. (Courtesy of Dr. T. A. Bailey).

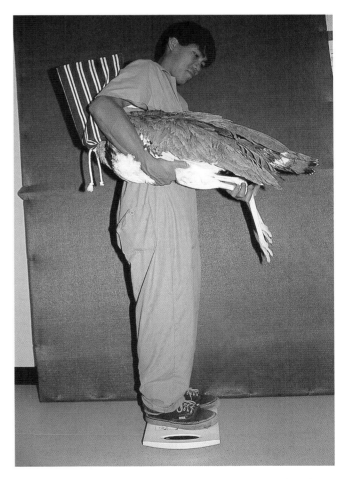

Fig. 2.12 Correct method of weighing a large bird such as this kori bustard (*Ardeotis kori*). (Courtesy of Dr. T. A. Bailey).

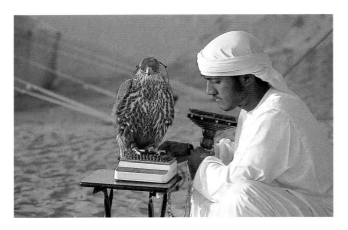

Fig. 2.13 A young Arab falconer weighing his falcon during the training season. A platform-type electronic balance fitted with plastic matting is ideal for weighing falcons.

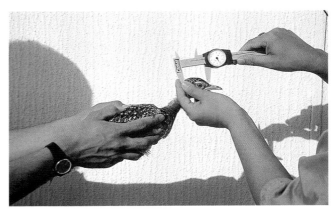

Fig. 2.14 Correct way of measuring the length of the skull in a rufous-crested bustard (*Eupodotis ruficrista*) using a Vernier measuring device. (Courtesy of Dr. T. A. Bailey).

much to commend them and are usually very accurate. They are particularly suitable for small birds and the weighing can be combined with restraining the bird for examination. When weighing birds of prey that are used for falconry, account has to be taken of any equipment that the bird is wearing, for example hood, jesses, bell, etc. Likewise, the weight of any transmitter must be deducted from the total value. When recording the weight of a bird, note should also be taken of whether it has recently fed and, in particular, in birds that have a crop, whether the crop contains food. The weight of a bird with a full crop can be significantly more than that of the same bird a few minutes earlier before it took food.

Systematic examination

This implies that a proper system is followed and this, in turn, reduces the risk of omitting a particular part of the examination or a particular procedure. Such omissions can produce complications or a false diagnosis in captive birds but has even more adverse repercussions when the examination is of a free-living bird that is subsequently released and there is not an opportunity to recapture it to rectify the omissions. Therefore a logical approach is needed that the clinician either follows automatically, because he/she is experienced, or should carry out following a written protocol or flow diagram. An example of an omission that can be significant is failure to check both that the bird has a preen gland and that the gland is functioning normally. This may be a key factor in ascertaining the cause of ill health and yet is a step that can be easily overlooked.

The preferred approach of the author to systematic clinical examination is to commence with the head of the bird and then to proceed down the body, examining wings, the body itself, the tail, the legs and the feet. At all stages, it is important to compare and contrast the right and left. Thus what may appear to be a swelling on the elbow joint of the left wing may prove to be a normal anatomical feature if the same swelling is found on the right elbow joint. However, caution must always be exercised, since bilateral skeletal abnormalities are not uncommon. At each stage, standard tests can be carried out on the particular part of the body that is being examined. Thus, for example, when the eyes are examined, the opportunity should be taken to check pupillary reflexes and possibly also to examine anterior chamber, lens, posterior chamber and retina with an ophthalmoscope. In the case of limbs (wings and legs) each joint should be flexed and extended, abducted and adducted.

Often the appearance of an organ or structure has to be correlated with function and this can present difficulties in the clinical examination. Different authors have their own approach; for example, some veterinary surgeons will include investigation of the sight of the bird, in particular checking that there is no obvious visual impairment during observation, and carry out examination of the eye when the bird is restrained. Others may delay assessment of visual function until after the physical examination. Locomotor performance is usually best assessed during the examination or at the end of examination. If, for example, a lesion of a leg or a wing is detected, the ability of the bird to stand, walk, run or fly is best assessed when all other tests have been done, since release during the examination may complicate other investigations. A swan with lead poisoning may exhibit weakness of the neck and find it difficult to hold its head erect. However, it will often mask this sign when it is aware of the close proximity of humans. The plantar surfaces of the feet must always be carefully checked, since small lesions such as early degenerative changes may be an important clue to the bird's ill health or provide useful background information on its management and care.

TABLE 2.1 Systematic examination of birds

Structure	Examination	Comments
Beak	Normal appearance, bilaterally symmetrical consistency normal. No evidence of damage or lesions	Normal morphology varies greatly according to the species of bird and its feeding habits
Nostrils (nares)	Equal in size and appearance. Presence or absence of discharge	
Buccal mucous membranes	Color normal. Absence of lesions. Normal appearance of associated structures such as glottis, etc.	Variation among different types of bird. Samples for diagnostic tests can be taken while the bird's beak is open
Ears	Discharge, foreign bodies, myiasis	Dampness of feathers may indicate discharge
Neck/crop	Swellings, impaction of crop, etc.	Esophagus and crop can be examined with endoscope and samples removed
Body (anterior/cranial)	Wounds, lesions, swellings, etc.	Combine with auscultation, palpation and percussion
Body (posterior/caudal)	As above	As above, combine with cloacal examination
Cloaca	Cloacal lips swollen. Seepage of urates/feces. Inflammation, calculus, egg	Digital and endoscopic examination of the cloaca is always advisable
Wings	Wounds, other lesions including fractures, dislocations, primary, secondary and covert feathers normal	Combine with function test (flight or similar)
Tail	Feathers intact, damaged, stress marks or other lesions	Combine with examination of preen gland
Preen gland	Present (absent in some birds). Swollen, normal/abnormal discharge, presence of oil	Gentle squeezing may result in production of secretion
Legs	As wings above	As wings above. Test function – ability of bird to stand, walk, run, etc.
Feet	Wounds, swellings or other lesions, especially bumblefoot (various stages)	

It is impossible to describe all the investigations that may be carried out during the course of systematic clinical examination. Birds vary greatly in size, in shape and in anatomy, and the extent to which a particular organ or structure is investigated may well be related to the presenting clinical signs or the owner's history. However, Table 2.1 lists some of the important features of clinical examination.

One of the most important characteristics of the class Aves is the presence of feathers, and the plumage must always be examined carefully. Feathers are of different types but the basic structure is the same. Feathers are composed of keratin but are subject to many insults and the appearance of the feathers and the molting pattern can be important indicators of health status. Care must always be taken when examining the plumage of birds that are exhibited or used for sport or some other such purpose. Damage can have an adverse effect on the bird and sour relations with clients.

Some aids to clinical examination are alluded to in Table 2.1. Others warrant mention. The clinical examination is primarily visual and tactile but much additional information can be gleaned by making use of the following:

- Auscultation using a stethoscope or a heart monitor
- Radiography
- Ultrasonography
- CT scan/MRI – if available
- Endoscopy – rigid or flexible – for examination (and, if necessary, sampling) via natural orifices or induced orifices (e.g. laparoscopy).

The taking of samples for laboratory examination is discussed elsewhere (see Ch. 3). However, brief mention should be made here, since sampling is an integral part of clinical examination. Samples that may be taken include feathers, ectoparasites, blood, urates/feces, exudates or material aspirated or removed by biopsy. It is important when planning clinical examination to have ready access to needles, syringes, sample collection bottles, etc. so that specimens can be collected satisfactorily during examination if the need arises.

Physiological data collection

Jaime Samour

Physiological data collection is an important aspect in the physical examination of an individual and, more specifically, monitoring the avian patient under general anesthesia (Fig. 2.15). There are three main physiological parameters for the assessment of the health status of an individual temperature, respiration and heart rate.

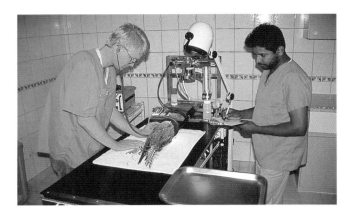

Fig. 2.15 A veterinary surgeon and his assistant examining a saker falcon prior to surgery. Physiological data collection is an important aspect in the physical examination and in monitoring patients under general anesthesia.

Temperature

The cloacal temperature in a clinically normal bird ranges between 40 and 41°C (105–107°F) but, as most practitioners would agree, this parameter has very limited diagnostic value.

Respiration rate

The respiration mechanism in birds is very similar to that in mammals. In both groups, the movements of the ribs and the sternum increase the diameter of the body cavities, commencing at the thoracic cavity followed by the abdominal wall. Therefore, the type of respiration in birds is thoracic–abdominal. Table 2.2 shows the normal respiration and heart rates of different species at rest and during restraint.

The respiration rate and type of respiration of a bird has to be assessed at close range within its transport cage, box or on the fist when the bird is at rest and, more importantly, prior to handling. Mechanical obstruction of the upper respiratory tract, such as is caused by trichomoniasis lesions or parasites of the genus *Syngamus*, will result in gasping, increased respiratory noise and, very often, fluttering of the skin immediately above the infraorbital sinuses.

In avian medicine, but in particular when dealing with falcons, the use of the 'stress or endurance test' has become increasingly popular for the assessment of air sacculitis associated with aspergillosis or *Serratospiculum* filarial worm infestation. This test involves assessing the respiration rate and type of respiration before and after the bird has been subjected to stress. To carry out this procedure in a falcon, the bird, with its hood on, should be allowed to rest for 5–10 min within the examination area at normal room temperature, and then the respiration rate/minute is estimated. The normal respiration rate of a falcon of over 900–1100 g at rest is between 15 and 20 per minute. The falcon is then allowed to fly suspended from the leash for an average of 30 seconds. A normal falcon should return to its original respiration rate within a period of 2–3 min. If the bird requires a longer period of time to return to normal, radiology or a more invasive diagnostic test such as endoscopy would be highly indicated. Endoscopy would be recommended if the falcon breathes with the beak open and if the type of respiration is laborious, deep and predominately abdominal.

During anesthesia, the respiration rate can be monitored by direct observation of the chest or abdomen of the bird or by using a respiratory monitor. Some of the monitors available on the market are not sensitive enough and they can only be used in large species since most of them need to be connected to endotracheal tubes. However, new sophisticated models are emerging that are sensitive enough to be used with face masks or endotracheal tubes

Bodyweight	Heart rate/min (resting)	Heart rate/min (restrained)	Respiration rate/min (resting)	Respiration rate/min (restrained)
25 g	274	400–600	60–70	80–120
100 g	206	500–600	40–52	60–80
200 g	178	300–500	35–50	55–65
500 g	147	160–300	20–30	30–50
1000 g	127	150–350	15–20	25–40
1500 g	117	120–200	20–32	25–30
2000 g	110	110–175	19–28	20–30

TABLE 2.2 Heart and respiration rates in clinically normal birds

Source: from: Harrison GJ, Ritchie BW (1994) Making distinctions in the physical examination. In: Ritchie BW, Harrison GJ, Harrison LR (eds) *Avian Medicine: Principles and Application*, pp. 144–175. Wingers Publishing, Lake Worth, FL.

and are fitted with an apnea alarm. In this respect, I use a respiration monitor[b] fitted with a sensor manufactured specifically for small birds and small laboratory animals and provided with an apnea alarm (Fig. 2.16). Table 2.3 shows heart and respiration rates in birds under isoflurane general anesthesia.

Heart rate

The heart rate in most avian species is too fast to be counted using a standard stethoscope. Therefore, this physiological parameter is normally obtained during anesthesia using an electrocardiogram (ECG) unit (Fig. 2.17) provided with 100 cm/min paper speed. The heart rate in birds is greatly affected by pain (Lawton, 1996), and therefore the use of an ECG machine is essential to monitor patients undergoing surgery under general anesthesia. The use of a hand-held ECG recorder[c] without leads was recently

described in conscious psittacine birds. This innovative device recorded accurate ECG tracings in awake and birds under isoflurane anesthesia (Lichtenberger et al., 2003). The use of hand-held ECG units can prove useful to monitor cardiac function in individuals representing an anesthetic risk.

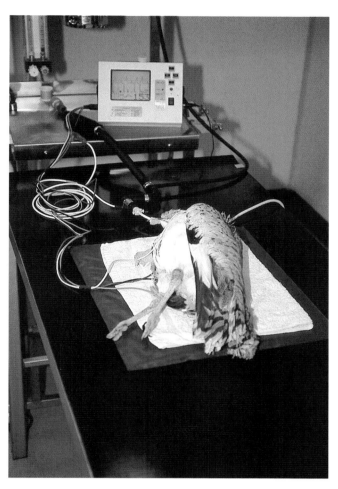

Fig. 2.17 An electrocardiogram (ECG) unit being used in a houbara bustard (*Chlamydotis undulata*) to monitor the depth of isoflurane anesthesia prior to surgery.

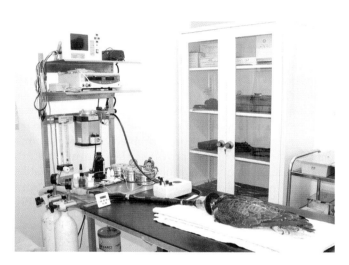

Fig. 2.16 A peregrine falcon (*Falco peregrinus*) under anesthesia, showing a respiration monitor. The sensor of the monitor is connected between the face mask and the anesthetic circuit (Eyres T piece). The main respiration monitor unit can be seen on the top of the table.

TABLE 2.3 Heart and respiration rates in birds under isoflurane anesthesia		
Species	**Heart rate/min**	**Respiration rate/min**
Budgerigar	600–700	55–75
Cockatiel	450–604	30–40
Pigeon	93.1 ± 5.4*	15–25
Parrot	120–780	10–20
Ostrich[†]	60–72	2–20

Source: *from: Korbel TJ, Milovanic A, Erhardt W et al. (1993) Aerosaccular perfusion with isoflurane – an anaesthetic procedure for head surgery in birds. *Proceedings of the European Association of Avian Veterinarians*, Utrecht, pp. 9–42; [†] from Bruning DF, Dolensek EP (1986) Ratite (Struthioniformes, Casuariiformes, Rheiformes, Tinamiformes and Apterygiformes). In: Fowler ME (ed.) *Zoo and Wild Animal Medicine*, 2nd edn, pp. 277–291. WB Saunders, Philadelphia.

REFERENCES

Lawton MPC (1996) Anesthesia. In: Beynon PH, Forbes NA, Harcourt-Brown NH (eds) *Manual of Raptors, Pigeons and Waterfowl*, pp. 79–88. British Small Animal Veterinary Association Ltd., Cheltenham.

Lichtenberger M, Swan T, Tilley L (2003) Recording an electrocardiogram in the conscious psittacine bird. *Proceedings of the European Association of Avian Veterinarians*, pp. 150–153, Tenerife.

Cage and environment

Peter McKinney

The health, welfare and breeding success of captive birds is directly related to the environment in which they are kept. Carefully managed aviaries tend to have fewer problems with disease, escape and injury. The pet parrot presents the greatest challenge, where basic cage design has not really changed for hundreds of years, exposing many, often endangered, parrots to years of unintentional neglect. Birds often develop behavioral problems and become obese because of the sedentary lifestyle.

Basic principles should be applied when we attempt to provide a home for any captive bird but welfare (i.e. the mental and physical health of the bird) should be our prime consideration.

Exercise

Every captive bird must have access to an exercise area. Young ratites require exercise to develop strong legs; falcons require a flying area to develop flight muscles and to reduce the incidence of pressure sores and pododermatitis (bumblefoot). Excessively long cages can be a problem for flying birds, as the bird may build up speed and accidentally collide with the wall of the aviary, resulting in serious injury. Some of the larger breeding establishments now house young falcons in circular cages so that the birds can fly without risk of injury in a corner. Although more expensive, this may be the cage design of the future.

Security

Captive birds depend on keepers for food, shelter and safety. Escapees do not always survive the harsh life in the wild and it is also the moral duty of the keepers not to release non-indigenous species. A double-door system is almost essential for most aviaries, but a compromise is to hang a cloth or plastic strips at the entrance. Before entering an aviary it is best to alert the birds to your presence as they may panic, resulting in injuries. Raptors kept in seclusion tend to be especially nervous, requiring special care during approach. Some species (e.g. goshawks, cockatoos) display serious intersex aggression and require a hiding area in the breeding aviaries. Other species are gregarious and can be maintained with minimal aggression provided adequate numbers of nest sites are installed (Fig. 2.18).

Aviaries should be safe from human and animal disturbance and pest free. Rats, mice and snakes can not only kill young birds but may disturb the adults, resulting in poor breeding results. The nesting area is especially vulnerable. Placing a sheet of Perspex behind a wall-mounted nest box is an excellent way to prevent predators climbing into the nest box. In this case the only way in is to fly in!

Especially in the tropics, but also in other areas, aviaries must be mosquito-proof, as many species develop pox carried by mosquitoes. Dogs and foxes can be a problem, requiring a solid wall around the aviary perimeter. Cats can also be a problem, but most birds get accustomed to them provided they do not disturb nesting areas. Many species of captive bird are valuable, so steps must be taken to protect the aviary from thieves and vandals. Security cameras are ideal, especially in combination with a guard dog!

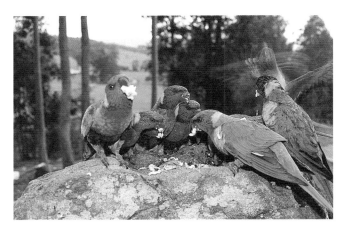

Fig. 2.18 Small psittacines can be kept in large groups with minimal aggression as long as enough nesting boxes are available.

Mental stimulation

For too long, the mental health of captive birds has been given low priority. The solitary pet parrot in a small cage is deprived of the basic activities of food seeking, bathing, courtship, flying, nest building and many more activities about which we may know very little. Toys for pet birds are now very popular with parrot owners and many birds also seem to benefit from radio and television, especially when the owner is not in the house. Captive gyrfalcons will play with tennis balls in the molting aviaries for hours on end. Food-seeking behavior may be stimulated by placing food at different sites and at irregular times in the aviary. This also encourages exercise. Parrots like to chew wood, and this activity can keep them active for hours and may also stimulate nesting behavior. Providing natural food can also stimulate birds in the captive environment.

Most captive birds appear to enjoy bathing, which provides a natural activity and improves feather quality (Fig. 2.19). Many larger collections operate a misting system for tropical birds, although care must be taken to avoid chilling. Shallow bathing sites are advised, as a wet bird may have difficulty getting out of a deep bath.

Aviary design

Aviary design must incorporate the needs of the species housed (Figs 2.20–2.31). Cold moist conditions can be detrimental to desert species and hot conditions may cause problems for temperate species and those from a cold climate. Excessively cold conditions are involved in the wing tip edema syndrome of raptors and in frostbite of toes for flamingoes. Translucent panels should be used to allow natural light exposure if enclosures are totally covered (i.e. seclusion). Alternatively, suitable artificial lighting should be provided. Providing and maintaining an adequate photoperiod within the aviary or cage is important. Extended lighting periods may result in disturbance of the reproductive cycle and molting, and may lead to feather plucking. Most species can be housed under a 12-hour lighting regime. However,

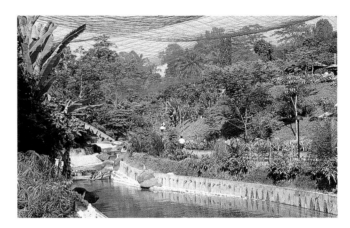

Fig. 2.20 Large, free-flying aviaries are becoming increasingly popular in zoological parks and bird gardens.

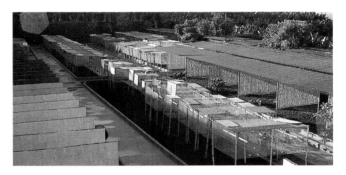

Fig. 2.21 Large-scale breeding aviaries have to be designed carefully and taking into consideration the basic needs of captive birds.

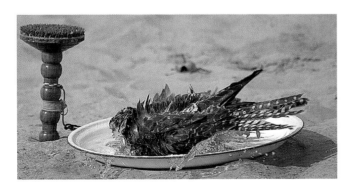

Fig. 2.19 During hot weather, falcons and many other avian species should have access to a water trough for bathing. This provides birds with a natural activity and improves feather quality. (Courtesy of Dr. J. Samour).

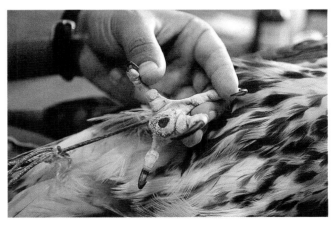

Fig. 2.22 Bumblefoot (pododermatitis) is a very common condition of captive falcons. This disease is frequently associated with the use of inadequate perches within molting rooms.

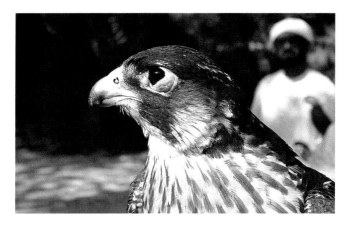

Fig. 2.23 A peregrine falcon (*Falco peregrinus*) displaying a typical pox lesion on the caudal commissure of the lower eyelid. In countries with a tropical climate, molting rooms should be fitted with windows covered with mosquito netting in order to prevent the transmission of diseases carried by mosquitoes, such as avian pox.

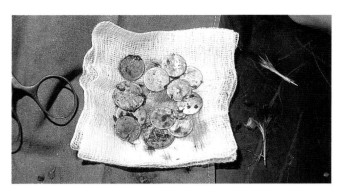

Fig. 2.26 In many countries around the world, waterfowl collections are kept on lakes or large ponds. However, in many bird gardens or zoological collections, ducks have access to smaller ponds where visitors have the habit of throwing coins and making a wish. The photograph shows a group of coins extracted surgically from the gizzard of a mallard duck (*Anas platyrhynchos*). The bird was presented with anorexia and hind leg paresis. The coins were detected by radiology. (Courtesy of Dr. J. Samour).

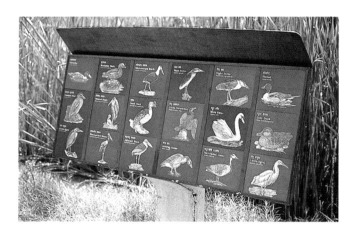

Fig. 2.24 Labels identifying the different birds housed in a large, multiple-species exhibit are essential in zoological parks and bird gardens. (Courtesy of Dr. J. Samour).

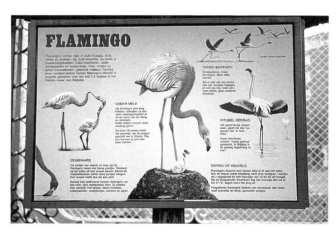

Fig. 2.25 Graphic displays containing biological data about individual species are also an important contribution to increase public awareness. (Courtesy of Dr. J. Samour).

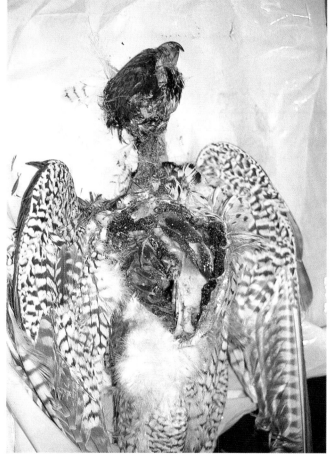

Fig. 2.27 This peregrine falcon was killed and partially eaten when a much larger saker/gyr hybrid falcon cut its leash within a molting room. Extreme care should be exercised when housing large, aggressive falcons together with smaller individuals. (Courtesy of Dr. J. Samour).

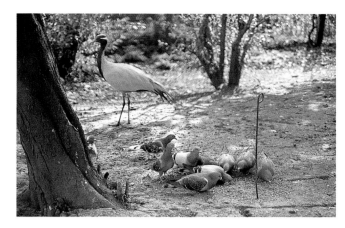

Fig. 2.28 In many bird gardens or zoological collections, large birds such as cranes and storks are housed in open paddocks. Pigeons and other birds, such as sparrows and starlings, very often flock to eat and drink water from this type of enclosure, representing a health hazard. Fine nylon netting used to roof the enclosures or specially designed water and feeding troughs could help to reduce this problem. (Courtesy of Dr. J. Samour).

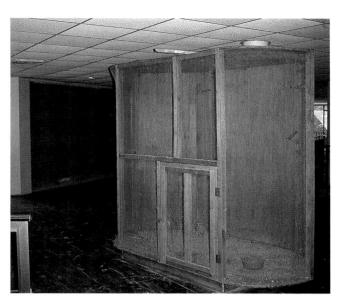

Fig. 2.29 Small, wooden and mesh cage located inside a closed bird pavilion. Birds housed in this type of cage do not have access to direct sunlight and wood is a very poor choice of material for building cages. (Courtesy of Dr. J. Samour).

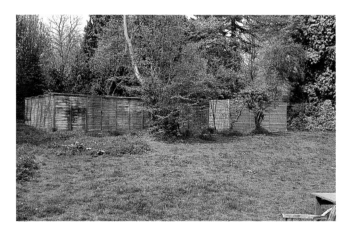

Fig. 2.30 Breeding aviaries for birds of prey on an English private farm. 'Secluded'-type aviaries are very popular among raptor breeders and are commonly built using wooden walls and fine nylon netting as roofing. (Courtesy of Dr. J. Samour).

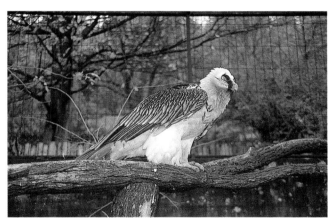

Fig. 2.31 Large raptors can be kept successfully in captivity for display or for breeding programs. However, large naturalistic aviaries are necessary in order to meet their requirements. The lammergeier (Gypaetus barbatus) in the picture has been provided with suitable perching surfaces such as large logs and a rockery to simulate as closely as possible its natural habitat. (Courtesy of Dr. J. Samour).

species under a breeding program should be exposed to 14–16 h of lighting.

In hot climates birds must be kept cool. In the Middle East, falcon aviaries often have an air conditioner at both ends as well as fans placed outside to direct cool air to the main perches. Most of the birds cool off by bathing (see Fig. 2.19) and then sitting near the fan. The unacclimatized falcons require air conditioning during the hotter months of the year.

In all aviaries and for all species, ventilation is very important. Clean air is essential for the welfare of captive birds and keepers alike. Poor ventilation predisposes to respiratory infections and I consider it a major con-

tributory factor in the development of aspergillosis in falcons.

A major problem with captive raptors is the development of bumblefoot (pododermatitis, Fig. 2.22). The cause is multifactorial but the type of perch is critical. In my experience, perches covered with Astroturf® or coconut matting are ideal. A choice of perches of different diameters should be provided for all species of birds that perch, especially passerines. In tropical areas, prevention of access by harmful insects such as mosquitoes will assist in preventing diseases such as avian pox (Fig. 2.23). Housing large aggressive species with smaller ones should only be attempted with great care (Fig. 2.27).

There is no magic formula for aviary design. Each species has its own requirements and each bird keeper will insist that his/her design is the best. A high level of public information is desirable (Figs 2.24, 2.25). We still have a lot to learn about housing birds and we should always strive to improve the welfare of birds in our care.

Clinical and diagnostic procedures

3

General principles

Judith C. Howlett

Accurate diagnosis of disease in the living bird depends upon a series of carefully carried out investigations. Observation of the sick or injured bird(s) should follow careful analysis of the history and other relevant records. Ideally the bird should be observed in its own surroundings without being aware of the observer. Clinical examination, which implies handling and restraint, follows observation. Once the bird is in the hand, it is possible to supplement clinical examination with a range of clinical diagnostic tests.

In this section, clinical diagnostic techniques that may be carried out routinely are discussed. They primarily involve the taking of blood or other samples for laboratory investigation.

The samples that are regularly taken from birds for diagnostic purposes are as follows:

- Feces
- Urates
- Blood
- Other 'normal' body products (e.g. semen)
- Biopsies
- Swabs
- Aspirates
- Feathers
- Skin scrapings.

Each of the samples above, plus others that are not listed, may be used for a variety of investigations. The tests to be carried out may dictate how the sample is taken, how it is preserved, how it is transported and how it is processed. It is therefore an important rule before taking samples to plan carefully and to be certain that appropriate materials and facilities are available. In recent years there has been an exponential increase in our understanding of the normal parameters of wild birds, particularly in captivity, and, as a result, interpretation of findings in samples has become easier and more reliable. Blood is the classic example. Techniques for the examination of avian blood have been improved beyond measure. Normal values for hematology and blood biochemistry have been established for many species and, even where these are not available, extrapolation from other species, particularly related ones, can be used successfully (Gascoyne *et al.*, 1994). There is a need to build a larger database on normal values of birds and therefore the taking of samples for diagnostic purposes, in addition to its role in diagnosis, may also assist in this respect.

The following rules apply generally to samples for clinical diagnostic investigation:

- As a general rule, be prepared to take blood and other samples from every avian case. It is better to be prepared to take samples and then be unable to do so than to have to subject a bird to subsequent handling because equipment and materials were not available on the first occasion. Have bottles, slides, specimen containers, etc. ready before clinical examination commences.
- Use the best-quality equipment, since poor samples can yield erroneous results. Anticoagulant bottles, for example, should be recently purchased and should have been stored properly, particularly in hot climates. Microscope slides should have been cleaned and polished beforehand.
- Follow standard techniques when sampling birds and ensure that this is performed efficiently and humanely. This may mean limiting how much blood is taken from a particular individual, especially if the bird is in poor condition. An in-house code of practice for sampling has much to commend it.
- Ensure that all samples taken are properly labeled and recorded. Various techniques may facilitate this; for example, the use of frosted glass microscope slides will facilitate labeling since this can be done with a pencil. Make sure that the slide is labeled on the same side as the sample. **Label bottles, not lids.** Such precautions are not only important from the point of view of prompt diagnosis and reducing the risk of transposing samples but may also be relevant if subsequently there is a court case or other inquiry into the circumstances of the case or the way in which samples were prepared.
- Monitor the bird carefully following sampling, not only because this is good practice in terms of the wellbeing of the bird but also because it may provide

further information on the condition of the bird – for example, prolonged bleeding time following blood sampling may be suggestive of dicoumarol poisoning.

- Be aware of the possible risks to human health when taking samples and follow appropriate guidelines. If, for example, a bird is believed to have a zoonotic infection (e.g. chlamydophilosis), take samples under a hood or ensure that those involved are wearing appropriate protective clothing. Do not expose staff – and certainly not owners – to hazards unnecessarily.

- Toxicology – assay of toxic or abnormally elevated substances in the blood (may overlap with biochemistry)
- Microbiology – detection of bacteria and other organisms in the blood and possible culture or passage to tissue culture or other animals
- DNA and chromosomal studies
- Blood gases (e.g. Po_2 and Pco_2 levels)
- Other.

Biomedical sampling

Judith C. Howlett

Table 3.14 (p. 66) sets out the protocol for collection, transportation and processing of all types of samples.

TABLE 3.2 Hemoresponses: influence of stress on blood cell counts

Blood component	Response
Erythrocytes (Hb, PCV/HCT)	Increased
Heterophils	Increased
Eosinophils	Decreased
Basophils	Increased
Lymphocytes	Decreased
Monocytes	Increased
Thrombocytes	Increased

Blood sampling

Jaime Samour, Judith C. Howlett

Blood from birds, like blood from mammals, can yield a surprising amount of valuable information. Techniques that can be carried out on blood include the following (Tables 3.1–3.4):

- Hematology – a qualitative and quantitative assessment of blood cells and other components
- Biochemistry – assay of various substances, normal and abnormal, in the blood
- Parasitology – detection of protozoal parasites or other blood parasites (e.g. microfilaria)

TABLE 3.3 Total white cell count and differential white cell count

Blood assessment	Associated conditions/infections
Heterophilia	Bacterial/fungal infections/inflammatory response
Heteropenia	Degenerative response
Monocytosis	Infection (tuberculosis, aspergillosis)
Lymphocytosis	Lymphoid leukosis
Eosinophilia	Parasites
Fibrinogen **increased**	Infection/inflammation/hemorrhage
Fibrinogen **decreased**	Liver failure
Blood film	Cell morphology/blood parasites

TABLE 3.1 Basic hematology principles

Tests and results	Conclusions
PCV/HCT, Hb and MCHC Relatively constant in mammals and birds	Therefore polycythemia, normochromic anemia and hypochromic anemia can be recognized in any adult mammal or bird without reference to species-specific reference ranges
RBC, MCV Variable in mammals and birds	But normocytic/macrocytic/microcytic anemias can be detected by knowing the normal MCV and Hb for the species under study
Thrombocyte count	When high, probability of disease also high
Fibrinogen	Raised in infections and inflammatory conditions

TABLE 3.4 Clinical evaluation: clinical value of absolute white cell counts

HETEROPHILS	
Increased	Infection, tissue damage, stress, some metabolic diseases, myeloid leukemia, etc.
Decreased	Degenerative response to infection, bone marrow damage, some deficiency diseases, aleukemic leukemia, viremia, etc.
LYMPHOCYTES	
Increased	Some infectious and metabolic diseases, lymphocytic leukemia, leukemoid reaction, etc.
Decreased	Stress, uremia, some malignancies, immunosuppressive conditions

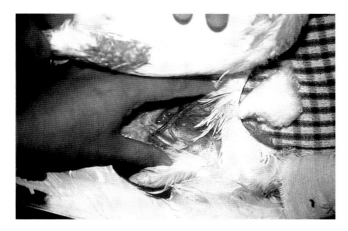

Fig. 3.1 The basilic vein (*vena cutanea ulnaris superficialis*) is probably the easiest site from which blood samples can be collected from birds. The photograph shows the raised basilic vein in a houbara bustard (*Chlamydotis undulata*) prior to blood sampling.

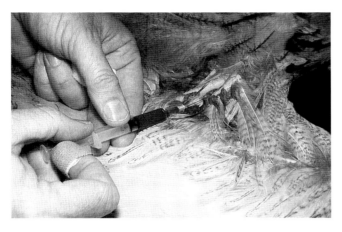

Fig. 3.2 Blood sample collection from a basilic vein (*vena cutanea ulnaris superficialis*) of a European eagle owl (*Bubo bubo*).

Each of these techniques may require specific sampling or preservation techniques and, as outlined earlier, this must be considered before the sample is taken. The development in recent years of micro-techniques has meant that relatively small samples can be accurately analyzed. This means that often one modest blood sample can be used for a variety of tests. However, care has to be taken to ensure that the right sample is preserved in the right anticoagulant (if appropriate) and that confusion does not occur.

Collection of blood samples

The total blood volume of a bird is approximately 10% of its bodyweight. Therefore a 30 g bird will have approximately 3 ml of blood of which, in a healthy bird, up to 10% (0.3 ml) can be safely removed without any detrimental effect. This volume has to be reduced in sick birds. It is possible to run a full hematology profile on 0.3 ml of blood.

Blood collected from a bird should be venous origin and in most birds can be taken from a basilic vein (*vena cutanea ulnaris superficialis*, Figs 3.1 and 3.2), which crosses the ventral surface of the humeral–radioulnar joint (elbow) immediately under the skin; or the jugular vein (*vena jugularis dextra*), usually the right, which is larger than the left (Figs 3.3 and 3.4); or the caudal tibial vein (*vena metatarsalis plantaris superficialis*), which is located on the medial side of the tibiotarsus above the tarsal joint

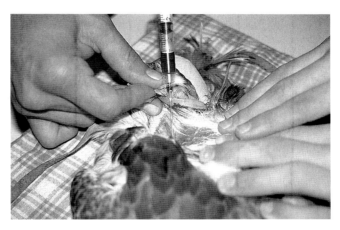

Fig. 3.3 Blood sample collection from the jugular vein (*vena jugularis dextra*) of a saker falcon (*Falco cherrug*).

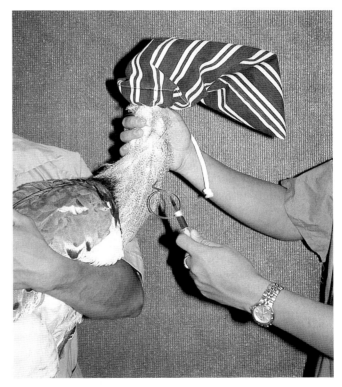

Fig. 3.4 Blood sample collection from the jugular vein (*vena jugularis dextra*), of a female kori bustard (*Ardeotis kori*). As a general rule, blood sampling from the jugular vein in birds is carried out on the right jugular vein, which is larger than that on the left side. A butterfly catheter attached to a syringe is being used for sample collection.

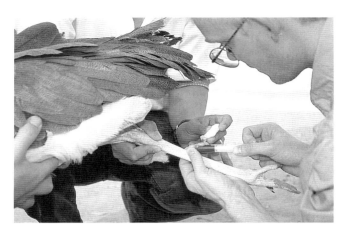

Fig. 3.5 Blood sample collection from a brachial (*vena cutanea ulnaris superficialis*) or caudal tibial vein (*vena metatarsalis plantaris superficialis*) of a kori bustard.

(Fig. 3.5). Samples can be collected from most species of birds under manual restraint and in the dorsal position. Other methods include clipping of a toenail, although blood from this site (from a capillary bed) often yields abnormal cell distributions and artifacts and should only be used when the other methods of collecting venous blood have failed. In smaller birds, where it is not possible to remove more than one drop of blood, this can be used to prepare a blood smear.

As an example, the technique for blood collection from the basilic vein for hematology analysis is described. While in the dorsal position, extend the right wing fully and prepare the medial aspect of the humeral area using cotton wool and surgical spirit. The application of pressure with the thumb at the proximal end of the humerus will raise the basilic vein, rendering it clearly visible running along the external lateral aspect of the humerus. A volume of 0.3–0.5 ml of blood can be obtained using 1 ml or 3 ml disposable syringes and 25 or 23 gauge × 5/8 in disposable needles, depending on the size of the bird. Bend the needle to an angle of about 25–30° and insert it gently into the vein. Begin collecting the sample but try to avoid exerting high negative pressure, since this will invariably cause the vein to collapse. It is highly recommended, while collecting the sample, to maintain steady pressure at the proximal end of the humerus to ensure a well defined vein. Bird skin is fairly delicate and damages easily. Bleeding and hematomas can easily occur, so care has to be taken with the technique, especially in small birds, in which the loss of a few drops of blood can have a significant effect on total blood volume. Collect samples into commercially available tubes containing the anticoagulant agent ethylene diamine tetra-acetic acid (EDTA; 1.5 mg/ml of blood) or lithium heparin tubes. EDTA samples are preferred for general hematological analysis, since it is not possible to estimate fibrinogen or to obtain an accurate white cell count on heparinized samples. In certain bird species (Corvidae, Gruidae, Struthionidae, Alcedinidae), mixing of blood with EDTA causes progressive hemolysis of the red cells and it is necessary to use lithium heparin as the anticoagulant.

Transportation of samples

All samples collected should be well-labeled, and sample submission forms should contain the following information:

- Name of owner
- Name/reference number of the bird
- Species, age and sex
- Clinical history, presenting signs, current treatments and differential diagnosis
- Date of sampling and time of collection
- Type of sample collected and, if applicable, anticoagulants used
- Details of site or sites from where the sample has been collected, if necessary for biopsies, etc., with a diagram
- Indication of tests or examination required
- Name of veterinary surgeon.

Note: If the samples are to be sent to a commercial laboratory it is necessary to pack them in compliance with local postal regulations.

Special considerations

- The containers should be secure, leakproof and protected from breakage, and also accessible to the staff receiving the sample.
- It is important that there is no contamination of documents enclosed or of anyone who comes into contact with the sample in the post office or in the laboratory.
- The sample should be sealed with waterproof tape to prevent any leakage.
- The container should be wrapped in an absorbable material such as cotton wool to soak up any potential leakage and help protect the container from any damage.
- The container should be double wrapped in leakproof plastic bags with the laboratory form attached in a separate bag.
- The sample should then be placed in a plastic clip-down container, or lightweight metal container, or cardboard or polystyrene box.
- The sample or samples should then be placed in a 'Jiffy' bag or other post-office approved packaging and correctly addressed.
- In the UK, for example, it is necessary to label the package with hazard tape 'PATHOLOGICAL SPECIMEN – FRAGILE WITH CARE': this can then be sent by first class post or dispatched by courier.

Processing of hematology samples

Hematology samples should be processed in the laboratory on the same day of collection if possible; if not then blood films should be made, air-dried at the time of collection. These will keep for up to 72 h without fixation, although it is essential that the films do not come into contact with any form of moisture. The techniques used to do full blood counts and fibrinogen are based on those used for mammals. Some modifications have been made to account for the fact that the red blood cells are relatively large and contain nuclei. It is useful to prioritize the order in which a sample is processed, when there is a limited sample volume available.

Priorities when processing a blood sample

- *A blood smear*: A small drop of blood on a microscope slide to make a smear. Stain immediately. This enables the morphology of the white blood cells (WBCs) and red blood cells (RBCs) to be examined.
- *PCV*: A filled capillary tube can be spun down and the packed cell volume (PCV) measured.
- *WBC*: 50 µl of blood into 0.95 ml of 1% ammonium oxalate solution.
- *Hemoglobin*: 20 µl of blood into 4 ml of 0.04% ammonia solution.
- *RBC*: 20 µl of blood into 4 ml red cell diluting fluid (formol–citrate solution) into a hemocytometer.

Hematology analyses

Jaime Samour, Judith C. Howlett

Hematology is the discipline of medical science that studies the blood and blood-forming tissues and is currently considered an integral part of clinical laboratory diagnostic support in avian medicine. Hematology assays seldom provide an etiological diagnosis but they remain, nevertheless, indispensable diagnostic tools to evaluate health and disease in individuals, for monitoring the response and progress of patients to therapeutic regimes, and to offer a prognosis.

The routine collection and processing of blood samples allows the evaluation of hematological responses to disease. In addition, the creation of hematology databases is important in establishing references values for various avian species. Significant advances have been made in the use of hematology assays in the differential diagnosis of pathological conditions in avian species in the past 15 years. This appears to have developed parallel to other areas such as nutrition, anesthesia, surgery and therapeutics.

The processing of hematology samples has also been enhanced in recent years. In the past, automatic analysis of avian blood samples was basically limited to total red cell counts using the cell counters that were available and making manual adjustments of the thresholds and current aperture settings (Coulter Counter ZF, Beckman Coulter Inc., Fullerton, CA). More recently, the analysis of avian blood samples has received a significant boost with the advent of more comprehensive and accurate automatic analytical systems based on laser flow cytometry (Cell Dyn 3500, Abbott Laboratories, Abbott Park, IL). This methodology is based on the measurement of scattered laser light, which fluctuates with the size of the cell, the complexity of the cell (e.g. overall shape, nucleus to cytoplasm ratio, granulation) and the size and shape of the nucleus after blood cells are exposed to a laser beam. This unit produces a graphic display containing a total optical white cell count, white cell differential count expressed in percentage and absolute values and total red cell count, hemoglobin measurement by the cyanmethemoglobin method, thrombocyte count, and white cell count by cell-lysing impedance measurement of cell nuclei (Fudge, 1995). However, the use of laser flow cytometric technology in avian species is not free from deficiencies.

There are certain pathological conditions in which the presence of enlarged thrombocytes, commonly referred to as megathrombocytes, in the blood film appears to be a characteristic hemoresponse. For instance, in the houbara bustard (*Chlamydotis undulata macqueenii*) the mean thrombocyte measurements in birds undergoing chronic inflammation (severe shoulder injury as a result of repeated crashing against wall of enclosure) were 9.22±0.21 µm length and 8.10±0.19 µm width compared with 5.47±0.12 µm length and 4.96±0.10 µm width in clinically normal birds (D'Aloia *et al.*, 1994). However, the mean diameter of lymphocytes in clinically normal houbara bustards is 7.7 µm (Samour *et al.*, 1994). It is therefore probable that a sample containing megathrombocytes would yield a high lymphocyte count under an automatic analytical system, as it would be impossible for even a sophisticated unit to differentiate between them. However, there are other species, such as the kori bustard (*Ardeotis kori*), in which the presence of large and small thrombocytes in the same blood film appears to be normal (Howlett *et al.*, 1995). When dealing with such species, the software would require some adjustments in order to differentiate these cells from lymphocytes. This would obviously imply the need to carry out extensive calibration based on repeated manual assessments on a significant number of samples.

Furthermore, in certain species it is relatively common to find large and small lymphocytes in the same blood film. This phenomenon has been observed in many psittacine species. Clinically normal kori bustards, for instance, demonstrated a mean diameter for small lymphocytes of 7.2±0.12 μm, whereas the mean diameter of large lymphocytes was 10.7±0.16 μm (Howlett *et al.*, 1995). Therefore, total white cell counts and white cell differentials counts cannot be accepted as reliable in every clinical case and in every species if the values have been estimated by laser flow cytometry. It is therefore highly recommended that these samples are re-evaluated using manual methods.

This section intends to combine the practicalities of a manual and an atlas by including hematological techniques and photographic identification of blood cells. The photographic section illustrates normal red cells, white cells and thrombocytes and includes some of the most common hemopathological responses (Figs 3.6–3.48).

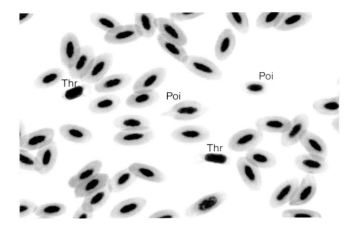

Fig. 3.8 Poikilocytes (Poi) and thrombocytes (Thr) of a saker falcon. (Modified Wright–Giemsa stain).

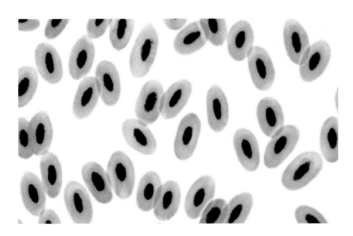

Fig. 3.6 Normal erythrocytes of a saker falcon (*Falco cherrug*). The erythrocytes in birds are oval in shape with oval nuclei containing dense chromatin clumps. (Modified Wright–Giemsa stain).

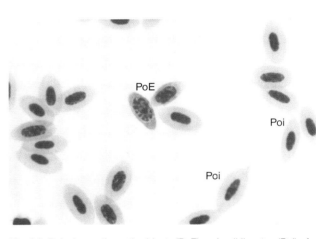

Fig. 3.9 Polychromatic erythroblasts (PoE) and poikilocytes (Poi) of a saker falcon. The size of the nucleus decreases and the amount of cytoplasm increases as the cells reach maturity. (Modified Wright–Giemsa stain).

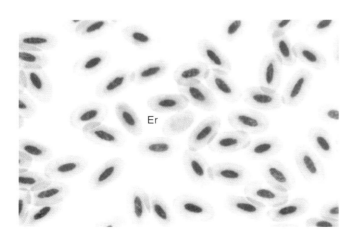

Fig. 3.7 An erythroplastid form (Er) of a saker falcon. The presence of a small number of anucleated erythrocytes is relatively normal during the examination of a blood film. (Modified Wright–Giemsa stain).

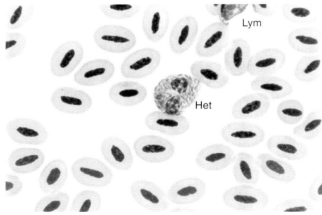

Fig. 3.10 Normal heterophil (Het) and normal lymphocyte (Lym) of a houbara bustard (*Chlamydotis undulata*). The avian heterophil is characterized by the presence of eosinophilic rod-shaped granules within the cytoplasm. (May–Grünwald–Giemsa stain).

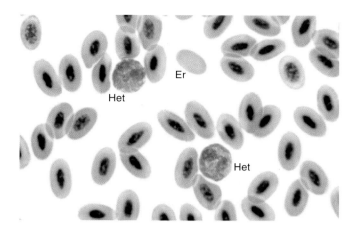

Fig. 3.11 Normal heterophils (Het) and an erythroplastid form (Er) of a saker falcon. (Modified Wright–Giemsa stain).

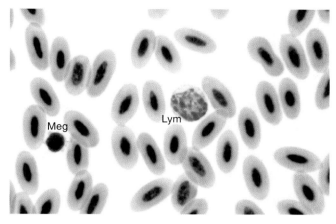

Fig. 3.12 Normal lymphocyte (Lym) and megathrombocyte (Meg) of a peregrine falcon (*Falco peregrinus*). The lymphocyte is a mononuclear cell, with a relatively large nucleus. These cells are often found compressed amongst two or three erythrocytes. (Mcdified Wright–Giemsa stain).

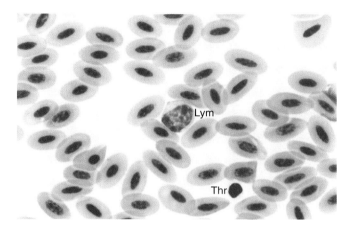

Fig. 3.13 Normal lymphocyte (Lym) and normal thrombocyte (Thr) of a saker falcon. Thrombocytes in birds are characterized by the presence of strongly basophilic nuclei, with a highly condensed chromatin and a vacuolated cytoplasm. (Modified Wright–Giemsa stain).

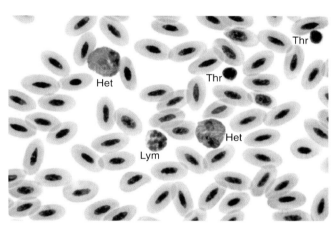

Fig. 3.14 Normal heterophils (Het), normal lymphocyte (Lym) and normal thrombocytes (Thr) of a saker falcon. (Modified Wright–Giemsa stain).

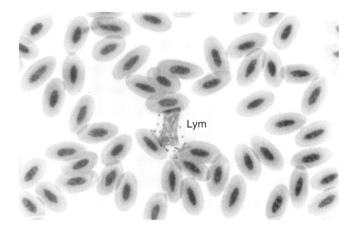

Fig. 3.15 A lymphocyte with azurophilic granules (Lym) of a saker falcon. These granules can be found in blood smears from healthy individuals. However, the presence of granules in the cytoplasm has been associated with viral diseases, in particular Newcastle disease. (Modified Wright–Giemsa stain).

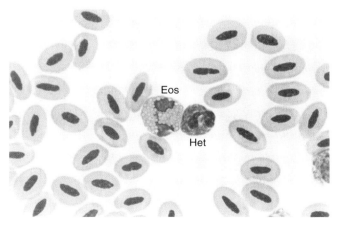

Fig. 3.16 Normal eosinophil (Eos) and normal heterophil (Het) of a kori bustard (*Ardeotis kori*). The eosinophil of this bustard species is characterized by the presence of large, symmetrical, round, red-brick-colored intracytoplasmic granules. (May–Grünwald–Giemsa stain).

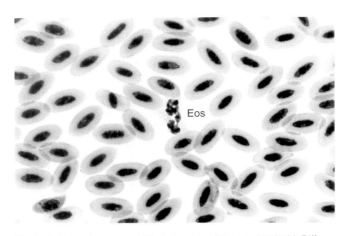

Fig. 3.17 Normal eosinophil (Eos) of a saker falcon stained with Diff Quick stain. The granules within the cytoplasm are not stained, giving the impression of numerous vacuoles.

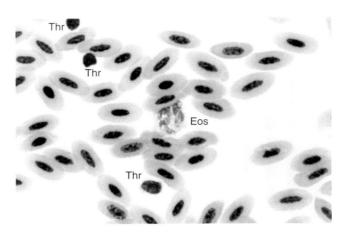

Fig. 3.18 Normal eosinophil (Eos) and normal thrombocytes (Thr) of a saker falcon stained with May–Grünwald–Giemsa stain. The granules are not stained, giving the false impression of vacuoles within the cytoplasm.

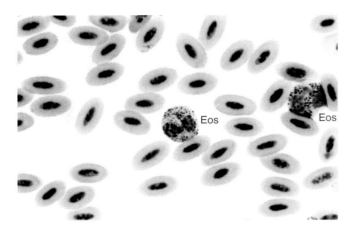

Fig. 3.19 Normal eosinophils (Eos) of a saker falcon. This staining method, as described in the text, provides an excellent granular definition making easy the positive identification of these cells. (Modified Wright–Giemsa stain).

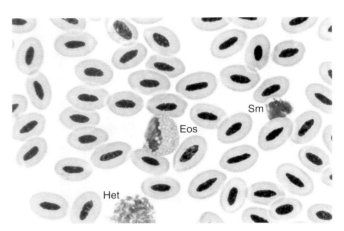

Fig. 3.20 Normal eosinophil (Eos), normal heterophil (Het) and a smudged cell (Sm) of a kori bustard. The so-called 'smudged cells' are very often the remains of the nuclei of damaged erythrocytes. This tends to occur during the preparation of the blood film as a result of mechanical damage. (May–Grünwald–Giemsa stain).

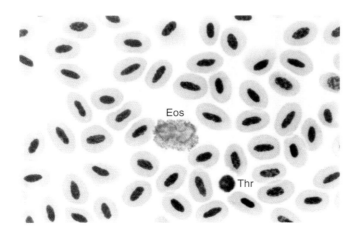

Fig. 3.21 A slightly disrupted eosinophil (Eos) and a normal thrombocyte (Thr) of a lesser sulfur-crested cockatoo (*Cacatua sulphurea*). The medium-sized round granules are pale blue in color. (May–Grünwald–Giemsa stain). The basophilic color of the eosinophil granules is characteristic of most psittacine birds.

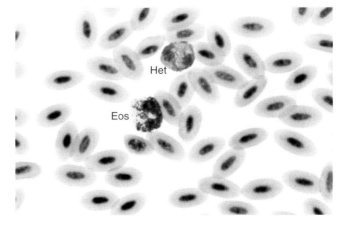

Fig. 3.22 Normal eosinophil (Eos) and normal heterophil (Het) of a peregrine falcon. (Modified Wright–Giemsa stain).

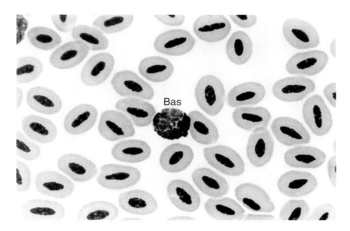

Fig. 3.23 Normal basophil (Bas) of a houbara bustard. The avian basophil is the smallest of the granulocytes and is characterized by the presence of strongly basophilic granules obscuring the cytoplasm and the nucleus of the cell. (May–Grünwald–Giemsa stain).

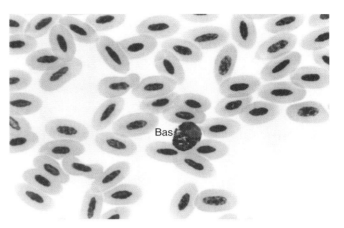

Fig. 3.24 Normal basophil (Bas) of a saker falcon. (Modified Wright–Giemsa stain).

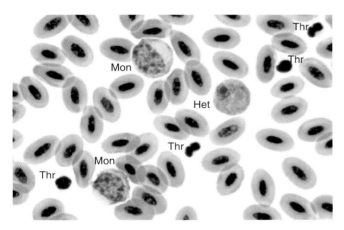

Fig. 3.25 Normal monocytes (Mon), normal heterophil (Het) and normal thrombocytes (Thr) of a saker falcon. The avian monocyte is characterized by its large size. The nucleus is commonly round or kidney-bean-shaped and the cytoplasm stains pale blue with a fine granular appearance and very often contains small to medium-sized vacuoles. (Modified Wright–Giemsa stain).

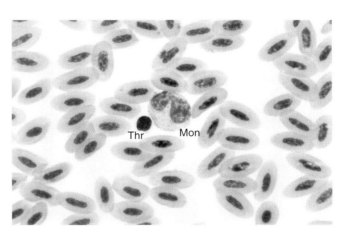

Fig. 3.26 Normal monocyte (Mon) and normal thrombocyte (Thr) of a saker falcon. (Modified Wright–Giemsa stain).

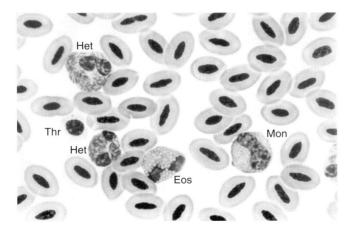

Fig. 3.27 Normal eosinophil (Eos), normal heterophils (Het), normal monocyte (Mon) and normal thrombocyte (Thr) of a kori bustard. (May–Grünwald–Giemsa stain).

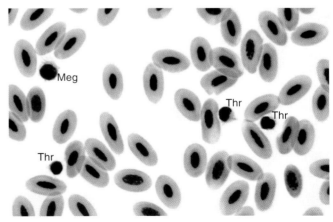

Fig. 3.28 Normal thrombocytes (Thr) and one megathrombocyte (Meg) of a saker falcon. (Modified Wright–Giemsa stain).

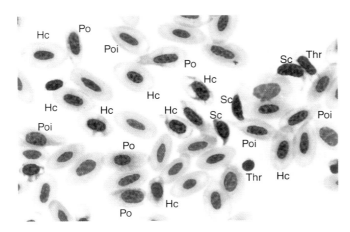

Fig. 3.29 Red cells from a saker falcon with severe anemia showing hypochromasia (Hc), poikilocytes (Poi), polychromasia (Po), a number of sickle cells (Sc) and some thrombocytes (Thr). (Modified Wright–Giemsa stain).

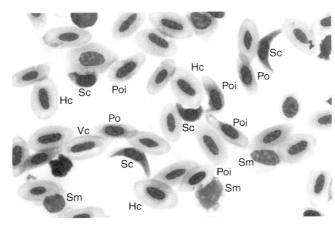

Fig. 3.30 A blood film from a saker falcon with severe sickle cell anemia showing many sickle cells (Sc), hypochromasia (Hc), poikilocytes (Poi), polychromasia (Po), vacuolation (Vc) and some smudged cells (Sm). (Modified Wright–Giemsa stain).

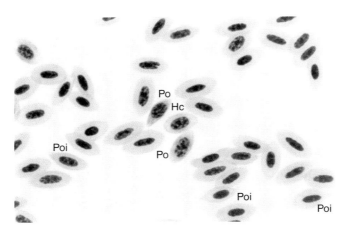

Fig. 3.31 Poikilocytes (Poi), polychromasia (Po) and hypochromasia (Hc) in a saker falcon. This bird was undergoing a moderate infection with the intracytoplasmic parasite *Babesia shortii*. (Modified Wright–Giemsa stain).

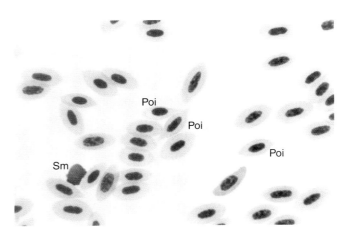

Fig. 3.32 Poikilocytes (Poi) and a smudged cell (Sm) of a saker falcon. (Modified Wright–Giemsa stain).

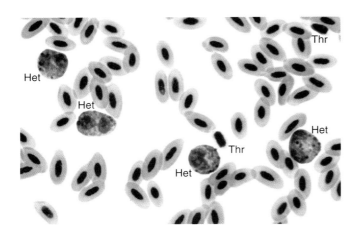

Fig. 3.33 Toxic heterophils (Het) and thrombocytes (Thr) of a peregrine falcon. Loss of lobulation (left shift) of the nucleus and degranulation. The granules are large round and strongly basophilic. (Modified Wright–Giemsa stain).

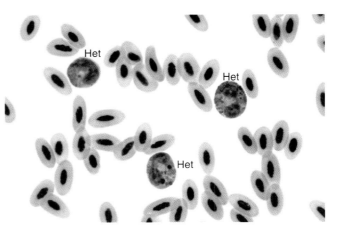

Fig. 3.34 Toxic heterophils (Het) of a gyrfalcon. Severe toxic changes including loss of lobulation (left shift) of the nucleus and severe degranulation. The granules are large round and strongly basophilic. The falcon was undergoing a severe infection with the fungus *Aspergillus fumigatus*. (Modified Wright–Giemsa stain).

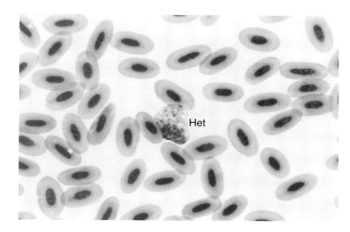

Fig. 3.35 Heterophil (Het) of a saker falcon with severe toxic changes. Severe degranulation and loss of lobulation (left shift) of the nucleus. (Modified Wright–Giemsa stain).

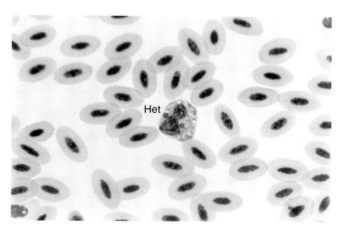

Fig. 3.36 Severe toxic changes in a heterophil (Het) of a gyrfalcon (*Falco rusticolus*). Severe degranulation and loss of lobulation (left shift) of the nucleus. (Modified Wright–Giemsa stain).

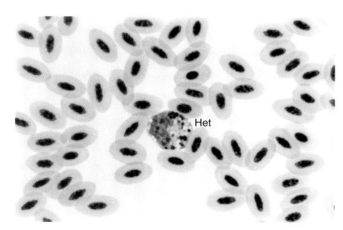

Fig. 3.37 Heterophil (Het) of a peregrine falcon with toxic changes. There is mild loss of granulation, loss of lobulation (left shift) and the large granules stained dark purple in color. (Modified Wright–Giemsa stain).

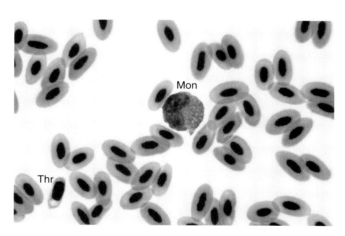

Fig. 3.38 A reactive monocyte (Mon) of a saker falcon. The cytoplasm is deeply basophilic and the nuclear chromatin is coarse. A thrombocyte (Thr) is also present. (Modified Wright–Giemsa stain).

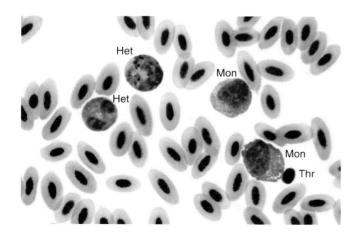

Fig. 3.39 Reactive monocytes (Mon), heterophils (Het) with toxic changes and a thrombocyte (Thr) of a saker falcon. The cytoplasm of the monocyte is deeply basophilic with few cytoplasmic vacuoles with a coarse nuclear chromatin. (Modified Wright–Giemsa stain).

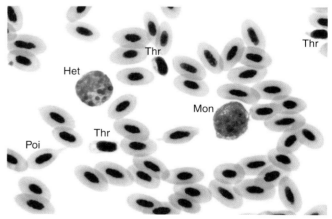

Fig. 3.40 Reactive monocyte (Mon), toxic heterophil (Het), thrombocytes (Thr) and poikilocyte (Poi) of a saker falcon. (Modified Wright–Giemsa stain).

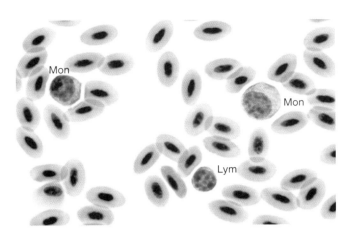

Fig. 3.41 Reactive monocytes (Mon) and reactive lymphocyte (Lym) of a saker falcon. The cytoplasm of the lymphocyte is basophilic and the nucleus is relatively large and round. (Modified Wright–Giemsa stain).

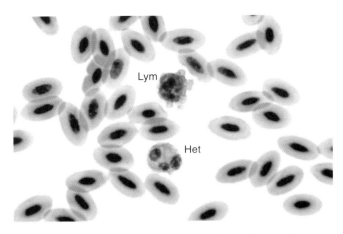

Fig. 3.42 Reactive lymphocyte (Lym) of a gyrfalcon. The cytoplasm is deeply basophilic with several cytoplasmic projections (scalloped cytoplasmic margin). The nucleus is round, centrally located and dark purple in color. A normal heterophil (Het) can also bee seen. (Modified Wright–Giemsa stain).

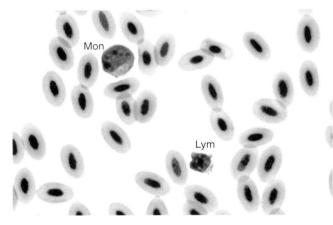

Fig. 3.43 Reactive monocytes (Mon) and reactive lymphocyte (Lym) of a saker falcon. (Modified Wright–Giemsa stain).

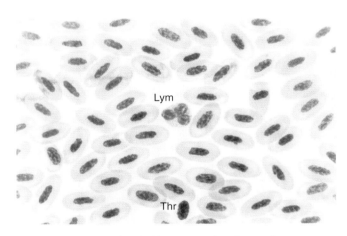

Fig. 3.44 Lymphocyte (Lym) with segmented nucleus and a thrombocyte (Thr) of a saker falcon. Bilobular or trilobular nuclear segmentation, referred to as clover-leaf-shaped nucleus, is a relatively rare occurrence in avian species and could be the result of an immune-mediated or chronic degenerative metabolic disease. (Modified Wright–Giemsa stain).

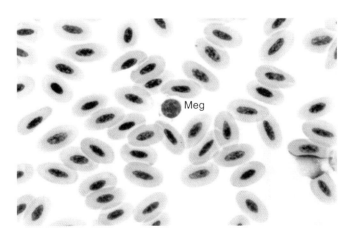

Fig. 3.45 Megathrombocyte (Meg) of a saker falcon. (Modified Wright–Giemsa stain). The presence of the so-called megathrombocytes is usually associated with chronic inflammation.

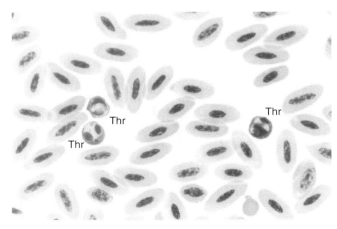

Fig. 3.46 Abnormal thrombocytes (Thr) of a saker falcon. This abnormality was related to a severe hepatic disorder. (Modified Wright–Giemsa stain).

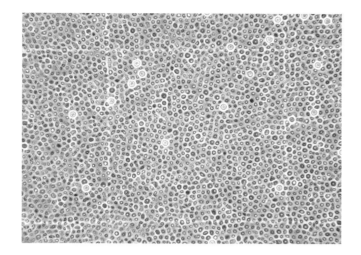

Fig. 3.47 Microscopic view of a loaded improved Neubauer counting chamber ready for leukocyte count. The white cells or leukocytes can be observed as white shiny cells under phase contrast microscopy. (400×).

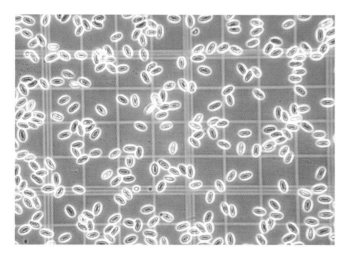

Fig. 3.48 Microscopic view of a loaded improved Neubauer counting chamber ready for erythrocyte count under phase contrast microscopy. Counting is usually conducted following the 'L' rule. Cells that touch the central line of the small squares to the left and bottom are counted. (400×).

Laboratory techniques

Red blood cell count (RBC × 10^{12}/l)

The total red blood cell count is in itself an important hematology assay but it is also essential for the estimation of the mean corpuscular volume (MCV) and the mean corpuscular hemoglobin (MCH). Many laboratories prefer to estimate RBC using an automatic system, as this is more precise than manual methods. The method described below refers to a manual technique.

Working solutions

BD Unopette™ 365851 red blood count manual hematology test (Becton Dickinson Co., NJ, USA)

The Unopette™ 365851 system is probably the most popular method used for manual red blood cell count in avian species. This system uses 10 μl of whole blood into 1.9 ml of 0.85% saline, resulting in a 1:200 dilution. The use of this system will not be described in this section.

The two other common systems used are based on using either Natt and Herrick's solution or formol citrate solution or Dacie's fluid, depending on whether the examination will be carried with or without phase contrast microscopy.

Natt and Herrick's solution for use without phase contrast microscopy

Ingredient	Amount
NaCl	3.88 g
Na_2SO_4	2.5 g
$Na_2HPO_4 \cdot 12H_2O$	2.91 g
KH_2PO_4	0.25 g
Formaldehyde 40%	7.5 ml
Methyl violet 2B	0.1 g
Distilled water	to 1000 ml

Note: Allow solution to stand overnight. Filter before use.

Formol-citrate solution (Dacie's fluid) for use with phase contrast microscopy

Ingredient	Amount
Formaldehyde 40%	10 ml
Trisodium citrate	31.3 g
Distilled water	to 1000 ml

Note: Refrigerate at 8–12°C.
Dacie's formol citrate solution is the least known diluting fluid but is the diluting fluid I use and recommend.

Materials and equipment

- 5 ml disposable sample tube with lid
- Automatic dispenser 0–50 ml
- Micropipette 20 μl and tip
- Roller mixer
- Plain microcapillary tube
- Petri dish (8.5 cm diameter)
- Filter paper (8.5 cm diameter)
- Swab sticks
- Distilled water
- Improved Neubauer hemocytometer and coverslip
- Microscope, preferably with phase contrast facility
- Laboratory tissues.

Method

Dispense 4 ml of formol citrate or Natt and Herrick's solution into sample tube. Pipette 20 μl of blood from sample, wipe the outside of pipette tip and dispense into the tube. Place tube on roller mixer for 3 min. Clean hemocytometer using a dry and clean, lint-free cloth or a tissue. Fix the coverslip firmly, making sure that Newton's rings (colored interference patterns) are present on either side of the counting chamber.

Take a small aliquot of the diluted sample using a capillary tube and fill the hemocytometer. Do not over- or underfill the chamber or allow any bubbles to be admitted during this process. Line a Petri dish with the filter paper and, using distilled water, wet the paper slightly. Break off two pieces from the swab sticks and place the pieces (6 cm long) on either side at the bottom of the Petri dish. Store the loaded hemocytometer on the sticks within the wetted Petri dish to avoid dehydration of the sample. Wait 5 min and count cells in 5×16 squares in the centre of the counting grid (80 small squares).

n = Number of cells counted, then: $\dfrac{n}{20}$ = RBC × 10^{12}/l.

Improved Neubauer counting chamber

The total red blood cell count is performed by counting the number of cells contained in the 25 groups of 16 small squares at the four corner and central squares in the central area of the chamber (Figs 3.49 and 3.50). These squares are separated by closely ruled triple lines, illustrated in the drawing as thick lines.

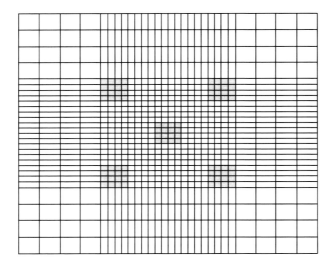

Fig. 3.49 Diagram of counting grid of the improved Neubauer hemocytometer. The 5 × 16 shaded squares are used for the red blood cell (RBC) count.

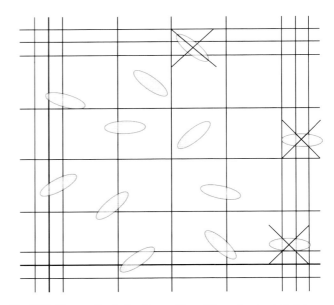

Fig. 3.50 Diagram illustrating the position of the cells counted. Area enlarged from Figure 3.49.

Counting system

Count cells that touch the center triple line (seen here as a thick line) of the ruling on the left and the bottom sides; do not count cells that touch the center triple line of the ruling on the right and the top sides.

Hemoglobin estimation (Hb g/dl)

In avian species, estimation of hemoglobin is hampered by the presence of nuclei in the erythrocytes. Hemoglobin estimation relies on the colorimetric measurement of hemoglobin released after the lysing of the erythrocytes. Hemoglobin can be estimated using automatic methods or manual methods. Commercial laboratories estimating hemoglobin using an automatic hematology analyzer have to take into consideration the photometric interference of the free nuclei after lysing of the erythrocyte. In the manual method, it is essential to remove the nuclei from the preparation, since its presence could yield unreliable results. The nuclei can be deposited by low-speed centrifugation but, since some hemoglobin remains attached to the nuclei, colorimetric readings are commonly low. This can be overcome by estimating hemoglobin as cyanmethemoglobin using alkaline Drabkin's cyanide–ferricyanide solution or as oxyhemoglobin using ammonia solution. In both cases, the estimation is carried out using a spectrophotometer at the absorbance reading of 540 nm. A calibration graph should be made using commercially available hemoglobin standards to express hemoglobin as oxyhemoglobin. Conversely, hemoglobin can be estimated directly as oxyhemoglobin using a commercially available hemoglobinometer. The method described below relies on the use of a hemoglobinometer or a colorimeter.

Materials and equipment

- Automatic dispenser 0–50 ml
- Five ml disposable sample tube with lid
- Micropipette 20 μl and tip
- Roller mixer
- Toothpicks
- Cuvette 10 mm²
- Laboratory lens tissue
- Hemoglobinometer.

Working solution

Ammonia solution

Ingredient	Amount
Ammonia solution (0.88 specific gravity)	4 ml
Distilled water	to 1000 ml

Note: Store in fridge at 8 – 12°C.

Method

Label sample tubes using a permanent marker. Use an automatic dispenser to transfer 4 ml of ammonia solution into sample tube. Wait for 5 min to allow working solution to reach room temperature. Aspirate 20 μl of whole blood from storage tube using micropipette, wipe side of pipette tip carefully using tissue and dispense on the side of sample tube. Avoid touching the distal opening of the pipette tip with the tissue as this will cause capillary shift of blood into the tissue. Avoid immersing the pipette tip into the diluting fluid. This is poor laboratory practice. Place sample tube in roller mixer and wait for 3 min. Decant approximately 3.5 ml of the diluted blood into cuvette. Remove cell nuclei jelly using toothpicks. Do not touch the clear reading walls of the cuvette with bare fingers. Clean clear reading walls of cuvette using laboratory lens tissue. Zero hemoglobinometer using ammonia solution as blank. Reading expressed as Hb g/dl.

HemoCue AB™ (Ängelholm, Sweden)

Method

Hemoglobin can also be estimated as azidemethemoglobin using a dedicated hemoglobinometer system (HemoCue AB, Sweden). This system includes reagent-preloaded microcuvettes and a photometer. The readings are carried out at 570 nm and 880 nm to compensate for turbidity within the sample.

Packed cell volume estimation (PCV%) hematocrit (Hct l/l)

Packed cell volume (PCV) is an important hematology assay since it provides an easy and objective way of estimating the number of erythrocytes in the sample. It is also essential for the calculation of the mean corpuscular volume (MCV) and mean corpuscular hemoglobin concentration (MCHC). In avian species, PCV is best estimated using the microhematocrit method described below. The use of plain microcapillary tubes is preferable, since the same tube can be used subsequently to estimate fibrinogen.

Materials and equipment

- Plain microcapillary tubes
- Cristaseal or any other suitable plastic sealant
- Microhematocrit centrifuge
- Microhematocrit reader.

Method

Fill microcapillary tube to approximately three-quarters of its length. Seal the dry end using the plastic sealer compound. Position the capillary tube correctly within rotor and centrifuge at 10 000 g for 5 min. Determine packed cell volume on hematocrit reader. Position the capillary tube on the acrylic holder of the reader. Align, at the distal end of the tube, the demarcation line between the sealing compound and the red blood cells with line A of the hematocrit reader. By sliding the tube holder to the right or to the left, align the marginal meniscus at the top of the plasma column with line B of the hematocrit reader. Position line C at the interface of the buffy layer and red cells and read hematocrit value on the scale (Fig. 3.51).

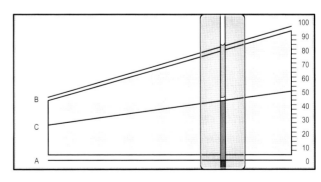

Fig. 3.51 Diagram of hematocrit reader illustrating the method for the estimation of the packed cell volume: PCV% - hematocrit: l/l.

Red cell indices

Mean corpuscular volume (MCV) is the expression of the average volume of individual erythrocytes calculated with the following formula:

$$MCV = \frac{PCV \times 10}{RBC} = MCV \text{ (femtoliters fl)}.$$

Mean corpuscular hemoglobin (MCH) is the expression of the average hemoglobin content of a single erythrocyte and is calculated with the following formula:

$$MCH = \frac{Hb \times 10}{RBC} = MCH \text{ (picograms (pg))}.$$

Mean corpuscular hemoglobin concentration (MCHC) is the expression of the volume within the erythrocyte occupied by the hemoglobin and is calculated with the following formula:

$$MCHC = \frac{Hb \times 100}{PCV} = MCHC \text{ (g/l)}.$$

White blood cell count (WBC × 10⁹/l)

Working solutions

BD Unopette™ 365877 eosinophil count manual hematology test (Becton Dickinson Co, NJ)

The Unopette™ 365877 system was originally developed for the estimation of eosinophils in human hematology but it has proved useful for determining the total white cell count in avian species. This system uses 25 μl of whole blood into 0.775 ml of 1% Phloxine B diluent resulting in a 1:32 dilution. This method will not be covered in this section.

Natt and Herrick's (for use without phase-contrast microscopy)

(See formula in RBC method above).

1% ammonium oxalate solution (for phase-contrast microscopy)

Ingredient	Amount
Ammonium oxalate	10 g
Distilled water	to 1000 ml

The method described below is based on the use of ammonium oxalate solution, which is the method I use and recommend.

Material and equipment

- 3 ml disposable sample tube with lid
- Automatic dispenser 0–50 ml
- Micropipette 100 μl and tip
- Roller mixer
- Plain capillary tube
- Petri dish (8.5 cm diameter)
- Filter paper (8.5 cm diameter)
- Swab sticks
- Improved Neubauer hemocytometer and coverslip
- Distilled water
- Microscope, preferably with phase contrast facility
- Laboratory tissues.

Method

Dispense 1.9 ml of 1% ammonium oxalate solution into sample tube. Pipette 100 μl of blood from sample, wipe the outside of pipette tip and dispense into the tube. Place tube on roller mixer for 3 min. Clean hemocytometer using a dry and clean, lint-free cloth or a tissue. Fix the coverslip firmly, making sure that Newton's rings (colored interference patterns) are present on either side of the counting chamber.

Take a small aliquot of the diluted sample, using a capillary tube, and fill the hemocytometer. Do not over- or underfill the chamber or allow any bubbles to be admitted during this process. Line a Petri dish with the filter paper and, using distilled water, wet the paper slightly. Break off two pieces from the swab sticks and place the pieces (6 cm long) on either side at the bottom of the Petri dish. Store the loaded hemocytometer on the sticks within the wetted Petri dish to avoid dehydration of the sample. Wait 5 min and count cells in 4 outer large squares of the counting grid (64 small squares) (Fig. 3.52).

n = number of cells counted, then: $\dfrac{n}{20}$ = WBC × 10⁹/l.

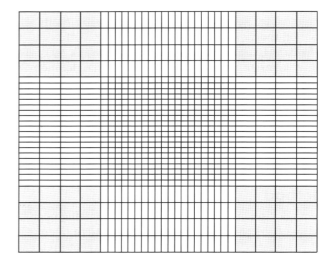

Fig. 3.52 Diagram of counting grid of the improved Neubauer hemocytometer. The four large shaded squares in the corners are used for the white cell (WBC) count.

Differential white cell count (%) and absolute number

For the differential white blood cell count and absolute white blood cell count, the film should be examined thoroughly under high power magnification (1000×) using oil immersion. The recommended topographic site is on the shoulder of the blood film, as this is the area where the blood cells are in one layer and are slightly segregated, thus facilitating examination.

In general terms, 100 white blood cells should be counted and classified according to the morphological and staining characteristics. Counting is usually carried out using a commercially available manual or electronic differential cell counter. The differential white blood cell count is expressed as a percentage of individual cell groups. The percentage of each cell group is then converted into absolute numbers by reference to the total WBC using the following formula:

$$\frac{\text{Percentage of white blood cell counted} \times \text{total WBC}}{100} = \text{absolute No} \times 10^9/l.$$

Fixation and staining of the blood film

It is commonly accepted that blood films can be prepared and be fixed and stained at a later date. This is incorrect: blood films should be, at least, fixed immediately after preparation, particularly if made in a hot and humid environment or under cold and freezing conditions. Blood films should never be exposed to direct sunlight, moisture of any kind or vapor from chemicals, formaldehyde in particular, as this would invariably affect cell morphology.

Fixation

In general, freshly prepared blood films should be immersed in absolute methanol within a Coplin jar for 5–10 min. This should be done immediately after preparation. Fixed blood films can then be stored within commercially available slide storage boxes and stained at a later date (e.g. under field conditions). Conversely, blood films can be stained immediately after fixation.

The importance of adequate fixation of blood films from avian species cannot be overemphasized. The intracytoplasmic granules of the heterophils and basophils are water-soluble; therefore, blood films should be adequately fixed before staining in order to preserve the integrity of these structures. A significant problem in avian hematology is the presence of smudged red cell nuclei as a consequent of hemolysis in poorly fixed blood films. This is one of the main reasons why clinicians and commercial laboratories are now inclined to use stains that are prepared in absolute methanol (e.g. Wright–Giemsa stain, Leishman stain) and are

used at full strength so films are fixed and stained at the same time. If you use absolute methanol within a Coplin jar for fixation in your laboratory, remember to replace it as soon as it begins showing chemical fatigue. This will depend on the number of slides fixed and the environmental conditions within the laboratory.

Staining

Most Romanowsky stains used for the staining of human and mammalian blood films are suitable for the staining of avian blood films. However, the results obtained with the various stains may be slightly different and the selection of stains is generally accepted as a matter of personal preference. Stains commonly used include Wright stain, Giemsa stain, Wright–Giemsa stain, Leishman stain, Wright–Leishman stain, May–Grünwald stain and May–Grünwald–Giemsa stain. I do not think that rapid stains on their own (e.g. Diff Quick, Rapid Diff) produce adequate quality for the differentiation of subtle blood cells structures and those of hematozoa. This is particularly important with respect to the morphological characteristics of the granulocytes.

Automatic slide stainers facilitate the staining of a relatively large number of blood films at the same time, producing consistent results and eliminating variations that may occur with manual techniques. Needless to say, this kind of equipment is relatively expensive to purchase and maintain and is more appropriate for high-volume commercial laboratories.

It is important that clinicians or laboratory technicians recall the basic principles of hematology when staining blood films. The pH of the stains should be checked each time new stock is prepared. Some stains, particularly those prepared from powder, should be adequately filtered. Glassware should be properly washed, rinsed with distilled water and dried thoroughly before use. Many of the common artifacts on blood films are due to careless preparation and improper methodology.

The staining method currently used and recommended by the author is a slightly modified Wright–Giemsa staining procedure, which is here described.

Working stain

Ingredient	Amount
Wright stain powder	3 g
Giemsa stain powder	0.3 g
Glycerol	5 ml
Absolute methanol	to 1000 ml (acetone free)

Note: Filter and store.

Method

Prepare thin blood smears. Place on staining rack. Flood smear with Wright–Giemsa stain, allow to stand for 3 min. Add equal amount of buffer Sørensen's pH 6.5–6.8, depending on batch stain. Mix gently by blowing using a pipette until metallic green sheen forms on the surface; allow to stand for 6 min. Rinse with buffer allowing to stand for 1 min for differentiation. Wash copiously with buffer. Wipe the back of smear with tissue to remove excess stain. Prop in rack until dry. (Note: this technique is modified from Campbell 1995.)

The placement of a coverslip using a commercially available mounting medium over the blood smear is optional. However, the mounting of blood films offers several advantages such as preventing scratching during transport, protection against damage during excessive manipulation (e.g. teaching material) and enhancing visualization for optimal examination and photography.

Morphological and staining characteristics of red blood cells, white blood cells and thrombocytes

Adequate knowledge of the morphology and staining characteristics of the different blood cells is of the utmost importance for the differentiation and classification of the different blood cells.

The most notable figure in the world of biological stains was Paul Ehrlich (1854–1915). He first invented a triacid stain that allowed differentiation and classification of white blood cells into the grouping widely used today. This stain was replaced by an eosin and methylene blue stain invented by Dimitri Leonidovich Romanowsky (1861–1921), which was subsequently modified by physicians such as Richard May (1863–1936), Gustav Giemsa (1867–

1948) and James Homer Wright (1871–1928). In general, the widely known 'Romanowsky stains' contain blue azure, which reacts with acid groups, including those of nucleic acids and proteins of the nucleus and cytoplasm, and eosin Y, which has an affinity for basic groups, in particular those of hemoglobin. When used in different avian species the slight variations observed may be the result of true species diversity or simply variations in the materials and methods used from individual to individual or from laboratory to laboratory. Table 3.5 outlines the morphological and staining characteristics of the different avian blood cells.

Preparation of the blood smear

Method

Blood films can be made from a drop of fresh non-anticoagulated blood directly from the tip of the syringe. Conversely, films can be made from blood stored in ethylene diamine tetra-acetic acid (EDTA) within 2–3 h after collection. There are two generally accepted methods for the preparation of blood films in hematology, the slide to slide technique and the coverslip to slide technique. The most popular method amongst avian clinicians is the coverslip to slide technique as blood red cell smudging is generally minimized.

Slide to slide technique

It is highly recommended to use one-end frosted microscopic slides to write down the ID of the sample

TABLE 3.5 Morphological and staining characteristics of the different blood cells

Blood cell	Morphological characteristics	Staining characteristics
Erythrocyte	**Mature cells**	**Mature cells**
	Medium size; oval, elongated shape; central oval, elongated nucleus	Cytoplasm: uniform pale orange to red pink. Nucleus: purple red, condensed, clumped chromatin
	Immature cells	**Immature cells**
	Smaller than mature cell; round to semi-oval; relatively larger nucleus	Polychromatic; pale to dark blue
Heterophil	Medium size; round shape; bilobed nucleus	Colorless cytoplasm; rod- to cigar-shaped, brick red to pale blue granules
Eosinophil	Medium size; round shape; bilobed nucleus	Pale blue cytoplasm; round to oval, brick red to pale blue granules
Basophil	Small size; round shape; unlobed nucleus	Pale blue cytoplasm; variable number of small, medium and large, dark red purple granules
Lymphocyte	Small to medium size; typically round to triangular shape; centrally positioned large, round nucleus; in general 25 cytoplasm:75 nucleus; coarsely condensed to highly condensed chromatin	Pale blue cytoplasm
Monocyte	Large size; typically round shape; eccentrically positioned kidney-shaped nucleus; in general 75 cytoplasm:25 nucleus; cytoplasm lace-like appearance, often medium size vacuoles, coarsely condensed chromatin	Cytoplasm pale blue to pale gray
Thrombocyte	Small; oval to rectangular shape; nucleus oval to rectangular	Cytoplasm colorless to pale blue; large vacuoles; nucleus highly condensed dark purple–red chromatin

using pencil. Wipe slides clean with a lint-free cloth or lens tissue. Use a plain microcapillary tube to withdraw a small amount of fresh nonanticoagulated blood directly from syringe tip or EDTA tube. Place a small drop of blood (2 µl) at one end of a slide. Select a spreader slide and position it in front of the drop of blood at an angle of about 45°. It is needless to say that the selected slide should be free from any indentation. To test this, pass the spreading edge over the edge of a finger nail. Move gently the spreader slide backwards to touch the drop of blood and allow the blood to run across the edge of the slide. Drive the slide gently forward with a steady but firm movement to create a uniform smear (Fig. 3.53). It is always good practice to make two good-quality blood films.

Coverslip to slide technique

The only significant difference between this method and the previous one consist on the following steps. Place a large rectangular coverslip over the drop of blood. Pull coverslip and the slide in opposite directions in a steady, but firm movement to create a uniform smear (Fig. 3.54).

Thrombocyte count (10⁹/l)

Method

Count thrombocytes while performing the differential white cell count. The absolute number of thrombocytes in the sample is subsequently calculated by using the following formula:

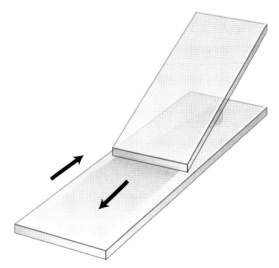

Fig. 3.53 Diagram illustrating the preparation of a blood smear using the slide to slide technique. Move spreader slide backwards to touch the drop of blood gently, allowing it to run across the edge of the slide. Move forward to make the smear. Move slowly if blood runs slowly; move fast if blood runs fast.

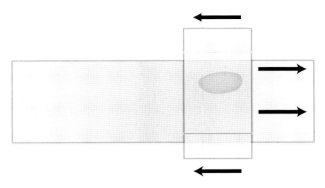

Fig. 3.54 Diagram illustrating the preparation of a blood smear using the coverslip to slide technique. Place coverslip on to drop of blood. Apply gentle pressure downward. Move slide and coverslip in opposite directions to make the smear.

$$\frac{\text{Number of thrombocytes counted}}{100} \times WBC = \text{Thrombocytes } 10^9/l.$$

Fibrinogen estimation (g/l)

Material and equipment

- Microcapillary tube rack for use in waterbath
- Microhematocrit centrifuge
- Water bath at 56°C ± 1°C
- Microcapillary tube holder
- Microscope with measuring eyepiece and stage Vernier scale
- Timer.

Method

After the measurement of the packed cell volume, place microcapillary tubes in the rack and immerse in waterbath at 56°C for 3 min. Make sure the entire plasma column is immersed. Remove capillaries and centrifuge again at 10 000 g for 5 min. Place in microcapillary tube holder and, using the measuring eyepiece and the stage Vernier of the microscope, take readings at the upper and lower limit of the protein layer and at the upper limit of the plasma column (Fig. 3.55).

The fibrinogen is estimated using the following formula:

$$\frac{B - A}{C - A} \times 100 = \text{fibrinogen (g/l)}.$$

Note: It is essential to perform this test on samples collected into EDTA, since the test is invalidated on samples stored in heparin or on samples containing clots.

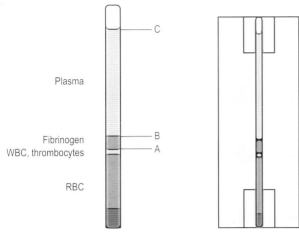

Fig. 3.55 On the left, the diagram shows the different measurements taken for the estimation of the fibrinogen; on the right, a modified microscope slide for holding the microcapillary tube during reading.

Age-related hematological changes

Age-related hematological findings were investigated in kori bustard (*Ardeotis kori*) chicks during their growth and development (Fig. 3.56). Blood samples were collected from 16 clinically normal chicks at 1 month intervals. The 10th sampling was actually obtained at 15 months of life.

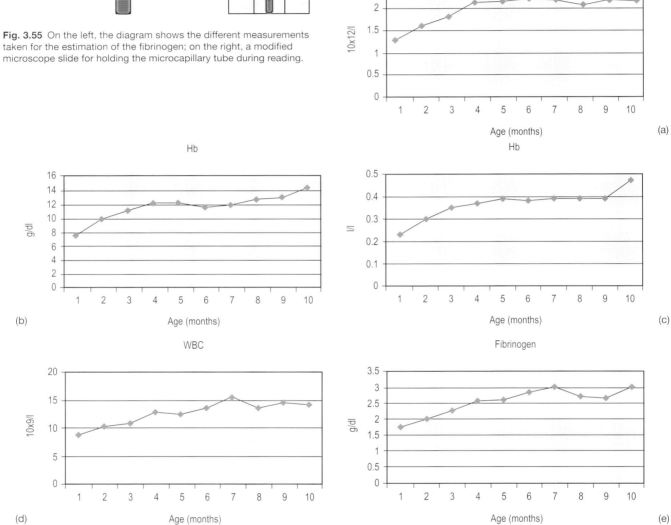

Fig 3.56 Age-related hematological findings in kori bustard (*Ardeotis kori*) chicks. (a) The RBC increased steadily for the first 4 months from $1.28 \pm 0.06 \times 10^{12}$/l at 1 month of age, increasing gradually up to the age of 4 months to $2.06 \pm 0.08 \times 10^{12}$/l. After this time, that RBC remained fairly constant. The RBC value at the age of 12–15 months was $2.08 \pm 0.06 \times 10^{12}$/l. (b) The HB value followed a similar pattern as for RBC with a value of 7.5 ± 0.2 g/dl at the age of 1 month, increasing to 12.1 ± 0.3 g/dl at 4 months of age. This value remained fairly constant until the age of 12 months, when it increased to 14.2 ± 0.4 g/dl. (c) The Hct value continued to increase steadily from 0.23 ± 0.7 l/l at 1 month of age, to 0.399 ± 0.9 l/l at 5 months of age and remained fairly constant until the age of 12–15 months when the value increased to 0.47 ± 0.9 l/l. (d) The WBC count at 1 month of age was $8.78 \pm 0.45 \times 10^9$/l, increasing to $15.6 \pm 0.7 \times 10^9$/l at 7 months then decreasing slightly to $14.5 \pm 0.5 \times 10^9$/l at 9 months of age. (e) The fibrinogen value was 1.76 ± 0.18 g/l at 1 month of age increasing steadily to 3.0 ± 0.2 g/l at the age of 7 months. Note: Redrawn from Howlett JC, Samour JH, Bailey TA, Naldo JL (1998) Age-related haematology changes in captive-reared kori bustards (*Ardeotis kori*). *Comparative Haematology International* 8: 26–30.

ACKNOWLEDGMENTS

The authors should like to thank the Editors of *Clinical Avian Medicine* (2006), Spix Publishing, for allowing the authors to reproduce parts of the Chapter on Diagnostic Value of Hematology.

REFERENCES

Campbell TW (1995) *Avian Hematology and Cytology*, pp. 3–19. Iowa State University Press, Ames, IA.

D'Aloia M-A, Samour JH, Howlett JC *et al.* (1994) Haemopathological responses to chronic inflammation in the houbara bustard (*Chlamydotis undulata macqueenii*). *Comparative Haematology International* **4**: 203–206.

Fudge AM (1995) Clinical application of laser flow cytometry to avian hematology analysis. In: *Proceedings of the Association of Avian Veterinarians*, Nashville, pp. 17–18.

Gascoyne SC, Bennet PM, Kirkwood JK, Hawkey CM (1994) Guidelines for the interpretation of laboratory findings in birds and mammals with unknown reference ranges: plasma biochemistry. *Veterinary Record* **134**: 7–11.

Howlett JC, Samour JH, D'Aloia M-A *et al.* (1995) Normal haematology of captive adult kori bustards (*Ardeotis kori*). *Comparative Haematology International* **5**: 102–105.

Samour JH, Howlett JC, Hart MG *et al.* (1994) Normal haematology of the houbara bustard (*Chlamydotis undulata macqueenii*). *Comparative Haematology International* **4**: 198–202.

FURTHER READING

Alonso JA *et al.* (1990) Hematology and blood chemistry of free-living young great bustards (*Otis tarda*). *Comparative Biochemistry and Physiology* **97a**: 611–614.

Averbeck C (1992) Haematology and blood chemistry of healthy and clinically abnormal great black backed gulls (*Larus marinus*) and herring gulls (*Larus argentatus*). *Avian Pathology* **21**: 215–223.

Campbell TW (1994) Hematology. In: Ritchie BW, Harrison GJ, Harrison LR (eds) *Avian Medicine: Principles and Application*, pp. 176–199. Wingers Publishing, Lake Worth, FL.

Clubb SL *et al.* (1990) Hematologic and serum biochemical reference intervals in juvenile eclectus parrots. *Journal of the Association of Avian Veterinarians* **4**: 218–225.

Clubb SL *et al.* (1991) Hematologic and serum biochemical reference intervals in juvenile cockatoos. *Journal of the Association of Avian Veterinarians* **5**: 16–21.

Clubb SL *et al.* (1991) Hematologic and serum biochemical reference intervals in juvenile macaws (*Ara* sp). *Journal of the Association of Avian Veterinarians* **5**: 154–162.

Dacie JV, Lewis SM (1995) *Practical Haematology*, 8th edn. Churchill Livingstone, Edinburgh.

D'Aloia M-A, Samour JH, Howlett JC *et al.* (1995) Normal haematology and age-related findings in rufous-crested bustards (*Eupodotis ruficrista*). *Comparative Haematology International* **5**: 10–12.

D'Aloia M-A, Samour JH, Bailey TA *et al.* (1996) Normal haematology of the white bellied (*Eupodotis senegalensis*), little black (*Eupodotis afra*) and Heuglin's (*Neotis heuglinii*) bustards. *Comparative Haematology International* **6**: 46–49.

Dein FJ (1986) Hematology. In: Harrison GJ, Harrison LR (eds) *Clinical Avian Medicine and Surgery*, pp. 174–191. WB Saunders, Philadelphia.

Dorrestein GM (1996) Cytology and haemocytology. In: Beynon PH, Forbes NA, Lawton MPC (eds) *Manual of Psittacine Birds*, pp. 38–48. British Small Animal Veterinary Association, Cheltenham.

Fudge AM (1996) Clinical hematology and chemistry of ratites. In: Tully TN, Shane SM (eds) *Ratites: Management, Medicine, and Surgery*, pp. 105–114. Krieger Publishing, Malabar.

Fudge AM (1997) Avian clinical pathology: hematology and chemistry. In: Altman RB, Clubb SL, Dorrestein GM, Quesenberry K (eds) *Avian Medicine and Surgery*, pp. 142–157. WB Saunders, Philadelphia.

Fudge AM (1998) Problem-oriented approach to blood panel interpretation. *Proceedings of the Association of Avian Veterinarians*, St Paul, pp. 285–299.

Fudge AM (1998) Avian cytology and hematology. *Proceedings of the Association of Avian Veterinarians*, St Paul, pp. 357–369.

Fudge AM (2000) *Laboratory Medicine: Avian and Exotic Pets*, pp. 1–8. WB Saunders, Philadelphia.

Gulland FMD, Hawkey CM (1990) Avian haematology. *Veterinary Annual* **30**: 126–136.

Harris DJ (2000) Clinical tests. In: Tully TN, Lawton MPC, Dorrestein GM (eds) *Avian Medicine*, pp. 43–51. Butterworth Heinemann, Oxford.

Hauska H, Gerlach H (1995) The development of the red blood cell pattern of growing parrot nestlings. In: *Proceedings of the 3rd Conference of the European Committee of the Association of Avian Veterinarians*, Jerusalem, pp. 178–182.

Hauska H, Gerlach H (1995) The development of the white blood cell pattern of growing parrot nestlings. In: *Proceedings of the 3rd Conference of the European Committee of the Association of Avian Veterinarians*, Jerusalem, pp. 183–186.

Hauska H, Redig PT (1997) Morphological changes in the white haemogram of raptors. In: *Proceedings of the 4th Conference of the European Committee of the Association of Avian Veterinarians*, London, pp. 205–208.

Hawkey CM, Samour JH (1988) The value of clinical hematology in exotic birds. In: Jacobson ER, Kollias GV Jr (eds) *Contemporary Issues in Small Animal Practice*, pp. 109–142. Churchill Livingstone, New York.

Hawkey CM, Samour JH, Ashton DG *et al.* (1983) Normal and clinical haematology of captive cranes (Gruiformes). *Avian Pathology* **12**: 73–84.

Hawkey C *et al.* (1990) Haematological changes in domestic fowl (*Gallus gallus*) and cranes (Gruiformes) with *Mycobacterium avium* infection. *Avian Pathology* **19**: 223–234.

Hernandez M (1991) Raptor clinical hematology. *Proceedings of the Association of Avian Veterinarians*, Vienna, pp. 420–433.

Hernandez M, Martin S, Fores P (1990) Clinical hematology and blood chemistry values for the common buzzard (*Buteo buteo*). *Journal of Raptor Research* **24**: 113–119.

Howlett JC (2000) Clinical and diagnostic procedures. In: Samour JH (ed.) *Avian Medicine*, pp. 28–50. Harcourt, London.

Howlett JC, Samour JH, Bailey TA *et al.* (1996) *Haemoproteus* in the houbara bustard (*Chlamydotis undulata macqueenii*) and the rufous-crested bustard (*Eupodotis ruficrista*) in the United Arab Emirates. *Avian Pathology* **25**: 4–55.

Howlett JC, Samour JH, Bailey TA, Naldo JL (1998) Age-related haematology changes in captive-reared kori bustards (*Ardeotis kori*). *Comparative Haematology International* **8**: 26–30.

Howlett JC, Bailey TA, Samour JH *et al.* (2002) Age-related hematologic changes in captive-reared houbara, white-bellied and rufous crested bustards. *Journal of Wildlife Diseases* **38**: 804–816.

International Council for Standardization in Haematology (1994) Guidelines for the evaluation of blood cell analysers including those used for differential leucocyte and reticulocyte counting and cell marker applications. *Clinical and Laboratory Haematology* **16**: 157.

Jain CJ (1993) *Essentials of Veterinary Hematology*, pp. 19–53. Lea & Febiger, Philadelphia.

Jennings IB (1996) Hematology. In Beynon PH, Forbes NA, Harcourt-Brown NH (eds) *Manual of Raptors, Pigeons and Waterfowl*, pp. 68–78. British Small Animal Veterinary Association, Cheltenham.

Jimenez A *et al.* (1991) Clinical haematology of the great bustard (*Otis tarda*). *Avian Pathology* **20**: 675–680.

Lane RA (1996) Avian hematology. In: Rosskopf W, Woerpel R (eds) *Diseases of Cage and Aviary Birds*, 3rd edn, pp. 739–772. Williams & Wilkins, Baltimore.

Lind PJ *et al.* (1990) Morphology of the avian eosinophil in raptors. *Journal of the Association of Avian Veterinarians* **4**: 33–38.

Maxwell MH (1993) Avian blood leucocyte responses to stress. *World Poultry Science Journal* **49**: 34–43.

Maxwell MH, Robertson GW (1995) The avian basophilic leukocyte: a review. *World Poultry Science Journal* **51**: 307–325.

Maxwell MH, Hocking PM, Robertson GW (1992) Differential leucocyte response to various degrees of food restriction in broilers, turkeys and ducks. *British Poultry Science* **33**: 177–187.

Merritt EL, Fritz CL, Ramsay EC (1996) Hematologic and serum biochemical values in captive American flamingos (*Phoenicopterus ruber ruber*). *Journal of Avian Medicine and Surgery* **10**:163–167.

Mikaelian I (1993) Variations circannuales des paramètres hématologiques de l'outarde houbara (*Chlamydotis undulata*). Professional thesis, Ecole Nationale Vétérinaire de Lyon, Université Claude Bernard, Lyon, France.

Mulley RC (1980) Hematology of the wood duck (*Chenonetta jubata*). *Journal of Wildlife Diseases* **16**: 271–273.

Palomeque J, Pinto D, Viscor G (1991) Hematologic and blood chemistry values of the Masai ostrich (*Struthio camelus*). *Journal of Wildlife Diseases* **27**: 34–40.

Peinado VI et al. (1992) Hematology and plasma chemistry in endangered pigeons. *Journal of Zoo and Wildlife Medicine* **23**: 65–71.

Pendl H (2001) Avian hematology for practitioners. *Proceedings of the Association of Avian Veterinarians*, Munich, pp. 387–400.

Samour JH, Peirce M (1996) *Babesia shortti* infection in a saker falcon (*Falco cherrug altaicus*). *Veterinary Record* **139**: 167–168.

Samour JH, D'Aloia M-A, Howlett JC (1996) Normal haematology of the saker falcon (*Falco cherrug*). *Comparative Haematology International* **6**: 50–52.

Samour JH et al. (1998) Normal haematology and blood chemistry of captive adult stone curlews (*Burhinus oedicnemus*). *Comparative Haematology International* **8**: 219–224.

Stewart JS (1989) Husbandry, medical and surgical management of ratites. *Proceedings of the Association of Avian Veterinarians*, Seattle, 119–122. Association of Avian Veterinarians, Bedford, TX.

Sturkie PD (1965) *Avian Physiology*, 2nd edn. Baillière Tindall & Cassell, London.

VanderHeyden N (1994) Evaluation and interpretation of the avian hemogram. *Seminars of Avian Exotic Pet Medicine* **3**: 5–13.

Villouta G, Hargreaves R, Riveros V (1997) Haematological and clinical biochemistry findings in captive Humboldt penguins (*Spheniscus humboldti*). *Avian Pathology* **26**: 851–858.

Biochemistry

Thomas A. Bailey

In this section, the biochemical tests that are commonly used to evaluate avian health are reviewed. Clinical signs in birds may be nonspecific and often only limited information is gleaned from the physical examination. Blood chemistry assays are a component of the clinical laboratory support that is required in the differential diagnosis of many diseases. Interpreting what a list of chemistry values from a sick bird really means can be confusing and, while biochemistry results are not usually diagnostic, they may be helpful in ruling out conditions or indicating the severity of organ pathology (Fudge, 1997). Relating changes in chemistry values to organ pathology is difficult, because with the exception of studies on pigeons by Lumeij (1987), there have been few detailed biochemical investigations in nondomestic avian species concerning tissue enzyme profiles, age-related changes and changes after experimental organ damage.

Sample collection and storage

Techniques for blood collection and the volume of blood that can safely be collected have already been discussed.

While the anticoagulant of choice for most laboratory tests is lithium heparin, there are some exceptions and the recommended samples that should be collected for different biochemical tests are listed in Table 3.6.

Normal biochemistry reference ranges

Published normal biochemistry ranges of blood enzymes, metabolites, electrolytes and trace elements for a selection of healthy adult and juvenile avian species are presented in Appendix 3. These values may prove useful for the interpretation of some laboratory findings. However, it is important for the reader to be aware that many of these 'normal' ranges are derived from single studies in captive collections, and for some species only small numbers of birds were involved. True population values can only be determined from larger samples that represent different diets, climates, housing environments, exercise levels, genders and age groups (Merritt et al., 1996). Unfortunately such studies are rare and avian veterinarians must make do with ranges derived from small numbers of birds.

In addition to seeing how many birds were sampled, in order to calculate a 'normal range', clinicians should critically assess what statistics were used to analyze the data. Unfortunately, many published reference ranges have been derived using inappropriate statistics. Many biochemistry data do not conform to a gaussian (normal) distribution and nonparametric statistics are needed to establish reference ranges (Lumeij, 1987; Lumeij et al., 1988a, 1988b). Reference ranges are established statistically to produce a 95% confidence interval. In the case of normally distributed data this is a 95% confidence interval of the mean; in the case of data that is not normally distributed, a 95% confidence interval of the median is more appropriate. What this means is that 5% (i.e. 1 in 20) of healthy birds will have values that fall outside a given 'normal' reference range.

The reader is recommended to consult the literature to gain a deeper insight into theories and pitfalls of establishing normal reference ranges (Lumeij, 1987; Lumeij et al., 1988a, 1988b; Hochleithner, 1994) and these days there are many statistics books that are intellectually digestible for nonstatisticians (Petrie and Watson, 1999; Petrie and Sabin, 2000).

Enzyme profiles

Table 3.7 reviews causes of increases in enzyme activities and also summarizes the tissue distribution of some enzymes in birds. This table may be of assistance in interpreting changes of plasma enzyme levels seen in clinical practice.

Elevations in plasma enzyme activities are related to leakage of enzymes from damaged cells (Lumeij, 1987;

TABLE 3.6 Recommended blood samples for avian biochemistry tests

Test	Plasma*	Serum	Other	Sampling comments
Alkaline phosphatase (ALKP)	√	√		
Alanine aminotransferase (ALT)	√	√		Hemolysis causes elevated activities
Ammonia			EDTA	Analyze samples immediately as ammonia is released by catabolism of many substances (e.g. urea)
Amylase	√	√		
Aspartate aminotransferase (AST)	√	√		
Bicarbonate	√	√		
Bile acids	√	√		Birds should be fasted for 12–24 h before sampling
Bilirubin	√	√		
Calcium	√	√		Calcium-binding anticoagulants (e.g. EDTA) will cause artificially low values
Chloride	√	√		
Cholesterol	√	√		
Creatin kinase (CK)	√	√		Citrate and fluoride inhibit CK activity
Copper	√			
Creatinine	√	√		
Delta-aminolevulinic acid dehydratase	√	√		
Gamma glutamyl transferase (GGT)		√	EDTA	Heparin interferes with test reactants and citrate, oxalate and fluoride artificially depress activity
Glutamate dehydrogenase (GLDH)	√	√		
Glucose	√	√		Analyze samples within 2 h to minimize effect of glycolysis by erythrocytes
Iron	√	√		Avoid hemolysis. Avoid citrate, oxalate and EDTA because they bind iron
Lactate dehydrogenase (LDH)	√	√		Hemolysis causes elevated activities
Magnesium	√			
Phosphorus	√	√		Avoid hemolysis. Citrate, oxalate and EDTA interfere with analysis
Potassium	√	√		Levels are elevated by hemolysis. Separate samples within minutes for accurate results. Hyperlipemia and hyperproteinemia cause artificially low values
Selenium		√		
Sodium	√	√		Hyperlipemia and hyperproteinemia cause artificially low values
Total protein	√	√		Plasma contains fibrinogen and in pigeons the concentration of total protein in plasma is higher than serum
Triglycerides	√	√		
Urea	√	√		
Uric acid	√	√		
Zinc		√		

*Plasma from lithium heparin tubes.

Lumeij *et al.*, 1988a). Interpretation of elevated plasma enzyme levels can only be performed if the enzyme profiles of various organs of the species under investigation are known, because the distribution of enzymes is markedly different between different organs and animal species. The clinical enzymology characteristics of many domestic mammals are well known but studies of enzyme patterns in avian tissues for diagnostic purposes have been limited to a few species (Cornelius *et al.*, 1958; Bogin and Israeli, 1976; Bogin *et al.*, 1976; Lumeij and Wolfswinkel, 1987; Lumeij *et al.*, 1988a, 1988b; Bailey *et al.*, 1999b).

It should be noted that not all elevations in plasma enzyme activities indicate a disease process, and tissue enzyme profiles can only serve as a rough guide to the interpretation of plasma enzyme activity. For example, although creatine kinase (CK) appears to be a specific and sensitive indicator of muscle cell damage in both

TABLE 3.7 Activity of enzymes in avian tissues and causes of increases in avian species

Enzyme	Activity in pigeon* and bustard[†] tissues	Causes of increase in avian species
ALT	Present in most tissues including the duodenum, pancreas, liver, proventriculus, heart and skeletal muscle	Nonspecific cell damage. Only rarely increased in avian liver disease
AST	Present in most tissues including liver, heart, skeletal muscle, brain, kidney, duodenum and pancreas. In bustards the highest levels are in the proventriculus, heart, skeletal muscle	Mainly liver (e.g. fatty liver), heart or muscle disease. Vitamin E/Se deficiency, IM injections. AST has a longer half-life than LDH and levels remain elevated for a few days longer after cellular damage has stopped
ALKP	Mostly in duodenum, kidney. Low levels in liver	Increased cellular activity, not necessarily damage. Higher in juveniles. Increases seen in egg-laying, fractures, neoplasia and infection
CK	Present in most tissues including the duodenum, pancreas, kidney, liver, proventriculus, skeletal muscle, heart muscle and brain	Muscle damage, IM injections, neuropathies, physical capture, surgery, vitamin E/Se deficiency, lead toxicity
GGT	Biliary and renal tubular epithelium	Not a sensitive indicator of hepatocellular damage
GLDH	Mitochondrial enzyme in most tissues. Liver, kidney and brain	Hepatocellular necrosis and severe liver disease
LDH	Present in most tissues including the duodenum, pancreas, skeletal muscle, heart muscle, liver, bone, kidney, red blood cells. Highest levels in bustards are in the proventriculus and heart muscle	Hemolysis and liver (e.g. fatty liver), heart or muscle disease, IM injections. This enzyme has a short half-life and concentrations decline rapidly after organ damage

* Lumeij 1987. † Bailey *et al.* 1999b.
Source: extracted and modified from Hochleithner, 1994, Fudge, 1997, Lumeij, 1987, Bailey *et al.*, 1999b.

mammals (Chalmers and Barrett 1982) and birds (Lumeij *et al.*, 1988a, 1988b), it is known that CK (and lactate dehydrogenase, LDH) levels dramatically increase in healthy bustards that are handled (Bailey *et al.*, 1997). Consequently, consideration should be given to previous episodes of handling when interpreting plasma CK and LDH values. Similarly, Dorrestein *et al.* (1986) induced muscle damage in pigeons by injecting doxycycline in the pectoral muscle and found good correlation between CK levels and the severity of the injury caused by the injection. When birds are known to have been recently injected intramuscularly elevated plasma CK, aspartate aminotransferase (AST) and LDH activity should be interpreted with caution. Other causes of biochemical artifacts are discussed in the accompanying tables and include bacterial contamination of samples, unseparated blood, hemolysis and various anticoagulants.

Metabolites and minerals

Analysis of metabolites in the blood provides information on the functional capacity of organs that are involved in different metabolic pathways. Commonly measured metabolites include plasma ammonia, bile acids, inorganic phosphate, urea and uric acid. The macrominerals (calcium, phosphorus, potassium, sodium and chloride) and microminerals (magnesium, zinc, iron, copper and selenium) also serve important metabolic functions and are crucial for maintenance, growth and reproduction. Tables 3.8 and 3.9 summarize causes of changes in metabolic and electrolyte tests in avian species. Once again, normal physiological variations need to be taken into account when interpreting plasma metabolite levels. Not all elevations indicate a disease process: for example, significantly elevated plasma

bile acid, uric acid and urea concentrations occur postprandially in raptors (Lumeij and Remple, 1991, 1992). Other physiological variations in metabolite levels are discussed in the accompanying tables.

Mineral deficiency or excess can cause disease, so animal health evaluation often requires the determination of mineral status. Mineral status can be determined by analysis of serum, bone, tissues (e.g. liver) and feed (Scheideler *et al.*, 1994). The normal mineral concentration ranges in the blood or tissues of healthy animals must be known to determine mineral status. Trace minerals, including copper, manganese, selenium and zinc function as accessory factors to enzymes and are required in small amounts in the diet (National Research Council, 1980, 1994). Trace minerals have been extensively studied in the blood and tissues of domestically farmed animals such as poultry and health examination of flocks frequently involves an assessment of mineral status. While the collection of blood samples is a practical and minimally invasive technique for screening nondomestic birds, further studies are warranted to correlate tissue (e.g. liver) and blood levels. For example, liver levels are considered to be the most reliable indicator of copper status in domestic species (Keen and Graham, 1989). Table 3.10 presents a summary of the physiology and effects of toxicity and deficiency in avian species of some minerals for which blood or tissue levels in birds have been published.

Vitamins

Vitamins are defined as natural food components that are present in minute quantities, are organic in nature and are essential for normal metabolism and health (Brue, 1994). They cause specific and characteristic deficiency

TABLE 3.8 Causes of changes in metabolic tests in avian species

Metabolite	Physiology	Causes of increase	Causes of decrease
Albumin	Albumin functions primarily as an osmotic pressure regulator and a transport protein and typically comprises 45–70% of avian serum protein. Accurate albumin determination can only be calculated through electrophoresis and many of the values presented in the appendices were determined by wet and dry chemistry assays and consequently should not be considered to provide an accurate measurement of albumin. Albumin levels should be assessed in context of the albumin:globulin ratio		Decreased synthesis due to chronic liver disease, chronic inflammation; increased loss due to renal disease, parasitism or overhydration
Ammonia	Most absorbed from the alimentary tract, some derived from protein catabolism in skeletal muscle. In healthy birds, ammonia is converted into uric acid and urea in the liver and blood levels are low	Decreased liver function Ammonia poisoning	
Amylase	Produced in the pancreas, liver and small intestine	Elevations associated with acute pancreatitis and enteritis	
Bile acids	Synthesized in the liver from cholesterol and act primarily as emulsifying agents in fat digestion and absorption. With the ingestion of food, bile is carried via the bile duct into the small intestine. Over 90% of bile acids are re-absorbed from the gastrointestinal tract and return via the portal circulation to the liver, where they are recycled. This is the 'enterohepatic cycle'. If liver function is impaired, bile acids are not properly reabsorbed and consequently the amount of excreted bile acids entering the circulation increases. Measurement of bile acid concentration is considered to be the most sensitive and most specific test available for determining liver dysfunction in birds and mammals	Reduced liver function (e.g. fatty liver disease), postprandial increase in some species	
Bilirubin	In birds the major bile pigment is biliverdin and biliverdin is not converted into bilirubin. Consequently, low or negligible concentrations are detected in the serum of healthy birds	Liver disease (rarely), chlamydophiliosis	
Calcium	Major constituent of bone. Involved in the transmission of nerve impulses, permeability and excitability of membranes, activation of enzyme systems, calcification of shells and contraction of the uterus before egg laying. Blood calcium levels directly linked to albumin levels. Calcium exists as three fractions in avian serum, as the ionized salt, as calcium bound to proteins and as complexed calcium (Stanford, 2003). The ionized calcium is physiologically active while the protein bound calcium is inactive. Consequently, the measurement of ionized calcium is currently considered to be the most accurate reflection of the calcium status of avian patients (Stanford, 2003)	Hyperproteinemia, dietary excess of vitamin D, dehydration, osteolytic bone tumor, ovulating hens	Hypocalcemic syndrome in some parrots, age-related in young birds, hypoalbuminemia
Cholesterol	Major lipid that is the precursor of steroid hormones and bile acids. Obtained from animal protein sources as well as being synthesized by the liver	Hypothyroidism Liver disease, bile duct obstruction, starvation, high fat diet, atherosclerosis	Liver disease Aflatoxicosis, low dietary fat, *Escherichia coli* endotoxemia
Creatinine	Derived from catabolism of creatine in muscle tissue and excreted by the kidneys. Does not provide an accurate assessment of avian renal function	Severe kidney damage, egg peritonitis, chlamydophiliosis, renal trauma, nephrotoxic drugs, feeding high-protein diets	
Delta-aminolevulinic acid dehydratase	Delta-aminolevulinic acid dehydratase (ALAD) is an enzyme that is affected by the presence of heavy metals. Blood ALAD levels are decreased in heavy metal toxicity		Heavy metal toxicity

Continued overleaf

TABLE 3.8 Causes of changes in metabolic tests in avian species *(continued)*

Metabolite	Physiology	Causes of increase	Causes of decrease
Glucose	Required as an energy source and must be maintained at adequate levels in the plasma. Blood levels maintained by the conversion of liver glycogen. All plasma glucose is filtered from the blood through renal glomeruli and reabsorbed in the tubules	Higher in many juvenile birds, circadian rhythm, increases after feeding, stress, diabetes mellitus	Hepatic dysfunction, septicemia, aspergillosis, neoplasia, anorexia
Phosphorus	Inorganic phosphorus is derived from the diet and is a major constituent of bone as well as playing a role in the storage, release and transfer of energy in acid–base metabolism. Elevations of phosphorus are uncommon in birds	Severe renal damage, hypervitaminosis D, nutritional hyperparathyroidism	Hypovitaminosis D, malabsorption, long-term glucocorticoid therapy
Total protein	Most plasma proteins are synthesized in the liver (not immunoglobulins and protein hormones). Proteins form the basis of organ and tissue structure	Chronic infections, lymphoproliferative disease, dehydration, in females normal increase before egg laying	Chronic hepatopathy, malabsorption, wasting diseases, blood loss, enteropathy, parasitism, renal disease, starvation, malnutrition, overhydration, age-related in young birds
Triglycerides	Major storage form of lipids and important energy source. Synthesized in the intestinal mucosa and liver from components of fat digestion	Egg-related peritonitis, hyperadrenocorticism, starvation of obese birds	
Urea	Formed by protein breakdown in the liver and excreted by glomerular filtration from the kidney. Tubular reabsorption occurs and is dependent on the state of hydration. In dehydrated birds urea is reabsorbed; in hydrated birds most filtered urea is excreted	Dehydration, urethral obstruction	
Uric acid	Major product of nitrogen catabolism. Synthesized in the liver and renal tubules and eliminated by secretion into the renal tubules. By the time plasma uric acid levels are elevated, significant tubular damage has occurred. Grain-eating birds have lower uric acid levels than carnivorous birds	Ovulation, postprandial increase hypovitaminosis-A-induced renal damage, dehydration, renal infection, renal intoxication, hypervitaminosis A, hypervitaminosis D_3, nephrotoxic drugs, gout (articular)	Juvenile birds have lower levels Severe liver disease

Source: extracted and modified from: Hochleithner, 1994; Fudge, 1997; Harris, 2000.

TABLE 3.9 Causes of changes in electrolyte tests in avian species

Metabolite	Physiology in avian species	Causes of increase	Causes of decrease
Chloride	Major extracellular anion. Osmotically active constituent of plasma. Changes rarely seen in avian samples	Dehydration	
Potassium	Only 2% of the body's potassium is in the extracellular fluid: the remaining 98% is kept within the cells by potassium pumps	Severe tissue damage Renal failure Adrenal disease Acidosis Dehydration Hemolytic anemia	Chronic diarrhea Diuretic therapy Alkalosis
Sodium	Present in extracellular fluid and responsible for determining extracellular fluid volume and osmotic pressure	Salt poisoning Excess water loss Decreased water intake	Renal disease Diarrhea Overhydration
Bicarbonate	Alterations of bicarbonate are characteristic of acid–base balance	Increase due to metabolic acidosis	Decrease due to metabolic alkalosis

Source: extracted and modified from Hochleithner, 1994.

TABLE 3.10 Physiology and effects of toxicity and deficiency in avian species of some minerals

Trace element	Physiology in avian species	Signs of toxicity	Signs of deficiency
Copper	Component of important enzymes and involved in hematopoiesis as well as in absorption and transfer of iron and hemoglobin synthesis. Serum copper levels are also useful in suspected cases of deficiency, as low levels are considered to be diagnostic. The normal range of copper in the blood of most healthy animals is between 50 and 150 µg/dl, although birds, fish and marsupials are characterized by copper levels that are half these values (Keen and Graham, 1989). Published sera levels of copper in birds include: kori bustards 67.8–101.6 µg/dl, ratites 15–28 µg/dl and Hispaniola amazons (*Amazona ventralis*) 6.5–18 µg/dl (Bailey *et al.*, 2004; Angel, 1996; Osofsky *et al.*, 2000)	Chick mortality, gizzard erosion and anemia. May induce selenium deficiency	Anemia, reduced feather pigmentation, bone demineralization, heart disorders, abnormal feather growth, and ataxia and paralysis of chicks
Selenium	Essential for enzyme activity and other biochemical processes. An essential component of glutathione peroxidase, which inhibits the formation of peroxidases	Poor reproductive performance, embryonic deaths and deformities	Simultaneous deficiency of selenium and vitamin E results in specific deficiency diseases
Zinc	Essential for enzyme activity and other biochemical processes. The most widely used method for assessing zinc status is the measurement of plasma levels (Keen and Graham, 1989). Typical plasma or serum levels of zinc in most species range from 50–150 µg/dl (Keen and Graham, 1989), while the normal range for zinc in Hispaniola amazons (*Amazona ventralis*) is 125–229 µg/dl (Osofsky *et al.*, 2000)	Leg paralysis and bone demineralization. High levels may result in secondary selenium deficiency	Embryonic abnormalities and reduced hatchability, scaling of the skin, poor feather development, impaired reproduction, shortened and thickened long bones and enlarged hock joints. Zinc absorption is reduced by high dietary levels of calcium and phytate phosphorus
Magnesium	Essential for normal physiological processes such as cellular respiration and enzyme activity and is involved in bone and egg shell formation	Altered bone calcification and mortality in young birds	Reduced hatchability, chick mortality and neuromuscular convulsions. Magnesium absorption is reduced by high dietary levels of calcium and phosphorus

Source: extracted and modified from Keen and Graham, 1989; Anderson *et al.*, 2002; National Research Council, 1994; Friend and Franson, 1999.

symptoms when they are limited in the diet. A summary of the physiology and effects of changes in vitamin levels in avian species is reported in Table 3.11.

The diagnosis of vitamin deficiencies in birds has tended to be diagnosed on the basis of clinical signs and response to supplementation. However, now that tests measuring vitamin levels in tissues and blood are becoming more widespread, the ability of veterinarians to diagnose deficiencies and to provide more rational supplementation will undoubtedly improve. Plasma vitamin E concentrations have been measured in a wide range of captive avian species (Gulland *et al.*, 1988; Dierenfeld 1989; Schweigert *et al.*, 1991; Dierenfeld and Traber, 1992; Dierenfeld *et al.*, 1993; Anderson *et al.*, 2002), but blood levels of other vitamins have not been so widely reported. Blood vitamin levels in some avian species are presented in Appendix 3.

Acid–base balance

The diagnosis of acid–base disturbances and electrolyte imbalances in humans and many domestic animals is well documented but little information has been published in birds. Venous heparinized blood is the sample most commonly used for blood gas analysis in birds and ideally determination should be carried out as rapidly as possible in-house. The advent of lower cost and portable units such as the I-STAT blood analyzer (Abbott Laboratories) makes blood gas a more practical analysis for clinicians. For assessment of acid base status pH, P_{CO_2} and HCO_3 levels are considered the most appropriate parameters (Martin, 1994). The assessment of the acid–base balance of sick birds is important when determining the most appropriate type of solution to use in fluid therapy. For example, lactated Ringer's

TABLE 3.11 A summary of the physiology and effects of changes in vitamin levels in avian species

Vitamin	Physiology in avian species	Causes and effects of changes in vitamin levels
A	Fat-soluble vitamin essential for growth and differentiation of epithelial tissues, mucopolysaccharide formation, stability of cell membranes, growth of bones and normal reproduction. Also improves the immune system. Stored in the liver and has the potential to act as a cumulative toxicant. Deficiencies can result from insufficient dietary fat, insufficient antioxidant protection or disorders that interfere with fat digestion or absorption. Liver disease may reduce the bird's ability to store vitamin A	**Deficiency** – Embryo mortality and abnormalities; susceptibility to respiratory infections; visual disorders; squamous metaplasia of mucous membranes; hyperkeratosis; decreased testis size and testosterone levels; urate deposits in the kidneys and ureters; egg binding; poorly formed eggs **Toxicity** – bone abnormalities; spontaneous fractures; conjunctivitis; enteritis; suppressed keratinization; internal hemorrhages; fatty liver and kidneys; secondary deficiencies of other fat-soluble vitamins
D_3	Fat-soluble vitamin essential for the absorption of calcium and consequently for normal bone and eggshell formation. It is destroyed by excess radiation with ultraviolet light and oxidation in the presence of rancidifying fatty acids. There are two forms of this vitamin, ergocalciferol (D_2), a plant derivative, and cholecalciferol (D_3), produced in the bird's body. Vitamin D_3 is synthesized in avian skin exposed to ultraviolet light and is 30–40 times more potent than vitamin D_2. A dietary source of vitamin D_3 is needed by animals that do not have access to ultraviolet light	**Deficiency** – thin, soft-shelled eggs; embryonic abnormalities and mortality; metabolic bone disease; leg weakness; seizuring; pathological bone fractures; poor feathering. Can be induced by high dietary vitamin A or E levels **Toxicity** – reduced fertility; decreased eggshell quality; soft tissue calcification; renal and artery calcification; bone demineralization; muscular atrophy
E	Fat-soluble vitamin that provides natural antioxidation protection for cells, fatty acids and other fat-soluble vitamins. Working in conjunction with vitamin E are several metalloenzymes that incorporate manganese, zinc, copper, iron and selenium. The selenium-containing glutathione peroxidase is the most important of these enzymes. Because of their similar activity, selenium and vitamin E tend to have a sparing effect on each other. Vitamin E is active in several metabolic systems, including cellular respiration, normal phosphorylation reactions, ascorbic acid synthesis, sulfur amino acid synthesis. It also has effects on immunity by increasing phagocytosis and antibody production, as well as stimulating macrophage and lymphocyte activity	**Deficiency** – low fertility; embryonic mortality; low hatchability; immunosuppression; testicular degeneration; and specific clinical abnormalities such as encephalomalacia, exudative diathesis and muscular myopathies. May be predisposed by giardiasis **Toxicity** – enlarged fatty livers; waxy feathers. High levels can cause secondary deficiency signs of bone demineralization or blood clotting failure if vitamins D_3 and K are marginal
K	Fat-soluble vitamin essential for normal blood clotting. It comes from three sources: green plants, bacteria and synthetic forms. The microbial synthesis in the intestinal tract is significant in most species. The requirements of this vitamin vary according to the extent to which different species use the synthesized vitamin K and to which they practice coprophagy. Destroyed by oxidation, alkaline conditions, strong acids, ultraviolet light and some sulfur drugs. Vitamin K also requires the presence of dietary fats and bile salts for absorption from the gut, so decreased pancreatic and biliary function can impair normal absorption	**Deficiency** – embryonic mortality; hemorrhaging; anemia; altered bone metabolism. Can be induced by high dietary levels of vitamins A or E or by prolonged antibiotic treatment **Toxicity** – high levels can cause chick mortality and anemia
B_1	Thiamine is a water-soluble vitamin essential for enzyme activity and cellular respiratory control as well as being involved in nerve activity. It is common in plant and animal food sources but generally at low concentration. Several compounds in nature possess antithiamine activity. These include amprolium, which inhibits thiamine absorption from the intestine, thiaminases, which are found in raw fish, and thiamine antagonists such as tannic acid. Thiamine is not stored in the body for a long time	**Deficiency** – embryonic mortality; muscular paralysis; ataxia; convulsions; neurological signs; organ atrophy **Toxicity** – not studied in birds. High levels in mammals can cause depression of the respiratory centre and blockage of nerve transmission
B_2	Riboflavin is a water-soluble vitamin essential for enzyme activity, carbohydrate utilization, cellular metabolism and respiration, uric acid formation, amino acid breakdown and drug metabolism. It is destroyed by ultraviolet light and alkaline solutions. Very little riboflavin is stored in the body and it is rapidly excreted	**Deficiency** – embryonic abnormalities and mortality; chick mortality; curled toe paralysis and other neuromuscular disorders; dermatitis; poor feather pigmentation; splayed legs; fatty liver **Toxicity** – not reported in birds. Toxicity not thought to be a risk because it is not well absorbed from the gut
B_6	Pyridoxine is a water-soluble vitamin involved in a number of enzyme systems as a coenzyme. It is required in all areas of amino acid utilization, the synthesis of niacin and the formation of antibodies. It is destroyed by oxidation	**Deficiency** – reduced hatchability; ataxia; neuromuscular disorders; perosis; hemorrhaging; gizzard erosion **Toxicity** – not reported in birds
B_{12}	Cyanocobalamin is a product of bacterial biosynthesis and therefore must be obtained by consuming a bacterial source or animal tissues that accumulate the vitamin. It is a critical component of many metabolic pathways and is involved in the synthesis of nucleic acids and protein	**Deficiency** – embryo abnormalities and mortality; chick mortality; gizzard erosion; poor feathering **Toxicity** – not reported in birds

TABLE 3.11 A summary of the physiology and effects of changes in vitamin levels in avian species *(continued)*

Vitamin	Physiology in avian species	Causes and effects of changes in vitamin levels
	as well as carbohydrates and fats. Most vitamin B_{12} in the body is found in the liver, with secondary stores in the muscles. Vitamin B_{12} is stored efficiently, with a long biological half-life of 1 year in humans	
Biotin	Water-soluble vitamin that is an active part of four different carboxylase enzymes in the body involved in the metabolism of energy, glucose, lipids and some amino acids. It is destroyed by strong acids and bases, oxidizing agents and the protein avidin in raw egg albumin. Biotin is widely distributed in foods at low concentrations. The synthesis of biotin by intestinal microflora may be important	**Deficiency** – embryo abnormalities and mortality; poor growth; dermatitis; perosis and leg abnormalities; fatty liver–kidney syndrome **Toxicity** – not reported in birds
Choline	Water-soluble vitamin that has four important metabolic functions: 1) as a component of phospholipids and therefore in maintaining cell integrity, 2) maturation of the cartilage matrix of bone, 3) fat metabolism in the liver, and 4) acetylated to form the neurotransmitter acetylcholine. While most animals synthesize choline, young animals cannot synthesize enough to meet the demands for growth	**Deficiency** – reduced hatchability; perosis and enlarged hocks; hepatic steatitis; fatty liver syndrome **Toxicity** – not reported in birds
Folic acid	Water-soluble vitamin involved in amino acid metabolism and bioconversion and in the synthesis of nucleotides. It is involved in red blood cell maturation, white cell production, functioning of the immune system, uric acid formation. It is also essential for normal growth. Some sulfur drugs increase folic acid requirements. Zinc deficiency can decrease the absorption of folic acid by reducing activity of the mucosal enzyme that creates an absorbable form of folic acid. Enzyme inhibitors are present in some foods such as cabbage, oranges, beans and peas	**Deficiency** – embryo abnormalities and mortality; perosis; macrocytic anemia; poor feathering; loss of feather pigmentation **Toxicity** – not reported in birds
Niacin	Water-soluble vitamin that is an important component of coenzymes NAD and NADP, which are involved in carbohydrate, fat and protein metabolism	**Deficiency** – dermatitis; perosis; stomatitis; enlarged hocks; anemia; digestive disorders; general muscular weakness **Toxicity** – coarse, dense feathering and anteriorly directed short legs in chickens
C	Ascorbic acid has not been demonstrated to be a required nutrient for most avian species. It is easily manufactured in the liver and kidneys of birds but biosynthesis can be inhibited by deficiencies of vitamins A, E and biotin. Ascorbic acid is involved in the synthesis of collagen, is an excellent antioxidant and can regenerate vitamin E	**Deficiency** – Signs of vitamin C deficiency have not been documented in birds
Pantothenic acid	Water-soluble vitamin that is a structural component of coenzyme A, one of the most critical coenzymes in tissue metabolism. As such it is involved in fatty acid biosynthesis and degradation, and the formation of cholesterol, triglycerides, phospholipids and steroid hormones. It is destroyed by heat, acids and bases	**Deficiency** – embryonic mortality; dermatitis; perosis; poor feathering; poor growth; fatty liver–kidney syndrome; ataxia; reduced semen volume and fertility **Toxicity** – not reported in birds

Source: adapted from Anderson, 1995; Brue, 1994; McWhirter, 1994.

solution is more appropriate in birds that are acidotic, while a 5% dextrose saline solution is more appropriate for birds with alkalosis (McKinney, 2003). Blood gas values for some avian species are presented in Appendix 3. Further work is warranted to establish reference ranges and interpretive guidelines in birds.

Age-related biochemistry changes

Investigations in many juvenile avian species including psittacines (Clubb *et al.*, 1990; Joyner and Duarte, 1994), storks (Montesinos *et al.*, 1997) and bustards (Bailey *et al.*,

1998a, 1998b, 1999a) have reported age-related changes in biochemistry values. These studies demonstrate significant differences in many chemistry values, including glucose, total protein, alkaline phosphatase (ALKP), AST, LDH and calcium, between healthy adult and juvenile birds. Calcium, total protein and AST levels tend to be significantly lower in the plasma of juvenile birds compared with adults. The requirement of protein, a major constituent of tissues, for growth may explain the low circulating levels in juvenile birds. High plasma ALKP is seen in juvenile birds and is considered to be associated with normal bone growth and development. As an example, Figs 3.57 and 3.58 show the changes in plasma calcium and ALKP in growing kori bustards.

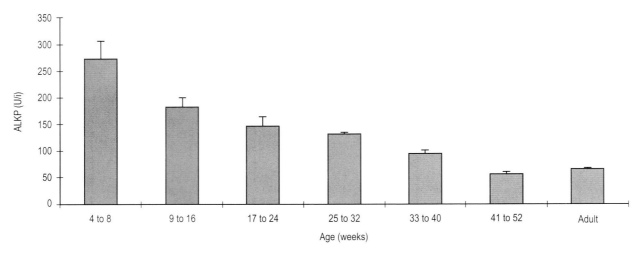

Fig 3.57 Plasma alkaline phosphatase levels (U/i) in kori bustards.

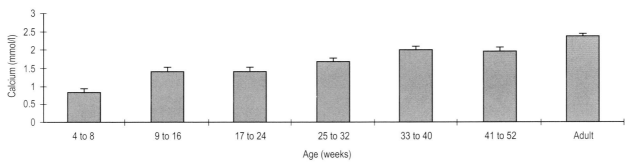

Fig 3.58 Plasma calcium levels (mmol/l) in kori bustards.

Urinalysis

Urinalysis is indicated if renal disease is suspected. Very few investigations have defined normal parameters of avian urine (Rosskopf *et al.*, 1986; Halsema *et al.*, 1988; Huchzermeyer, 1998; Tschopp *et al.*, 2007). Tissue enzyme studies have shown that avian kidney tissues contain high concentrations of glutamate dehydrogenase (GLDH), gamma glutamyl transferase (GGT), alkaline phosphatase (AP), CK, LDH, AST and ALT (Lumeij and Wolfswinkel, 1987, Lumeij *et al.*, 1988a, Bailey *et al.*, 1999b). In mammals it is known that after renal damage these enzymes are largely excreted via the urine (Keller, 1981) and biochemical analysis of avian urine may be a valid diagnostic assay that warrants more consideration than it has received to date.

The main problem with birds is collecting uncontaminated samples. Ostriches are the only bird to deposit urine separately from their feces, which enables the collection of clean samples of urine without being contaminated with feces containing protein (Huchzermeyer, 1998; Mushi *et al.*, 2001). Under experi–

mental conditions, samples have been collected from pigeons fitted with a cloacal cannula or from birds placed in holding cages with mesh floors, the samples from whom could be collected on to plastic sheeting. Transient polyuria can be induced in many species by administering water by crop tube and, in some groups of birds, such as raptors, collection of urine in a clinical setting is a comparatively straightforward technique (Tschopp *et al.*, 2007). In falcons, a normal *mute* (intestinal and urinary tract output in raptors) consists of a dark black center (feces) surrounded by a pure chalky white urate mass, sometimes with a larger ring of clear urine. The liquid (urine) part of a fresh mute can readily be aspirated, centrifuged and the supernatant analyzed using either a commercial dip stick or a standard biochemistry analyzer. Tschopp *et al.* (2007) found increased levels of GGT and total protein in sick falcons compared with healthy falcons (Table 3.12). Reference values of urinalysis in healthy falcons are presented in Appendix 3. Sometimes the only laboratory evidence of renal disease may be the presence of casts and urine sediment. Therefore samples should be carefully examined for the presence of these.

TABLE 3.12 Urinalysis in avian species

Parameter	Normal physiology	Causes of change in avian species
Color and consistency	Urine usually clear, exceptions include ratites and Anseriformes, which have opaque, cloudy urine	The color of the urine can change after ingestion or injection with water-soluble vitamins (e.g. vitamin B). Lead intoxication can cause chocolate-milk-colored urine and urates. Severe liver disease (e.g. Pacheco's disease virus, chlamydophiliosis, falcon herpes virus) can increase the secretion of biliverdin, resulting in lime green urine and urates
Specific gravity	Varies with the state of hydration. Measured with a refractometer. Values of 1.005–1.020 are considered normal	Any disease characterized by polyuria and polydipsia. Increased water loss without increased solute loss results in a low specific gravity and occurs in intravenous fluid therapy, hyperthyroidism, liver disease, pituitary neoplasia and glucocorticoid therapy
pH	Most pet birds have a urinary pH between 6.0–8.0. pH is related to the diet: carnivores tend to have acidic urine and granivores more alkaline urine	Birds with urine pH less than 5.0 are considered acidotic
Urinary protein	Trace protein, probably because of fecal contamination, can be detected in the urine of the majority of birds	In raptors protein levels have been reported as being twice as high in urine from sick birds (aspergillosis, parasitic diseases, lead toxicosis, amyloidosis) compared with healthy birds
Glucose	Avian urine should not normally contain glucose. Trace levels may be detected in normal birds because of fecal contamination	In raptors glucose levels have been reported as being higher in urine from sick birds (aspergillosis, parasitic diseases, lead toxicosis, amyloidosis) compared with healthy birds
Blood	Commercial test strips can differentiate between hematuria and hemoglobinuria	Blood in the urine may originate from the cloaca, urinary, reproductive or alimentary tracts. The diet should be taken into consideration: most raptors are positive for blood because of their meat diet
GGT	Avian kidney tissues have been shown to have high activity of many enzymes, including GGT	In raptors increased levels of GGT have been reported in urine from sick birds (aspergillosis, parasitic diseases, lead toxicosis, amyloidosis), whereas serum GGT levels were in normal range for these birds. More work is needed on the clinical significance of urinary enzymes
Chloride	Chloride levels in urine depend mainly on the concentration of sodium chloride in food and also on the state of hydration, which is influenced by climatic factors	Very few studies are available on chloride levels in the urine of birds. Urinalysis results from farmed healthy ostriches showed that ranges of chloride were much higher (up to 400 times higher) than values in falcons

Source: extracted and modified from Hochleithner, 1994; Tschopp et al., 2007.

REFERENCES

Anderson S (1995) Bustard micronutrient review. NARC External Report No. 4.

Anderson SJ, Dawodu A, Patel M et al. (2002) Plasma concentrations in six species of bustards (Gruiformes: Otididae). Journal of Wildlife Diseases 38: 414–419.

Angel CR (1996) Serum chemistries and vitamin D metabolites in ostriches, emus, rheas and cassowaries. International Conference on Improving our Understanding of Ratites in a Farming Environment, Manchester, pp. 122–124.

Bailey TA, Wernery U, Naldo J, Samour JH (1997) Concentrations of creatine kinase and lactate dehydrogenase in captive houbara bustards (Chlamydotis undulata macqueenii) following capture. Comparative Haematology International 7: 113.

Bailey TA, Wernery U, Howlett J et al. (1998a) Normal blood chemistry and age-related changes in the white-bellied bustard (Eupodotis senagalensis), with some clinical observations. Comparative Haematology International 8: 61–65.

Bailey TA, Wernery U, Howlett J et al. (1998b) Age-related plasma chemistry changes in the buff-crested bustard (Eupodotis ruficrista gindiana). Journal of Veterinary Medicine 45: 635–640.

Bailey TA, Wernery U, Howlett J et al. (1999a) Age-related plasma chemistry changes in houbara (Chlamydotis undulata) and kori bustards (Ardeotis kori). Journal of Wildlife Diseases 35: 31–37.

Bailey TA, Wernery U, Howlett J, John A, Raza H (1999b) Diagnostic enzyme profile in houbara bustard tissues (Chlamydotis undulata macqueenii). Comparative Haematology International 9: 36–42.

Bailey TA, Silvanose CD, Combreau O, Howlett JC (2004) Normal blood concentrations of copper, magnesium and zinc in stone curlew and five species of bustards in the United Arab Emirates. Proceedings of the European Association of Zoo and Wildlife Veterinarians Meeting, Ebeltoft, pp. 297–301.

Bogin E, Israeli B (1976) Enzyme profile of heart and skeletal muscles, liver and lung of roosters and geese. Journal of Veterinary Medicine 23: 152–157.

Bogin E, Avidar Y, Israeli B (1976) Enzyme profile of turkey tissues and serum. Journal of Veterinary Medicine 23: 858–862.

Brue RN (1994) Nutrition. In: Ritchie BW, Harrison GJ, Harrison LR (eds) Avian Medicine and Surgery: Principles and Applications, pp. 63–95. Wingers Publishing, Lake Worth, FL.

Chalmers GA, Barrett MW (1982) Capture myopathy. In: Hoff GL, Davis JW (eds) Noninfectious Diseases of Wildlife, pp. 84–89. Iowa State University Press, Ames, IA.

Clubb SL, Schubot RM, Joyner K et al. (1990) Hematologic and serum biochemical reference ranges in juvenile macaws, cockatoos and eclectus parrots. Proceedings of the Association of Avian Veterinarians, Phoenix, pp. 58–59. Association of Avian Veterinarians, Bedford, TX.

Cornelius CE, Bishop J, Switzer J et al. (1958) Serum and tissue transaminase activities in domestic animals. Cornell Veterinarian 49: 116–126.

Dierenfeld ES (1989) Vitamin E deficiency in zoo reptiles, birds, and ungulates. Journal of Zoo and Wildlife Medicine 20: 3–11.

Dierenfeld ES, Traber MG (1992) Vitamin E status of exotic animals compared with livestock and domestics. In: Packer L, Fuchs J (eds) Vitamin E in Health and Disease, pp. 345–370. Marcel Dekker, New York.

Dierenfeld ES, Sheppard CD, Langenberg J et al. (1993) Vitamin E in cranes: reference ranges and nutrient interactions. Journal of Wildlife Diseases 29: 98–102.

Dorrestein GM, De Bruijne JJ, Buitelaar MN (1986) Bioavailability, tissue distribution, muscle injury and effects on serum enzyme activity after parenteral administration of doxycycline to pigeons. PhD thesis, University of Utrecht, Netherlands.

Friend M, Franson JC (1999) *Field Manual of Wildlife Diseases*. US Department of the Interior and US Geological Survey. Wildlife Health Center, USA.

Fudge A (1997) Avian clinical pathology: hematology and biochemistry. In: Altman RB, Clubb SL, Dorrestein GM, Quesenberry K (eds) *Avian Medicine and Surgery*, pp. 142–157. WB Saunders, Philadelphia.

Gulland FMD, Ghebremeskel K, Williams G, Olney PJS (1988) Plasma vitamins A and E, total lipid and cholesterol concentrations in captive jackass penguins (*Spheniscus demersus*). *Veterinary Record* **123**: 666–667.

Halsema WB, Alberts H, deBruijne JJ, Lumeij JT (1988) Collection and analysis of urine in racing pigeons (*Columba livia domestica*). *Avian Pathology* **17**: 221–225.

Hochleithner M (1994) Biochemistries. In: Ritchie BW, Harrison GJ, Harrison LR (eds) *Avian Medicine and Surgery: principles and applications*, pp. 223–245. Wingers Publishing, Lake Worth, FL.

Huchzermeyer FW (1998) *Diseases of ostriches and other ratites*, p. 48. Agricultural Research Council, Onderstepoort, Republic of South Africa.

Joyner KL, Duarte JPS (1994) Hematology and serum biochemistry values in captive juvenile yellow-naped amazons (*Amazona auropalliata*). *Proceedings of the Association of Avian Veterinarians*, Reno, pp. 185–188.

Keen CL, Graham TW (1989) Trace elements. In: Kaneko JJ (ed.) *Clinical Biochemistry of Domestic Animals* pp. 753–795. Academic Press, Harcourt Brace Jovanovich, San Diego, CA.

Keller P (1981) Enzyme activities in the dog: tissue analyses, plasma values, and intracellular distribution. *American Journal of Veterinary Research* **42**: 575–582.

Lumeij JT (1987) A contribution to clinical investigative methods for birds, with special reference to the racing pigeon, *Columba livia domestica*. PhD thesis, University of Utrecht, The Netherlands.

Lumeij JT, Remple JD (1991) Plasma urea, creatinine and uric acid concentrations in relation to feeding in peregrine falcons (*Falco peregrinus*). *Avian Pathology* **20**: 79–83.

Lumeij JT, Remple JD (1992) Plasma bile acid concentrations in response to feeding in peregrine falcons (*Falco peregrinus*). *Avian Diseases* **36**: 1060–1062

Lumeij JT, Wolfswinkel J (1987) Tissue enzyme profile of the budgerigar, *Melopsittacus undulatus*. In: A contribution to clinical investigative methods for birds, with special reference to the racing pigeon, *Columba livia domestica*, pp. 71–78. PhD Thesis, University of Utrecht, Netherlands.

Lumeij JT, de Bruijne JJ, Slob A, Rothuizen J (1988a) Enzyme activities in tissues and elimination half-lives of homologous muscle and liver enzymes in the racing pigeon (*Columba livia domestica*). *Avian Pathology* **17**: 851–864.

Lumeij JT, Meidam M, Wolfswinkel J *et al*. (1988b) Changes in plasma chemistry after drug-induced liver disease or muscle necrosis in racing pigeons (*Columba livia domestica*). *Avian Pathology* **17**: 865–874.

McKinney PA (2003) Clinical applications of the I-Stat blood analyser in avian practice. *Proceedings of the European Association of Avian Veterinarians*, Tenerife, pp. 341–345.

McWhirter P (1994) Malnutrition. In: Ritchie BW, Harrison GJ, Harrison LR (eds) *Avian Medicine and Surgery: principles and applications*, pp. 842–861. Wingers Publishing, Lake Worth, FL.

Martin L (1994) pH, P_aCO_2, electrolytes and acid–base status. In: *All You Really Need to Know to Interpret Arterial Blood Gases*, pp. 107–129. Lippincott Williams & Wilkins, Baltimore.

Merritt EL, Fritz CL, Ramsay EC (1996) Hematologic and serum biochemical values in captive American flamingos (*Phoenicoterus ruber ruber*). *Journal of Avian Medicine and Surgery* **10**: 163–167.

Montesinos A, Sainz A, Pablos MV, Mazzucchelli F, Tesouro MA (1997) Hematological and plasma biochemical reference intervals in young white storks. *Journal of Wildlife Diseases* **33**: 405–412.

Mushi EZ, Binta MG, Isa JW (2001) Biochemical composition of urine from farmed ostriches (*Struthio camelus*) in Botswana. *Journal of the South African Veterinary Association* **72**: 46–48.

National Research Council (1980) *Mineral Tolerance of Domestic Animals*. National Academy Press, Washington, DC.

National Research Council (1994) *Nutrient Requirements of Poultry*, 9th edn. National Academy Press, Washington, DC.

Osofsky A, Jowett PL, Hosgood G, Tully T (2000) Normal blood concentrations for lead, zinc, iron and copper in Hispaniolan amazons (*Amazona ventralis*). *Proceedings of the Association of Avian Veterinarians*, Portland, pp. 243–244.

Petrie A, Sabin C (2000) *Medical Statistics at a Glance*. Blackwell Science, Oxford.

Petrie A, Watson P (1999) *Statistics for Veterinary and Animal Sciences*. Blackwell Science, Oxford.

Rosskopf WJ, Woerpel RW, Lane RA (1986) The practical use and limitations of the urinalysis in diagnostic pet avian medicine: with emphasis on the differential diagnosis of polyuria, the importance of cast formation in the avian urinalysis and case reports. *Proceedings of the Association of Avian Veterinarians*, Miami, pp. 61–73.

Scheideler SE, Wallner-Pendleton EA, Schneider N, Carlson M (1994) Determination of baseline values for skeletal (leg bone) growth, calcification and soft tissue mineral accretion. *Proceedings of the Association of Avian Veterinarians*, Reno, pp. 111–120.

Schweigert FJ, Uehlein-Harrell S, Hegel GV, Wiesner H (1991) Vitamin A (retinol and retinyl esters), α-tocopherol and lipid levels in plasma of captive wild mammals and birds. *Journal of Veterinary Medicine* A **38**: 35–42.

Stanford M (2003) Measurement of ionised calcium in African grey parrots (*Psittacus erithacus*): the effect of diet. *Proceedings of the European Association of Avian Veterinarians*, Tenerife, pp. 269–275.

Tschopp R, Bailey, TA, Di Somma A, Silvanose C (2007) Urinalysis as a non-invasive procedure in *Falconidae*. *Journal of Avian Medicine and Surgery*, **21**(1):1–7.

FURTHER READING

Harris DJ (2000) Clinical tests. In: Altman RB, Clubb SL, Dorrestein GM, Quesenberry KE (eds) *Avian Medicine and Surgery*, pp. 43–51. WB Saunders, Philadelphia.

Lumeij JT, de Bruijne JJ (1987) Enzyme activities in pigeon tissues. In: A contribution to clinical investigative methods for birds, with special reference to the racing pigeon, *Columba livia domestica*, pp. 46–55. PhD Thesis, University of Utrecht, Netherlands.

Lumeij JT, Remple JD, Remple CJ, Riddle KE (1998) Plasma chemistry in peregrine falcons (*Falco peregrinus*): reference values and physiological variations of importance for interpretation. *Avian Pathology* **27**: 129–132.

Stanford M (2003) Measurement of 25-hydroxycholecalciferol in captive grey parrots (*Psittacus e. erithacus*). *Veterinary Record* **153**: 58–59.

Aspirates

Judith C. Howlett

Aspirates can yield valuable information that may assist in diagnosis. Examples of sites in birds from which aspirates may be taken include swollen joints (synovial fluid) plus purulent exudates or transudates in the body cavity.

Aspirates should not be taken until the patient has been fully evaluated. This may involve investigations such as radiography. The taking of an aspirate can prove hazardous, since it usually involves the use of a needle, and therefore every precaution must be taken to minimize the risk of further damage to the bird. Sometimes it is possible to monitor the passage of a needle for aspiration using radiography or other imaging techniques. Usually, however, aspiration has to be performed 'blind', in which case great care has to be taken (Figs 3.59–3.62).

The equipment for aspiration of fluid or semifluid material from a lesion in a bird consists essentially of a syringe and needle. From time to time a Vacutainer

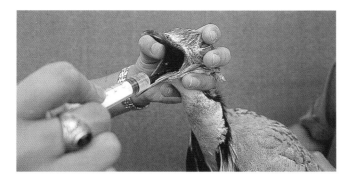

Fig. 3.59 Aspirates from the choana or the oropharynx can be obtained from small, medium-sized or large birds using a sterile lacrimal cannula attached to a syringe. Aspirates from these areas are very useful for protozoology studies.

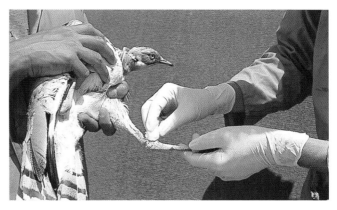

Fig. 3.61 The hock joint is disinfected prior to the collection of an aspirate from the swollen joint of a houbara bustard (*Chlamydotis undulata*).

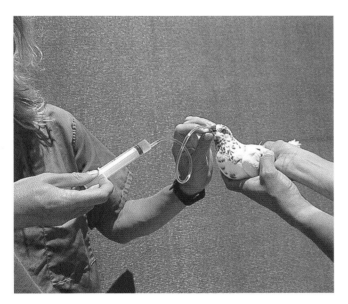

Fig. 3.60 A catheter is being used to obtain a crop aspirate from a domestic pigeon (*Columba livia*).

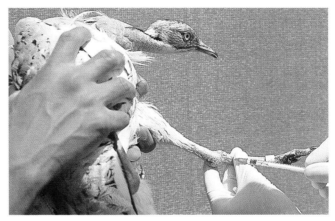

Fig. 3.62 A 25-gauge needle attached to a tuberculin syringe is ideal for joint aspirates.

can be used but in general this is not recommended, since it can cause damage and rapid evacuation of fluid from a lesion may have systemic effects. In most cases, the aim of aspiration is to remove a small quantity of material for laboratory investigation. Total aspiration – for example, draining a fluid-filled cyst – is best performed subsequently when the likely etiology and topography of the lesion is clear. The choice of needle and syringe size for aspiration depends upon a number of factors, including individual preference. As a general rule, if a small sample is needed, then a small syringe (1 ml) should be used. The needle should be as short as possible, provided that it is compatible with obtaining the sample. Too long a needle may inadvertently damage other tissues, particularly if the bird moves. The size of needle required is debatable. A narrow-gauge needle will cause less tissue damage. There will be less danger of leakage, once the needle is

removed. However, this has two main disadvantages: 1) if the material being aspirated is semisolid or contains aggregates of solid material, these may either block the needle or perhaps not be aspirated, thus giving a false picture on laboratory examination; and 2) when the material is drawn up into the needle (and even more so if it is subsequently ejected through the needle) there is a danger, as in hematology, that cells are lysed and artifacts appear. A wide-gauge needle is the opposite of the above and is, in my opinion, generally to be preferred. As a general rule, a 23–25 gauge needle is likely to be appropriate for aspiration of samples from birds.

Methods of aspirating also vary. I recommend bold, but careful, insertion of the needle for a few millimeters, then application of pressure by drawing back the plunger on the syringe. Changes in direction can then be made to the needle until fluid or other material is aspirated. If this fails to work, the syringe and needle may need to be withdrawn and either inserted into another area or perhaps a wider-bore needle used.

Once an aspirate has been obtained in the needle, a decision has to be made as to how best to deal with this. As with hematology, there are many options – smears for examination of cells, culture for bacteria or fungi, biochemical and other tests if the sample is sufficiently large, etc. Again it is wise to have a flow diagram and a triage system.

It must be remembered that, even if aspiration appears to be unsuccessful, this is not necessarily the case. The tip of the needle or, possibly, even the terminal few millimeters may contain material from the lesion. For this reason, if aspiration appears to be unsuccessful, the needle should nevertheless be used for laboratory tests. If bacteriological culture is deemed the most important investigation, then the tip of the needle can be used to plate out directly on to blood agar or other media. A preferable technique, not only for bacteriology but for other investigations also, is to remove the needle and to flush through a small volume (0.1 ml maximum) of sterile saline to wash out the tip of the needle and to flush any material that may be present. This can be used to prepare a smear on a slide or the fluid (ideally plus cells) can be placed in a small ampoule for tests.

Following aspiration the patient should be carefully monitored, in particular for signs of leakage through the needle hole, and appropriate prophylactic treatment may be necessary (e.g. antibiotics if damage has been caused to a joint or elsewhere).

Swabs

Christudas Silvanose

The term 'swab' implies the use of a specific piece of equipment to remove the sample (Figs 3.63 and 3.64). Other techniques can also be used (e.g. washings, brushings and scrapings) and will be discussed under Biopsies, below.

Swabs can be taken for a variety of purposes including bacteriology, mycology, virology, mycoplasmology and cytology.

There are two important considerations when collecting a swab:

- The type of swab that is used
- The area that is swabbed.

The type of swab can very greatly influence the results and thus the action to be taken. There are many types of swab and, while the majority consists essentially of a wooden or metal (e.g. aluminum) stick and a cotton-based tip, there are many variants. The swabs most likely to be used in avian practice are:
- Dry cotton wool swabs
- Cotton wool swabs in transport medium (e.g. Stuart's transport medium)

- Alginate-coated swabs
- Any of the above designed specifically for pediatric use or for sampling narrow orifices (e.g. nasopharyngeal swabs).

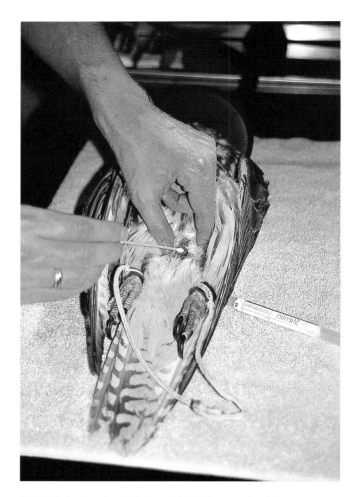

Fig. 3.63 A cloacal swab being collected from a saker falcon (*Falco cherrug*) under isoflurane anesthesia.

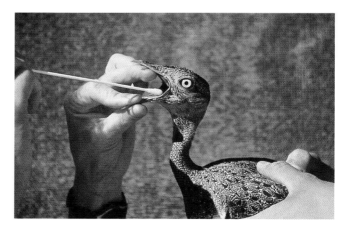

Fig. 3.64 Oropharyngeal swabs can be collected relatively easily from a live buff-crested bustard (*Eupodotis ruficrista*).

TABLE 3.13 Protocol for the collection, transportation and processing of samples for virology investigations

Specimen	Investigation	Transportation	Medium method
Swab from oropharynx, cloaca, choana, nose, conjunctiva, liver and lung	Direct microscopy Culture	Cellmatics™ viral transport pack (Difco), at 2–10°C (35.6–50°F)	Electron microscopy Embryonated egg culture, cell culture

Note: Identification tests include electron microscopy, hemagglutination, hemadsorption, cytopathic changes and antigen–antibody reaction.

Each of the above has some advantages. Under most circumstances, dry cotton wool swabs are satisfactory, particularly if the sample is being taken from an extensive lesion (see below) and is likely to be plated or processed rapidly in-house. Sometimes the efficacy of such dry swabs, in terms of picking up organisms and the latter surviving, is enhanced if the dry swab is first immersed in sterile saline. Swabs in transport medium are to be preferred when samples are not to be examined immediately and particularly when proper storage may be difficult (e.g. in field work or in countries where refrigeration and other facilities are not available). Again, there are many types of transport medium, each with its own particular features, but in general it can be assumed that Stuart's transport medium will prove satisfactory for the storage of many types of bacterium for substantial periods of time. Transport media are also available for more specific purposes, such as transportation of suspect viruses or mycoplasmas. Even if a transport medium is used, every care must be taken to store and transport samples carefully (Table 3.13). They should be handled gently (not dropped or shaken) and, in general, are best kept at normal refrigerator temperature (4°C (39.2°F)) until processing can be carried out.

Collection of microbiological swabs

For consistent laboratory results it is important to avoid errors, including:

- Sampling from the incorrect site
- Nondiagnostic sample
- Contamination of the swab from environmental factors (e.g. accidentally touching the swab)
- Sampling during antibiotic therapy
- Using inappropriate materials, including the wrong transport medium, etc.
- Contact with inhibitory chemicals (i.e. disinfectants).

The different recommended protocols for the collection, transportation and processing of samples are outlined in Table 3.14.

Antibiotic sensitivity tests are set out in Table 3.15.

Upper respiratory tract

Sampling is recommended if a bird is presenting any of the following signs:

- Pharyngitis
- Coughing
- Sneezing
- Oral odor.

Swab any obvious oral lesions, but otherwise swab the choanal slit.

Method

The bill or beak may be opened manually with the fingers or by using gauze bandage on the upper and lower beak. In some birds with a strong bite, such as psittacines, an oral metal speculum can be used, or a towel acts as a soft gag.

Nasal discharges are not necessarily good samples – even if the discharge is associated with upper respiratory tract infection. (Microscopic examination may show the discharge to be full of bacteria.) Ocular or conjunctival swabs are not always of clinical value. Ocular signs in upper respiratory tract infections are often due to *Chlamydophila* or *Mycoplasma* spp.; therefore, sample the choana.

A noninvasive method to sample sinuses is to instill sterile normal saline into the nares. Allow the saline to permeate through the sinuses; drainage will occur through the choanal slit. Swab this site as described previously.

Lower gastrointestinal tract

It is best to sample very fresh feces for culture; a cloacal swab may be collected as an alternative. This may not represent the lower gastrointestinal tract, as the cloaca may be dry and relatively devoid of bacteria. The swab should be inserted having first been wetted with sterile saline or Ringer's solution; this can help with the insertion as well as with the recovery of organisms. With regard to the size of swab, it may be beneficial to use a 'small' swab such as an 'ENT' swab with diminutive patients.

TABLE 3.14 Protocols for the collection, transportation and processing of samples

Specimen	Investigation	Transportation	Medium/method
MYCOLOGY INVESTIGATIONS			
Skin scraping	Direct microscopy	Sterile container at 4–10°C (39.2–50°F)	Smear with 10% potassium hydroxide or lactophenol aniline blue preparation (KOH)
Culture		Stuart media Saline swab Sterile container at 4–10°C	Sabouraud's agar, dermatophyte agar
Tissue	Direct microscopy	Sterile container at 4–10°C	Smear with 10% KOH preparation for soft tissue and 20% KOH for hard tissue
	Culture	Stuart media Sterile container at 4–10°C	Sabouraud's agar for fungi Yeast–mold agar for *Candida* spp. Brain–heart infusion agar for *Histoplasma capsulatum* and *Coccidioides immitis*
Swab	Direct microscopy	Saline swab at 4–10°C	Smear with lactophenol aniline blue or normal saline preparation Smear with India ink preparation for *Cryptococcus neoformans*
	Culture	Stuart media Saline swab at 4–10°C	Sabouraud's agar for fungi Yeast-mold agar for *Candida* spp. Brain–heart infusion agar for *Histoplasma capsulatum* and *Coccidioides immitis*
Feathers	Direct microscopy Culture	Sterile container at 4–10°C Sterile container at 4–10°C	Smear with 20% KOH preparation Sabouraud's agar, dermatophyte agar
Aspirated fluid, bronchial wash	Direct microscopy	Sterile container at 4–10°C	Smear with lactophenol aniline blue or normal saline preparation
	Culture	Stuart media Sterile container at 4–10°C	Sabouraud's agar for fungi Yeast-mold agar culture for *Candida* spp. Brain–heart infusion agar for *Histoplasma capsulatum* and *Coccidioides immitis*
Liver, lung, other organs and intestine	Direct microscopy	Saline swab Sterile container at 4–10°C	Smear with 10% KOH or lactophenol aniline blue or normal saline preparation
	Culture	Stuart media Saline swab Sterile container at 4–10°C	Sabouraud's agar for fungi Yeast–mold agar culture for *Candida* spp. Brain–heart infusion agar for *Histoplasma capsulatum* and *Coccidioides immitis*
Animal feed	Culture	Sterile container at 4–10°C	Sabouraud's agar or Czapek agar
ENVIRONMENT SCREENING			
	Culture	Air-settled plates at 4–10°C	Sabouraud's agar or Czapek agar
PROTOZOOLOGY INVESTIGATIONS			
Feces and cloacal swab	Direct microscopy	Normal saline at 20–30°C (68–86°F)	Smear with normal saline preparation for trophozoites Smear with Lugol's iodine or Dobell and O'Connor's iodine solution for *Amoeba* cysts Potassium dichromate incubation for *Coccidia* oocysts
	Culture	Normal saline at 20–30°C	Balamuth media for *Amoeba* spp. Unipath or Clausen's media for *Trichomonas* spp.
Oropharyngeal and choanal swabs	Direct microscopy	Normal saline at 20–30°C	Smear with normal saline preparation for trophozoites Smear with Lugol's iodine or Dobell and O'Connor's iodine solution for *Amoeba* cysts
	Culture	Normal saline at 20–30°C	Balamuth media for *Amoeba* spp. Unipath or Clausen's media for *Trichomonas* spp. Cell culture or embryonated egg cultures for *Toxoplasma gondii*
Blood	Direct microscopy Culture	EDTA or double oxalate ACD or CPD	May–Grünwald–Giemsa-stained smear NNN or Tobie's or Wenyon's media for *Trypanosoma* spp. Broth containing serum, erythrocytes, inorganic salts, amino acids and various growth factors for *Plasmodium* spp. Cell or embryonated egg cultures for *Toxoplasma gondii*
BACTERIOLOGY INVESTIGATIONS			
Aspirated fluid and bronchial wash	Direct microscopy	Flame fixed smear	Gram stained smear Fluorescent microscopy for *Chlamydophila* spp. Ziehl–Neelsen's staining technique for *Mycobacterium* spp.
	Mycobacterium spp. Aerobic culture	Amies charcoal media at 4–10°C	Loewenstein–Jensen media Blood agar and MacConkey or EMB agar

TABLE 3.14 Protocols for the collection, transportation and processing of samples (continued)

Specimen	Investigation	Transportation	Medium/method
	Anaerobic culture	Amies charcoal media	RCM, *Clostridium* agar and blood agar with anaerobic incubation
	Chlamydophila culture	Spencer and Johnson media at 4–10°C	Cell culture
	Mycoplasma culture	PPLO broth or Trypticase soy broth with bovine, 2SP and calf serum, at 4–10°C	*Mycoplasma* media
	Haemophilus spp. culture	Amies charcoal media at 20–25°C (68–77°F)	Chocolate agar with X, Y factor and 10% carbon dioxide incubation
Swab	Direct microscopy	Saline swab	Gram-stained smear
		Flame-fixed smear	Fluorescent microscopy for *Chlamydophila* spp Ziehl–Neelsen's staining technique for *Mycobacterium* spp.
	Mycobacterium spp. Aerobic culture	Amies charcoal media at 4–10°C	Loewenstein–Jensen media Blood agar and MacConkey or EMB agar
	Anaerobic culture	Amies charcoal media	RCM, *Clostridium* agar and blood agar with anaerobic incubation
	Chlamydophila culture	Spencer and Johnson media at 4–10°C	Cell culture
	Mycoplasma culture	PPLO broth or trypticase soy broth with bovine, 2SP and calf serum, at 4–10°C	*Mycoplasma* media
	Haemophilus spp. culture	Amies charcoal media at 20–25°C (68–77°F)	Chocolate agar with X, Y factor and 10% carbon dioxide incubation
	Campylobacter spp.	Cary–Blair transport media at 4–10°C	*Campylobacter*-selective media or Butzler's selective media APW and TCBS for *Vibrio* spp. *Campylobacter* incubation
Post-mortem samples: liver, lung and other organs	Direct microscopy	Saline swab	Gram-stained smear
		Flame fixed smear	Fluorescent microscopy for *Chlamydophila* spp. Ziehl–Neelsen's staining technique for *Mycobacterium* spp.
	Mycobacterium spp. Aerobic culture	Amies charcoal media	Loewenstein–Jensen media Blood agar and MacConkey or EMB agar
	Anaerobic culture	Amies charcoal media	RCM, *Clostridium* agar and blood agar with anaerobic incubation
	Chlamydophila culture	Spencer and Johnson media at 4–10°C	Cell culture
	Mycoplasma culture	PPLO broth or trypticase soy broth with bovine, 2SP and calf serum, at 4–10°C	*Mycoplasma* media
	Haemophilus spp. culture	Amies charcoal media	Chocolate agar with X, Y factor and 10% carbon dioxide incubation
	Campylobacter spp.	Cary–Blair transport media	*Campylobacter* selective media or Butzler's selective media APW and TCBS for *Vibrio* spp. *Campylobacter* incubation
Swab from egg shell	Aerobic culture	Amies charcoal media	Blood agar and MacConkey or EMB agar
	Anaerobic culture	Amies charcoal media	RCM, *Clostridium* agar and blood agar with anaerobic incubation
Infertile egg contents	Direct microscopy	Sterile container	Gram-stained smear
		Flame-fixed smear	Fluorescent microscopy for *Chlamydophila* spp.
	Aerobic culture	Amies charcoal media	Blood agar and MacConkey or EMB agar
	Anaerobic culture	Amies charcoal media	RCM, *Clostridium* agar and blood agar with anaerobic incubation
	Chlamydophila culture	Spencer and Johnson media at 4–10°C	Cell culture
	Mycoplasma culture	PPLO broth or trypticase soy broth with bovine, 2SP and calf serum	*Mycoplasma* media
Animal feed	Aerobic culture	Amies charcoal media	Blood agar and MacConkey or EMB agar
	Anaerobic culture	Amies charcoal media	RCM, *Clostridium* agar and blood agar with anaerobic incubation
Swab from incubators and hatchers	Aerobic culture	Amies charcoal media at 4–10°C	Blood agar and MacConkey or EMB agar
	Anaerobic culture	Amies charcoal media	RCM, *Clostridium* agar and blood agar with anaerobic incubation

Candida/yeast identification tests include germ tube test, API 20 C Aux, MUAG Candi test and Uni–Yeast–Tek wheel.
Bacterial identification tests include analytical profile index (API), Kligler's iron agar (KIA) reactions/triple sugar iron agar (TSI) cytochrome oxidase activity, catalase, coagulase/staphylase, and agglutination with specific antisera.

TABLE 3.15 Antibiotic sensitivity tests

Antibiotics	Concentration	Isolates
Amoxicillin	25 µg	All pathogenic Gram-negative and -positive bacteria
Amoxicillin–clavulanic acid	30 µg	All pathogenic Gram-negative and -positive bacteria
Ampicillin	10 µg	Gram-positive pathogenic bacteria
Ampicillin	30 µg	Gram-negative pathogenic bacteria
Carbenicillin	100 µg	*Pseudomonas* spp. and other Gram-negative pathogens
Chloramphenicol	10 µg	Gram-negative pathogenic bacteria
Chloramphenicol	30 µg	Gram-negative pathogenic bacteria
Enrofloxacin	25 µg	All pathogenic Gram-negative and -positive bacteria
Erythromycin	15 µg	All pathogenic Gram-positive bacteria
Gentamicin	10 µg	All pathogenic Gram-negative and -positive bacteria
Piperacillin	100 µg	*Pseudomonas* spp. and other Gram-negative pathogens
Penicillin-G	1 unit	Gram-positive pathogenic bacteria
Penicillin-G	2 units	Gram-negative pathogenic bacteria
Sulfamethoxazole	25 µg	All pathogenic Gram-negative and -positive bacteria
Sulfonamide	300 µg	*Pseudomonas* spp. and other Gram-negative pathogens
Tetracycline	30 µg	All pathogenic Gram-negative and -positive bacteria
Ticarcillin	75 µg	*Pseudomonas* spp. and other Gram-negative pathogens

Antibiotic sensitivity tests include media–nutrient agar, Mueller–Hinton agar, blood agar, Method–Kirbey–Bauer's disc diffusion, metheselene technique, and broth dilution technique.

FURTHER READING

Fudge AM (1996) Avian microbiology. In: Rosskopf WJ Jr, Woerpel RW (eds) *Diseases of Cage and Aviary Birds*, 3rd edn, pp. 795–806. Williams & Wilkins, Baltimore.

Gaskin JM (1988) Microbiologic techniques in avian medicine. In: Jacobson ER, Kollias GV Jr (eds) *Contemporary Issues in Small Animal Practice*, pp. 159–175. Churchill Livingstone, New York.

Koneman EW, Allen SD, Janda WM *et al.* (1992) Introduction to microbiology part 1: the role of the microbiology laboratory in the diagnosis of infectious diseases. Guidelines to practice and management. In: *Color Atlas and Textbook of Diagnostic Microbiology*, 4th edn, pp. 1–46. JB Lippincott, Philadelphia.

Koneman EW, Allen SD, Janda WM *et al.* (1992) Diagnosis of infections caused by viruses, *Chlamydophila*, *Rickettsia* and related organisms. In: *Color Atlas and Textbook of Diagnostic Microbiology*, 4th edn, pp. 966–1048. JB Lippincott, Philadelphia.

Van Cutsem J, Rochette F (1991) Diagnostic methods. In: Van Cutsem J, Rochette F (eds) *Mycoses in Domestic Animals*, pp. 23–43. Janssen Research Foundation, Beerse, Belgium.

Crop and airsac flushing

Judith C. Howlett

Crop flushing

Examination of crop aspirate may be indicated in birds with a history of vomiting, excessive regurgitation or other crop abnormalities. This is done by carefully inserting a sterile round-ended plastic or rubber tube through the bird's mouth and esophagus into the crop. The tube should pass freely without resistance, so as to avoid any physical damage to the esophagus or crop. It helps to have the bird's head and neck extended straight during the procedure to assist in the passing of the tube; one can usually physically palpate the tube in the esophagus to check that it is in the right place. The crop content can be gently aspirated into a sterile syringe attached to the other end of the tube. Care should be taken not to use too much pressure as this can cause damage to the crop mucosa. A crop wash can be made, flushing the crop with a small amount of sterile 0.9% saline and immediately aspirating the fluid for cytological examination using the previously mentioned technique.

Airsac flushing

Campbell (1995) describes wash samples as aspiration techniques in which a small amount of sterile 0.9% saline is infused into an area and immediately reaspirated in an attempt to get a cytological sample from areas where sampling is difficult or that provide a small cellular field. For example, tracheal washes can be performed on birds suspected of having upper respiratory tract disease. The flushing may be carried out on an anesthetized or well restrained nonanesthetized patient. A plastic catheter small enough to pass down the trachea is inserted via the open glottis (care being taken not to contaminate the tip in the oral cavity). In larger birds the plastic catheter can be passed through an inserted sterile endotracheal tube.

The tube is passed to the level of the thoracic inlet near the syrinx. If the bird is still conscious, an oral speculum should be used in birds capable of biting the tube. The bird should be held horizontally and a small amount of sterile saline (1.0–2.0 ml/kg) should be quickly infused into the area and immediately reaspirated to complete the wash sample.

Similar techniques can be used to collect cytological samples of the lower respiratory tract, which may prove helpful in the diagnosis of chlamydophiliosis, aspergillosis or bacteria causing airsac infections. Airsac cytology samples can also be collected if the bird is undergoing endoscopy examination.

REFERENCE

Campbell TW (1995) *Avian Hematology and Cytology*, 2nd edn, pp. 47–69. Iowa State University Press, Ames, IA.

FURTHER READING

Fudge AM (1996) Avian cytology. In: Rosskopf WJ Jr, Woerpel RW (eds) *Diseases of Cage and Aviary Birds*, 3rd edn, pp. 806–820. Williams & Wilkins, Baltimore.

Ectoparasites

Judith C. Howlett

The more commonly found arthropod ectoparasites affecting the skin and feathers of birds are mites, but lice, fleas, ticks and flies may also be seen. The symptoms can include feather damage and loss, skin irritation, pruritus, etc. Some of the more common are detailed in Table 3.16. Methods of determining whether ecto-parasites are present are detailed below in the section on Skin Scrapings and Feathers.

FURTHER READING

Arends JJ (1997) External parasites and poultry pests. In: Calnek BW (ed.) *Diseases of Poultry*, 10th edn, pp. 785–813. Mosby–Wolfe, London.

Coles BH (1985) *Avian Medicine and Surgery*, pp. 240–242. Blackwell Science, Oxford.

Greve JH (1996) Parasites of the skin. In: Rosskopf WJ Jr, Woerpel RW (eds) *Diseases of Cage and Aviary Birds*, 3rd edn, pp. 423–426. Williams & Wilkins, Baltimore.

Malley AD, Whitbread TJ (1996) The integument. In: Beynon PH, Forbes NA, Harcourt-Brown NH (eds) *Manual of Raptors, Pigeons and Waterfowl*, pp. 129–139. British Small Animal Veterinary Association, Cheltenham.

Skin scrapings and feathers

Judith C. Howlett

The integument of avian species is generally much thinner and more delicate than that of mammals. It is attached to muscles in only a few places but has extensive attachments to the skeleton (e.g. feet and skull). As with mammals it consists of three layers: the epidermis, the dermis (containing connective tissue, blood vessels, nerve endings, feather follicles and feather-erecting muscles) and the subcutis (containing fat). The subcutis and dermis do not contain much elastic fiber and therefore are not very elastic and tear easily.

Skin scrapings are carried out to determine whether fungal or parasitic (mite) infections of the superficial skin layers are present (see the section on Ectoparasites). The sample should be taken from a suspected area, although severely traumatized areas of skin should be avoided.

Taking a skin scraping

For superficial scrapings

- Moisten the skin with cotton wool soaked in mineral oil
- Tense the skin between finger and thumb
- The skin can then be gently scraped with a dull scalpel blade – include scrapings from the edge of a lesion.

For deeper scrapings (some mites dwell in the subcutis)

- Moisten the area to be scraped with a little 10% potassium hydroxide (KOH)
- Tense the skin between finger and thumb
- Gently (remembering that avian skin is quite delicate) scrape the lesion until pinpoints of blood appear.

In both cases transfer the material collected on to a glass slide and cover with a coverslip (or put into a suitable container). Too much material on the slide will make identification more difficult. Gentle warming helps the KOH to clear the keratin and debris so that a systematic search can be made for parasites and fungal spores. The KOH helps 'clear' the parasite, making the features more identifiable. The slide can be examined under the microscope on low power. Alternatively the skin scraping can be placed in a Petri dish with 70% ethanol.

Examination of feathers

Identification of ectoparasites can prove difficult, as detailed clinical examination can fail to confirm the presence of ectoparasites. It may be necessary to take feather and/or feather stub samples to investigate whether arthropods such as mites are in residence.

Place feathers or feather stubs in sodium hydroxide 10% in a V-bottomed container such as a 30 ml Universal container; keep at 37°C (98.6°F) overnight. Microscopic

TABLE 3.16 Arthropod ectoparasites

Order	Description	Species	Symptoms	Identification
Lice (Mallophaga)	Biting or chewing lice	*Columbicola columbae* – slender louse *Menopon latum* – large body louse *Menacanthus*	Pin holes in feathers and irregular edges, skin irritation	Finding the lice or eggs in the feathers; can often be seen crawling off an anesthetized bird
Fleas		*Ceratophyllus gallinae* *Echidnophaga gallinacea*	Irritation, restlessness, not often seen	Finding eggs or larvae in nesting sites
Ticks *Argasidae* *Ixodidae*	Soft ticks Hard ticks		Irritation, loss of condition In severe cases in small birds death through blood loss	Identification of parasite
Mites	Red or roost mites	*Dermanyssus* spp.	Skin irritation and feather damage. In severe cases the blood sucking can lead to severe anemia and even death of the host	May be seen at night when it feeds; it leaves the bird to lay its eggs. Check caging/housing during the day
	Fowl mites	*Ornithonyssus* spp.	As above	Adult form large, when engorged are bright red and can be seen with the naked eye; they remain on the host permanently
	Quill mites	*Syringophilus* spp.	Skin irritation and feather damage/rot. Inhabit the inside of the feather shaft and are difficult to see	Can be seen under a microscope ×40
	Burrowing mite Depluming mite Scaly leg mite	*Knemidocoptes* spp.	Skin irritation and feather damage. Inhabits the skin at the base of the quill. Honeycomb lesions are produced: can cause severe crusty lesions of legs and feet as a result of burrowing	Skin scrapings
	Harvest mite	*Trombicula* spp.	Blistering can occur around the point of the mite's attachment to the skin	
	Itch mite	*Myialges* spp.	Pruritic dermatitis, hyperkeratosis, scab and scurf formation	Skin scrapings
Louse fly, 'flat flies' (*Hippoboscidae*)		Cause irritation and may transmit blood parasites (e.g. *Haemoproteus* spp.). May cause blood loss in small birds	Flat parasitic flies that stay in the plumage	
Mosquitoes (*Culicidae*)	*Hemiptera* spp.	Biting, also transmit blood parasites and avipoxvirus in warm countries		
Gnats (*Simulidae*)		Transmit *Leucocytozoon* spp. infection		
Blow flies (*Tachinidae*)		Attracted to open wounds	Myiasis	

examination of the sediment should reveal ectoparasites or body parts against nondescript material. Alternatively, the affected feather can be placed in 70% ethanol and examined under low power.

When feathers and stubs are placed in a sealed plastic envelope for at least 24 h, the parasites tend to migrate from the feathers and become caught in the folds of the envelope. The ectoparasites can be examined through the plastic under low power on the microscope.

Feather stubs should also be examined, as some species of mite live in the shaft of the feather. For quill mites, the shaft can be split lengthways and placed in 70% ethanol and examined as above. Further examination of the skin and feather pulp cavity includes the following (see details in the next section on Biopsies).

- **Skin**: cytology, culture and biopsy of the skin is indicated in cases of dermatitis. Impression smears – inflammation, neoplasia, bacteria and fungi
- **Feather pulp cavity**: cytology of pulp cavity for bacteria and fungi, and smears regarding inflammatory processes within the pulp.

FURTHER READING

Coles BH (1985) *Avian Medicine and Surgery*. Blackwell Science, Oxford.

Fisher M (1995) Elementary mycology and parasitology. In: Lane DR, Cooper B (eds) *Veterinary Nursing*, pp. 333–355. Elsevier Science, Oxford.

Greve JH (1996) Parasites of the skin. In: Rosskopf WJ Jr, Woerpel RW (eds) *Diseases of Cage and Aviary Birds*, 3rd edn, pp. 423–426. Williams & Wilkins, Baltimore.

Griener EC, Ritchie BW (1994) Parasites. In: Ritchie BW, Harrison GJ, Harrison LR (eds) *Avian Medicine: Principles and Application*, pp. 1007–1029. Wingers Publishing, Lake Worth, FL.

King AS, McLelland J (1984) The integument. In: King AS, McLelland J (eds) *Birds: Their Structure and Function*, 2nd edn, pp. 23–42. Baillière Tindall, London.

Malley AD, Whitbread TJ (1996) The integument. In: Beynon PH, Forbes NA, Harcourt-Brown NH (eds) *Manual of Raptors, Pigeons and Waterfowl*, pp. 129–139. British Small Animal Veterinary Association, Cheltenham.

Wallis AS (1996) Skin conditions. In: Beynon PH, Forbes NA, Harcourt-Brown NH (eds) *Manual of Raptors, Pigeons and Waterfowl*, pp. 246–253. British Small Animal Veterinary Association, Cheltenham.

Biopsies

Judith C. Howlett

The taking of biopsies is an increasingly important part of avian diagnostic medicine. In this section, the term 'biopsying' will be used not only for the surgical excision or removal by punching or drilling of a piece of tissue but also for the collection of exfoliated samples by brushing, washing, scraping or taking impression smears (touch preparations).

A whole range of organs and tissues of birds can be biopsied, and a list of these is given in Table 3.17. Information on biopsy techniques is also provided.

When biopsies involving sensitive tissues are taken, the bird will need to be anesthetized or local analgesia used (with caution). The site of biopsy requires careful thought and planning. Often the assistance of other techniques is needed, such as radiography or ultrasound, to ascertain the optimum location for sampling. A biopsy needs to be sufficiently deep to provide the relevant information for the pathologist but not so deep that, for example, the wall of an organ is perforated. The center of a lesion

TABLE 3.17 Biopsy sites and techniques in birds

Organ/tissue	Technique(s)	Comments
Skin, including feather follicles	Surgical excision or skin biopsy punch. Needle biopsy. Scraping. Plucking of feathers may provide small numbers of cells	Avoid aggressive pre-operative disinfection, which may affect biopsy. Postoperative treatment of biopsy wound may be necessary
	Exfoliative	Particularly useful if lesion is ulcerated
Muscle and fat (external)	Surgical excision. Needle biopsy	Bleeding often marked but rarely of consequence
Oral cavity and cloaca	Surgical excision. Exfoliative	Some lesions (e.g. cloacal papillomas) bleed heavily. Electrosurgical excision or cryosurgery will minimize hemorrhage but may damage the biopsy
Upper gastrointestinal tract	Biopsy forceps. Flexible (sometimes rigid) endoscope. Exfoliative	Avoid overinflation of stomach with air: sample rugae
Lower intestinal tract (colon and rectum)	Biopsy forceps. Flexible or rigid endoscope. Exfoliative	
Kidney	Rigid endoscope	
Female reproductive tract (oviduct)	Biopsy forceps. Rigid or flexible endoscope. Exfoliative	Approach *per vaginam* or via laparoscopy
Male reproductive tract (testes)	Surgical excision or needle biopsy. Biopsy forceps. Exfoliative	Approach internal testes via laparoscopy
Respiratory tract (lung)	Biopsy forceps. Rigid endoscope	Approach usually via trachea. Supplementary air supply may be needed in birds through abdominal airsacs. Laparoscopic or intercostal approach in pigeons
Respiratory tract (avian airsac)	Biopsy forceps. Needle biopsy. Surgical excision. Exfoliative	Approach via laparoscopy
Liver	Needle (suction) biopsy. Punch biopsy	Bleeding may be a problem
Bone	Needle biopsy. Bone punch (trephine). Surgical excision	Bone punches are expensive

Exfoliative = collection by brushing, washing or taking of impression smears (touch preparations).

TABLE 3.18 Handling and processing of biopsies from birds

Type of biopsy	Procedure	Comments
Surgical excision (total) or incision (partial removal)	Touch preparations on glass slides, then: 1) half in 10% buffered formal saline (BFS) or other fixative for histopathology and/or electron microscopy, 2) half kept fresh for microbiology and other procedures	Choice of fixative will depend upon techniques to be followed. Heavily keratinized material (e.g. from reptiles) may need to be softened before histological processing
Skin biopsy punch	As above	As above. Can be used for horn following drilling
Biopsy forceps	Lifted out of forceps cup using a 23 gauge needle and placed on lens tissue moistened with sterile saline. Selected biopsies can then either be submitted fresh for microbiology or (still wrapped in lens tissue) fixed in 10% BFS or other fixative	These samples are small, easily damaged and easily lost. They should be counted, dealt with rapidly, kept moist and not handled unnecessarily. Recommend affixing samples to pieces of cucumber
Needle biopsy	Flushed out with sterile saline or fixative on to moistened lens tissue and then processed as above	The sample is small, sometimes very friable and easily lost
Bone biopsy punch	As above	Decalcification is usually necessary

may provide relatively little information because, for example, it consists primarily of ulcer or necrotic material. In such a case, a biopsy should be taken from the periphery. Biopsies from neoplasms usually need to be taken from near the center of the lesion, however, since too superficial a biopsy may yield only surrounding connective tissue. On the other hand, the center of a tumor may be necrotic. When taking a biopsy the aim is to obtain sufficient tissue of the right quality to make a diagnosis or to assess progress of a pathological lesion. Irrelevant material, such as blood clot and debris, can prove misleading.

Handling and processing of samples must be carried out proficiently. Particular care has to be taken if the biopsy material is needed fresh, for example for microbiology, biochemistry or clinical tests, as well as for fixing for light or electron microscopy. In such circumstances, multiple biopsies should be considered. It is also wise to prepare an impression smear of a sample before it is fixed. A suggested approach to handling and processing is given in Table 3.18.

There are dangers in taking biopsies. Birds may be damaged because an organ or tissue is perforated, because there is hemorrhage, because there is further infection or neoplastic cells or because tissue damage results in chronic changes. The bird must be carefully assessed beforehand and monitored following sampling.

Cytology

John E. Cooper, Christudas Silvanose

Cytology is the study of cells and has an important role in avian medicine:

- In its own right, as a rapid and inexpensive technique that can be used in the clinic and in the field (Latimer *et al.*, 1988; Campbell, 1993, 1995; Harrison and Campbell, 1994; Corr *et al.*, 2002)
- As an adjunct to other disciplines, especially histopathology but also bacteriology and parasitology (Cooper, 1994; Rosenthal *et al.*, 2004).

Cytology can either provide a diagnosis itself or supplement/complement one made using other methods.

The key to successful cytological investigation is accurate sampling and tissue preparation (Pinches, 2005a, 2005b, 2005c). As in hematology (itself a form of cytology), the essential prerequisite is a monolayer (Hawkey and Dennett, 1989). A useful analogy is an egg, where the yolk is the nucleus, the albumen the cytoplasm. In cytological preparations, the cells should be like a fried egg – well spread and thin.

Sampling and processing

Specimens from birds for cytological examination can be conveniently divided initially into:

- Fluids, such as serous exudates of peritoneal effusions, which are best taken by syringe/needle and then spread on a slide in a similar way to blood
- Solids, such as the cut surfaces of a tumor or granuloma, which are best sampled either in situ or following removal (Cooper, 1994) as imprints ('touch preparations' or impression smears), having first reduced the amount of blood on the cut surface by blotting on filter paper
- Samples from oropharynx, trachea, nares and cloaca, which are collected by sterile swab and rotated/rolled on to a slide
- Washed samples, which require cytocentrifugation to increase smear cellularity.

TABLE 3.19 Some staining techniques in avian hematology

Stain	Use	Comments
Romanowsky stains e.g. Giemsa, Wright's, Wright–Giemsa, May–Grünwald–Giemsa	All cell types including blood. Will also stain organisms such as hemoparasites and *Chlamydophila*	Best to air-dry. Variable results depending on type of stain and skill of technician. Stained preparations retain color if kept in dark
Commercial quick stains e.g. Diff-Quik®, Rapid Diff®, Hemacolor®, Aviacolor®	Most cell types but especially blood and bone marrow	No fixation needed. Rapid – can be examined within a few minutes. Stained preparations tend to fade
Gram's	Bacteria. Myelin	Standard procedure
Ziehl–Neelsen (Z–N)	*Mycobacterium* spp. Other acid-fast organisms e.g. *Cryptosporidium*	Modified Z–N (Macchiavello's) will detect *Chlamydophila* and some mycoplasmas
Sudan III or oil red	Detection of fat (lipid)	Useful because in histological sections the fat has been removed and cannot therefore be demonstrated directly
New methylene blue	Fungal hyphae. Fibrin. Certain bacteria	Can combine with other stains e.g. eosin
Neat stain (eosin and methylene blue)	General cells and other structures	

TABLE 3.20 Categories of structures

Cell/structure	Comments
Normal host cells	May show an increase in numbers (e.g. lymphoid hyperplasia of the spleen, proliferation of epithelium) or be present in abnormal sites (e.g. heterophilic infiltration of the liver)
Abnormal host cells	May be indicative of pathology but may also be artifacts due to poor sample collection, transportation or processing
Pathological host cells	Pathological host cells may show discrete individual changes (e.g. degeneration, vacuolation, metaplasia, neoplasia) or be part of a pattern involving different types of cell. The size of cells may be important (measure with graticule and compare with cells of known size, e.g. erythrocytes). Giant cells and inclusion bodies may be a feature
Extrinsic cells	These are cells that are not derived from the host (patient) but may be relevant to diagnosis (e.g. parasites, inhaled material, foreign bodies)
Contaminants	Be wary of plant and other contaminants, especially when working in the field when several samples are being collected or processed at the same time – transportation of cells can occur

At least two preparations, preferably more, should always be taken, even if not all are stained and examined. It is far better to have an excess of preparations than to rely on only one smear and to have misgivings about sending it to a colleague for a second opinion and thus risk its being lost or broken.

Fixation may or may not be necessary or desirable, depending on the staining technique to be used. If in doubt, if the sample is to be processed within 24 h it should be air-dried – but be prepared that this can cause crenation of cells. Various stains can be employed (Table 3.19).

Microscopy may reveal five main categories of structure (Table 3.20).

Unstained preparations can also be of value. Wet mounts may demonstrate (for example) ciliated host cells or parasites while an unstained smear may reveal fat (adipocytes) or cholesterol crystals.

Important pathological changes, detection of which may require examination of many fields and involve several cell types, include:

- Acute inflammation
- Chronic inflammation
- Nonmalignant proliferation
- Malignant proliferation (neoplasia).

Inflammatory (acute and chronic) and neoplastic responses are sometimes confused. Some examples, with means of differentiation, are given in Table 3.21.

General points

- Always try to quantify cellularity. Remember that some cells, e.g. epithelium, exfoliate more readily than do others, e.g. fibroblasts. Numbers of cells may, therefore, vary depending upon the type involved
- Record all findings, even if, at the time, they appear to be irrelevant.

Although interpretation is based primarily upon clinical/post-mortem history coupled with analysis of cytological findings, it is *vital* to compare the latter with results of other investigations, e.g. microbiology, hematology, clinical chemistry and, possibly, histopathology and electron microscopy.

TABLE 3.21 Type of cytological response

Response	Cell type	Significance/Comments
Inflammatory	Heterophils (normal)	Acute inflammation
	Heterophils (degenerate)	Infection, usually bacteria
	Mixed heterophils, lymphocytes, etc.	Chronic or subacute infection
	Macrophages in abundance (sometimes giant cells)	Fungal, *Mycobacterium*, foreign-body reactions
Neoplastic	General features: populations of similar cells with individual differences, including variable nuclear:cytoplasmic ratio, prominent nuclei and nucleoli, sometimes abnormal/multiple nuclei Increase in mitotic index	
	Spindle-shaped cells that exfoliate poorly	Sarcoma
	Round/oval cells, often in patterns	Carcinoma
	Round/oval cells, lymphoblast-like	Lymphoid neoplasm (e.g. leukemia)
	Mixed cells (but with neoplastic features)	Poorly differentiated neoplasm
	Squamous epithelial cells in large numbers but few features of neoplasia	Papilloma (or tissue hyperplasia)

Interpretation

Correct interpretation requires:

- A sound knowledge of normal host cell morphology and normal appearance of microorganisms and metazoan parasites
- An understanding of pathological changes, especially at the cellular level, e.g. pyknosis, karyorrhexis, inclusion-body formation
- An appreciation of the limitations of cytological techniques and of our poorly developed understanding of the relevance of some changes, especially in nonmammalian species.

Interpretation is based on:

- Clinical/post-mortem history
- Analysis of cytological findings by microscopy (NB. always use low power first).

Examples of avian cytological findings

These are illustrated in Figures 3.65–3.88.

ACKNOWLEDGMENTS

We are grateful to Dr Ravi Seebaransingh (The University of the West Indies) for his helpful comments on an early draft of this section. We thank numerous colleagues, past and present, in Arabia, Europe, Africa and the Caribbean who have participated in our studies and shared interests in avian cytology. The images used in this section are reproduced with permission from: Bailey TA, *Diseases and Medical Management of Houbara Bustards and Other Otididae*, published by the National Avian Research Center, PO Box 45553, Abu Dhabi, United Arab Emirates.

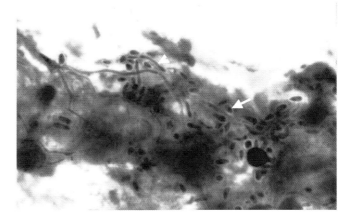

Fig. 3.65 Smear from the oral cavity of a Heuglin's bustard (*Neotis heuglinii*) showing *Candida* sp. with budding cells (arrow) and hyphae (arrowhead) formation. (May–Grünwald–Giemsa stain, 1000×).

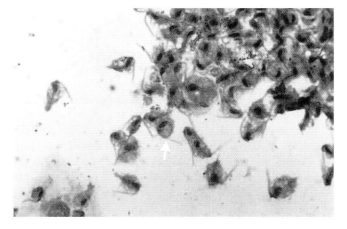

Fig. 3.66 *Trichomonas gallinae* (arrows) in a smear from the oral cavity of a kori bustard (*Ardeotis kori*). (May–Grünwald–Giemsa stain, 1000×).

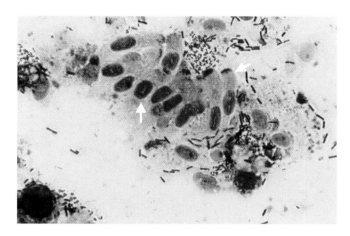

Fig. 3.67 Smear from the intestinal contents of a kori bustard with a heavy infestation of endoparasites showing abnormal exfoliation of columnar epithelial cells (arrows). (May–Grünwald–Giemsa stain, 1000×).

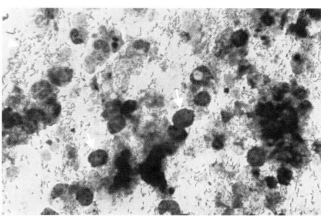

Fig. 3.68 Smear from the nares of a houbara bustard (*Chlamydotis undulata*) showing acute inflammatory response that reveals predominantly heterophils (arrows) and bacterial rods. (Neat stain, 1000×).

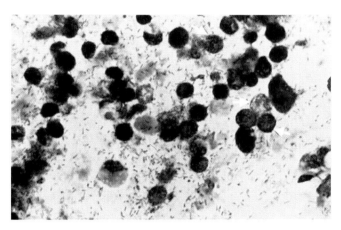

Fig. 3.69 Smear from the nares of a houbara bustard showing a chronic active inflammatory response that reveals mixed inflammatory cells (arrows), predominantly macrophages and bacterial rods. (Neat stain, 1000×).

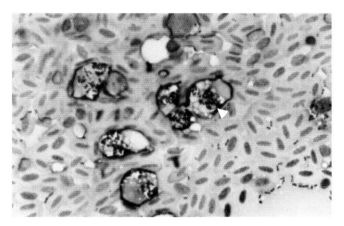

Fig. 3.70 Lung imprint of a houbara bustard with chronic bacterial pneumonia showing macrophages with phagocytosed bacteria (arrowhead). (Neat stain, 1000×).

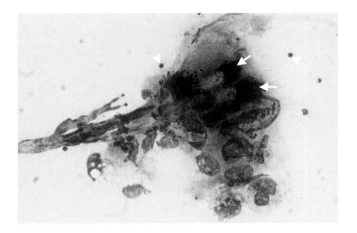

Fig. 3.71 Lung imprint of a stone curlew (*Burhinus oedicnemus*) showing conidiophores (arrowheads) and conidiospores (arrows). *Aspergillus fumigatus* was isolated. (Neat stain, 1000×).

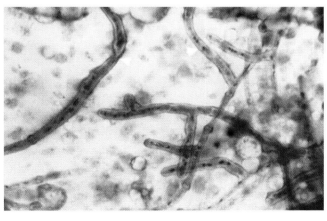

Fig. 3.72 Lung imprint of a gyrfalcon (*Falco rusticolus*) showing hyphae (arrowheads). *Aspergillus fumigatus* was isolated. (Neat stain, 1000×).

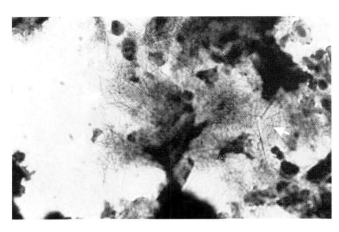

Fig. 3.73 Aspirate from the synovial aspirate fluid of a kori bustard showing urate crystals (arrows) and revealing articular gout. (Neat stain, 1000×).

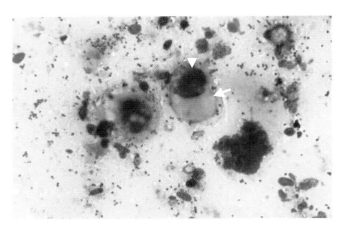

Fig. 3.74 Smear from a pox lesion showing squamous epithelial cells with large cytoplasmic vacuoles (arrow) that force the cell nucleus to the periphery of the cell (arrowhead). (Neat stain, 1000×).

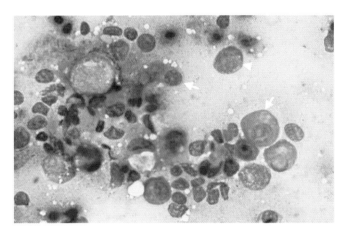

Fig. 3.75 Impression smear from the spleen of a houbara bustard with septicemic pox, showing plasma cells (arrows) and increased numbers of immature lymphocytes (arrowhead). (Neat stain, 1000×).

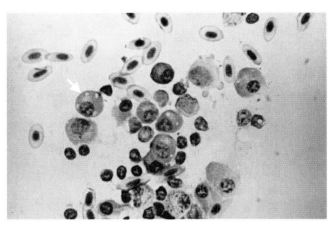

Fig. 3.76 Spleen imprint of a kori bustard showing a marked increase of plasma cells (arrow) suggestive of a reactive spleen. (Neat stain, 1000×).

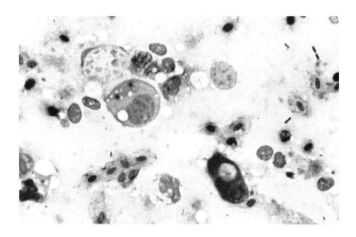

Fig. 3.77 Spleen imprint of a houbara bustard showing vacuolated plasma cells with karyorrhexis (arrow) due to septicemic pox. (Neat stain, 1000×).

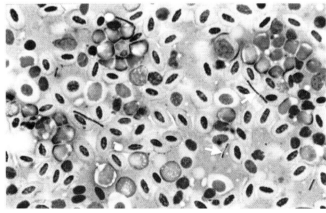

Fig. 3.78 Spleen imprint of a houbara bustard that died of an acute septicemic bacterial infection, showing chains of bacteria (arrows). (Neat stain, 1000×).

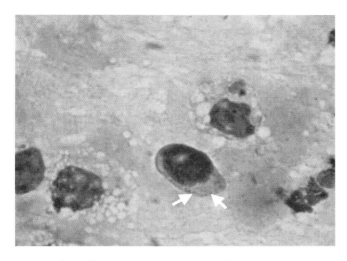

Fig. 3.79 Smear from the airsac biopsy of a gyrfalcon showing inclusions (arrowed) indicative of a *Chlamydophila* infection. (Neat stain, 1000×).

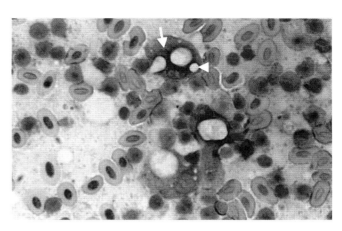

Fig. 3.80 Liver imprint smear from a houbara bustard with avian leukosis, showing hepatocytes with cytoplasmic basophilia (arrow) and vacuolation (arrowhead). (Neat stain, 1000×).

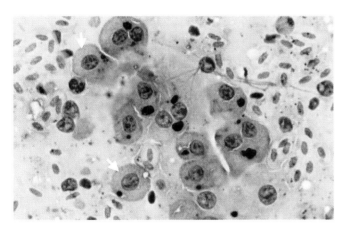

Fig. 3.81 Cytology imprint smears from normal kidney showing renal epithelial cells with abundant cytoplasm and round to oval slightly eccentric nucleus (arrows). (Neat stain, 1000×).

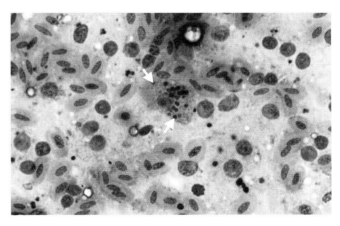

Fig. 3.82 Kidney imprint from a houbara bustard showing renal cells with iron pigment (hemosiderin) (arrowed). (Neat stain, 1000×).

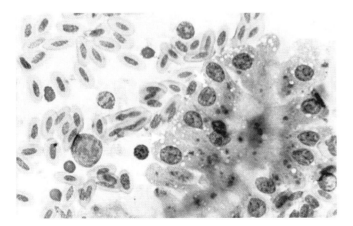

Fig. 3.83 Kidney imprint smear from a houbara bustard, showing vacuolated renal cells (arrows) due to septicemic pox. (Neat stain, 1000×).

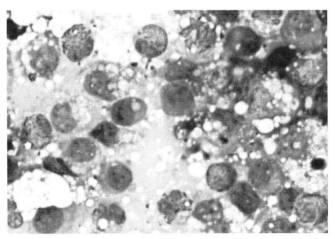

Fig. 3.84 Smear from the airsac biopsy of a peregrine falcon (*Falco peregrinus*) with airsacculitis, showing mixed inflammatory cells including heterophils and macrophages. (Neat stain, 1000×).

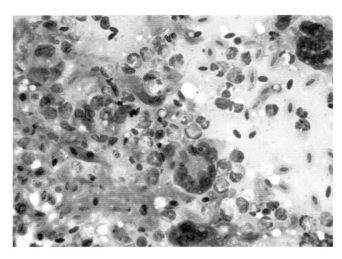

Fig. 3.85 Smear from the airsac biopsy of a gyrfalcon with aspergillosis, showing heterophils, macrophages, multinucleated giant cells and fungal spores. (Neat stain, 1000×).

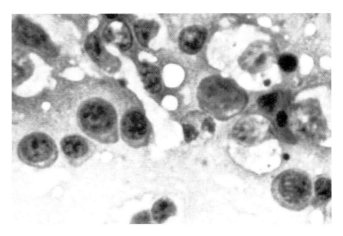

Fig. 3.86 Liver imprint smear from a gyr/peregrine hybrid falcon with mycobacteriosis showing, reactive mononuclear cells with deep basophilia. (Neat stain, 1000×).

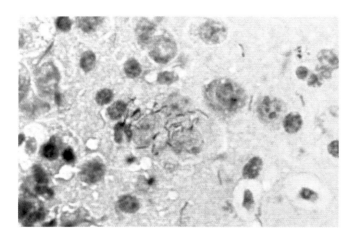

Fig. 3.87 Liver imprint smear from a hybrid falcon (gyr × peregrine) with mycobacteriosis, showing acid-fast rods. (Ziehl–Neelsen stain, 1000×).

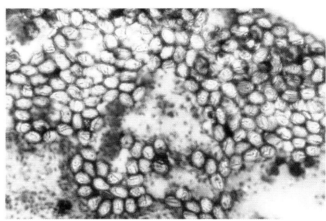

Fig. 3.88 Smear from the airsac biopsy of a peregrine falcon with serratospiculosis, showing *Serratospiculum* sp. ova. (Neat stain, 100×).

REFERENCES

Campbell TW (1993) Cytodiagnosis in raptor medicine. In: Redig PT, Cooper JE, Remple JD, Hunter DB *Raptor Biomedicine*, pp. 11–14. University of Minnesota Press, Minneapolis.

Campbell TW (1995) *Avian Hematology and Cytology*, 2nd edn. Iowa State University Press, Ames, IA.

Cooper JE (1994) Biopsy techniques. *Seminars in Avian and Exotic Pet Medicine* **3**: 161–165.

Corr SA, Maxwell M, Gentle MJ, Bennett D (2002) Preliminary study of joint disease in poultry by the analysis of synovial fluid. *Veterinary Record* **152**: 549–554.

Harrison GJ, Campbell TW (1994) Cytology. In: Ritchie BW, Harrison GJ, Harrison LR (eds) *Avian Medicine: Principles and Application*. Wingers Publishing, Lake Worth, FL.

Hawkey CM, Dennett TB (1989) *A Colour Atlas of Comparative Veterinary Haematology*. Wolfe, London.

Latimer KS, Goodwin MA, Davis MK (1988) Rapid cytologic diagnosis of respiratory cryptosporidiosis in chickens. *Avian Diseases* **32**: 826–830.

Pinches M (2005a) First steps in cytology; non inflammatory cell types. *UK Vet* **10**(5): 78–81.

Pinches M (2005b) First steps in cytology; the examination, and beyond. *UK Vet* **10**(4): 89–92.

Pinches M (2005c) Increasing information yield in cytology. *UK Vet* **10**(3): 96–98.

Rosenthal KL, Morris DO, Mauldin EA *et al.* (2004) Cytologic, histologic, and microbiologic characterization of the feather pulp and follicles of feather-picking psittacine birds: a preliminary study. *Journal of Avian Medicine and Surgery* **18**: 137–143.

FURTHER READING

Silvanose CD, Bailey TA (2006) Bustard diagnostic cytology. In: Bailey TA (ed.) *Diseases and Medical Management of Houbara Bustards and other Otididae*, Ch 7. National Avian Research Center, Abu Dhabi.

Teachout DJ (2005) Cytological sample analysis and interpretation. National Wildlife Rehabilitators' Association, USA. *Topics in Wildlife Medicine. Clinical Pathology* **1**: 43–45.

Radiography

Jesus Naldo

Radiography is an essential practical procedure in avian medicine that is applicable to the diagnosis of musculoskeletal disorders and diseases of the celomic cavity. It is one of the most important diagnostic tools because of the availability of rapid interpretation and the ability to perform it on patients of different sizes. It is useful as a primary diagnostic technique and also as an adjunct to other procedures, such as endoscopy and hematology, in making a differential diagnosis. In addition, radiography can prove valuable for the monitoring of progression of diseases and in evaluating the efficiency of therapeutic regimens. Radiological techniques in avian practice have made great progress with the introduction of high frequency ultralight radiographic units, cassettes with high definition screens, fast films and automatic developers. With the advent of safe and efficient inhalation anesthetic agents, such as isoflurane, radiography in birds is now an uneventful procedure.

X-ray unit

In avian radiography the X-ray unit should have a kVp setting ranging from 45 to 75, although in most cases a kVp of 50–55 is used. Most portable X-ray units have this capacity and are capable of producing between 15 and 35 mA. By using modern intensifying screens, good radiographs can be produced with 15–20 mA and exposure time of 0.04–0.2 seconds.

Portable units are most widely used in general veterinary practice and are suitable for avian radiography. They possess a number of advantages, which include:

* They are less expensive than other types of unit
* They can operate from a 13 A or 15 A electrical point
* They can be easily taken to pieces and transported by car
* They are light and easily maneuvered.

Screens, cassettes, films

High-definition or fine-grain screens in cassettes are now more widely used in avian practice than nonscreen films because of the following features:

* They produce more fine detail than fast screens
* They require less amperage than nonscreen film but more amperage than fast screens.

Rare earth intensifying screens with single-emulsion films will give detailed results. However, they require longer exposure time compared with double-emulsion film-cassette combinations.

The choice of film depends on the detail required in the radiograph and the nature of the examination. There are three types of screen film:

* Standard – a fine-grain medium-speed film that is good for use with high-definition intensifying screens. Excellent for avian radiography and extremities of larger species
* Fast – the speed is almost twice than that of standard. Good for veterinary radiography
* Ultrafast – needs shorter exposure time, suitable for use in veterinary radiography but has a short storage life.

Restraint and positioning

Adequate restraint for radiography is critical if high-quality diagnostic radiographs are to be obtained. Physical restraint is stressful and there is a high probability of worsening the condition of the bird and causing dislocations or even bone fractures. More importantly, with physical restraint there is an increased possibility of radiation exposure to staff.

Inhalation anesthesia with isoflurane (IsoFlo, Abbott Laboratories) is the safest method of restraining birds (see details in Ch. 4). Prior to radiographic examination, birds are anesthetized with a combination of isoflurane and oxygen administered by a face mask. Birds under anesthesia for more than 15 min are intubated with an uncuffed endotracheal tube. Anesthesia is induced with 5% isoflurane and maintained with 2–3% isoflurane combined with oxygen at 0.5 l/min.

Until recently, anesthesia was not recommended in contrast studies of the gastrointestinal tract because it may lead to cessation of gastrointestinal motility. However, studies by Lennox and Crosta (2005) showed no significant differences in the progression of barium sulfate between radiographs collected with isoflurane and manual restraint alone.

Positioning of the patient is very important in order to produce a good diagnostic radiograph. Survey radiographs of the whole body in the ventrodorsal and lateral projections are taken of each bird. Detailed radiograph of an extremity (head, neck, wing, foot) is taken when indicated. Perfect positioning for a whole-body projection can be achieved with the following procedure (Baumgartner, 1991; McMillan, 1994; Harcourt-Brown, 1996; Krautwald-Junghanns, 1996; Romagnano, 1997; Smith and Smith, 1997; Krautwald-Junghanns and Trinkaus, 2000).

In the **ventrodorsal view** (Fig. 3.89):

* The bird is placed on dorsal recumbency
* The keel should be superimposed over the vertebral column

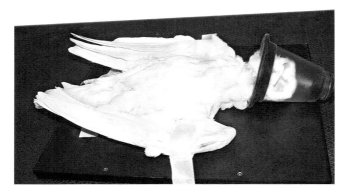

Fig. 3.89 Positioning technique for ventrodorsal body radiograph of a little corella (*Cacatua sanguinea*) under isoflurane anesthesia. Both wings are slightly extended and secured with masking tape. The legs are pulled backwards and secured with masking tape on the tarsometatarsus. The bird is taped directly to the cassette.

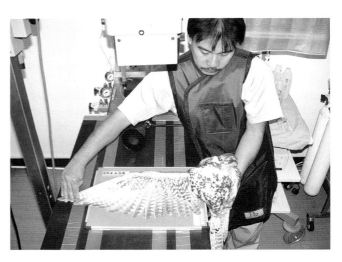

Fig. 3.91 Positioning technique for craniocaudal radiograph of the wing of a saker falcon (*Falco cherrug*) under isoflurane anesthesia. The bird is held with the wing fully extended and the head to the side.

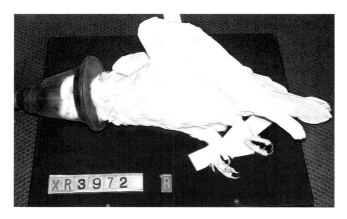

Fig. 3.90 Positioning technique for lateral body radiograph of a little corella under isoflurane anesthesia. Both wings are extended dorsally and secured with masking tape. The legs are pulled caudally and secured with masking tape on the tarsometatarsus. The bird is taped directly to the cassette.

- Both wings are slightly extended laterally and secured with masking tape
- Both legs are pulled backwards, positioned symmetrically and secured with masking tape on the tarsometatarsus
- Center the primary beam over the patient at the point of the sternum, and collimate to reduce scatter.

In the **lateral view** (Fig. 3.90):

- The bird is usually placed in left to right lateral recumbency
- The hip and shoulder joints should be superimposed
- The wings should be extended dorsally, with the lower wing placed slightly cranial to the upper wing to permit differentiation of right from left

- The upper wing is secured with masking tape across the carpometacarpal joints
- Foam padding should be placed in between the wings to prevent overextension
- Both legs can be extended caudally or the dependent leg can be positioned cranially to the contralateral leg and secured at the tarsometatarsus with masking tape
- The X-ray beam is centered on the midline cranial to the caudal tip of the sternum.

In addition to the ventrodorsal and lateral radiographs of an extremity, detailed radiographs of the wing and foot can be achieved with the following procedures.

In the **craniocaudal view** (Fig. 3.91):

- A craniocaudal view of the wing may be beneficial particularly to evaluate fractures of the wing or damage to the clavicle, coracoid, scapula or humerus
- Have an adequately protected technician hold the bird with the affected wing fully extended and head to the side
- True craniocaudal positioning results in superimposition of the antebrachial bones and all digits. This projection can also be achieved in an oblique position, which permits separation of the radius and ulna as well as the alular digits
- Evidence of the pectoral muscles extending toward the humerus indicates the ventral surface of the wing.

In the **'stressed' view** (Fig. 3.92):

- A detailed radiograph of the wing in 'stressed' position may be beneficial to evaluate fractures or damage to the humerus, clavicle, coracoid or scapula
- The bird is placed on dorsal recumbency

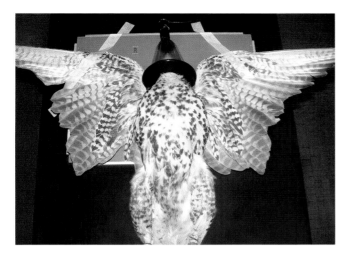

Fig. 3.92 Positioning technique for stressed radiograph of the wings of a saker falcon under isoflurane anesthesia. The bird is placed on dorsal recumbency. The legs are pulled backwards and secured with masking tape on the tarsometatarsus. The wings are extended and 'stressed' cranially and secured with masking tape on the metacarpals.

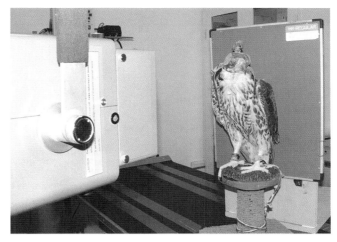

Fig. 3.94 Positioning technique for a survey radiograph of a peregrine falcon in a standing position. The bird is placed standing on a custom-built stand or perch. A cassette is placed on a holder positioned as closed as possible to the bird. This technique is used for birds that cannot be anesthetized; however, its use offers only limited diagnostic value.

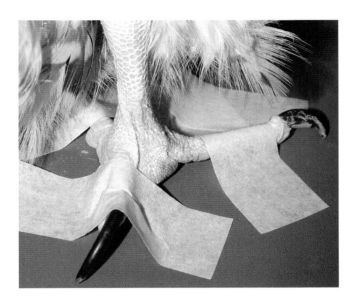

Fig. 3.93 Positioning technique for caudoplantar radiograph of the foot of a peregrine falcon (*Falco peregrinus*) under isoflurane anesthesia. The bird is placed on ventral recumbency over a rolled towel. The foot is positioned with the plantar surface as close as possible to the cassette. All digits are secured with masking tape. Center the primary beam at the point of the metatarsophalangeal joint of digit 1.

- Both legs are pulled backwards, positioned symmetrically and secured with masking tape on the tarsometatarsus
- Both wings are fully extended laterally, 'stressed' cranially, positioned symmetrically and secured with masking tape on the metacarpals.

In the **caudoplantar view** (Fig. 3.93):

- A caudoplantar view of the foot is beneficial to evaluate the digits, metatarsophalangeal joints and sesamoid bone between the metatarsophalangeal

joint of digit 2 and the flexor tendons in some raptor species. It is particularly useful in assessing chronic bumblefoot infection
- The bird is placed on ventral recumbency over a rolled towel
- The foot is positioned with the plantar surface as close as possible to the cassette
- All digits are secured with masking tape
- Center the primary beam at the point of the metatarsophalangeal joint of digit 1 (hallux).

Survey radiographs of hooded birds of prey that cannot be anesthetized for a particular reason (e.g. anesthetic risks – recently fed, too stressed, dyspneic, etc. – or simply because the owner has refused anesthesia) can be taken with the bird standing on a perch. The diagnostic value of this technique is very limited and it can be used only on selected cases, e.g. some musculoskeletal disorders, lead pellets or fragments in the ventriculus, impaction, and detection of a passive induced transponder (PIT).

In the **standing position** (Fig. 3.94):

- Radiographs can be obtained in the ventrodorsal or lateral positions
- A cassette should be placed on the holder or stand positioned as close as possible to the patient
- Rotate the head of the radiographic machine to center the horizontal beam over the patient and collimate to reduce scatter
- Maintain the required exposure settings (Table 3.22).

Conventional radiography

Most radiographs included in this section were taken with a portable radiographic unit (ATOMSCOPE HF 80, Mikasa X-ray Co. Ltd, Tokyo, Japan). This unit has

TABLE 3.22 Avian radiographic techniques – conventional radiography

Subject	Bodyweight (g)	kV	mA	Time (s)	FFD (inches)
Whole body, proximal limbs	2500–3500	60	15	0.04	26
Head, distal limbs	2500–3500	55–60	15	0.04	23.5–26
Whole body	1400–1500	55–60	15	0.04	23.5
Whole body	800–1300	55	15	0.04	23.5
Whole body	<800	50	15	0.04	23.5
Extremities – head, feet, wing	1000–1500	55	15	0.04	23.5
Extremities – head, feet, wing	<1000	50	15	0.04	23.5

Radiographs were recorded on standard double emulsion films (MG-SR, Konica Medical Film, Japan) in high definition screens in cassettes (HR-Regular, Veterinary X-Rays, UK).
kV, kilovoltage; mA, milliampere – the ATOMSCOPE HF 80 portable X-ray equipment has a constant setting of 15 mA; FFD, focal to film distance.

TABLE 3.23 Avian radiographic techniques – magnification radiography

Subject	Bodyweight (g)	kV	mA	Time (s)	OFD (inches)	FFD (inches)
Whole body	1400–1500	55–60	15	0.04	12	20
Whole body	800–1300	55	15	0.04	12	20
Whole body	<800	50	15	0.04	12	20
Extremities – head, feet, wing	1000–1500	55	15	0.04	12	20
Extremities – head, feet, wing	<1000	50	15	0.04	12	20

Radiographs were recorded on standard double emulsion films (MG-SR, Konica Medical Film, Japan) in high definition screens in cassettes (HR-Regular, Veterinary X-Rays, UK).
kV, kilovoltage; mA, milliampere – the ATOMSCOPE HF 80 portable X-ray equipment has a constant setting of 15 mA; FFD, focal to film distance, OFD, object to film distance.

an X-ray tube voltage of 50–80 kV, fixed 15 mA current and exposure time of 0.02–1.98 s. Screen films (MG-SR, Konica Medical Film, Tokyo, Japan) and cassettes (HR-Regular, Veterinary X-Rays, Beaconsfield, UK) were used. The exposure settings for conventional radiography used in our hospital are described in Table 3.22.

Magnification radiography

Magnification or augmented radiography will enhance visualization of special areas of interest (e.g. the infraorbital sinus, limbs, joints). The cost of magnification is a reduction in the spatial resolution or image sharpness, which is inversely proportional to the degree of magnification (Tell *et al.*, 2003). The exposure settings for magnification radiography used in our hospital are described in Table 3.23.

Indications:

- Evaluating the nature and extent of craniofacial soft tissue or musculoskeletal abnormalities
- Evaluating sinuses
- Evaluating ocular and ear abnormalities
- Evaluating limbs and joints.

Table top technique (Fig. 3.95):
- The film cassette is placed on the top of the table
- The object to film distance (OFD) is increased by placing the patient on Styrofoam blocks

- The focal to film distance (FFD) is decreased by lowering the tube housing closer to the film cassette.

Radiographic contrast study

Contrast studies may be performed for the examination of the following:

- Organ size
- Organ shape
- Organ position
- Abnormal contents
- Outline of an organ against neighboring organs
- Determination of organ function
- Thickness and condition of the wall of hollow structures.

Gastrointestinal contrast studies

Indications:

- Chronic regurgitation
- Persistent diarrhea
- Constipation
- Abnormal palpation
- Abdominal enlargement
- Abnormalities in the gastrointestinal tract observed on survey radiographs.

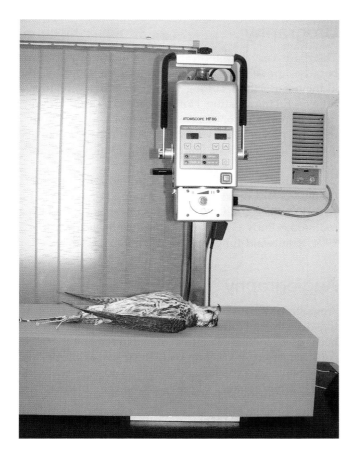

Fig. 3.95 Positioning technique for obtaining a magnified view of the head of a peregrine falcon. The object to film distance (OFD) was 8″ and the focal to film distance (FFD) was 20″. The OFD was increased by placing the falcon on a Styrofoam block.

The **common techniques** used in avian gastrointestinal tract contrast radiography include:

- Gastrointestinal contrast with 25–45% barium sulfate administered directly into the esophagus at a dosage of 20 ml/kg bodyweight. The contrast medium will be in the proventriculus and ventriculus within a few minutes and will reach the intestines in 30–60 min

(Table 3.24). If the area of interest is the lower gastrointestinal tract, the contrast medium can be administered directly to the ventriculus (Krautwald-Junghanns and Trinkaus, 2000)

- Double contrast with 25% barium sulfate (positive contrast medium) in a dosage of 10 ml/kg bodyweight given either orally or cloacally. Air (negative contrast medium) is introduced immediately after the administration of barium sulfate at 20 ml/kg bodyweight. This technique is useful for demonstration of the thickness and condition of the wall of the gastrointestinal tract and for demonstration of the cloaca (Krautwald-Junghanns and Trinkaus, 2000)
- Iohexol, a nonionic, low-osmolar, water-soluble, iodinated contrast medium, may be used as an alternative to barium sulfate suspension for gastrointestinal tract contrast studies. It should be used in suspected cases of intestinal perforation because iodine is less likely than barium sulfate to cause peritonitis. If aspirated, iohexol is absorbed from the celomic cavity with minimal tissue reaction. Iohexol has a rapid transit time through the avian gastrointestinal tract when compared with barium. However, iohexol studies often produce uneven luminal coverage and bubbles (Smith and Smith, 1997; Romagnano and Love, 2000).

Radiographic abnormalities that may be defined by gastrointestinal contrast studies (McMillan, 1994) include:

- Change in location, size or shape of abdominal organs
- Differentiation between the gastrointestinal tract and other organs
- Increased or decreased motility
- Increased or decreased luminal diameter
- Mucosal irregularities
- Filling defects
- Changes in wall thickness
- Extravasation of contrast media
- Dilution of contrast with mucous or fluid.

Subject	Stomach	Small intestines	Large intestines	Cloaca
Canary	5	10–15	15–30	30–90
Indian hill mynah	5	10–15	15–30	30–90
Racing pigeon	5–10	10–30	30–120	120–240
Hawk	5–15	15–30	30–90	90–360
Budgerigar	5–30	30–60	60–120	120–240
African gray parrot	10–30	30–60	60–120	120–130
Amazon parrot	10–60	60–120	120–150	150–240
Pheasant	10–45	45–120	120–150	150–240

TABLE 3.24 Barium sulfate transit times

Time in minutes for barium sulfate administered by crop gavage to reach and fill various portions of the gastrointestinal tract.
Source: modified from McMillan MC (1994) Imaging techniques. In: Ritchie BW, Harrison GJ, Harrison LR (eds) *Avian Medicine: Principles and Application*, pp. 246–326. Wingers Publishing, Lake Worth, FL.

Positive pressure insufflation contrast radiography

In an anesthetized, intubated bird, airsacs can be insuf–flated manually to increase total airsac area, thus using air as a negative contrast medium to improve visualization of internal organs and their borders on radiographs (Figs 3.96 and 3.97) (Sherrill *et al.*, 2001).

- Once anesthetized, birds are intubated with a semiflexible silicone endotracheal tube and maintained at a surgical plane of anesthesia
- A rebreathing circuit fitted with a ventilation bag (1 liter) and a manometer (units in cmH$_2$O) is used.
- Whole body radiographs are taken without and then with positive pressure insufflation (PPI)
- PPI at 20 cm H$_2$O pressure was applied manually to the ventilating bag of a closed rebreathing circuit while radiograph is taken.

Urography

There are very few indications for urography in birds because gross and histological characteristics of the kidney cause the resulting images to provide relatively little useful information. However, it can be used to define renal dimensions or masses. Indications for urography include polyuria/polydipsia and nonspecific clinical signs of leg paresis or joint swelling (Smith and Smith, 1997).

For urogenital tract contrast radiography the agent used is 70–80% organic iodine compound or a compound with 300–400 mg iodine/ml with a dosage of 700–800 mg iodine/kg bodyweight given intravenously (McMillan, 1994; Krautwald-Junghanns and Trinkaus, 2000).

Angiography

Angiography could be an important diagnostic tool for the detection of cardiovascular disease in birds. It has been used in the diagnosis of aneurysm of the right coronary artery in a white cockatoo (*Cacatua alba*) (Vink-Nooteboom *et al.*, 1998) and atherosclerosis of the aorta and brachiocephalic arteries in a severe macaw (*Ara*

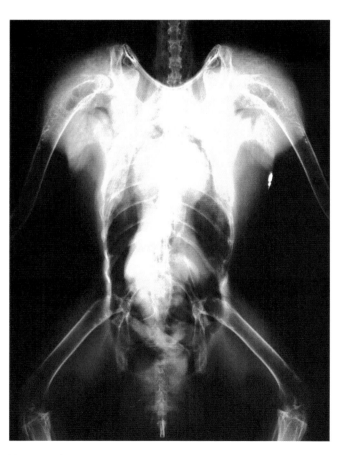
(a)

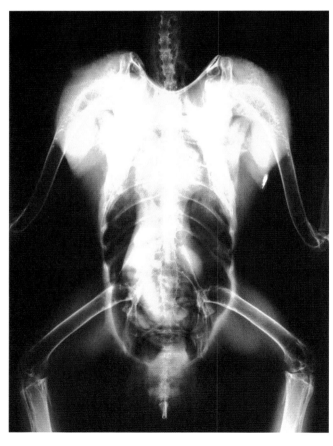
(b)

Fig. 3.96 (a) Ventrodorsal survey radiograph and (b) ventrodorsal positive-pressure insufflation (PPI) radiograph of an anesthetized, intubated saker falcon. Note enhanced visualization of internal structures, including the thoracic and abdominal airsacs, as a result of PPI.

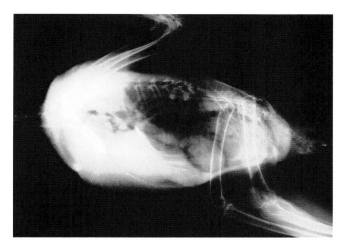
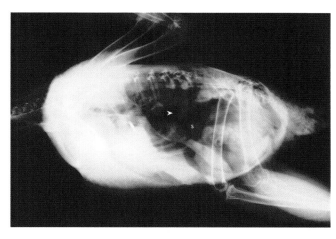

(a)

(b)

Fig. 3.97 (a) Lateral survey radiograph and (b) lateral PPI radiograph of an anesthetized, intubated saker falcon. Note enhanced visualization of internal structures, including the spleen (s) and thoracic and abdominal airsacs, as a result of PPI. A large, focal radiodense mass can be observed along the caudal thoracic airsac field (arrow).

severa) (Phalen *et al.*, 1996). Fluorescein angiography was used to examine the blood supply of the eyes of various raptors (Korbel *et al.*, 2000).

Myelography

Abnormalities that can be detected by myelography include spinal cord compression, spinal trauma, or space occupying masses. Patients must be anesthetized for this procedure. A 25 gauge spinal needle is carefully inserted at the thoracosynsacral junction and 0.8–1.2 ml/kg of nonionic iodinated material is injected into the subarachnoid space (Harr *et al.*, 1997). Alternatively, contrast material can be injected directly into the cerebellar medullary cistern (McMillan, 1994).

Radiographic interpretation

A systematic approach to film interpretation is important in order to reach a correct diagnosis. In evaluating films do not just focus on the most obvious lesion and perhaps overlook more subtle changes. A useful technique is to first assess the film for overall quality from a technical viewpoint, then work sequentially through each body system. I use an organ-by-organ system approach,

proceeding from cranial to caudal, evaluating the head and neck, skeletal system, respiratory, cardiovascular, gastrointestinal, other celomic organs and genitourinary systems.

Silverman (1990) recommends the following analysis:

- Skeletal – skull, spine, pectoral girdle, pelvic girdle, wings, legs
- Cardiovascular – heart, greater vessels
- Respiratory – nasal sinuses, mouth, trachea, syrinx, lungs, airsacs
- Gastrointestinal – mouth, crop, esophagus, proventriculus, ventriculus, intestines, cloaca
- Genitourinary – pelvic region, kidneys, abdomen, cloaca
- Accessory organs – liver, spleen.

The radiographs are scrutinized according to the following criteria (Baumgartner, 1991):

- Size of the organ
- Density of organs and parts of organs
- Structure of organs
- Evaluation of the contents of the gastrointestinal tract.

Abnormal radiographic findings and their indications are given in Table 3.25. Figs 3.98–3.125 illustrate some abnormal radiological findings.

TABLE 3.25 Abnormal radiographic findings	
Radiological signs	**Indications**
RESPIRATORY SYSTEM	
Increased radiodensity of the tracheal lumen (tracheal masses)	Hypovitaminosis A
	Bacterial infection (pseudomoniasis)
	Mycotic infection (aspergillosis)
	Parasitic infection (trichomonosis)
	Pox virus infection
	Foreign bodies (seeds)
	Endotracheal tube injury
Displacement or abnormal position of the trachea	Presence of abnormal masses in the ventral cervical area
Increased radiodensity of the tracheal rings or wall of the tracheobronchial syrinx	Calcification of the trachea or tracheobronchial syrinx in older birds
Mottled tracheobronchial syrinx shadow with overdistension of the abdominal airsacs (air trapping)	Stenosis due to a mycotic granuloma on the tracheobronchial syrinx, pseudomoniasis or trichomonosis
Overdistension of the axillary portion of the clavicular airsacs	Stenosis of the lower respiratory tract
Homogeneous increased radiodensity of the lung field	Bacterial pneumonia

TABLE 3.25 Abnormal radiographic findings *(Continued)*

Radiological signs	Indications
Nonhomogeneous increased radiodensity of the lung field	Mycotic pneumonia
Irregular, focal dense areas in the lungs	Mycotic, mycobacterial granuloma
Increased radiodensity in the heart–lung area often concentrated around the main bronchus	Chronic bronchitis
	Chronic bronchopneumonia
Increased radiodensity and rounding of the caudal lung field	Congestion of the caudal part of the lung in chronic disease
Thickening of the airsac walls (cavern formation)	Chronic mycotic infection
Increased radiodensity of the airsac walls	Due to crystalline deposits or calcification of the airsac walls
Homogeneous increased radiodensity of the thoracic and abdominal airsacs	Fat deposits on the airsacs
	Airsacculitis of uncertain origin (bacterial, viral, chlamydophilic or mycotic infections)
Nonhomogeneous increased radiodensity of the thoracic and abdominal airsacs	Chronic mycotic airsacculitis
	Mycotic or mycobacterial granuloma
Solitary or multiple, focal increased radiodensities in the thoracic and abdominal airsacs	Abscesses
	Neoplasia
Rounding of the caudal parts of the abdominal airsacs	Chronic airsacculitis
Compression of the thoracic and abdominal airsac field	Seen as secondary to mass lesions in the caudal celomic cavity (distension of the alimentary tract, neoplasms or egg binding)

GASTROINTESTINAL SYSTEM

Thickening of the wall of the esophagus/crop and proventriculus	Vitamin A deficiency (often associated with an enlarged kidney shadow)
	Chronic inflammation due to *Candida* spp. infection or a worm infection
Distension and/or impaction of the crop	Overeating of grit
	Improper hand rearing technique
	Ingestion of foreign materials
	Secondary to enlarged thyroids
	Lead toxicity
	Obstruction in the proventriculus, ventriculus and upper intestines
Dilatation of the gastrointestinal tract	Neurogenic infections
	Neurotoxic poisons
	Food impaction
	Ileus of the distal segments
Dilatation of the proventriculus	Bacterial infection
	Mycotic infection
	Parasitic infection
	Heavy metal toxicity
	Impaction
	Foreign body
	Normal baby bird
Thickening of the proventricular wall	Parasitic infection
Severe dilatation of the proventriculus, retarded passage, thinning of the proventricular walls and atrophy and deformation of the ventriculus	Proventricular dilatation disease
	Candidiasis
Gas-filled dilatation of the ventriculus	Lead toxicosis
	Newcastle disease
Thickening of the wall of the ventriculus	Newcastle disease
Excessive grit in the ventriculus and intestines	Deficiency disease or disturbance in the crop, ventriculus or intestines
Heavy metal particles that are visible as radiopaque foreign bodies in the ventriculus	Lead shot
	Paint flakes
	Wire
Dorsocranial or dorsocaudal displacement of the ventriculus	Enlarged liver
Ventrocranial or ventrocaudal displacement of the ventriculus	Enlarged kidney, spleen or gonad
Ventrocranial displacement of the ventriculus	Enlarged intestinal loops
	Egg in the oviduct
	Ovarian cysts
Gas-filled intestines	Bacterial infection
	Functional ileus
	Luminal or extraluminal mass obstruction
	Aerophagia secondary to severe respiratory distress, heavy metal toxicity or gas anesthesia
Dilatation of the duodenal loop or any other loop of the intestine with increased radiodensity	Massive prepatent worm infection
	Bacterial or mycotic infection
	Pancreatitis
	Neoplasia
	Luminal or extraluminal mass obstruction
Dilatation of the cloaca	Cloacitis
	Neoplasms
	Cloacolith
	Proventricular dilatation disease
	Retained soft shell egg

TABLE 3.25 Abnormal radiographic findings *(Continued)*

Radiological signs	Indications
	Traumatic dilatation
	Idiopathic dilatation
	Liver and spleen
Decreased hepatic radiopacity	Hepatic lipidosis
Focal irregularities of the hepatic contour	Granulomatous lesions
Reduced size of the liver shadow (microhepatia). The liver shadow is separated from the heart in the hourglass shadow	Generalized emaciation Poor nutrition Pesticide toxicity May occur normally in macaws
Enlarged liver shadow	*Chlamydophila psittaci* infection Tuberculosis Pacheco's disease Herpesvirus hepatitis Other viral diseases Neoplasia Metabolic diseases Parasitic diseases
Ground-glass appearance of the entire celomic cavity. The lungs and airsacs are compressed (ascites)	Liver cirrhosis Hemochromatosis Neoplasia Congestive heart failure Viral infections Bacterial endocarditis and myocarditis
Severe spleen enlargement	*Chlamydophila psittaci* infection (accompanied with airsacculitis and lung consolidation) Tuberculosis Yersiniosis Neoplasia
Enlarged spleen shadow with enlargement of the liver and kidneys	Tuberculosis Viral diseases Urogenital system
Radiodense crystalline deposits in the kidneys	Renal gout Dehydration Chronic bacterial infection
Enlarged kidney shadows with or without increased density	Neoplasia Cysts *Chlamydophila psittaci* infection Bacterial diseases Metabolic diseases Post-renal obstruction Heavy metal toxicity
Enlargement of the cranial pole of the kidney	Kidney enlargement as above Adrenal enlargement Gonadal enlargement
Increased density without enlargement of the kidneys	Gout Dehydration Vitamin A deficiency
Egg in the oviduct	Egg binding if combined with specific symptoms (weakness, pressing, dyspnea) Salpingitis
An area of increased density caused by fragmented egg shell dorsal and caudal to the intestinal mass	
Diffused increase in radiodensity of the caudal celomic cavity and no differentiation of various organs is possible (abdominal effusion)	Ovarian neoplasia Egg yolk related peritonitis Cardiovascular system
Increased apex to base dimension, enlarged vascular structures, prominence to the left atrial segment, abnormal shape of the heart shadow (cardiomegaly)	Valvular disease Endocarditis Chronic anemia Compression from extrinsic masses Hemochromatosis
Globoid enlargement of the heart shadow	Pericardial effusion that may be due to *Chlamydophila psittaci* infection, polyomavirus, tuberculosis, polyomavirus, sarcocystosis or neoplasia
Enlargement and/or increased radiodensity of the heart shadow	Pericarditis Epicarditis Marked fatty deposition
Alteration of the heart's shape and contour (dilatation of one chamber)	Maybe genetic abnormality
Not well defined shadow of the cranial end of the heart	Bronchitis Bronchopneumonia

TABLE 3.25 Abnormal radiographic findings *(Continued)*

Radiological signs	Indications
Reduced size of the heart shadow (microcardia). May have radiolucent gap between heart and liver	Hypovolemia Nutritional inadequacy
Calcification of major vessels and lung fields	Arteriosclerosis (in very old psittacines and birds of prey)

SKELETAL SYSTEM

Radiological signs	Indications
Increased radiodensity of the infraorbital sinus. Osteolytic changes may be present on the surrounding bones	Rhinitis Sinusitis
Decreased skeletal radiodensity, deformities of the long bones, ribs and spine, and/or fractures of the metaphyses	Metabolic bone disease (osteoporosis, osteomalacia, rickets, fibrous osteodystrophy, nutritional secondary hyperparathyroidism) Twisting and bending deformities of the long bones
Multiple osteolytic and sclerotic changes in the medullary cavity of the long bones	Mycobacterial infections
Homogeneous increased in medullary bone density (polyostotic hyperostosis)	In female birds prior to egg production
Irregular increased in medullary bone density	Pathological high estrogen level associated with laminated eggs, gonadal tumors or cysts Osteomyelitis
Increased bone radiodensity associated with periosteal proliferation and swelling of surrounding soft tissue	
Collapsed joint space, periarticular proliferation of bone and soft tissue swelling	Arthritis
Arthritic and osteolytic changes of the digits, joints and tarsometatarsus	Septic bumblefoot

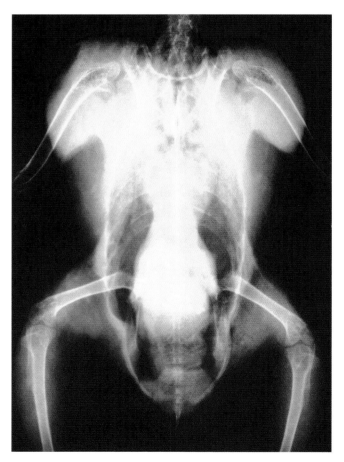

(a)

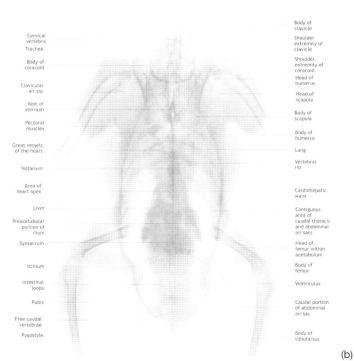

(b)

Fig. 3.98 (a) Ventrodorsal radiograph of the body of a normal blue-fronted Amazon parrot (*Amazona aestiva*). (b) Digitized picture of the same bird to illustrate the different body parts.

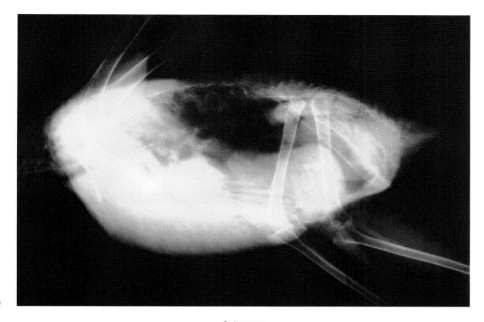

(a)

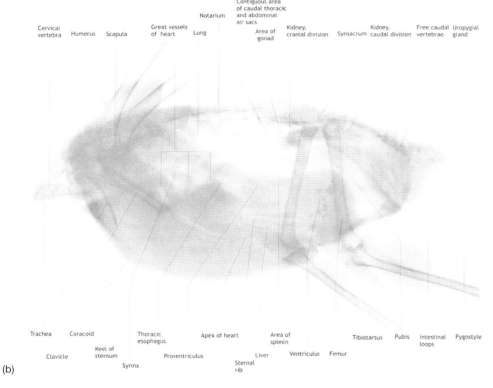

Cervical vertebra | Humerus | Scapula | Great vessels of heart | Notarium | Lung | Contiguous area of caudal thoracic and abdominal air sacs | Area of gonad | Kidney, cranial division | Synsacrum | Kidney, caudal division | Free caudal vertebrae | Uropygial gland

Trachea | Coracoid | Clavicle | Keel of sternum | Syrinx | Thoracic esophagus | Proventriculus | Apex of heart | Sternal rib | Area of spleen | Liver | Ventriculus | Femur | Tibiotarsus | Pubis | Intestinal loops | Pygostyle

(b)

Fig. 3.99 (a) Lateral (Le-Rt) radiograph of the body of a normal blue-fronted Amazon parrot. (b) Digitized picture of the same bird to illustrate the different body parts.

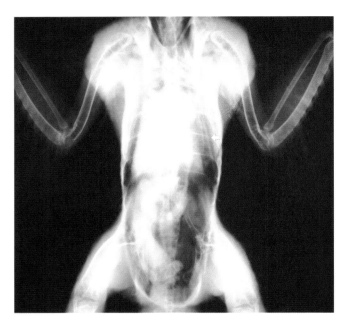

Fig. 3.100 Lateral survey radiograph of a little corella showing a large quantity of radiopaque material (grit) in the ventriculus.

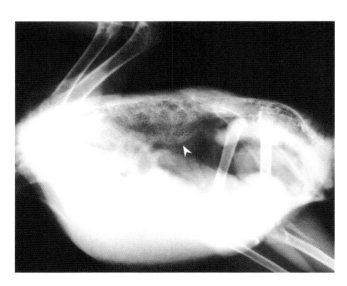

Fig. 3.101 Ventrodorsal survey radiograph of a violet touraco (*Musophaga violacea*) showing a unilateral homogeneous increased radiopacity affecting the left cranial thoracic airsac (arrow). Air trapping is evident in the left caudal thoracic and abdominal airsac field. The typical hourglass cardiohepatic waist is not evident in this species.

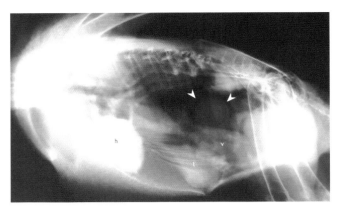

Fig. 3.103 Lateral survey radiograph of a saker falcon showing an enlarged spleen (arrows) visible on the dorsal aspect of the ventriculus (v). The heart (h) and liver (l) shadows are reduced in size. Note the radiolucent gap between the heart and liver. Severe spleen enlargement could be due to viral or bacterial (tuberculosis, chlamydophilosis) diseases or lymphoma.

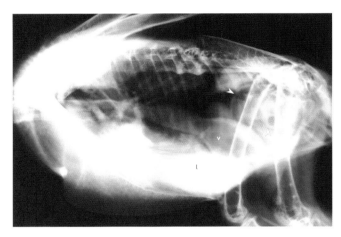

Fig. 3.104 Lateral survey radiograph of a gyr/saker hybrid falcon (*Falco rusticolus–Falco cherrug*) showing gaseous distension of the ventriculus (v) and intestinal loops (arrows). The thickened ventriculus is displaced caudodorsally by the enlarged liver (l). This bird presented with a history of reduced appetite, chronic vomiting and progressive weight loss. This case of severe gastroenteritis was the result of a bacterial infection.

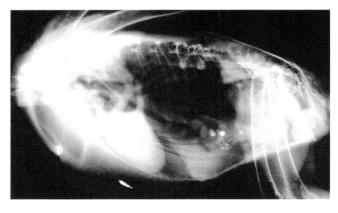

Fig. 3.105 Lateral survey radiograph of a saker falcon showing a lead pellet in the ventriculus. The falcon was fed a collared dove (*Streptopelia decaocto*) shot the previous day using a 12-bore shotgun.

Fig. 3.102 Lateral survey radiograph of a gray parrot (*Psittacus erithacus*) that presented with dyspnea. There is increased consolidation of the lung field, which is consistent with pneumonia (arrow).

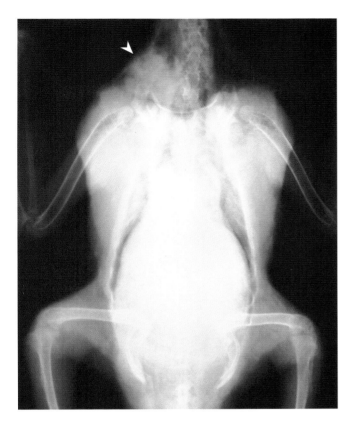

Fig. 3.106 Ventrodorsal survey radiograph of an eclectus parrot (*Eclectus roratus*) presented because of severe dyspnea, abdominal swelling and green urates. An extensive diffused radiopacity across the hepatic and peritoneal celomic cavities is present. The bird was suffering from ascites associated with severe amyloidosis affecting mainly the liver. Ascites is the accumulation of serous fluids in one or various celomic cavities. There are food particles present in the crop (arrow).

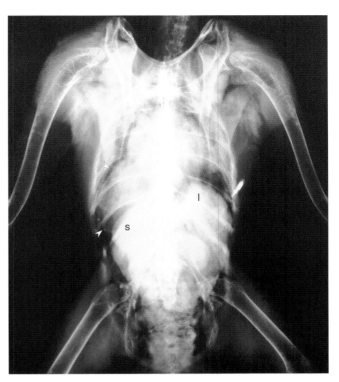

Fig. 3.108 Ventrodorsal survey radiograph of a saker falcon showing an enlarged liver (l) and spleen (s) and a large radiodense mass (arrows) along the right cardiohepatic waist. On post-mortem examination the mass was found to be an encapsulated aspergilloma. Histopathological examination revealed severe amyloid deposits in the liver.

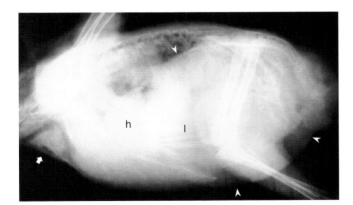

Fig. 3.107 Lateral survey radiograph of the same bird as in Fig. 3.106. A large soft-tissue shadow is present in the caudal celomic cavity (arrowheads) and the lungs and airsacs are massively compressed. Ascites associated with severe liver congestion is the result of increased portal venous hydrostatic pressure and decreased portal venous colloid osmotic pressure. The boundaries of the heart (h) and liver (l) shadows are not well defined. There are food particles present in the crop (arrow). Note the deformation of the caudal synsacrum.

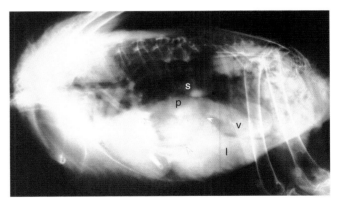

Fig. 3.109 Lateral survey radiograph of the same falcon as in Fig. 3.108. Arrows indicate the margins of the radiodense mass. The enlarged liver (l) caused the caudodorsal displacement of the ventriculus (v). The enlarged spleen (s) can be observed on the dorsal aspect of the proventriculus (p).

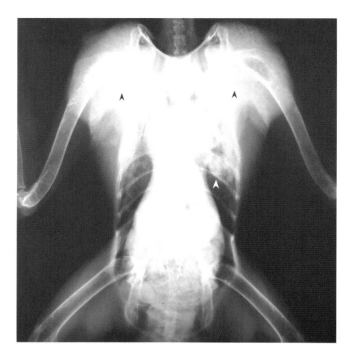

Fig. 3.110 Ventrodorsal survey radiograph of a saker/gyr hybrid falcon with aspergillosis that was presented because of poor flight performance and dyspnea. A large, focal radiodense mass can be observed along the left cardiohepatic margin (white arrow). There is a loss of air space in both clavicular airsacs (black arrows).

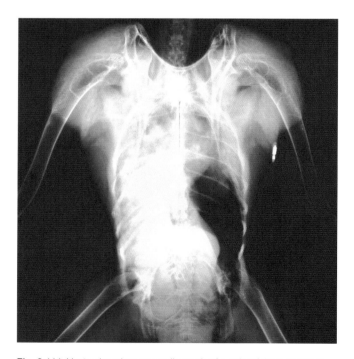

Fig. 3.111 Ventrodorsal survey radiograph of a saker falcon showing a severe, unilateral airsacculitis affecting the right thoracic and the abdominal airsacs.

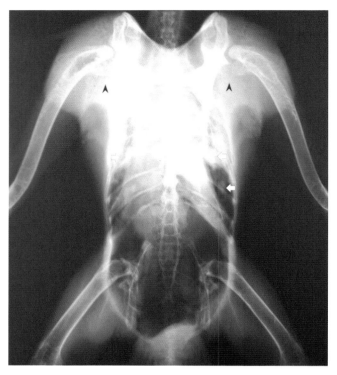

Fig. 3.112 Ventrodorsal survey radiograph of a gyrfalcon presented with a history of severe dyspnea, reduced appetite, poor flight performance and light green urates. The radiograph shows severe air trapping of the caudal thoracic and abdominal airsac field, probably due to mechanical obstruction of the ostia pulmonare. Multifocal radiodense masses are present in the thoracic airsac and lung field (arrows). The heart, liver and other organs cannot be differentiated and there is a loss of air space in both clavicular airsacs (arrowheads).

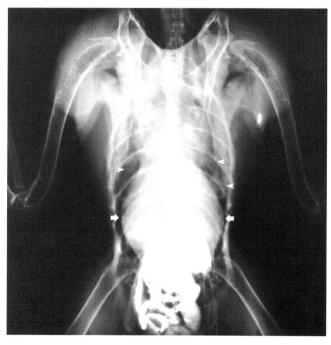

Fig. 3.113 Ventrodorsal gastrointestinal contrast radiograph of a saker falcon taken 3 h after barium sulfate was administered by stomach gavage. The liver (arrows) is massively enlarged and there are multifocal radiodense masses present in the thoracic airsac and lung field (arrowheads).

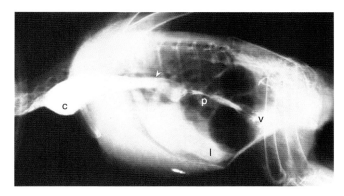

Fig. 3.114 Lateral gastrointestinal contrast radiograph of a saker/gyr hybrid falcon taken 15 min after barium sulfate administration. There is massive dilatation of the caudal thoracic and abdominal airsacs displacing the ventriculus (v) caudodorsally. c, crop; arrow, thoracic esophagus; p, proventriculus; l, liver.

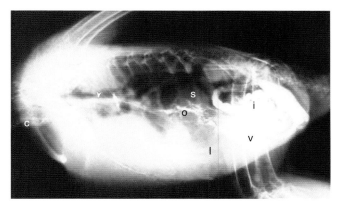

Fig. 3.115 Lateral gastrointestinal contrast radiograph of a saker falcon taken 90 min after barium sulfate administration. The massively enlarged liver (l) has displaced the ventriculus (v) and intestinal loops (i) caudodorsally. The spleen (s) is also enlarged. c, crop; arrow, thoracic esophagus; p, proventriculus.

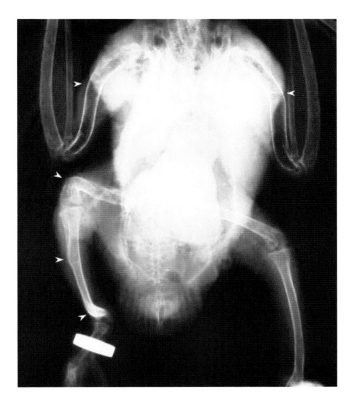

Fig. 3.116 Ventrodorsal radiograph of a 1-year-old vasa parrot (*Coracopsis vasa*). Deformity of the spine, bowing of most of the long bones (arrows) and pathological fracture on the right femur due to metabolic bone disease.

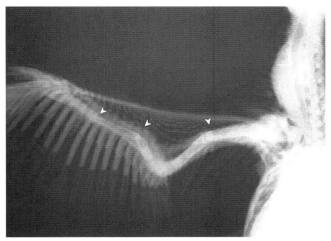

Fig. 3.117 Metabolic bone disease in a young Bonelli's eagle (*Hieraaetus fasciatus*) being reared on a meat-only diet. Bowing with pathological fractures of the humerus, radius and ulna. The overall bone density is decreased and the cortical outlines of the long bones are barely visible. (Courtesy of Dr. T. A. Bailey).

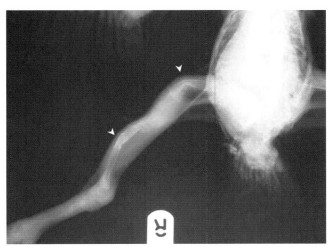

Fig. 3.118 The same bird as in Fig. 3.117. Bowing with pathological fractures of the femur and tibiotarsus. (Courtesy of Dr. T. A. Bailey).

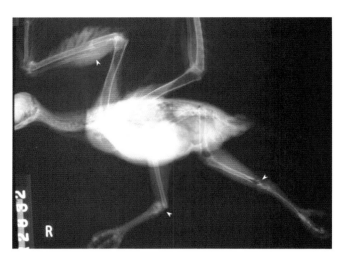

Fig. 3.119 Lateral radiograph of a common kestrel (*Falco tinnunculus*) showing a high energy, comminuted fracture of the right radius and ulna, and distal tibiotarsi (arrows). Note the soft tissue swelling around the fracture site on the wing.

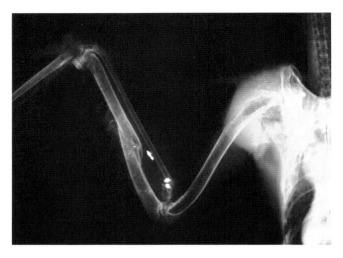

Fig. 3.120 Ventrodorsal radiograph of the wing of a lanner falcon (*Falco biarmicus*) showing lead fragments of different sizes embedded in the radius, ulna and shoulder region. Note the callus formation on the ulna and radius.

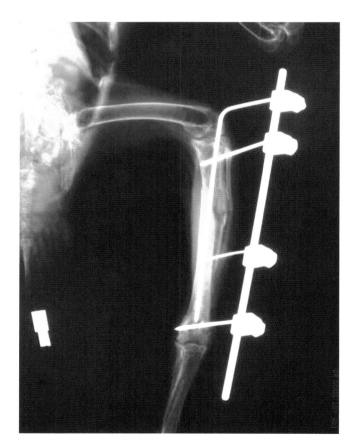

Fig. 3.121 This saker/gyr hybrid falcon was admitted with a high-energy, comminuted fracture of the proximal tibiotarsus. This is the most common type of fracture encountered in clinical practice with captive raptors. Fractures on this bone tend to occur in newly tethered birds and during training exercises. The fracture was repaired using an IM-ESF tie-in technique utilizing an IM pin inserted in a normograde fashion from the tibial crest, three positive-profile threaded pins placed in the proximal and distal fragments and tie-in using a bar and clamps.

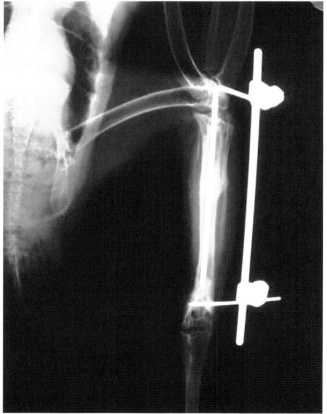

Fig. 3.122 A low-energy, transverse fracture of the proximal tibiotarsus in a Barbary falcon (*Falco pelegrinoides*). The fracture was repaired using an IM-ESF tie-in technique utilizing an IM pin inserted in a normograde fashion from the tibial crest and a single positive-profile threaded pin placed in the distal fragment and tie-in using a bar and clamps.

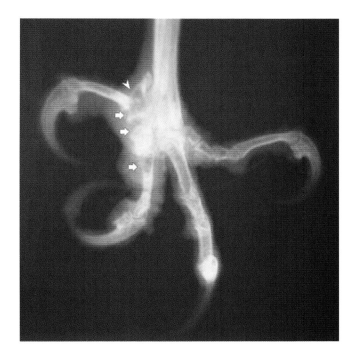

Fig. 3.123 Craniocaudal radiograph of the foot of a saker falcon with severe bumblefoot infection showing soft tissue swelling and marked osteolytic changes of the trochlea of the tarsometatarsus, first metatarsal bone (arrowhead) and proximal phalanges of digits I and II (arrows).

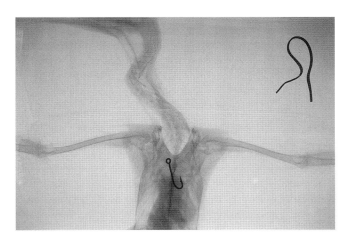

Fig. 3.125 A ventrodorsal view of a seagull with a fishing hook lodged in the proventriculus. The bird was presented with a piece of fishing line protruding through the mouth. The bird died immediately after the radiograph was obtained, probably as a result of severe weight loss, dehydration and septicemia.

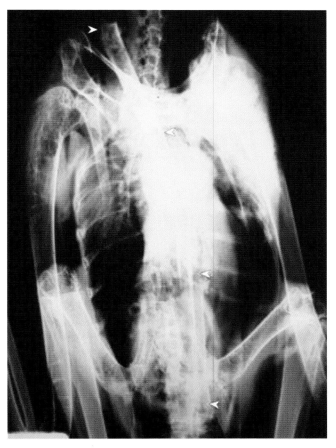

Fig. 3.124 A ventrodorsal survey radiograph of a short-toed snake-eagle (*Circaetus gallicus*). Note the presence of the entire limb of the prey (probably a long-legged wader), with the proximal femur occupying the thoracic inlet extending up to the caudal part of the thoracic esophagus. The tibiotarsus occupies the proventriculus and ventriculus. Then it folds at the intertarsal joint. The tarsometatarsus and the digits occupy the ventriculus, proventriculus and caudal part of the thoracic esophagus (arrows). (Courtesy of J. G. de la Fuente, A. L. Sánchez and the Faculty of Veterinary Medicine, León).

Krautwald-Junghanns ME, Trinkaus K (2000) Imaging techniques. In: Tully TN, Lawton MPC, Dorrestein GM (eds) *Avian Medicine*, pp. 52–73. Butterworth-Heinemann, Oxford.

Lennox AM, Crosta L (2005) The effects of isoflurane anaesthesia on gastrointestinal transit time. *Proceedings of the European Association of Avian Veterinarians*, Arles, pp. 207–210.

McMillan MC (1994) Imaging techniques. In: Ritchie BW, Harrison GJ, Harrison LR (eds) *Avian Medicine: Principles and Application*, pp. 246–326. Wingers Publishing, Lake Worth, FL.

Phalen DN, Hays HB, Filippich LJ *et al.* (1996) Heart failure in a macaw with atherosclerosis of the aorta and brachiocephalic arteries. *Journal of the American Veterinary Medical Association* **209**: 1435–1440.

Romagnano A (1997) Radiology. In: *Proceedings of the Association of Avian Veterinarians*, Reno, pp. 551–561.

Romagnano A, Love NE (2000) Imaging interpretation. In: Olsen GH, Orosz SE (eds) *Manual of Avian Medicine*, pp. 391–423. Mosby, St Louis.

Sherrill J, Ware LH, Lynch WE *et al.* (2001) Contrast radiography with positive-pressure insufflation in northern pintails (*Anas acuta*). *Journal of Avian Medicine and Surgery* **15**: 178–186.

Silverman S (1990) Basic avian radiology. *Proceedings of the Association of Avian Veterinarians*, Phoenix, pp. 334–338.

Smith BJ, Smith SA (1997) Radiology. In: Altman RB, Clubb SL, Dorrestein GM, Quesenberry K (eds) *Avian Medicine and Surgery*, pp. 170–199. WB Saunders, Philadelphia.

Tell L, Silverman S, Wisner E (2003) Imaging techniques for evaluating the head of birds, reptiles and small exotic mammals. *Exotic DVM* **5**(2):31–37.

Vink-Nooteboom M, Schoemaker NJ, Kik MJ *et al.* (1998) Clinical diagnosis of aneurysm of the right coronary artery in a white cockatoo (*Cacatua alba*). *Journal of Small Animal Practice* **39**: 533–537.

REFERENCES

Baumgartner R (1991) Radiology in birds. *Proceedings of the European Association of Avian Veterinarians*, Vienna, pp. 405–409.

Harcourt-Brown NH (1996) Radiology. In: Beynon PH, Forbes NA, Harcourt-Brown NH (eds) *Manual of Raptors, Pigeons and Waterfowl*, pp. 89–97. British Small Animal Veterinary Association, Cheltenham.

Harr KE, Kollias GV, Rendano V *et al.* (1997) A myelographic technique for avian species. *Veterinary Radiology Ultrasound* **38**: 187–192.

Korbel RT, Nell B, Redig PT *et al.* (2000) Video fluorescein angiography in the eyes of various raptors and mammals. *Proceedings of the Association of Avian Veterinarians*, August 30–September 1, Portland, Oregon, pp. 89–95.

Krautwald-Junghanns ME (1996) Avian radiology. In: Rosskopf W, Woerpel R (eds) *Diseases of Cage and Aviary Birds*, pp. 630–663. Williams & Wilkins, Baltimore.

FURTHER READING

Coles BH (1988) Radiographic examination. In: Price CJ (ed.) *Manual of Parrots, Budgerigars and other Psittacine Birds*, pp. 25–34. British Small Animal Veterinary Association, Cheltenham.

Douglas SW, Williamson HD (1980) *Principles of Veterinary Radiography*, 3rd edn, pp. 10–53. Baillière Tindall, London.

Krautwald ME, Tellhelm B, Hummel GH *et al.* (1992) *Atlas of Radiographic Anatomy and Diagnosis of Cage Birds.* Paul Parey, Berlin.

Rubel GA, Isenbugel E, Wolvekamp P (1991) *Atlas of Diagnostic Radiology of Exotic Pets.* WB Saunders, Philadelphia.

Silverman S (1990) Advanced avian radiographic interpretation. *Proceedings of the Association of Avian Veterinarians*, Phoenix, pp. 339–342.

Image-intensified fluoroscopy

Thomas A. Bailey, Antonio Di Somma, Celia G. Martinez

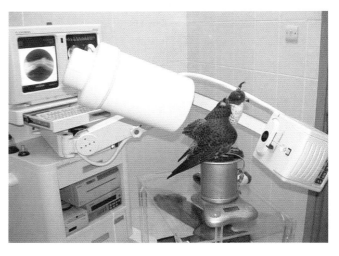

Fig. 3.126 Falcon with a dropped wing standing on a perch for fluoroscopy examination. Trained falcons that are hooded will quietly stand on a perch while fluoroscopy investigations are undertaken. Fluoroscopy is useful in the preliminary screening of cases without using anesthesia.

Fluoroscopy is a technique for continuous or intermittent X-ray monitoring. Fluoroscopy uses X-rays to produce real-time video images. After the X-rays pass through the patient, instead of using film they are captured by a device called an image intensifier and converted into light. This light is then captured by a TV camera and is displayed on a video monitor. The advantage of fluoroscopy over conventional radiography is that X-ray images may be viewed directly without taking and developing X-ray photographs. This allows 'real-time' observation of certain dynamic body processes, such as food moving through the digestive tract, and is also useful in certain surgical and diagnostic procedures. Additionally, examinations may be recorded on to videotape for review at a later stage.

In human medicine fluoroscopy is routinely used for intraoperative localization of patient anatomy and surgical instrument position. By providing this information, it facilitates improved accuracy and reduced surgical exposure for a wide variety of procedures. Fluoroscopy is especially useful for identifying the presence of restricted or blocked passages in the hollow organs of the body.

Fluoroscopy equipment

The fluoroscopy images that illustrate this section were taken with a Premier Mini-C-arm Imaging System (FluoroScan Imaging Systems Inc., USA) (Fig. 3.126). The FluoroScan Premier radiography system works at greatly reduced levels of radiation exposure and scatter, although lead aprons should always be worn by operators. The radiography beam of this system is tightly collimated and heavily filtered. It is designed to operate at a tube current of 0.1 mA or less. The FluoroScan system has a number of features that enable images of different qualities to be viewed by varying the number of video frames that are averaged (called noise suppression). The lowest noise suppression settings are desirable for cinematic viewing, which is important for motion studies. Higher suppression settings are required for high quality still images. Figure 3.127 shows the difference in quality between two noise suppression settings.

Trained falcons that are hooded will quietly stand on a perch while fluoroscopy investigations are undertaken (Fig. 3.126) while a Perspex table is used to perform fluoroscopy examinations on anesthetized birds (Fig. 3.128).

Fluoroscopy in birds

Although fluoroscopy is not widely used in avian medicine, owing to the cost of the units, it is considered to be an important way of monitoring the motility of the avian gastrointestinal tract (McMillan, 1994), in particular to screen and evaluate proventricular dilation disease in psittacines (Storm and Greenwood, 1993; Romagnano and Love, 2000). Specifically, it has been used in contrast studies of the psittacine gastrointestinal tract (Taylor *et al.*, 1999; Vink-Nooteboom *et al.*, 2003), locating string foreign bodies in a juvenile umbrella cockatoo (*Cacatua alba*) (Oglesbee and Sreinohrt, 2001), diagnosing megacloaca in a Moluccan cockatoo (*Cacatua moluccensis*) (Graham *et al.*, 2004), investigating proventricular obstruction in an eclectus parrot (*Eclectus roratus*) (De Voe *et al.*, 2003), and as a research tool to investigate the effects of metoclopramide on gastrointestinal tract motility in Hispaniolan parrots (*Amazona ventralis*) (Bowman, 2002). Fluoroscopy is also likely to be a useful technique

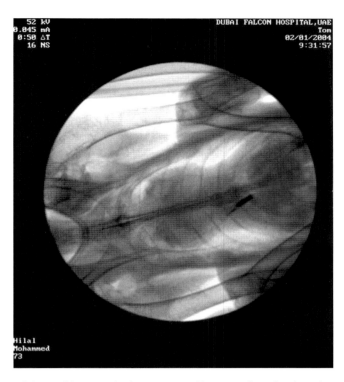

(a)

(b)

Figs 3.127 Falcon, anteroposterior projection. Hepatomegaly. In the sequence it is possible to see the improvement of image quality using the noise suppression feature. Note the grainy quality of the image with no noise suppression (a) and the improved quality using noise suppression (b).

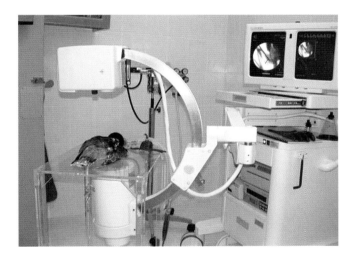

Fig. 3.128 A Perspex table may be used to perform fluoroscopy examinations on anesthetized birds.

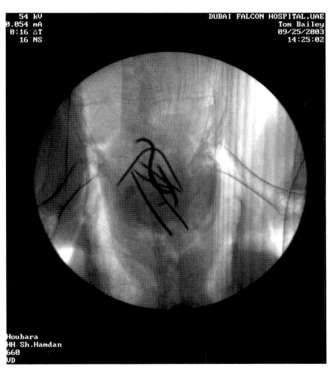

Fig. 3.129 Houbara bustard (*Chlamydotis undulata*), anteroposterior projection. Radio-opaque particles (wire) in the ventriculus.

in avian obstetrics, particularly in the investigation of dystocia and egg retention. In our hospital we have found fluoroscopy useful to screen birds for ventricular foreign bodies (Fig. 3.129) including lead pellets, hepatomegaly (Figs 3.127 and 3.130), esophageal granulomas (Fig. 3.131) and consolidated granulomas of the lower respiratory tract (Fig. 3.132). Fluoroscopy is also helpful in the workup of suspected fractures and has the advantage that the bird does not have to be restrained to make a preliminary diagnosis (Fig. 3.126). Intraoperative imaging

is useful during orthopedic surgery to assist in the realignment of fractures and placement of orthopedic implants (Figs 3.133–3.135), to monitor bone healing and to check the placement of intraosseous (IO) catheters

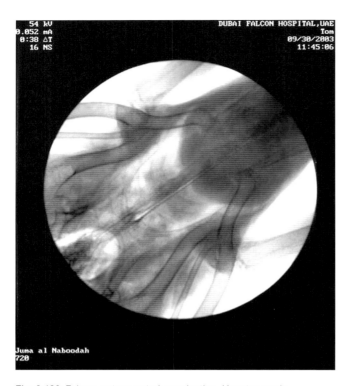

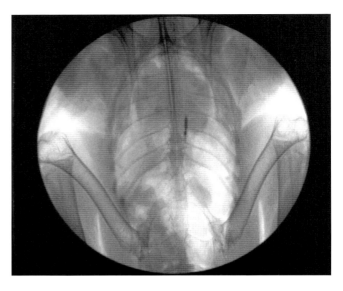

Fig. 3.132 Falcon, anteroposterior projection. Asymmetrical shadow over the airsacs, asymmetrical irregular area of increased density in the lungs. Aspergillosis.

Fig. 3.130 Falcon, anteroposterior projection. Hepatomegaly. Histopathology of liver biopsies confirmed amyloidosis.

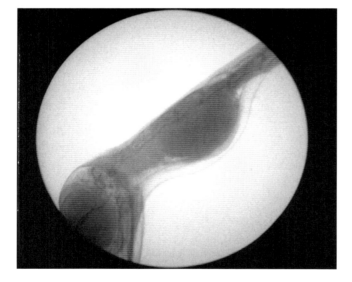

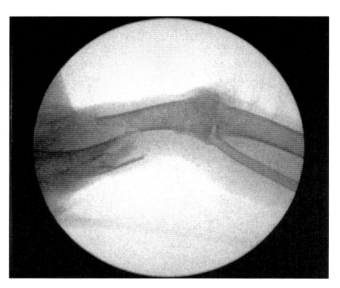

Fig. 3.133 Falcon, anteroposterior projection. Fractured humerus.

Fig. 3.131 Houbara bustard, lateral projection. Soft tissue radiodensities in the esophagus due to *Trichomonas* sp. infection.

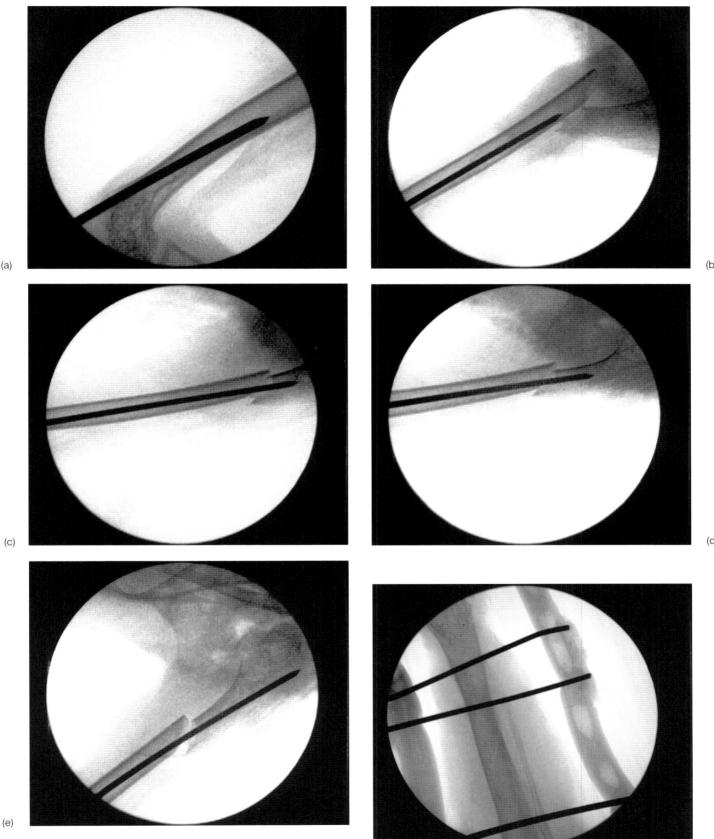

(a)

(b)

(c)

(d)

(e)

Fig. 3.134 (a–e) The use of fluoroscopy intraoperatively is useful for the placement of orthopedic implants during fracture repair. This sequence shows the placement of an intramedullary pin in the femur of a falcon.

Fig. 3.135 Falcon, anteroposterior projection. Repair of fractured tibiotarsus using type II external fixators.

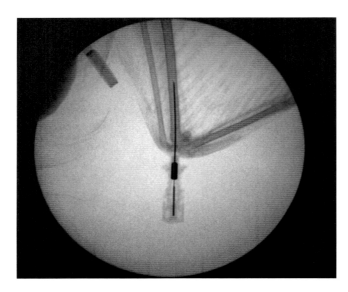

Fig. 3.136 Fluoroscopy provides a very rapid way of checking the placement of intraosseous catheters.

(Fig. 3.136). In our experience fluoroscopy does not provide sufficiently fine-resolution images for detecting early pathological changes in the lower respiratory tract.

Investigations of the avian gastrointestinal tract using fluoroscopy

Diseases involving the gastrointestinal tract are common in birds and indications for barium follow-through examination include: acute or chronic vomiting and diarrhea that is not responsive to treatment, abnormal survey radiographic findings suggestive of an obstructive pattern, unexplained organ displacement, loss of abdominal detail suggesting perforation, hemorrhagic diarrhea, a history of ingestion of foreign material and chronic unexplained weight lost (McMillan, 1994). Fluoroscopy images obtained at appropriate intervals give

information regarding transit time (e.g. delayed transit time in cases of foreign body obstruction) and video contrast fluoroscopy has been used to demonstrate abnormal gastrointestinal tract motility and uncoordinated gastric contractions in parrots with proventricular dilatation disease (Degernes *et al.*, 1999).

There is considerable species and individual variation in the barium transit time of the gastrointestinal tract in birds and it is important to be aware of normal times for a given species. Table 3.26 summarizes the times and location of the contrast media passing through the gastrointestinal tract of falcons, hawks and parrots. Figure 3.137 shows retention of barium in the ceca of a houbara bustard (*Chlamydotis undulata macqueenii*) 30 h after administration, a normal finding in this species. Fig. 3.138 shows barium in the gastrointestinal tract of a stone curlew (*Burhinus oedicnemus*), a species that is susceptible to gastric candidiasis. In contrast, delayed gastric transit time can be an indication of candidiasis in this species. The transit time depends on the species' diet, size and length of the digestive tract (Tully *et al.*, 2000). It is also influenced by numerous other factors, such as age, nutritional status, pathological conditions, stress and medications (McMillan, 1994). If the administration of the contrast medium is preceded by prolonged fasting, then its passage is initially accelerated down to the ventriculus, but there is an increased transit time through the rest of the gastrointestinal tract, prolonging the elimination of the contrast medium (Krautwald-Junghanns *et al.*, 1992).

Survey radiographs should always be taken before beginning contrast study (McMillan, 1994; Krautwald-Junghanns, 1996). This is of particular importance for the demonstration of radiodense heavy metal particles, since such particles could be disguised by the contrast agent (Krautwald-Junghanns *et al.*, 1992). Additionally, the patient's gastrointestinal tract should be empty before contrast administration, because food and fecal material can mimic or obscure lesions (Lennox *et al.*, 2000). Regurgitation of the contrast medium may occur in severely stressed birds, predisposing the patient to aspiration pneumonia. Because of the risk of aspiration, contrast study is contraindicated in comatose or laterally

TABLE 3.26 Comparative data of barium gastrointestinal tract transit times in falcons, hawks, and Amazon parrots

Time	Falcons	Hawks	Amazon parrots
0 min	Crop	Crop	Crop
1–3 min	Crop/stomach/intestines		
10 min		Crop/stomach	Crop
15 min	Crop/stomach/intestines	Stomach	Stomach
30 min	Crop/stomach/intestines/cloaca	Small intestine	Stomach
1 h	Stomach/intestines/cloaca	Large intestine	Small intestine
2 h	Intestines/cloaca	Cloaca	Large intestine
4 h	Intestines/cloaca	Cloaca	Cloaca
8 h	Cloaca	Empty	Empty

Martinez C. G. *et al.* (2007).

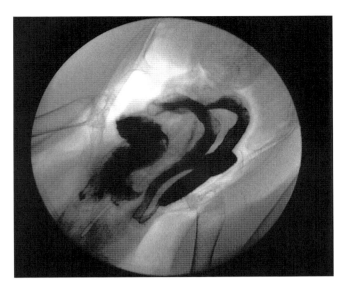

Fig. 3.137 Houbara bustard, ventrodorsal projection. Gastrointestinal contrast with barium sulfate, at 30 h. In the houbara bustard contrast media is retained in the ceca from 6–30 h onwards.

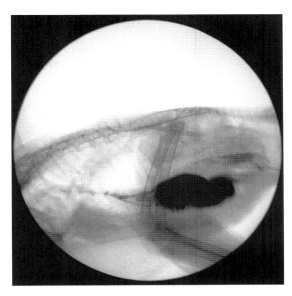

Fig. 3.138 Stone curlew (*Burhinus oedicnemus*), lateral projection. Gastrointestinal contrast with barium sulfate. Stone curlews are susceptible to gastric candidiasis and delayed gastric transit time can be an indication of candidiasis in this species.

recumbent birds and in those with respiratory depression (Smith and Smith, 1997). In our hospital falcons are fasted for 12 h before performing gastrointestinal tract contrast study fluoroscopy.

The dose of barium sulfate used varies depending on the species and presence or absence of a crop, and ranges from 0.025–0.05 ml/g bodyweight, with the lower dose range used in larger species. Lesions in the mucosa are best identified by using a higher dose, while a lower dose can be used if the intention is to simply identify borders of the gastrointestinal tract (Krautwald-Junghanns, 1996). If an inadequate dose is used the gastrointestinal tract will not be distended completely (Burk and Feeney, 1996). We use a dose of 25 ml/kg barium sulfate administered directly into the crop in falcons. The image sequence is 1–3 min after administration of contrast media followed by 15 min, 30 min, 1 h, 2 h, 4 h and 8 h intervals. Dorsoventral and lateral views should be taken to determine the exact location of the barium in the gastrointestinal tract. Manual restraint for radiography or fluoroscopy is very likely to decrease gastric motility, as the procedure produces at least some degree of excitement, fear and struggling (Lennox et al., 2000). Consequently, evaluation of gastrointestinal transit time is best accomplished in a nonanesthetized, nonrestrained bird using fluoroscopy, or 'standing' radiographs collected using a lateral beam on an adapted, perching bird. Falcons that we see in our hospital are trained for falconry and hooded birds such as these will quietly stand on a perch while fluoroscopy investigations are undertaken. This is a low stress technique, much easier to follow without needing anesthesia and with no risk

for the falcons. Other species that cannot be handled in this way can be examined in cardboard boxes or in small Perspex cages fitted with perches. Figure 3.139 show a sequence of images in a falcon before being given barium and after administration at 1–3 min, 15 min, 30 min, 1 h, 2 h, 4 h and 8 h.

In healthy falcons a quick initial passage of the contrast media to the ventriculus and intestines is generally observed. Slower passage of contrast medium from the crop to the ventriculus has been seen in healthy falcons that are stressed. Contractions of the crop are visualized and boluses of contrast medium passing through the esophagus towards the proventriculus are also easily identified. There appears to be a wide range of transit times even in healthy falcons and some normal birds can have a delayed emptying of the crop (Garcia-Martinez, personal communication). In other avian species stress affects the transit time of the media through the gastrointestinal tract. A slow or prolonged passage of contrast medium occurs in large seed-eating birds, young birds, obese birds and when the stomach is congested or distended with food, as well as in stressed and sedated or anesthetized birds (Krautwald et al., 1992; McMillan, 1994; Krautwald-Junghanns, 1996; Tully et al., 2000).

Certainly the most useful roles of fluoroscopy in avian medicine are in the investigation of gastrointestinal disorders and intraoperative imaging during orthopedic surgery. The reduction of patient stress, a result of the minimal handling needed and the speed of examination result in a more realistic interpretation structural and functional changes of the alimentary tract in disease. With experience, it should be possible to detect more

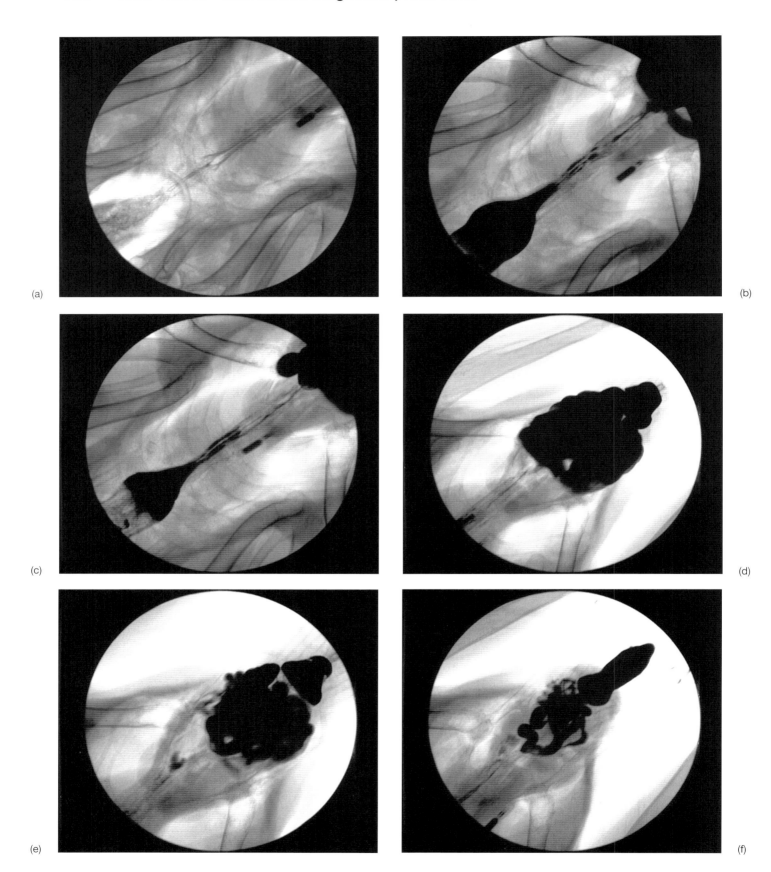

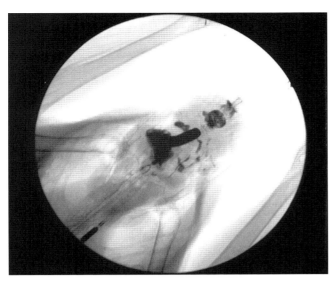

(g)

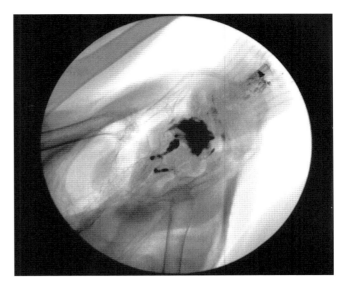

(h)

Figs. 3.139 Series of images before and after administration of barium: (a) before administration; (b) at 1–3 min; (c) at 15 min; (d) at 30 min; (e) 1 h; (f) 2 h; (g) 4 h; and (h) 8 h after administration in a falcon.

subtle changes in gastrointestinal tract function or to screen birds for early signs of wasting disease. The use of fluoroscopy in the placement of implants during orthopedic surgery allows procedures to be carried out rapidly and enables the surgeon to align fractures with great precision. In mammals fluoroscopy has been used in the diagnosis of cardiac disease and this is an area of avian medicine that may warrant further investigation.

REFERENCES

Bowman MR, Part JA, Ziegler LE, O'Brien R (2002) Effects of metoclopramide on the gastrointestinal tract motility of Hispaniolan parrots (*Amazona ventralis*). *Proceedings of the American Association of Zoo Veterinarians* **1**: 117–117.

Burk RL, Feeney DA (1996) *Small Animal Radiology and Ultrasonograph – a diagnostic atlas and test*, 2nd edn. WB Saunders, Philadelphia.

Degernes LA, Fisher PE, Diaz DE (1999) Gastrointestinal scintigraphy in psittacines. *Proceedings of the Association of Avian Veterinarians*, New Orleans, pp. 93–94.

De Voe R, Degernes L, Karli K (2003) Dysplastic koilin causing proventricular obstruction in an eclectus parrot (*Eclectus roratus*). *Journal of Avian Medicine and Surgery* **17**: 27–32.

Garcia-Martinez C, Bailey TA, Di Somma A (2007) Radiography and image-intensified fluoroscopy of barium passage through the gastrointestinal tract of falcons. *Proceedings of the European Association of Avian Veterinarians*, Zurich, pp. 508–511.

Graham JE, Tell LA, Lamm MG, Lowenstine LJ (2004) Megacloaca in a Moluccan cockatoo (*Cacatua moluccensis*). *Journal of Avian Medicine and Surgery* **18**: 41–49.

Krautwald ME, Tellhelm B, Hummel G et al. (1992) *Atlas of Radiographic Anatomy and Diagnosis of Cage Birds*. Paul Parey, Berlin.

Krautwald-Junghanns ME (1996) Avian radiology. In: Rosskopf WJ, Woerpel RW (ed.) *Diseases of Cage and Aviary Birds*, pp. 630–663. Williams & Wilkins, Baltimore.

Lennox AM, Crosta L, Buerkle M (2002) The effects of isoflurane anesthesia on gastrointestinal transit time. *Proceedings of the Association of Avian Veterinarians*, Monterey, pp. 53–55.

McMillan MC (1994) Imaging techniques. In: Ritchie BW, Harrison GJ, Harrison LF (eds) *Avian Medicine: Principles and Application*, pp. 246–326. Wingers Publishing, Lake Worth, FL.

Oglesbee B, Sreinohrt L (2001) Gastrointestinal string foreign bodies in a juvenile umbrella cockatoo. *Compendium Continuing Education for the Practicing Veterinarian* **23**: 946–946.

Romagnano A, Love NE (2000) Imaging interpretation. In: Olsen GH, Orosz SE (eds) *Manual of Avian Medicine*, pp. 419. Mosby, St Louis.

Smith BJ, Smith SA (1997) Radiology. In: Altman RB, Clubb SL, Dorrenstein GM, Quesenberry K (eds) *Avian Medicine and Surgery*, pp. 170–199. WB Saunders, Philadelphia.

Storm J, Greenwood AG (1993) Fluoroscopic investigation of the avian gastrointestinal tract. *Journal of Avian Medicine and Surgery* **7**: 192.

Taylor M, Dobson H, Hunter B et al. (1999) The functional diagnosis of avian gastrointestinal disease – an update. *Journal of Avian Medicine and Surgery* **20**: 85.

Tully TN, Lawton MPC, Dorrestein GM (2000) *Avian Medicine*. Butterworth Heinemann, Oxford.

Vink-Nooteboom M, Lumeij JT, Wolvekamp WT (2003) Radiography and image-intensified fluoroscopy of barium passage through the gastrointestinal tract in six healthy Amazon parrots (*Amazona aestiva*). *Veterinary Radiology and Ultrasound* **44**: 43–48.

FURTHER READING

Ivey E, Knox V (2002) Effects of metoclopramide on alimentary tract motility in psittacines birds. *Proceedings of the Association of Avian Veterinarians*, Monterey, pp. 57–59.

Ultrasonography

M.-E. Krautwald-Junghanns, M. Pees

Although there are limiting factors for the use of ultrasound in birds (the small size of the objects, limited coupling possibilities and anatomical peculiarities, above all the airsac system), due to the technical progress over the last years, ultrasonography in birds has become a valuable and important diagnostic tool. Today, various studies on the use of ultrasonography have been published covering the examination of the heart, the liver, the spleen as well as the gastrointestinal and urogenital system. There are still limitations in comparison to mammal medicine but, for some indications, especially the examination of the cardiovascular and the urogenital system, ultrasonography provides unique information. For some disease processes (e.g. pericardial effusion) it is even the only definite possibility for intra vitam diagnosis.

Whereas the sonographic presentation of the inner organs in healthy birds may sometimes be difficult, the situation in diseased birds is often completely different. Organ enlargements, displacement of the airsacs and fluid accumulations facilitate the coupling of the transducer and improve the image quality.

Technical equipment

The small size of the organs and – concerning echocardiography – high heart rates make special demands on the technical equipment and limit the use of older ultrasound devices in avian medicine.

The following requirements should be met when using ultrasound in birds:

- Electronic probes with small coupling surfaces (microcurved probes are preferable)
- Probes with examination frequencies of at least 7.5 MHz
- Internal hard disc for storage of images and motion loops, or the possibility to record on video tape.

The size of the probe is critical, especially in small birds. Best results are obtained using scanners developed for human pediatric medicine as well as for operative or gynecological use (Fig. 3.140). For small birds, a stand-off might be useful for the examination.

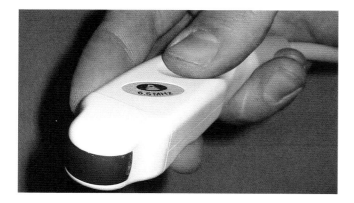

Fig. 3.140 A transducer for ultrasonographic examination in birds should have small coupling surfaces. This microcurved probe with a frequency of 7.5 MHz is ideal for the examination in birds up to a body mass of 1000 g.

For birds up to 1000 g body mass, a scanner frequency of 7.5 MHz is recommended for proper visualization of the cardiac structures. Higher frequencies may be beneficial but lead to a decrease in frame rate and maximum examination depth. Recording of digital motion loops or video sequences is recommended since the assessment and morphometry can be done after the examination without stress for the bird.

For echocardiographic examinations, the following points are important:

- A minimum of 100 frames per second
- A Doppler function (color and spectral Doppler)
- An electrocardiography (ECG-) trigger function.

The high frame rate is necessary to get images from defined cardiac stages as systole and diastole. In birds with heart rates up to 600 beats per minute, meaning 10 beats per second, a frame rate of 100 images/s provides 10 images per cardiac cycle. Although there is only limited experience with the use of Doppler in birds, ultrasound devices used for cardiology should provide both spectral Doppler and color Doppler function – these techniques will become more important in the future. The trigger function is useful to correlate cardiac images and measurements with certain stages of the ECG, therefore being able to identify the corresponding cardiac stage (end-diastolic and end-systolic).

Patient preparation, approaches and examination procedure

Since the filled gastrointestinal tract may disturb the penetration of the ultrasound waves and therefore the visualization of organs beyond the intestines (especially with the ventromedian approach, see below), birds should be fasted before examination. For psittacines, 2–4 h are recommended; pigeons should be fasted for 12 h and raptors up to 48 h.

In general, no anesthesia is necessary for the ultrasonographic examination. For the examination of the circulatory system, stress may be problematic for the interpretation of the results in awake birds, but on the other hand, anesthesia may also affect the heart rate and contractility. Therefore, for B-mode examinations, anesthesia is recommended only for stress-sensitive birds, but spectral Doppler examinations should be done under general anesthesia to reduce the influence of handling and fixation to the blood velocity.

The patient may be held by an assistant or by the owner either in dorsal or lateral (using the flank area) recumbency or in a standing position. In patients with clinical signs of cardiac disease or dyspnea, dorsal recumbency may cause severe circulatory problems and therefore should be avoided. Generally, it is advisable

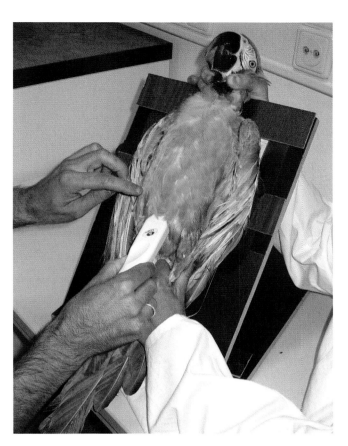

Fig. 3.141 Ventromedian approach, blue and gold macaw (*Ara ararauna*). The transducer is coupled in the median behind the sternum. A fixation device is used to hold the bird in an upright position.

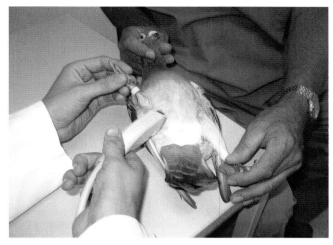

Fig. 3.142 Parasternal approach, pigeon (*Columba livia*). For this approach, the leg is pulled either backwards or forwards. It is only possible in birds with enough space between the last rib and the pubic bones.

to hold the bird as upright as possible. Fixation devices (Fig. 3.141) might be helpful.

Because of the anatomy of the avian patient, the possibilities of placing the transducer in contact with the skin are limited. Since intimate contact between the transducer and skin is necessary for optimal image quality, there are only two approaches suitable: the ventromedian approach behind the sternum and the parasternal approach behind the last rib. The ventromedian approach is the main approach. The transducer is coupled in the median directly behind the caudal end of the sternum (Fig. 3.141). The parasternal approach is usable in birds with sufficient space between the last rib and the pelvic bones, e.g. pigeons and some raptor species. The scanner is coupled on the right side of the bird, because on the left side the gizzard might disturb the penetration of the ultrasound waves. The leg is pulled either backwards or forwards and the probe has to be pressed slightly to the body wall to compress the underlying airsacs (Fig. 3.142).

Feathers impede the contact between scanner and skin and therefore reduce the image quality. Whether they have to be plucked or if it is sufficient to part them depends on the species. In pigeons, chickens and birds of prey, some feathers normally have to be plucked. In most psittacines on the other hand, separating the feathers is sufficient in most cases. For the ventromedian approach, in psittacines a featherless area behind the sternum (breeding spot) can be used. In waterfowl, plucking of the feathers should be done very carefully because they might lose their ability to swim. Finally, sufficient quantities of a commercially available water-soluble acoustic gel should be applied to ensure a good contact between transducer and skin. These gels are well tolerated and can be removed from feathers and skin easily.

In ultrasonographic diagnostics, assessment of the results is much more subjective and much more dependent on personal experience and personal examination technique than in radiography. Therefore, for the routine ultrasonographic evaluation, a fixed pattern for the examination should be used. A recommended method for the examination of the celomic cavity is to start with the evaluation of the liver followed by the heart, the gastrointestinal and finally the urogenital system.

With the ventromedian approach, the transducer is directed cranially to visualize the liver tissue (Fig. 3.143). After identifying the liver, the transducer is swept from lateral to medial, until the whole liver has been examined. If indicated ultrasound-guided liver biopsies may be taken.

For examination of the heart, the transducer is directed craniodorsally until the heart is identified – the liver works as an acoustic window. When the heart has been visualized, the transducer is swept laterally, to examine section by section. First the sagittal view (perpendicular to the sternum) is examined, afterwards the transducer is rotated 90° to have a second plane of view. Before

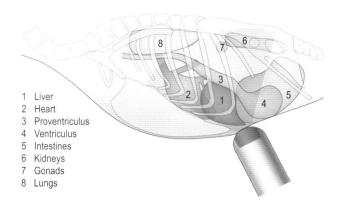

1 Liver
2 Heart
3 Proventriculus
4 Ventriculus
5 Intestines
6 Kidneys
7 Gonads
8 Lungs

Fig. 3.143 Ventromedian approach, schematic view. The homogenous tissue of the liver serves as an acoustic window to visualize the heart.

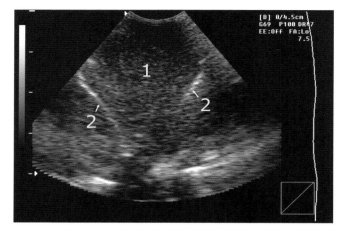

Fig. 3.144 Sonographic examination, ventromedian approach, African gray parrot (*Psittacus erithacus*), normal liver. The liver tissue (1) is delicately granulated and of average echogenicity. The borders between the liver lobes are visible as hyperechoic lines (2).

taking measurements, the probe has to be adjusted until the maximum extent of the ventricles is shown. With the parasternal approach, additional transverse sections of the heart can be obtained.

The transducer is swept to the left side to start the examination of the gastrointestinal tract. The gizzard is easy to identify due to its large muscles and its large content of grit stones in granivorous birds. The proventriculus can be seen occasionally on the right side; the small intestines can only be demonstrated clearly with high examination frequencies (at least 10 MHz). Furthermore the peristalsis of the small intestines can be recognized; the cloaca is seen in the caudal abdomen.

Finally the urogenital system lying behind the intestines is examined starting with the presentation of the kidneys. The kidneys should be scanned in a cross-section to identify the tissue (see below). After identification, the whole extent of the organ can be demonstrated in a longitudinal section. The presentability of the testes and the ovary depends on the status of sexual activity, immature and inactive gonads are normally not visible in the ultrasound image.

Organs and organ systems

Liver

The most frequent indication for the ultrasonographic examination of the liver is an enlargement of the hepatic silhouette in the radiographic examination. The ultrasonographic appearance of the liver parenchyma is of average echogenicity and coarsely granular, but with a uniform texture throughout (Fig. 3.144). The edges of the liver appear sharp but, since only parts of the liver can be assessed at the same time, measurements of the liver size

are difficult. Intrahepatic vessels are sometimes visible as anechoic channels. In birds with a gallbladder, this is a smooth, clearly defined, round or oval structure with thin walls and anechoic contents. It is located caudally to the right liver lobe.

In birds with liver disease, common alterations found in the ultrasonographic examination include:

- Enlarged (or reduced) size
- Irregular, swollen edges (Fig. 3.145)
- Decreased or increased echogenicity of the parenchyma or focal parenchymal lesions
- Dilated and/or congested liver vessels (Fig. 3.145)
- Liver cysts (sharply defined, anechoic mass with marked posterior acoustic enhancement)
- Fluid (e.g. ascites) in the celomic cavity (Fig. 3.145)

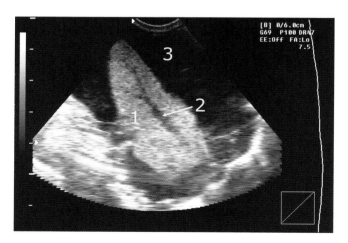

Fig. 3.145 Sonographic examination, ventromedian approach, African gray parrot. The liver (1) is swollen; dilated vessels (2) are visible and ascites (3) is present.

TABLE 3.27 2D echocardiography, important measured and calculated parameters in birds (mean ± SD)

Parameter	Ventromedian approach Psittacus erithacus erithacus (Pees et al., 2004)	Amazona spp. (Pees et al., 2004)	Cacatua spp. (Pees et al., 2004)	Diurnal raptors* (Boskovic et al., 1999)	Parasternal approach Pigeons (Schulz, 1995)
Body mass (g)	493±55	353±42	426±162	720±197	434±52
LEFT VENTRICLE					
Length systole (mm)	22.5±1.9	21.1±2.3	19.0±1.3	14.7±2.8	17.9±1.0
Length diastole (mm)	24.0±1.9	22.1±2.2	19.9±1.6	16.4±2.7	20.1±1.4
Width systole (mm)	6.8±1.0	6.7±1.2	6.4±1.7	6.3±1.1	5.2±0.4
Width diastole (mm)	8.6±1.0	8.4±1.0	8.3±1.5	7.7±1.2	7.4±0.6
Width fractional shortening (%)	22.6±4.4	22.8±4.2	25.6±7.0	Not given	27.2±4.5
RIGHT VENTRICLE					
Length systole (mm)	9.2±1.4	9.4±1.8	10.3±1.2	12.7±2.7	Not given
Length diastole (mm)	11.5±1.9	10.3±1.3	11.3±2.3	13.9±2.5	9.9±0.8
Width systole (mm)	2.8±0.9	3.1±0.7	2.3±0.0	2.1 ± 0.6	Not given
Width diastole (mm)	4.8±1.1	5.2±1.3	3.5±0.5	2.5±0.8	4.0±0.5
Width fractional shortening (%)	40.8±11.9	34.1±3.7	33.3±10.3	Not given	Not given
INTERVENTRICULAR SEPTUM					
Thickness systole (mm)	2.9±0.5	2.2±0.1	1.9±0.3	1.9±0.6	3.8±0.1
Thickness diastole (mm)	2.5±0.3	2.1±0.4	1.7±0.4	1.9±0.5	3.3±0.2

* Including Buteo buteo, Accipiter nisus, Accipiter gentilis, Milvus milvus.

Focal lesions are easy to identify, because they interrupt the uniform appearance of the liver parenchyma. Neoplastic alterations often appear as focal echogenic areas, whereas necroses often produce hypoechoic areas. The identification of diffuse parenchymal lesions (e.g. fatty liver alterations) is more difficult. Although the echogenicities of inflammation, neoplasia, calcification and granuloma are different, it is not possible to predict the histological nature of a lesion from the ultrasonographic appearance. Only tentative diagnoses are possible and biopsy is required for the definitive diagnosis. Ultrasound-guided biopsies may be taken easily from defined regions of the liver parenchyma according to the procedure in mammals.

Circulatory system

The great advantage of ultrasound in examining the avian heart is the presentation of the inner structures and therefore the possibility to assess both the morphological and the functional status. However, because of the anatomical peculiarities of the avian heart, the protocol (standardized views) recommended for echocardiography in mammals cannot be used in birds. M-mode, a valuable tool for assessment of wall thickness and contractility in mammals, is not useful in birds, since the avian heart is only visualized in longitudinal and semitransverse views. To date, B-mode (2D echocardiography) in birds

is an established examination technique and reference values have been reported for several species (Table 3.27). Also, Doppler echocardiography has been tested successfully in birds. Flow patterns could be shown in color mode and velocities could be measured in the areas of the atrioventricular openings and the aortic root. Systematic examinations and reference values using pulsed-wave spectral Doppler are available for some species whereas the use of color Doppler is only documented in some case reports.

The body mass and the external palpable sternal length are useful parameters to set the measurements in relation to the bird's size. An ECG should be derived to trigger the cardiac images to an end-systolic and end-diastolic stage.

B-mode (2D echocardiography)

Using two-dimensional (2D) echocardiography, the inner structures of the heart can be assessed subjectively and by taking measurements (Figs 3.146–3.148). The size of the ventricles, the wall thickness of the interventricular septum and the contractility of the ventricles are important parameters to evaluate the cardiac morphology and function. Additionally, the left atrioventricular (AV) valves, the aortic valves and the right muscular AV valve can be assessed depending on the image quality. Signs of congestion (hydropericardium, ascites and congestion of liver vessels) are easy to recognize.

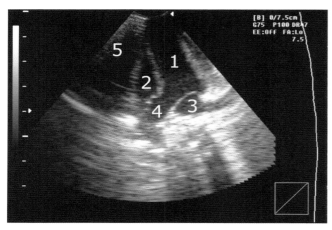

(a)

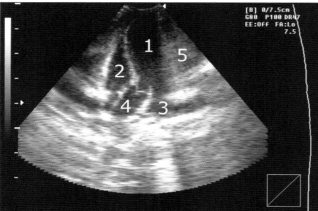

(b)

Fig. 3.146 Sonographic examination, ventromedian approach, European buzzard (*Buteo buteo*), normal heart. (a) systole, (b) diastole. The left (1) and right (2) ventricle as well as the left atrium (3) are visible. The valves of the aortic root (4) are closed during diastole, whereas during systole, the atrioventricular valves are closed. 5, liver tissue.

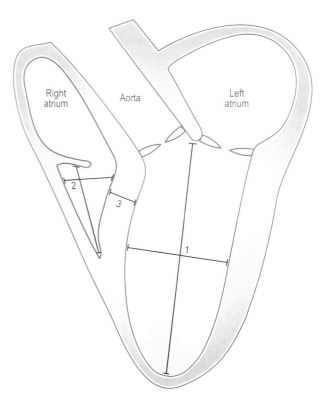

Fig. 3.147 Schematic view of the avian heart, horizontal view, measurement points. Reference values are given in Table 3.27 for the length and the width of the left ventricle (1), the right ventricle (2) and the interventricular septum (3).

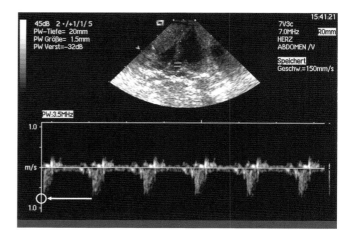

Fig. 3.148 Sonographic examination, ventromedian approach, spectral Doppler, carrion crow (*Corvus corone*), normal heart. Within the two-dimensional image, a gate shows the area for the spectral Doppler measurements. The velocity is shown against the time, in this case approx. 80 cm/s (yellow line).

Measurements are taken from the 2D image following the 'inner edge method'. Besides the size, the contractility (fractional shortening, FS) of the ventricles is of special importance. It is calculated using the formula FS [%] = (diastolic value − systolic value) × 100/diastolic value). Because of the sickle moon shape of the right ventricle in the avian heart, the contractility of this chamber is much higher than that of the left one.

Doppler echocardiography

Spectral Doppler is used for determining the velocity of the blood flow (inflow, outflow), which is displayed as a 2D graph against time (Fig. 3.148). Reference values are available for the diastolic inflow into the left and right ventricle and the systolic outflow into the aorta (Table 3.28).

Color Doppler shows the velocity of the blood flow in colors overlying the 2D image (Fig. 3.149). It can be used for positioning of the gate for spectral Doppler echocardiography but has also been reported to be useful in detecting valvular insufficiencies and aneurysms. Since the frame rate decreases considerably in most ultrasound devices when using color Doppler, its value is limited in avian echocardiography at present.

In birds with cardiovascular disease, common alterations found in the ultrasonographic examination include:

TABLE 3.28 Velocities of intracardial blood flow in some bird species (anesthetized)

Parameter	Amazona spp. (Pees et al., 2005)	Ara spp. (Carrani et al., 2003)	Cacatua galerita (Carrani et al., 2003)	Psittacus erithacus (Carrani et al., 2003)	Falco spp. (Straub et al., 2001)	Buteo buteo (Straub et al., 2001)
Diastolic inflow left ventricle (m/s)	0.18±0.03	0.54±0.07	0.32±0.15	0.39±0.06	0.21±0.03	0.14±0.01
Diastolic inflow right ventricle (m/s)	0.22±0.05	Not given	Not given	Not given	0.21±0.04	0.14±0.02
Systolic outflow aortic root (m/s)	0.83±0.08	0.81±0.16	0.78±0.19	0.89±0.13	0.95±0.07	1.18±0.05

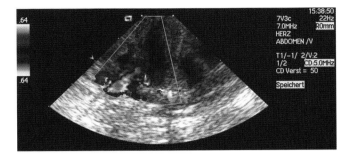

Fig. 3.149 Sonographic examination, color Doppler, ventromedian approach, carrion crow, normal heart. The outflow into the aorta is shown as blood flowing away from the transducer (blue).

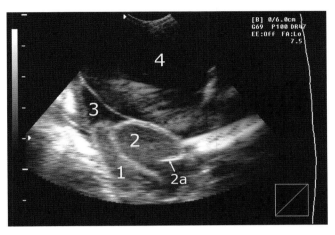

Fig. 3.150 Sonographic examination, ventromedian approach, African gray parrot, right-sided cardiac insufficiency. The right ventricle (2) is larger than the left ventricle (1), the muscular atrioventricular valve (2a) is thickened. Pericardial effusion (3) and ascites (4) are present.

- Arrhythmias
- Enlarged (or reduced-size) ventricles (Fig. 3.150)
- Increased or decreased thickness of the walls
- Increased or decreased contractility of the ventricles
- Alterations of the myocardium or the endocardium
- Alterations of the pericardium, including pericardial effusion (Figs 3.150, 3.151)
- Alterations of the valves (thickening, insufficiency) (Fig. 3.150)
- Increased or decreased cardiac blood flow velocities
- Ascites and liver congestion (Figs 3.150, 3.152).

The most frequent pathological echocardiographic findings are hydropericardium and hypertrophy/ dilatation of the right ventricle. Both alterations are often caused by right-sided congestive heart failure. In these cases, the right ventricle is often nearly as large as the left one; the walls are significantly thickened. In birds with hydropericardium, an anechoic area is visible between the heart and the pericardium. Increase in blood pressure in the large circulatory cycle often leads to liver congestion (dilated liver vessels visible) and to ascites. Hypertrophy of the right muscular AV valve is often associated with hypertrophy of the right ventricle. Alterations of the left ventricle are seen less frequently. They may be combined with thickened atrioventricular valves indicating valvular damage and insufficiency. Left-sided congestive heart failure is normally combined with right-sided alterations due to congestion in the small circulatory cycle.

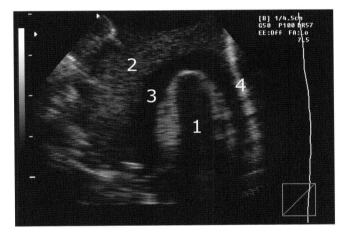

Fig. 3.151 Sonographic examination, ventromedian approach, African gray parrot, chlamydophiliosis. Pericardial effusion (3) is visible as anechoic area between the heart (1) and the liver (2). 4, sternum.

Gastrointestinal tract

The gizzard is easy to identify because of its large muscles and its large content of grit in granivorous birds. Because of the total reflexion, a typical acoustic shadowing can be seen behind the gizzard (Fig. 3.152). The proventriculus can be demonstrated when enlarged whereas the identification of the normal-sized organ is difficult. The

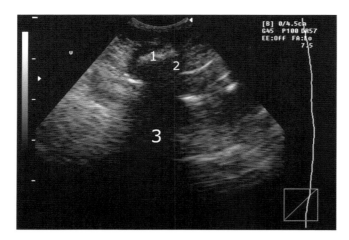

Fig. 3.152 Sonographic examination, ventromedian approach, monk parakeet (*Myiopsitta monachus*), normal gizzard. The content of the gizzard is hyperechoic (1), whereas the muscular wall is hypoechoic (2). Because of the total reflections of the grit, there are no structures visible beyond the gizzard (acoustic shadowing, 3).

intestines are assessable only with probes that have a frequency of at least 10 MHz. With these probes, the wall layers and the content can be demonstrated (Fig. 3.153). Peristalsis can be also recognized with lower frequencies. The cloaca is easily demonstrated in the caudal abdomen. A retrograde filling of the cloaca with fluid may help to assess the mucosa.

In birds with gastrointestinal disease, common alterations found in the ultrasonographic examination include:

● Increased or decreased peristalsis
● Enlarged or reduced size of the organs
● Increased wall thickness, e.g. due to inflammation.

Since there have still been no studies of the use of ultrasound for the examination of the gastrointestinal tract in diseased birds, assessment is based on the subjective experience of the examiner. Therefore, at present, the value of ultrasound for the examination of the gastrointestinal tract in birds is limited in comparison to other imaging techniques.

Urogenital system

Because of its anatomy, the reproductive tract in the avian species is not as easy to examine as in mammals. The gastrointestinal tract and the airsacs impede the examination. At the moment, sex determination with ultrasonography is only possible in female birds with large follicles or eggs present or in larger birds such as ratites with the use of intracloacal scanners.

In birds with urogenital tract disease, common changes found at ultrasonographic examination include:

● Organ enlargements, including signs of neoplastic alteration (necrotic areas) (Figs 3.154–3.157)
● Cystic alterations of the ovary and the kidneys (Fig. 3.156)
● Eggs without calcified shell (Fig. 3.158)
● Eggs with broken calcified shell
● Thickening of the oviduct (inflammatory processes) (Fig. 3.159)
● Inflammation products within the oviduct (laminated eggs) (Fig. 3.159).

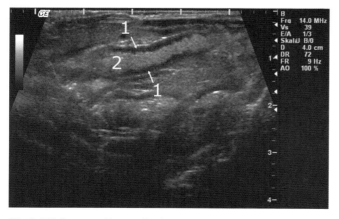

Fig. 3.153 Sonographic examination, ventromedian approach, channel-billed toucan (*Ramphastos vitellinus*), enteritis. Different layers of the thickened wall (1) are visible. 2, intestinal content. (Courtesy of I. Kiefer, Leipzig).

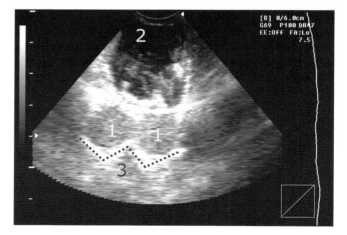

Fig. 3.154 Sonographic examination, ventromedian approach, African gray parrot (*Psittacus erithacus*), nephrosis due to toxicosis. The increased size of the kidneys (1) is visible, ascites (2) is present. 3, W-shaped reflection of the vertebral column and the pelvic bones.

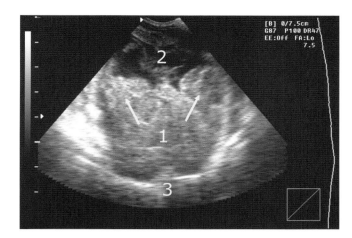

Fig. 3.155 Sonographic examination, ventromedian approach, yellow-crowned amazon (*Amazona ochrocephala*), kidney neoplasia. The kidney tissue (1) forms a solid mass of inhomogeneous echogenicity. Other organs are displaced (arrows); ascites (2) is present. 3, W-shaped reflexion of the vertebral column and the pelvic bones.

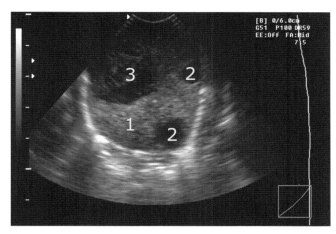

Fig. 3.156 Sonographic examination, ventromedian approach, little corella (*Cacatua sanguinea*), kidney cysts and kidney bleeding. The cysts (2) are visible as anechoic areas within the kidney tissue (1). The bleeding was demonstrated as an anechoic area containing movable hyperechoic structures (coagula).

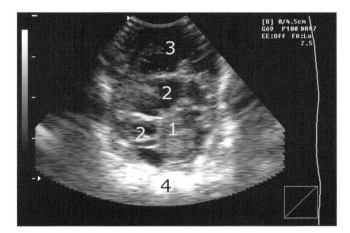

Fig. 3.157 Sonographic examination, ventromedian approach, budgerigar (*Melopsittacus undulatus*), testicular neoplasia. The neoplasia is presented as a solid mass (1) with several anechoic areas (2, necroses). 3, ascites; 4, reflection of the vertebral column.

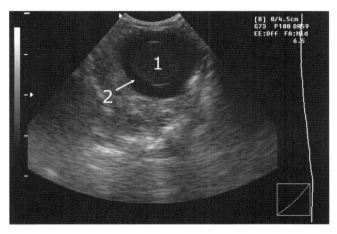

Fig. 3.158 Sonographic examination, ventromedian approach, peach-faced lovebird (*Agapornis roseicollis*), uncalcified egg. The yolk (1) is demonstrated as a central area of average echogenicity; the albumin (2) presents as an anechoic area around the yolk. This case is not a pathological alteration but a normal stage of egg development.

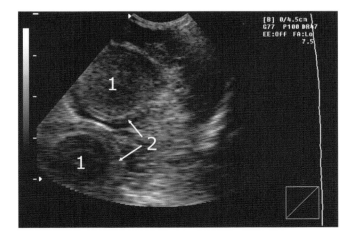

Fig. 3.159 Sonographic examination, ventromedian approach, African gray parrot, laminated egg. The wall of the oviduct (2) is thickened, the content (1) is demonstrated with alternating echogenicity ('onion-layers').

Kidneys

Sonographic demonstration of the normal kidney by transcutaneous ultrasonography is not possible in most cases. This is because of its position along the vertebral column, within the depressions of the pelvis and the surrounding abdominal airsacs. However, in cases of kidney enlargement, the airsacs are distended and it is possible to visualize the kidneys. Both the size and the parenchyma can be assessed without difficulty, not only in large birds but also in smaller ones (e.g. budgerigars). In cross-section (with the plane of the beam perpendicular to the spinal column), the kidneys are visualized lying in a W-shaped total reflexion caused by the pelvic/spinal bones (Figs 3.154, 3.155). In this view, the kidneys can be compared to one another. In this section view of the kidneys they appear as round to oval, and their size can be measured. By turning the transducer about 90°, the kidneys can be examined in their long axis (longitudinal to the spinal column). The echotexture of the enlarged inflamed kidneys is homogenous and rather anechoic, with no recognizable inner structure. Neoplasms are visible as voluminous and often rounded single masses, frequently with diffuse inhomogeneous echotexture and hypoechoic areas (Fig. 3.155). Cysts of the kidneys are easy to detect by means of ultrasound. They appear sonographically as clearly defined, rounded anechoic structures (Fig. 3.156), often with marked distal acoustic enhancement. If a differentiation between renal and ovarian cysts is not possible, an ultrasound-guided puncture of the fluid-filled cavities can be performed and the fluid can be examined.

Uric acid depositions and/or calcifications cause reflections (increased echogenicity); the renal tissue appears more inhomogeneous. However, diagnosis of renal gout by means of ultrasound is difficult: other techniques (radiology, endoscopy, blood chemistry, biopsy) should be taken into account before making a diagnosis.

Gonads

Sonographic demonstration of testes is only successful in the case of highly sexually active birds. The parenchyma of this organ shows a delicately granulated structure of average echogenicity. Neoplasia, inflammatory processes and other changes, in conjunction with enlargement of the organ, are observable sonographically. Neoplastic tissue is often presented as a rounded single mass that is demarcated from surrounding structures (Fig. 3.157). However, it is not possible to associate the masses definitely with the testes. Ultrasound-guided biopsy for histopathology is possible but difficult (risk of internal bleeding).

Ovary

Sonographic demonstration of the ovary is successful in most active hen birds with a bodyweight of more than 70 g. The picture of active ovaries is characterized by the presence of follicles of different sizes representing various stages of development. Developing follicles are first seen as round areas with an indistinct, anechoic or hypoechoic inner structure. In advanced stages of development the follicles exhibit the more echoic content of yolk. More distally in the oviduct, in the magnum, the ova exhibit a distinct separation between the echogenic yolk and a surrounding poorly echoic perimeter of albumin. The hyperechoic shell, added in the uterus, is easily recognizable.

Ovarian neoplasias are distinctly demonstrable by means of sonography. Accompanied by massive enlargement of the affected organ, the well defined structures appeared as large rounded masses of mixed echogenicity, seen as marked focal or diffuse inhomogeneous echo-

texture. Because of their massive extension, the origin of the tumors cannot be determined. Ovarial cysts appear sonographically as clearly defined, rounded anechoic compartments, showing the phenomenon of distal acoustic enhancement.

Oviduct

Irrespective of its functional state, the unchanged oviduct is often sonographically indistinguishable from the surrounding abdominal structures (intestines). The active oviduct can be distinguished because of the presence of eggs and the lack of contractility (in comparison to the intestines).

Advanced inflammatory processes of the oviduct are recognizable by increased thickness of the oviduct wall. If laminated eggs are present, their echogenicity depends on the kind of effusion. Mostly, laminated eggs are presented with changing hypo- and hyperechoic areas around a central point. This is due to the different densities of the deposited material, which gives the laminated egg the sonographic appearance of onion layers (Fig. 3.159).

Sometimes, cysts of the rudimentary right oviduct may be detected. They show the same sonographic picture as ovarian cysts. Abnormal eggs are detected most frequently in suspected cases of egg binding. Thin-shelled or noncalcified eggs (Fig. 3.159), malformed eggs and eggs with destroyed shells are sonographically assessable. Because of their high echogenicity, roughness of the eggshell cannot be demonstrated in most cases.

Other organs

Spleen

Because of the position of the spleen, the parasternal approach is preferable for the examination. Sonographic demonstration of the normal organ is not possible. In birds with splenomegaly it might be identified as a round or oval structure of average echogenicity. Differentiation between neoplastic and inflammatory changes is difficult.

Eye

Ultrasonography of the avian eye is useful for diagnosis of ocular changes, especially when direct visualization of the inner eye is not possible, for instance in cases of opacity of the lens. A-mode ultrasonography is mainly used for biometry of the eyeball. 2D B-mode ultrasonography supplies more information about ocular structures and pathological changes in the eye. After application of local anesthetic the transducer can be placed directly on the cornea. Acoustic gels are only required if the transducer is placed on the closed eyelids. The anterior chamber and the vitreous are physiologically free of echogenic structures. See Further reading for detailed information on ultrasonographic examination of the avian eye.

REFERENCES

Boskovic M, Krautwald-Junghanns ME, Failing K *et al.* (1999) Möglichkeiten und Grenzen echokardiographischer Untersuchungen bei Tag- und Nachtgreifvögeln (Accipitriformes, Falconiformes, Strigiformes). *Tierärztliche Praxis* **27**: 334–341.

Carrani F, Gelli D, Salvadori M *et al.* (2003) A preliminary echocardiographic initial approach to diastolic and systolic function in medium and large parrots. *Proceedings of the Association of Avian Veterinarians*, Tenerife, pp. 145–149.

Pees M, Straub J, Krautwald-Junghanns ME (2004) Echocardiographic examinations of 60 African grey parrots and 30 other psittacine birds. *Veterinary Record* **155**: 73–76.

Pees M, Straub J, Schumacher J *et al.* (2005) Pilotstudie zu echokardiographischen Untersuchungen mittels Farb- und pulsed-wave-Spektraldoppler an Blaukronenamazonen (*Amazona ventralis*) und Blaustirnamazonen (*Amazona a. aestiva*). *Deutsche Tierärztliche Wochenschrift* **112**: 39–43.

Schulz M (1995) Morphologische und funktionelle Messungen am Herzen von Brieftauben (*Columbia livia* forma domestica) mit Hilfe der Schnittbildechokardiographie. Doctoral thesis, Justus Liebig-Universität, Gießen.

Straub J, Pees M, Schumacher J, Krautwald-Junghanns ME (2001) Doppler-echocardiography in birds. *Proceedings of the Association of Avian Veterinarians*, Munich, pp. 92–94.

FURTHER READING

Enders F (1995) Beitrag zur sonographischen Diagnostik von Lebererkrankungen der Vögel unter besonderer Berücksichtigung röntgenologischer Befunde. Doctoral thesis, Justus Liebig-Universität, Gießen.

Gumpenberger M, Korbel RT (2001) Comparative aspects of diagnostic imaging in avian ophthalmology using ultrasonography and computed tomography. *Proceedings of the Association of Avian Veterinarians*, Munich, pp. 99–102.

Hofbauer H (1997) Beitrag zur transkutanen Ultraschalluntersuchung des aviären Urogenitaltraktes. Doctoral thesis, Justus Liebig-Universität, Gießen.

Krautwald-Junghanns ME, Schulz M, Hagner D *et al.* (1995) Transcoelomic two-dimensional echocardiography in the avian patient. *Journal of Avian Medicine and Surgery* **9**: 19–31.

Krautwald-Junghanns ME, Stahl A, Pees M *et al.* (2002) Sonographic investigations of the gastrointestinal tract of granivorous birds. *Veterinary Radiology and Ultrasound* **43**: 576–578.

Pees M, Straub J, Krautwald-Junghanns ME (2003) Echocardiographical examinations of healthy psittacine birds under special consideration of the African Gray parrot. *Proceedings of the Association of Avian Veterinarians*, Tenerife, pp. 161–167.

Riedel U (1991) Ultrasonography in birds. *Proceedings of the Association of Avian Veterinarians*, Vienna, pp. 190–198.

Advanced anatomical imaging

Paolo Zucca, Mauro Delogu, Fabio Cavalli

Any sufficiently advanced technology is indistinguishable from magic.

Arthur C. Clarke, Profiles of the Future

Advanced clinical imaging methods are one of the most important noninvasive diagnostic tools available in avian medicine. Although these play an important role in the care and management of the avian patient, only radiography and ultrasound are used on a regular basis in veterinary medicine. In fact, very few veterinary centers are equipped with computed tomography (CT) or magnetic resonance imaging (MRI) because of the high cost of purchasing and maintaining these units. Because of the scarcity of CT or MRI equipment in veterinary practice, there appears to be a lack of knowledge on standard image file formats associated with these advanced diagnostic units. The result of every clinical investigation with an advanced diagnostic device such as CT or MRI, or simpler ultrasound apparatus is a certain number of digital image files (see below). Digital imaging and communications in medicine (DICOM) imaging format is the standard in human medicine for storing and communicating such images and will also become the standard for veterinary medicine in the near future. Every veterinarian should know how to open and to get additional information from these images. However it is difficult to move directly from the use of classical (analog and film-based) radiography to the new diagnostic imaging tools (digital and filmless) without acquiring a basic knowledge of image manipulation (Zucca *et al.*, 2007a, 2007b). For this reason this short section focuses on DICOM and the other most commonly used image file formats, giving an iconographic overview of the different advanced diagnostic tools and their potential application in avian medicine, with special reference to CT and MRI.

The DICOM standard

The DICOM standard, originally created as a reference standard for digital imaging and communication in medicine by the American College of Radiology and the National Electrical Manufactures Association (NEMA), is maintained by several NEMA multidisciplinary DICOM standard committees. These committees exist to create and maintain international standards for the communication of biomedical, diagnostic and therapeutic information in those medical disciplines that use digital images and associated data (Bighood *et al.*, 1997; NEMA Strategic Document, 2004). One of the DICOM standards defines a file format for the distribution of images and people refer to image files that are compliant with part 10 of the DICOM standard as DICOM format files (NEMA PS 3–10, 2004). A DICOM image set is completely different from any other image file because it contains a header (which includes information about the patient's name, the examination data, who performed the examination, the diagnostic tools used, the type of scan, the image dimensions and the information related to the diagnostic procedure) as well as all the image data. These images cannot be seen if a DICOM viewer program is not installed on the computer. There are several good freeware programs on the Internet that allows you to open images, make three-dimensional representations, refer every set of DICOM images (see Downloads, links and further reading, below) and start using veterinary telemedicine and telereferring. For further details about the DICOM standard, see the NEMA Diagnostic Imaging and Therapy System Division homepage (http://medical. nema.org/). An interactive DVD for self-teaching of DICOM image manipulation in avian medicine has recently been developed (Zucca *et al.*, 2007a, 2007b).

Image file formats and their use in veterinary medicine

There are several file formats available for saving and transferring medical images. They seem quite similar but they are not. The use of one format or another can dramatically modify the quality of the images you store. Furthermore, almost every standard allows choice among different levels of compression. When you acquire or modify images for diagnostic purposes you should try to obtain the highest definition your system can support. The second step is to choose carefully the best image format for your purposes (Table 3.29). The Joint Photographic Experts Group (JPEG) format was conceived to reduce the file size of images as much as possible without visibly affecting their quality. It is the first-choice format for any photographic-like true-color image, including radiographs. This standard allows files to contain 16.7 million colors and it is one of the most commonly used formats for storing medical images and radiographs and posting on the Internet.

The Tagged Image File Format (TIFF) standard, on the other hand, is an uncompressed format. This means that it retains the highest level of information possible, but the files are very large. Several CT and MRI units have dedicated software that allows scans to be saved in DICOM format with a copy of the same files in JPEG or TIFF. If you do not have to post files via the Internet, TIFF guarantees you improved postacquisition processing. It is important to emphasize that this standard saves the whole image without any loss of information. The Portable Network Graphic (PNG) standard is a lossless compression format, which means that an image with many colors saved as a PNG image will not lose any quality when uncompressed. However, files are bigger in size than JPEGs. The Graphics Interchange Format (GIF) is almost never used in diagnostic imaging. It is more suited for web design or for exchanging low-resolution (usually 72–90 dpi) images via e-mail. Finally always remember that you cannot recover what is lost; i.e. if you save an image in the wrong format or at low definition you lose details and these details are lost forever, even if you subsequently save the image again at higher definition using a better format (Zucca *et al.*, 2007a, 2007b).

Avian medicine requires a good anatomical knowledge of the patient under treatment and this process takes a long time to acquire with the classic education methods such as dissection and standard radiographs (Zucca *et al.*, 2007a). An avian veterinarian has more than 10 000 species of birds as potential patients and their morphological and functional variability is greater than that among the different breeds of domestic animal. Furthermore, avian veterinarians sometimes treat rare or endangered species for which few anatomical and physiological data are available. The use of noninvasive investigative methods such as CT or MRI could represent an important contribution not only to the care of the single patient but also to avian conservation in the widest meaning of the term. A shareware CT and/or MRI scan database in a DICOM format of selected avian species could represent a great source of information for students interested in improving their knowledge in the avian medicine field and for colleagues working with rare, endangered or simply less well known avian species (Zucca *et al.*, 2007a). The daily use of advanced diagnostic units does not necessarily require a practice to own an expensive CT or MRI unit. The avian veterinarian could benefit greatly simply through real time consultation of a virtual anatomical atlas of the avian species under treatment, stored on a CD or on the practice's computer. After the 'DNA bank', avian veterinarians should start thinking of an 'avian image bank', which could represent an important contribution to the diagnostic procedures, education and conservation related to avian species.

Examples of avian advanced Imaging findings

These are illustrated in Figures 3.160–3.180.

Technical details

The ultrasound study in Figure 3.160 was made using a new-generation hand-held echography unit (My Lab 30, ESAOTE, Genoa, Italy). CT scans were obtained using a 16-slice CT unit (Aquilion 16, Toshiba Medical Systems, Japan) and 0.5 mm thick slices were made, with 5 mm table increments (pitch 1.4); images were reconstructed every 0.5 mm. 120 kV, 250 mA. All digital images (obtained in DICOM format) were stored and then processed with 3D imaging software (Vitrea2, Vital Image, Minnetonka, MI) on an independent workstation. Figure 3.167 (right) was produced using the Stack View package for CT/

Image format file	Size
JPEG (Joint Photographic Experts Group)	436 kb (at lower compression)
TIFF (Tagged Image File Format)	6.72 Mb
PNG (Portable Network Graphic)	4.74 Mb
GIF (Graphics Interchange Format)	1.26 Mb (256 colors)

TABLE 3.29 Differences in size of the same image (15×11.22 cm – definition at 300 dpi) in different image file formats

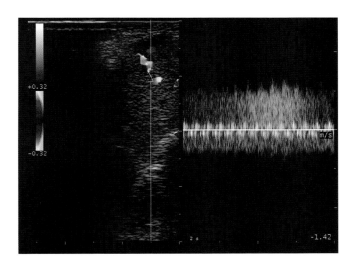

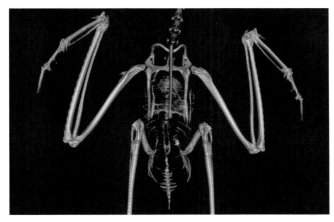

Fig. 3.160 Eurasian buzzard (*Buteo buteo*), adult, live specimen, echo Doppler of a hepatic vessel. The file has been exported in a DICOM format using a new-generation hand-held echography unit (My Lab 30, ESAOTE, Genoa, Italy). Modified with permission from Zucca *et al.* 2007a.

Fig. 3.162 Mediterranean herring gull, adult, live specimen, CT scan, 3D representation of the skeleton, detail of the wings, thorax and abdomen, ventral view.

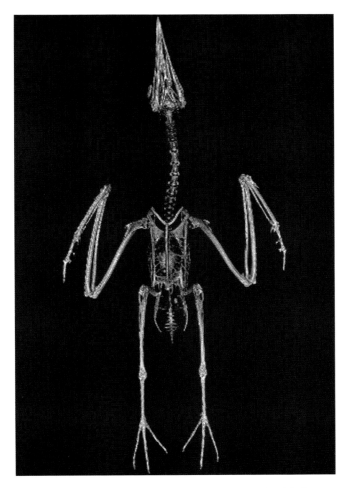

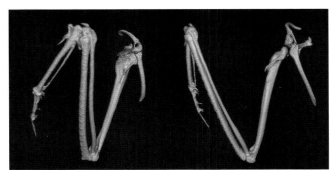

Fig. 3.163 Mediterranean herring gull, adult, live specimen, CT scan, 3D representations of the left thoracic girdle and wing, bony layer, lateral and dorsal view.

Fig. 3.161 Mediterranean herring gull (*Larus cachinnans*), adult, live specimen, CT scan, 3D representation of the full skeleton, ventral view.

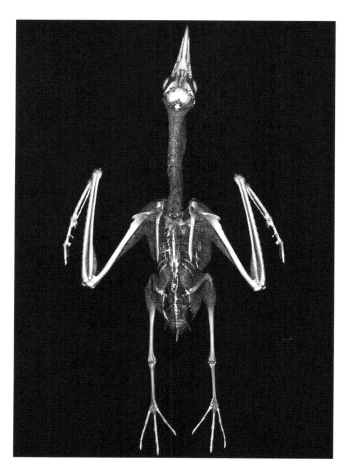

Fig. 3.164 Mediterranean herring gull, adult, live specimen, CT scan, 3D representation of the superficial muscular layer, dorsal view.

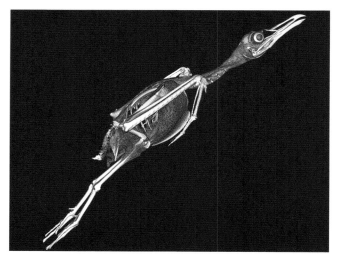

Fig. 3.165 Mediterranean herring gull, adult, live specimen, CT scan, 3D representation of the superficial muscular layer, right lateral view.

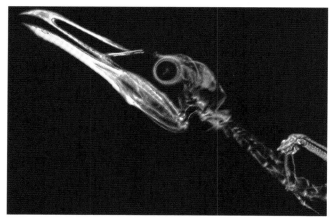

(a)

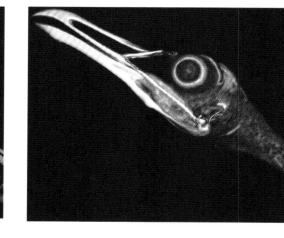

(b)

(c)

Fig. 3.166 (See overleaf)

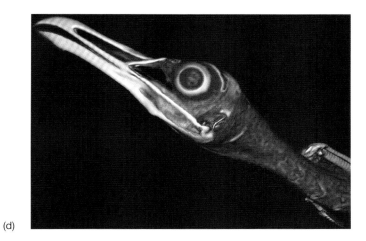

(d)

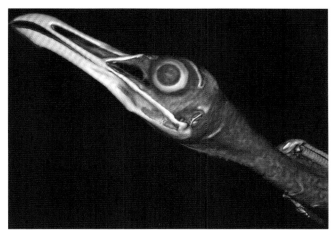

(e)

Fig. 3.166 Mediterranean herring gull, adult, CT scan, 3D representation of the head and neck. The set of images shows how, by changing the software settings to highlight different tissues and the air/threshold values for rendering, it is possible to move from the bony layer (a) to the external muscular layer (e), passing through the different tissues (b, c, d).

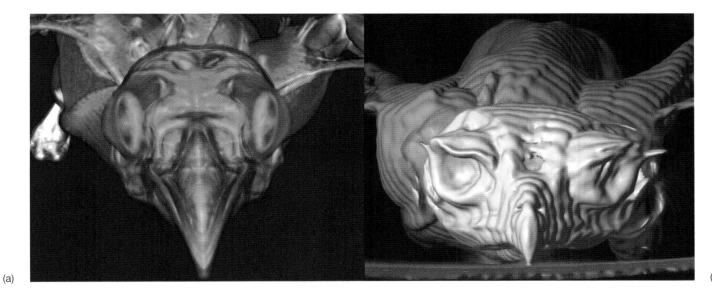

(a)

(b)

Fig. 3.167 (a) Hooded crow (*Corvus corone cornix*), adult, live specimen, CT scan, 3D representation of the head combining both image and shading values of bony and muscular layers for rendering, frontal view. (b) Tawny owl (*Strix aluco*), adult, dead specimen, CT scan, 3D surface representation of the head, frontal view. The two images were made from two studies with two different CT scan spiral units (16-slice vs 1 slice); the interslice thickness for the hooded crow was 0.5 mm while for the tawny owl it was 2 mm. Furthermore, the latest-generation digital imaging program used to make the 3D representation of the hooded crow, Vitrea 2, allowed a better definition during the 3D rendering process. In fact, the 'waves' of the tawny owl almost disappear in the image of the crow. In addition, the examination of a dead and a live specimen makes a significant difference to the image quality.

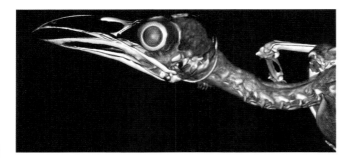

(a)

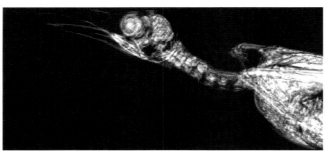

(b)

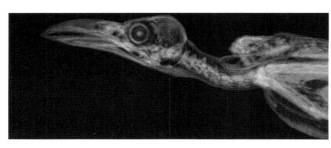

(c)

Fig. 3.168 Hooded crow, adult, live specimen, CT scan, 3D representation of the left side of the head. Changing the air/threshold and using different standard settings for different tissues available from the analytical software, it is possible to highlight different tissue layers of the same anatomical area. In (a), using a 'tissue/muscle' setting it is possible to distinguish the muscular tissue (yellow) from the brain and the eye, which are brownish. (b) was made using the 'vascular' setting and it is possible to appreciate the anatomical areas with higher vascularization, while (c) allows the external muscular structure to be visualized under the dermal layer.

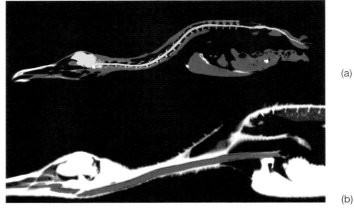

(a)

(b)

Fig. 3.169 Mediterranean herring gull, adult, live specimen, CT scan, 2D slices of the full body, sagittal view. (a) Anatomical study of the central nervous system. The brain and the spinal cord are highlighted in yellow. Note the two distinct enlargements of the spinal cord at the cervical and lumbosacral level. In flying birds, the cervical enlargement is greater than the lumbar (King and McLelland, 1984). (b) Same specimen, same view, anatomical study of the trachea highlighted in pink. The specialization of the avian forelimb greatly influences the length of the neck and consequently of the trachea. To compensate the increased resistance of air flow, birds show an increased tracheal radius (about ×1.3) compared to mammals (King and McLelland, 1984).

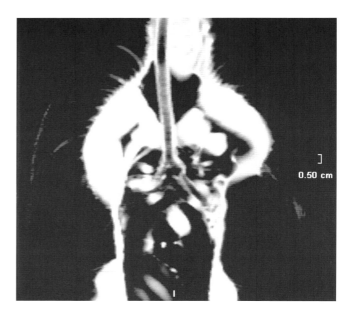

Fig. 3.170 Mediterranean herring gull, adult, live specimen, CT scan, 2D slices of the full body, axial view. Details of the trachea, the syringeal bulla, the primary bronchus and the lungs.

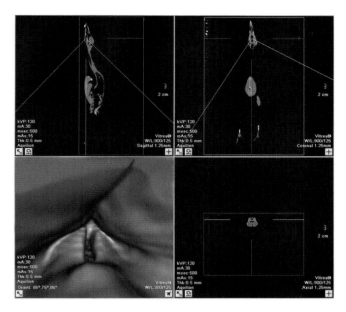

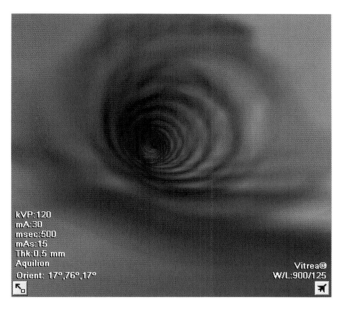

Fig. 3.171 Mediterranean herring gull, adult, live specimen, CT scan, 3D rendering of the internal organs and cavities – a virtual voyage inside the body. The three 2D views of the larynx, sagittal, axial and coronal and its 3D reconstruction. The yellow lines show the exact location and direction of the virtual larynx–oral cavity. The observer is positioned on the tongue facing the larynx.

Fig. 3.172 Mediterranean herring gull, adult, live specimen, CT scan, 3D rendering of the internal cavities – a virtual voyage inside the trachea, full screen. The observer is positioned at about half way along the trachea, heading towards the thoracic inlet.

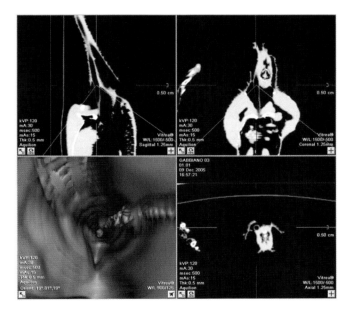

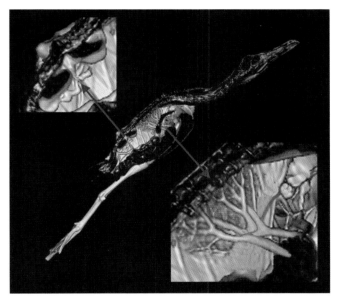

Fig. 3.173 Mediterranean herring gull, adult, live specimen, CT scan, 3D rendering of the internal cavities – a virtual voyage inside the trachea, as in Fig. 3.172 but at a lower tracheal level, about the thoracic inlet. The shadows of the bony structures and the internal organs are reflected on the internal walls of the trachea. It is possible to see part of the syrinx at the bottom of the 3D reconstruction. See also yellow lines for the exact location and direction of the observer's view.

Fig 3.174 Mediterranean herring gull, adult, live specimen, CT scan – a virtual voyage inside the body, 3D rendering of the celomic cavity. Sagittal section of the body and 3D reconstruction of the internal organs of the left side of the body. Top left, enlargement the left kidney (highlighted in green); bottom right, enlargement of the left lung with the primary and secondary bronchi and the parabronchi. On the right side of the box the left subclavian artery is visible.

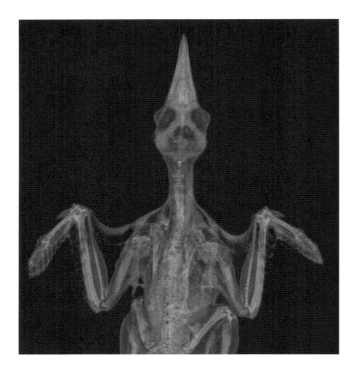

Fig. 3.175 Hooded crow, adult, live specimen, CT scan, 3D representation of the head, neck and forelimb, dorsal view. A proper balance among different parameters such as air/threshold, a reduced slice thickness and the combination of both image and shading values for rendering allows the finest details to be visualized, such as the patagium membranes.

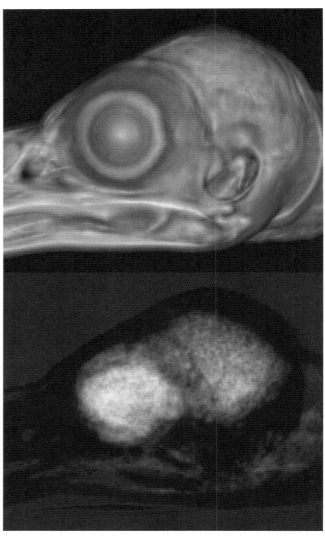

Fig. 3.177 Hooded crow, adult, live specimen, CT scan, 3D rendering, lateral view of the head, detail of the ocular area and the brain case. The two images are exactly the same: the only difference is the software settings, which are 'tissue/muscle' for the upper image and 'vascular' for the lower image, in which it is possible to appreciate the most highly vascular anatomical areas, represented by the brain and the eye.

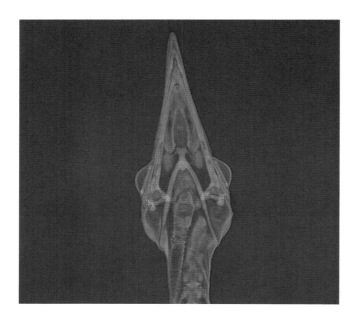

Fig. 3.176 Hooded crow, adult, live specimen, CT scan, 3D representation of the head and the neck, ventral view; software settings on 'tissue/muscle'. The quadrates and the hyoid bone are well defined and it is possible to see the tongue, the larynx, the trachea and the esophagus.

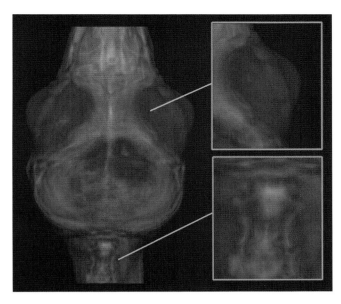

Fig. 3.178 Hooded crow, adult, live specimen, CT scan, 3D rendering of the head, dorsal view. The upper inset shows an enlargement of the scleral ossicles or scleral ring, while in the lower inset it is possible to clearly see the occipital area with the atlas and its articulation with the second cervical vertebrae. On either side are the epibranchial ends of the hyoid, which articulates with the occipital area of the brain case.

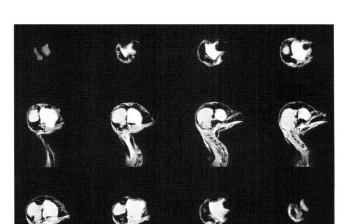

Fig. 3.180 Tawny owl, adult, dead specimen, MRI, sagittal view of the head, multislice presentation. The central nervous system appears in yellow, while the enormous ocular area is colored pale blue. Note the different orientation angle of the brain compared to that of the herring gull.

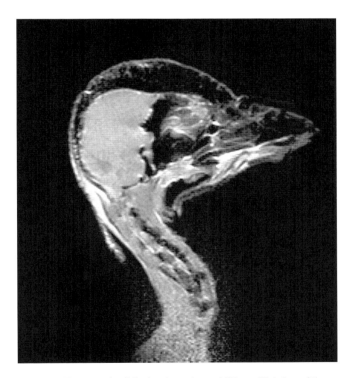

Fig 3.179 Tawny owl, adult, dead specimen, MRI, sagittal view of the head.

MRI images on an independent workstation (EasyVision Release 5.2 system of Philips Medical Systems, Philips, Einthoven, Netherlands). MRI scans were obtained using a 1.5 T unit (Intera, Philips, Einthoven, Netherlands) slice thickness 2.00, interslice gap 0.2, using spin-echo and gradient-echo sequences, while Figures 3.179 and 3.180 were made using a freeware DICOM imaging program (MRIcro).

Downloads, links and further reading

Applications and DICOM viewers–analyzers

- *Osiris* was developed by the Digital Imaging Unit (UIN) of the Service for Medical Computing (SIM) of the Radiology Department of the University Hospital of Geneva, Switzerland. Link at http://www.sim.hcuge.ch/osiris/01_Osiris_Presentation_EN.htm
- *Osirix* was developed by the Department of Radiology, David Geffen School of Medicine, University of California, Los Angeles, CA. This is an open source project image processing software dedicated to DICOM images produced by medical equipment and confocal microscopy. The software is developed in Objective-C on a Macintosh platform under the OS X operating system. Link at: http://www.osirix–viewer.com
- *ezDICOM* (Chris Rorden *et al.* – Windows) is designed to display most medical images: MRI, CT, radiographs and ultrasound. All versions of ezDICOM can automatically detect and open Analyze, DICOM, Genesis, Interfile, Magnetom, Somatom and NEMA images. Link at http://www.psychology.nottingham.ac.uk/staff/cr1/ezdicom.html
- MRIcro (Chris Rorden – Windows and Unix) can view Analyze, DICOM, ECAT, Genesis, Interfile, Magnetom, Somatom and NEMA images and

convert them to the popular Analyze format. Link at http://www.psychology.nottingham.ac.uk/staff/cr1/mricro.html

- Adobe Photoshop Plugin (public domain) for ACR/NEMA import (works with NIH Image also). Link at David A. Clunie web page: http://www.dclunie.com/dicom-plugin/
- DICOM Import Component for QuickTime (Escape). Link at: http://www.escape.gr/dicom/

Archive of DICOM images on the web

- Sébastien Barré has a nice archive of DICOM images (human medicine). Link at http://www.barre.nom.fr/medical/samples/index.html

Self-teaching tutorial for DICOM standard in avian medicine on DVD

- Zucca P, Delogu M, Pozzi-Mucelli R *et al.* (2007b) *The Bird of Prey Anatomical Project DVD*, see References.

Veterinary informatics

- AVI – Association for Veterinary informatics. Link at: http://www.avinformatics.org/index.htm

ACKNOWLEDGMENTS

We would like to thank Dr. Dino Scaravelli, Ichthyopathology and Aquaculture Centre, University of Bologna, Italy, for commenting on the manuscript.

REFERENCES

Bighood WD, Horii SC, Prior FW *et al.* (1997) Understanding and using DICOM, the Data Interchange Standard for Biomedical Imaging. *Journal of the American Medical Informatics Association* **4**: 199–212.

King AS, McLelland J (1984) Birds, their structure and function. Baillière Tindall, London.

NEMA Strategic Document (2004) Digital imaging and communications in medicine (DICOM), version 4.0. National Electrical Manufacturers Association, Rosslyn, VA.

NEMA PS 3–10 (2004) Digital imaging and communications in medicine (DICOM). Part 10: Media storage and file format for media interchange. National Electrical Manufacturers Association, Rosslyn, VA.

Zucca P, Pozzi-Mucelli R, Gelli D, Delogu M (2007a) Advanced clinical anatomy imaging. In: Samour JH, Naldo LJ (eds) *Atlas of Anatomy and Clinical Radiology of Birds of Prey: including advanced interactive anatomical imaging.* Elsevier, London, pp. 261–273.

Zucca P, Delogu M, Pozzi-Mucelli R, Cova M *et al.* (2007b) The Bird of Prey Anatomical Project DVD. In: Samour JH, Naldo LJ (eds) *Atlas of Anatomy and Clinical Radiology of Birds of Prey: including advanced interactive anatomical imaging.* Elsevier, London, (ISBN: 0702028029).

FURTHER READING

Bartels T, Krautwald-Junghanns ME, Portmann S *et al.* (2000) The use of conventional radiography and computer-assisted tomography as instruments for demonstration of gross pathological lesions in the cranium and cerebrum in the crested breed of the domestic duck (*Anas platyrhynchos*). *Avian Pathology* **29**: 101–108.

Fleming GJ, Lester NV, Stevenson R *et al.* (2003) High field strength (4.7 T) magnetic resonance imaging of hydrocephalus in an African grey parrot (*Psittacus erithacus*). *Veterinary Radiology and Ultrasound* **44**: 542–545.

Gumperberger M, Henninger W (2001) The use of computed tomography in avian and reptilian medicine. *Seminars in Avian and Exotic Pet Medicine* **10**: 174–180.

Gumpenberger M, Korbel R (2001) Ultrasonographic and computer tomographic examinations of the avian eye. *Proceedings European Association of Veterinary Diagnostic Imaging*, Paris, pp. 18–21.

Krautwald-Junghanns ME, Kostka VM, Dorsch B (1998) Comparative studies on the diagnostic value of conventional radiography and computed tomography in evaluating the heads of psittacine and raptorial birds. *Journal of Avian Medicine and Surgery* **12**: 149–157.

Krautwald-Junghanns ME, Schuhmacher F, Sohn HG (1998) Examination of the lower respiratory tract of Psittacines and Amazoniae varieties by means of reconstructed computer X-ray tomography. 1: Examination of healthy parrots. *Tierärztliche Praxis Ausgabe Kleintiere–Heimtiere* **26**: 61–70.

Orosz S, Toal R (1992) Tomographic anatomy of the golden eagle. *Journal of Zoo and Wildlife Medicine* **23**: 39–46.

Smith RD, Williams M (2000) Applications of informatics in veterinary medicine. *Bulletin of the Medical Library Association* **88**: 49–51.

Talbot RB (1991) Veterinary medical informatics. *Journal of the American Veterinary Medical Association* **199**: 52–57.

Van der Linden A, Verhoye M, Van Auderkerke J *et al.* (1998) Non-invasive in vivo anatomical studies of the oscine brain by high resolution MRI microscopy. *Journal of Neuroscience Methods* **81**: 45–52.

Endoscopy

Jaime Samour

Endoscopy (Greek: *endon* = within + *skopein* = to examine) is the direct visual inspection of any cavity of the body and organs using an endoscope (Table 3.30). Endoscopy was first used in avian medicine as a means of determining the sex of monomorphic species. One of the earliest reports concerning the use of an endoscope for sex determination in birds during the 1940s and 1950s was made by Dr W. M. P. Hauser in 1977. Dr Hauser, a physician from Tacoma, WA, was a devoted and passionate aviculturalist. On his farm he kept and bred cranes, waterfowl and gallinaceous birds. In this report, he described the technique of cloacal examination using a hand-held, battery-operated otoscope commonly used in human practice. During the late 1960s and 1970s, human otoscopes and proctoscopes were used by field biologists and zoologists for sex determination in penguins through cloacal examination (Ainley, 1970; Le Resche, 1971; Sladen, 1978). Bailey (1953) was probably the first to report the use of an otoscope inserted into the body through a small incision in order to determine sex and assess reproductive status. Subsequently, endoscopic examination of the gonads through a small laparotomy

TABLE 3.30 Common endoscopy applications in avian medicine

Application	Anatomical site
Otoscopy or auriscopy	External auditory canal
Rhinoscopy	Cranial sinuses
Pharyngoscopy	Oropharynx
Tracheoscopy	Trachea
Ingluvioscopy	Crop
Esophagoscopy	Esophagus
Gastroscopy	Proventriculus, ventriculus
Celoscopy/laparoscopy	Celomic cavity
Cloacoscopy	Cloaca

and the use of otoscopes became an established procedure in avian medicine (Risser, 1971; Ingram, 1977, 1978, 1980; Harlin, 1996). However, it was not until 1977 that the first report on sex determination in avian species using rigid endoscopes appeared in the literature (Satterfield and Altman, 1977). The technique was based on the use of endoscopes fitted with a rigid rod-lens system and the illumination was provided through a fiberoptic cable attached to a powerful light source. Nowadays, endoscopy is a very well established medical procedure in avian medicine as a diagnostic technique and for sex determination of monomorphic species (Bush, 1978, 1980; Bush et al., 1978; Harrison, 1978, 1986; Satterfield, 1980; Burr et al., 1981; McDonald, 1982, 1987, 1996; Jones et al., 1984; Kollias, 1988; Taylor, 1989, 1990, 1992, 1994; Samour, 1991).

Equipment and instrumentation

Hand-held battery-operated otoscopes and tubular endoscopes are still favored by many practitioners. These represent a more modest investment and offer the advantage that they can be used under field conditions. However, rod–lens endoscopy technology is far superior, providing a higher-resolution image, a wider angle of view and increased illumination. Moreover, high-quality still photography and video imaging are more viable propositions through rod–lens endoscopes, although this is also possible with some of the most sophisticated tubular endoscopes.

Great advances have been made in the past 15 years in the production of endoscopy equipment suitable for avian use. The choice of equipment is directly related to the different applications and the size of the avian patient. Table 3.31 lists equipment and instruments for avian endoscopy.

Clinical and surgical applications

Clinical examination

Indications for clinical endoscopy examination are given in Table 3.32. The different techniques for endoscopic examination of the avian patient are facilitated by the existence of airsacs, the cloaca and, in most species, a crop. Rigid endoscopes are ideal for examining the celomic cavity, the upper digestive and respiratory systems and the cloaca. Flexible endoscopes are also useful and offer several advantages over rigid endoscopes in the clinical examination of the upper digestive and respiratory tracts. For instance, the retrieval of foreign objects from the gizzard of birds such as penguins, waterfowl and birds of prey is greatly facilitated by using a flexible endoscope. Hand-held battery-operated otoscopes and tubular endoscopes are ideal for examination of the upper digestive and respiratory systems and the cloaca in the most common cage and aviary birds (Fig. 3.181). Proctoscopes or vaginoscopes, commonly used in human medicine, fitted with fiberoptic lighting are the instruments of choice for cloacal examination in penguins, waterfowl and ratites.

Surgical applications

There is a vast range of surgical procedures carried out in human medicine that use endoscopy techniques, thus minimizing trauma and recovery time. In avian medicine, the benefits of conducting surgery through endoscopes are just beginning to be explored. However, some advances have been made in recent years. The removal, with the aid of endoscopy, of *Serratospiculum seurati* adult filarial worms from the celomic cavity of falcons (Figs 3.182 and 3.183) is routinely practiced in falcon hospitals in the United Arab Emirates (Samour, 1996). Many avian practitioners treat lesions of aspergillosis, on the airsacs or the celomic cavity, topically using antifungal agents in addition to parenteral therapy (Figs 3.184 and 3.185). Subsequently, the lesions are removed through endoscopy (N. Forbes and K. Riddle, personal communication; J. Samour, unpublished data). Other conditions are illustrated in Figs 3.186–3.190.

Growing concern has been expressed in many countries around the world about the use of hybrid falcons in the sport of falconry. It has been suggested that a hybrid falcon could accidentally escape and cross-breed with free-living birds of closely related species. Hybrid falcons 75% gyr (*Falco rusticolus*) and 25% saker (*Falco cherrug*), and 50% peregrine (*Falco peregrinus*) and 50% gyr are among the most popular used in falconry. There have been several independently confirmed cases of cross-breeding between accidentally released hybrids and

Equipment	Specifications	Description
DIAGNOSIS AND EXAMINATION		
Rigid endoscope (selfoscope)	1.2, 1.7 mm outer diameter	67–114 mm working length; 0° and 30° angle of view
Rigid endoscope (needlescope, arthroscope)	1.9, 2.2, 2.5, 2.7, 3, 4, 5 mm outer diameter	170–190 mm working length; 0° and 30° angle of view
Flexible endoscope	1.6, 2.4, 3, 3.5, 5 mm outer diameter	200, 255, 365, 380, 450 mm working length; 0° angle of view; 0.6, 1.2, 2.2 mm working channel
Proctoscopes	12, 18, 21 mm outer diameter	100–120 mm working length
Fiberoptic cable	1800, 2300 mm length	1–3.5 mm fiber bundle diameter
Light source	Halogen or xenon high-intensity light; lamps 150, 250, 300, 400 W	Adjustable light intensity, standby lamp, endoflash
Second viewer or teaching attachment		Rigid or flexible attachment to allow viewing by second operator
PHOTOGRAPHY AND VIDEO IMAGING		
Still camera	35 mm SLR camera, automatic	Camera adaptor for rigid and flexible endoscopes
Video camera	Camera controller; PAL and NTSC color systems; lens 21–38 mm focal distance	Camera adaptor for rigid and flexible endoscopes
Color video monitor	9, 14, 20″ screen; resolution 450–700 lines	Full-size image, 4 or 16 split, thermo sublimations print system
Color video printer	S-VHS or Betacam SP video recorder	Video recorder
Biopsy and surgery		
Operating rigid endoscopes	2.7, 5, 10 mm diameter, straight, obliquely offset or right-angled eyepiece endoscopes	250–300 mm working length; 0° angle of view; 1.8–5 mm working channel
Rigid instruments	Biopsy forceps, grasping forceps, injector, scissors, needle holder, clamps	Conventional, bipolar
Flexible instruments	Biopsy forceps (fenestrated, ellipsoid, alligator), cytology brush, grasping forceps (basket, sharp-toothed), injector	Conventional
Irrigation and suction pump	Irrigation and suction tubes	Vacuum 65 kPa ±10%, pressure 200 kPa ±10%, aspiration capacity 3.5 l/m
Radiosurgery system	3.8 or 4.0 MHz dual radiofrequency unit, foot pedal, monopolar and bipolar leads	
Laser system	Diode and CO_2 units, 400 and 600 μm conical and flat-tipped diode laser fibers, semirigid CO_2 laser ceramic probes	
Cleaning and maintenance		
Automatic cleaning and disinfecting units		For rigid and flexible endoscopes
Automatic maintenance units		For flexible endoscopes
Trays	Disinfecting, sterilization, storage	For rigid endoscopes
Brushes	Cleaning	Working channels for rigid and flexible endoscopes

Endoscopy examination	Indication
Otoscopy or auriscopy	Ectoparasites, foreign bodies, infections
Rhinoscopy	Trichomonosis, candidiasis, other infections
Pharyngoscopy	Trichomonosis, candidiasis, general infections, foreign bodies
Tracheoscopy	Trichomonosis, aspergillosis, gapeworms, foreign bodies
Ingluvioscopy	Trichomonosis, foreign bodies, general infections, retained pellets (mostly birds of prey)
Esophagoscopy	Trichomonosis, foreign bodies
Gastroscopy	Foreign bodies, impactions
Celoscopy/laparoscopy	Sex determination, assessment of gonadal activity, monitoring of gonadal cycle, age determination, retrieval of *Serratospiculum* spp. filarial worms, diagnosis and treatment of *Aspergillus* spp. lesions, diagnosis of tuberculosis and neoplasm, surgery, biopsies, general clinical diagnosis
Cloacoscopy	Sex determination, impactions, uroliths, prolapse, infections

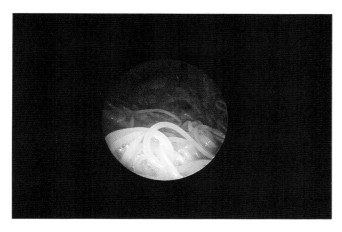

Fig. 3.181 Large number of *Serratospiculum seurati* filarial worms in the caudal thoracic airsac of a saker falcon (*Falco cherrug*).

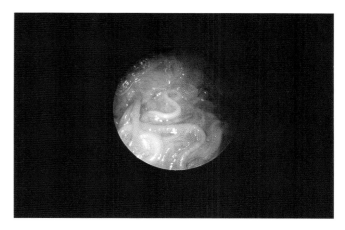

Fig. 3.182 *Serratospiculum seurati* filarial worms 7 days after treatment. Most of the worms are dead or decomposing. Note the yellow-green fluid surrounding the worms. Temporary airsacculitis may occur post-treatment as a direct result of the death of a large number of these filarial worms.

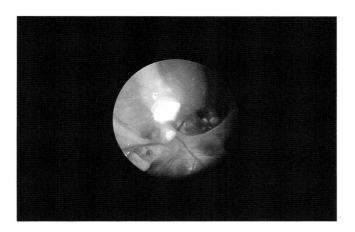

Fig. 3.183 Typical *Aspergillus fumigatus* plaques within the celomic cavity of a peregrine falcon (*Falco peregrinus*).

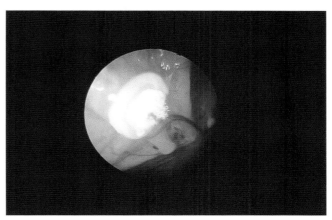

Fig. 3.184 Close-up of a sporulating plaque of *Aspergillus fumigatus*.

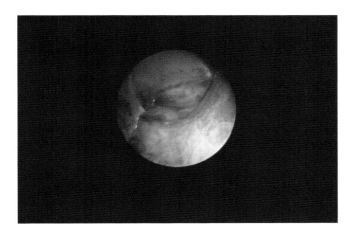

Fig. 3.185 Airsacculitis in a gyrfalcon (*Falco rusticolus*) associated with *Aspergillus flavus* infection.

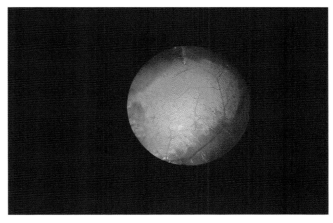

Fig. 3.186 Mild pneumonia in a saker falcon (*Falco cherrug*). Note the congestion at the ventral area of the lung.

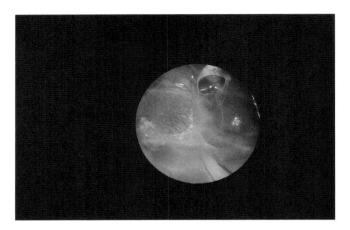

Fig. 3.187 Severe pneumonia in a peregrine falcon. Most of the lung shows extensive congestion.

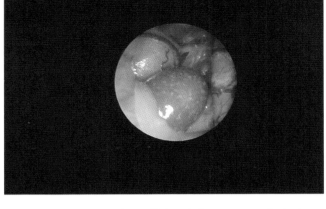

Fig. 3.188 An enlarged spleen with 'mottled' appearance of a houbara bustard (*Chlamydotis undulata*). Structural changes of the spleen have often been observed in clinically normal individuals of this species during routine endoscopy examinations. Part of an intestinal loop is visible above the spleen.

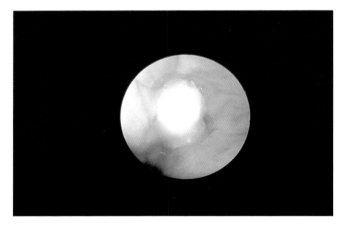

Fig. 3.189 Large caseous mass in the esophagus of a kori bustard (*Ardeotis kori*) produced by *Trichomonas gallinae*.

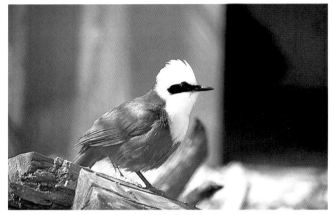

Fig. 3.190 One of the most important factors determining the success of avian captive breeding programs is the housing of 'true' pairs, since many species, such as this white-crested laughing thrush (*Garrulas leucolophus*), do not show sexual dimorphism.

free-living falcons in both North America and Europe. Vasectomy has been carried out in adult male domestic pigeons (*Columba livia*) using endoscopy techniques (J. Samour, unpublished data). This surgical procedure consisted of simply sectioning and removing a 10–20mm section of the *vas deferens* of adult, mature birds. In the adult bird, the identification and sectioning of the *vas deferens* is relatively easy, in particular during the breeding cycle. Great care has to be exercised during the manipulation of the surgical instruments (e.g. biopsy forceps) because of the close proximity of the vas deferens to the ureter and common iliac vein. Recently, a technique to vasectomize immature Japanese quails (*Coturnix coturnix japonica*) was described (Jones and Redig, 2003). The single-entry endoscopy-assisted technique consisted in sectioning the *vas deferens* at its proximal end as it leaves the epididymis, where there is no close association with the ureter, using a biopsy forceps. The *vas deferens* was then gently separated from the ureter by pulling carefully and completely

sectioned in the middle by gentle traction. Surgical techniques to sterilize male and female birds through celiotomy have been previously described by Bennett (1993) and Heidenreich (1997). Endoscopy-guided surgical procedures to sterilize male (Jones and Redig, 2003) and female birds have also been described (Pye *et al.*, 2001a, 2001b; Lierz, 2004; Hernandez-Divers, 2005; Lierz and Hafez, 2005). It is now possible, for instance, to perform a salpingohysterectomy or a vasectomy in birds using one-, two- or three-point entry. A single-entry technique involves the use of an endoscope, commonly a 2.7mm telescope, inserted through an operating sheath. When the *vas deferens* has been detected, a flexible biopsy forceps is then introduced through the port of the sheath and directed towards the surgical site. With this technique, the surgeon holds the sheath and endoscope with one hand while manipulating the forceps with the other one. Using the two-point entry technique, the operator holds the endoscope with one hand while manipulating the electrosurgical unit or surgical instruments with the other one at a different entry point. Using the three-point surgical entry technique, the endoscope can be placed on a sand bag or handled by an assistant while the operator manipulates the surgical instruments and the electrosurgical unit (Lierz, 2004; Hernandez-Divers, 2005; Lierz and Hafez, 2005), which have been inserted via different surgical sites. Endoscopes can also be held in position using a custom-made or commercially available angle-poise device.

Experimental trials have been carried out recently sterilizing male birds through endoscopy-assisted injections directly into the testes using zinc gluconate neutralized by arginine (Wilson *et al.*, 2004). Two different doses, a high and a lower, were tried in this study. The authors found undesirable effects, including mortality, associated with the high dose. The lower dose did not produce any undesirable effects but there was histological evidence suggesting the retention of reproductive ability (Wilson *et al.*, 2004). There is an obvious need for further research with this and other novel chemical products that may become available in the future.

One of the most popular surgical applications using an endoscope is endoscopy-guided collection of biopsies (Taylor, 1994; McDonald, 1996). A novel endoscopy-assisted testicular biopsy technique was recently described in Psittaciformes as a means of assessing fertility (Crosta *et al.*, 2002). A similar endoscopy-assisted testicular biopsy technique involving aspiration and cytology to assess the reproductive status in male swift parrots (*Lathamus discolor*) has also been described (Gartrell, 2002). Both techniques may prove useful for establishing the reproductive potential of individuals in captive breeding programs. The indications and different techniques for the collection of biopsies are covered earlier in this chapter.

Other endoscopic surgical techniques in the avian patient include the removal of tracheal foreign bodies (Clayton and Ritzman, 2005) and *in situ* suction of impacted and removal of soft-shelled eggs within the oviduct (Crosta and Timossi, 2005).

Sex determination of monomorphic species

Celoscopy (laparoscopy) for sex determination

The preoperative considerations for celoscopy in the avian patient are similar to those for general surgery. A full clinical examination is essential, in addition to information relating to age, diet, housing and general management. Old and obese birds improperly housed and fed on inadequate diets are high anesthetic risks and individuals from the Falconiformes and Psittaciformes are particularly so. Figures 3.191–3.198 indicate some of the difficulties in avian sex determination.

The selection of anesthetic technique varies according to the species and the circumstances confronting the avian practitioner. Injectable anesthetic agents have been successfully used in over 10 000 endoscopy examinations in over 350 different avian species (Jones *et al.*, 1984; J. Samour, unpublished data). The anesthetics and anesthetic combinations used include ketamine hydrochloride, ketamine hydrochloride in combination with xylazine hydrochloride, and alphaxalone-alphadolone. This last has been the anesthetic of choice for

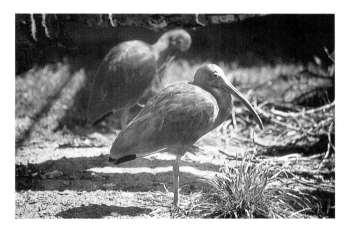

Fig. 3.191 Many species such as ibises and flamingoes are kept in bird gardens or zoological collections in flocks. In a small or large flock, it is also essential to maintain an adequate sex ratio to ensure breeding success.

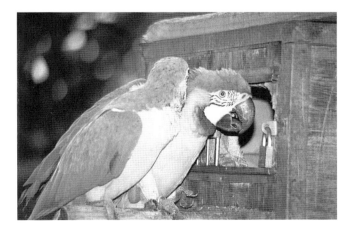

Fig. 3.192 Traditionally, many species in captivity have been sexed by observing behavioral patterns between individuals such as grooming and feeding. In the case of a 'true' pair, the male will usually groom and feed the female. However, if the 'pair' is formed by individuals of the same sex one individual will very often assume the dominant role, giving a wrong impression. (Courtesy of Mr. P. McKinney).

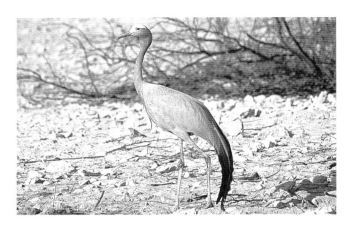

Fig. 3.193 Cranes have an elaborate courtship display that includes a ritual dance accompanied by a series of calls. This intrinsic behavioral pattern has been used to pair cranes in captivity. On many occasions this method for sexing cranes has proved wrong. The housing of two individuals of the same sex can induce one of the individuals to assume the dominant role. The male Stanley crane (*Anthropoides paradisea*) shown in this illustration was housed together with another, much smaller male. They were both seen attempting copulation, nest building and even sitting on the nest to incubate. Three weeks after the 'failed incubation period' the keeping staff inspected the nest and found one toy soldier, two paper wrappings and one stone. The 'pair' of cranes had been sexed 3 years previously using the size of the birds and their courtship display.

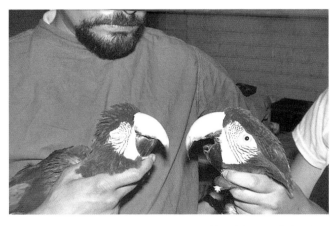

Fig. 3.195 Two adult red and green macaws (*Ara chloroptera*) showing significant difference in size. Using traditional criteria, the smaller bird could be a female while the larger individual could be the male. They were surgically sexed after spending 3 unfruitful years together. They were found to be both females.

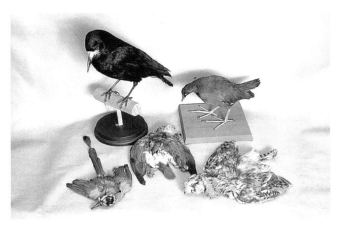

Fig. 3.194 A significant amount of the published information on sexual dimorphism in birds, including plumage appearance, weights and measurements, is based on data from skins and preserved specimens in museum collections. Some of this data may have come from a surprisingly small amount of reference material.

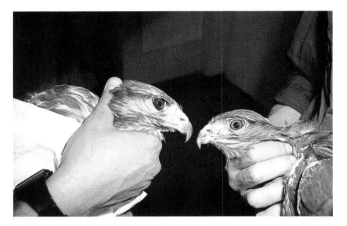

Fig. 3.196 The two common buzzards (*Buteo buteo*) illustrated in the photograph appear to be of different sexes. Note the differences in size and eye coloration. When surgically sexed both individuals were found to be females despite the fact that there was a difference of more than 800 g between them.

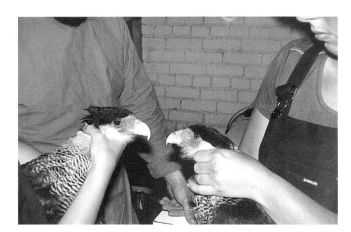

Fig. 3.197 The two common caracaras (*Polyborus plancus*) in the photograph had been housed together for more than 8 years. Surgical sexing showed that both individuals were males. Note the significant difference in size between the two specimens.

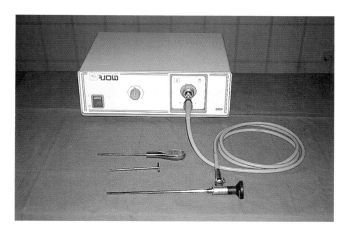

Fig. 3.198 Basic equipment for avian endoscopy. Light source, fiberoptic cable, rigid rod–lens endoscope, trocar and cannula.

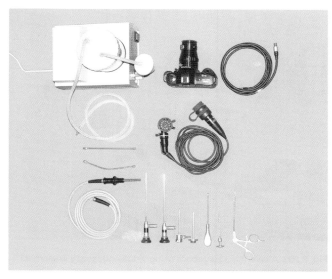

Fig. 3.201 Materials, instruments and equipment commonly used for minor endoscopy-assisted surgical procedures and biopsies, including equipment for still photography and video endoscopy.

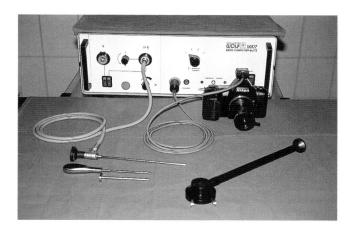

Fig. 3.199 Endoscopy equipment required for still endophotography. Light source provided with an electronic flash, fiberoptic cable, rigid rod–lens endoscope, trocar and cannula, camera with adaptor for endoscope connected to light source, second viewer or teaching attachment.

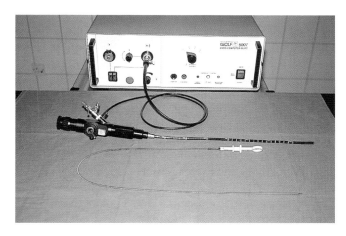

Fig. 3.200 Flexible endoscopes are useful tools for the retrieval of foreign bodies from the crop and stomach of birds. They may also prove useful for internal surgical procedures.

long-legged birds such as cranes, storks and flamingoes, and other species such as touracoes, vultures and hornbills (Samour *et al.*, 1984a). Gaseous anesthetic agents are also routinely used in birds. Currently, isoflurane is the preferred agent of many avian practitioners (Harlin, 1996; Lawton, 1996; McDonald, 1996; Rosskopf and Woerpel, 1996). This anesthetic agent offers several advantages when used with the avian patient, including a high safety margin, rapid induction and fast recovery. When a practitioner is confronted with a large number of birds for sex determination weighing 1 kg or more, such as large macaws, cranes, flamingoes and ibises, the use of alphaxalone–alphadolone is highly recommended.

In birds weighing less than 250 g the use of a small operating table 250 mm long, 150 mm wide and 100 mm high is recommended. The top is made of Perspex molded to accommodate the body of the bird and the sides are made of aluminum, finishing in an 'L'-shaped base 10 mm wide. The table is placed on a heating pad at 37°C (98.6°F). This provides a suitable temperature of around 28°C (82.4°F) through heat conduction. Larger birds can be laid on a towel placed directly on the heating pad. Figures 3.199–3.201 illustrate the equipment commonly used for avian endoscopy.

The avian patient is positioned in right lateral recumbency with the wings folded in the normal anatomical position. The left leg is fully extended forward and the lateral aspect of the abdomen is prepared for surgery. The area should be plucked of all feathers and scrubbed and disinfected with a suitable disinfectant agent. A sterile drape should be placed over the bird. Transparent drapes offer the advantage of allowing the

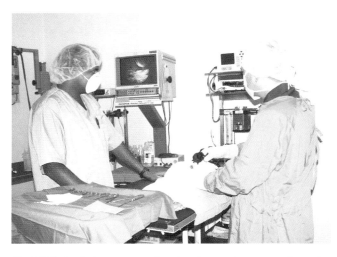

Fig. 3.202 A veterinary surgeon is using video endoscopy equipment to visualize the airsac system of a falcon. Note the numerous filarial nematodes of the genus *Serratospiculum* present on the airsac wall.

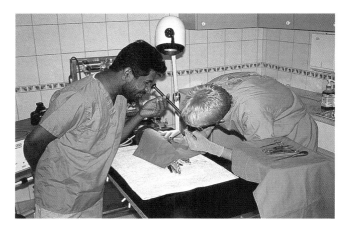

Fig. 3.204 A veterinary surgeon conducting an endoscopy examination on a bird. A second viewer or teaching attachment is being used to show a pathological condition to an assistant.

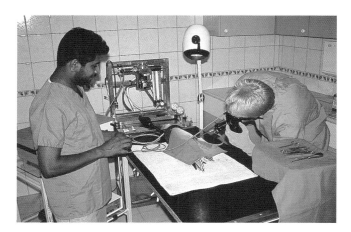

Fig. 3.205 The veterinary surgeon should be prepared to obtain photographs during routine endoscopy examinations since these can be important records of pathological findings.

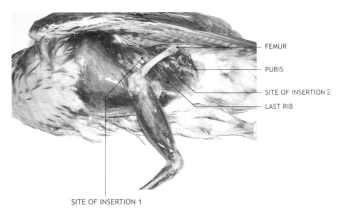

FEMUR
PUBIS
SITE OF INSERTION 2
LAST RIB
SITE OF INSERTION 1

Fig. 3.203 External reference points for the insertion of the trocar and cannula for general endoscopy examination.

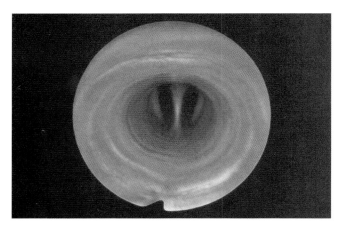

Fig. 3.206 An endoscopy view of the normal trachea and the tracheobronchial syrinx in a saker falcon (*Falco cherrug*). The tracheobronchial syrinx is an anatomical site commonly affected with aspergillosis, pseudomoniasis and trichomonosis infections. The examination of these anatomical sites is imperative with patients presenting with dyspnea, stridor and wet rale.

surgeon to observe the surgical reference points clearly, in contrast to conventional cloth-type drapes. The surgical approach varies according to the species. When the left leg is fully extended, it is possible to identify a triangle formed by the last rib, the proximal femur and the cranial edge of the pubis. The surgical approach recommended for most species is the proximal area of this triangle. This approach is particularly recommended in birds with a large ventriculum, such as birds of prey. Several other techniques have been proposed by many different authors and these have been adequately covered by Taylor (1994). Figure 3.202 outlines external reference points for avian endoscopy and Figures 3.203–3.206 illustrate the procedure in progress.

Endoscopy examination of the gonads has been carried out in individuals weighing between 28 g and 12 kg (J. Samour, unpublished data). The size of the endoscope should be directly related to the size of the bird. For instance, in small birds weighing less than 100 g an endoscope of 1.9 mm diameter is suitable, while in larger birds weighing 500 g a 3 mm endoscope is more appropriate. In large birds, such as cranes, flamingoes and storks, a 5 mm endoscope is ideal. A small incision (of the same diameter as the endoscope to be used) is made in the skin. The trocar and cannula are then inserted into the cavity. The role of the assistant restraining the anesthetized bird is extremely crucial at this point, in particular when using conventional cloth-type drapes. The bird has to be held square on the table with the back completely straight. Any change of the positioning could result in an accident when the trocar is driven into the cavity. As a practical rule, the trocar and cannula should be inserted at a 45° angle to the table and 45° to the back of the bird. Blunt-ended trocars are preferable in avian endoscopy. A common accident for beginners, and even experienced practitioners, is to lose the sense of direction and puncture the liver or, more commonly, the ventriculus. This may happen if the assistant has

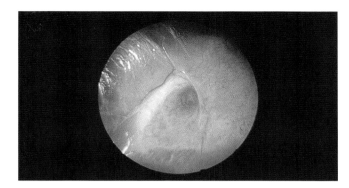

Fig. 3.209 Ostium of the cranial thoracic airsac in a houbara bustard.

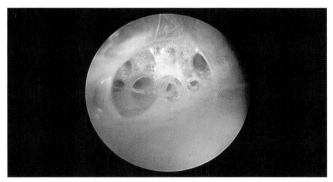

Fig. 3.210 Ostium of the caudal thoracic airsac in a gyrfalcon

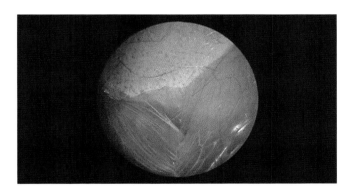

Fig. 3.207 An anterior upper view of the caudal thoracic airsac. The lung can be seen at the cranial end of the airsac.

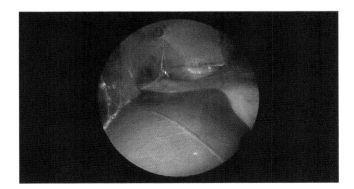

Fig. 3.208 A posterior lower view of the caudal thoracic airsac. Part of the liver can be seen partially covering the ventriculus in a clinically normal peregrine falcon.

inadvertently rotated the bird in either direction or the surgeon has not been able to identify correctly the reference points for the surgical approach. The latter is a very common occurrence with obese birds. When the instruments are correctly placed, the trocar is withdrawn and the endoscope is inserted through the cannula. It is a poor practice to introduce the telescope without the aid of the cannula since the fragile seal or the lens at the terminal end of the telescope could be damaged. In addition, the use of the cannula offers the advantage of allowing the operator to introduce and withdraw the telescope repeatedly for cleaning.

If the endoscope is correctly placed, the surgeon should be looking into the caudal thoracic airsac (Figs 3.207 and 3.208). Cranially, it should be possible to see the lung ventrally to the left, the ventriculus partially covered by the liver, and, to the right, the wall of the left abdominal airsac. Figures 3.209 and 3.210 are cranial thoracic airsac views. The attention should be directed to the abdominal airsac for the examination of the gonads. In most species, only the left ovary is functional in the female bird. In contrast, both testes are present in

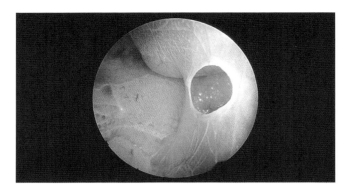

Fig. 3.211 A small perforation has been made on the wall of the abdominal airsac in order to examine and obtain a photograph of the immature ovary in a houbara bustard as part of a research project.

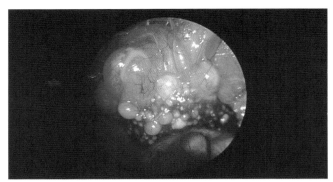

Fig. 3.214 Melanistic ovary of a lesser sulfur-crested cockatoo (*Cacatua sulphurea*) at the onset of the breeding season. Note the small and medium-sized developing follicles.

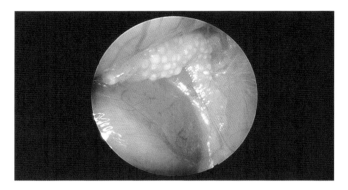

Fig. 3.212 Kidney, adrenal gland and immature ovary of an 8-month-old stone curlew (*Burhinus oedicnemus*). Note the V shape of the immature gonad.

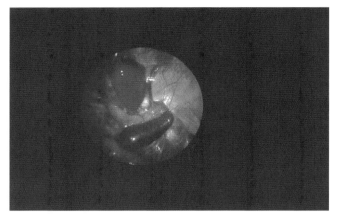

Fig. 3.215 Melanistic and inactive testis of a lesser sulfur-crested cockatoo outside the breeding season.

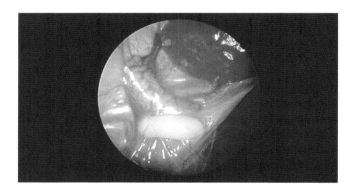

Fig. 3.213 Kidney, adrenal gland and immature testis of an 8-month-old stone curlew.

the male bird. The gonads (Figs 3.211–3.215) are usually located at the anterior base of the cranial lobe of the kidney, forming a triangle with the adrenal gland at the front. One of the greatest advantages of sex determination by direct visualization of the gonads is that it is possible to gather other useful information in addition to determining the sex of the bird. The gonads undergo dramatic seasonal changes throughout the year. Changes in the size, color and appearance of the gonads are all important key features for the assessment of reproductive status. The gonads of some avian species, such as cockatoos, toucans, touracoes and many others, are pigmented as a result of melanin deposits. Immature and sexually inactive individuals of these species display a wide range of gonad coloration, from pale-gray, pale blue-green and pale-green through dark metallic green to black. The color of the gonads changes with seasonally related morphological changes. For instance, the weight of the testes in a male bird may increase 10–500 times (Johnson, 1986). In a particular study, the seasonal developmental changes of the ovary were monitored in houbara bustards (*Chlamydotis undulata*) using photography and assigning a particular score according to the different structural anatomical features (Figs 3.216–3.217) (J. Samour, unpublished data).

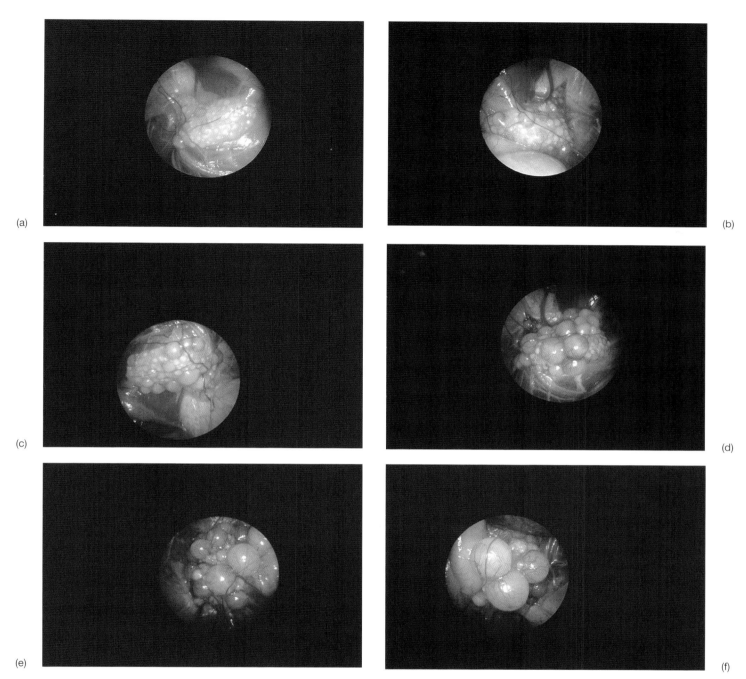

Fig. 3.216 Developmental sequence of the ovary in a houbara bustard throughout the breeding season. Endoscopy assessment of gonadal development was carried out through morphological changes and a score was given on a scale from 0 to 5. Blood samples were also collected, parallel to the endoscopy study, to determine changes in hormonal levels. The birds were examined every month, from February to July. (a) Score 0. Ovary small, triangular in shape, follicles very small, small fatty deposits. (b) Score 1. Ovary small, triangular in shape, early ovarian activity, at least 1 follicle 3 mm in diameter, small fatty deposits. (c) Score 2. Larger ovary, rectangular in shape, increased ovarian activity, at least three 5 mm diameter follicles, ovarian stroma still visible. (d) Score 3. Larger, rectangular in shape, several 5–10 mm diameter follicles, stroma partially visible. (e) Score 4. Larger, cluster appearance, several 10–15 mm diameter follicles, stroma not visible. (f) Score 5. Large, cluster appearance, several 15–25 mm diameter follicles, stroma not visible.

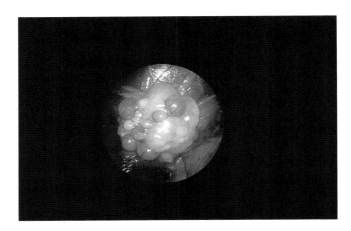

Fig. 3.217 Ovary of a houbara bustard displaying typical signs of follicular regression at the end of the breeding cycle.

Cloacoscopy for sex determination

Cloacoscopy (cloacal examination) has proved to be a useful technique to determine the sex of penguins (Samour *et al.*, 1983) and young ratites (Samour *et al.*, 1984b). In the case of penguins, the bird is held upside down with its head and neck between the knees of, and its back towards, the seated operator. The legs and wings are restrained by a handler. While holding the tail, the operator inserts the lubricated proctoscope into the cloaca to a depth of 65 mm in king (*Aptenodytes patagonica*), 40 mm in gentoo (*Pygoscelis papua*) and 25 mm in Humboldt (*Spheniscus humbolti*), rockhopper (*Eudyptes crestatus*) and blackfooted (*Spheniscus demersus*) penguins. The obturator is then withdrawn and the dorsal wall of the cloaca carefully examined. The avian cloaca is divided into four different regions, the proctodeum, urodeum, coprodeum and colorectum. The examination is directed towards the urodeum. Around the midline of this area, there are two pairs of papillae. The inner pair make up the ureteric papillae, which are similar in length and morphology in both sexes. The outer pair represent the openings of the vasa deferentia. In the male bird, these papillae are well developed and the same size as the inner pair. In contrast, in the female bird, the papillae of the outer pair are smaller and substantially shorter. Additionally in females, the oviductal opening is clearly visible on the left side of the urodeum. During the laying season, the mucous membrane around the opening of the oviduct is swollen and pink–red in color.

The technique for sex determination in young ratites is very similar to that for penguins. The bird is restrained in a similar way and the choice of proctoscopes is related to the size of the bird. Through the proctoscope, the operator will easily be able to identify the phallus in males. At this age it is not possible to identify the oviductal opening of young female birds. Therefore, in females, the sex is established only by the absence of the phallus. In monomorphic species, such as rheas and emus, and in juvenile and subadult individuals of dimorphic species such as ostriches, sex determination is carried out through digital examination of the cloaca (Samour *et al.*, 1984; Fowler, 1996).

REFERENCES

Ainley DG (1970) PhD. thesis, Johns Hopkins University.

Bailey RE (1953) Surgery for sexing and observing gonad condition in birds. *Auk* **70**: 497–499.

Bennett RA (1993) A review of avian soft tissue surgery. *Proceedings of the Association of Avian Veterinarians*, Nashville, pp. 65–71.

Burr EW, Huchzermeyer FW, Riley AE (1981) Laparoscopic examination to determine sex in monomorphic avian species. *Journal of the South African Veterinary Association* **52** (1) 45–47.

Bush M (1978) Laparoscopy in zoological medicine. *Journal of the American Veterinary Medical Association* **9**: 1081–1087.

Bush M (1980) Laparoscopy in birds and reptiles. In: Harrison RM, Wildt DE (eds) *Animal Laparoscopy*, pp. 186–197. Williams & Wilkins, Baltimore.

Bush M, Kennedy S, Wildt DE, Seager SWJ (1978) Sexing birds by laparoscopy. *International Zoo Yearbook* **18**: 197–199.

Clayton LA, Ritzman TK (2005) Endoscopic-assisted removal of a tracheal seed foreign body in a cockatiel (*Nymphicus hollandicus*). *Journal of Avian Medicine and Surgery* **19**: 14–18.

Crosta L, Timossi L (2005) Imaging techniques in avian obstetrics. *Proceedings of the European Association of Avian Veterinarians*, Arles, pp. 301–306.

Crosta L, Gerlach H, Bürkle M, Timossi L (2002) Endoscopic testicular biopsy in Psittaciformes. *Journal of Avian Medicine and Surgery* **16**: 106–110.

Fowler ME (1996) Clinical anatomy of ratites. In: Tully TN, Shane SM (eds) *Ratite Management Medicine and Surgery*, pp. 1–11. Krieger Publishing Company, Malabar, FL.

Gartrell BD (2002) Assessment of the reproductive state in male swift parrots (*Thamus discolor*) by testicular aspiration and cytology. *Journal of Avian Medicine and Surgery* **16**: 211–217.

Harlin RW (1996) Otoscopic sexing. In: Rosskopf W Jr, Woerpel RW (eds) *Diseases of Cage and Aviary Birds*, 3rd edn, pp. 697–698. Williams & Wilkins, Baltimore.

Harrison GJ (1978) Endoscopic examination of avian gonadal tissue. *Veterinary Medical Small Animal Clinician* **73**: 479–484.

Harrison GJ (1986) Endoscopy. In: Harrison GJ, Harrison LR (eds) *Clinical Avian Medicine and Surgery*, pp. 224–244. WB Saunders, Philadelphia.

Hauser WMP (1977) Game bird breeders. *Aviculturists, Zoologists and Conservationists Gazette* **26**: 6–10, 10–11.

Heidenreich M (1997) *Birds of Prey: Medicine and Management*, pp. 196–199. Blackwell Science, Oxford.

Hernandez-Divers SJ (2005) Minimally invasive endoscopic surgery of birds. *Journal of Avian Medicine and Surgery* **19**: 107–120

Ingram KA (1977) Laparotomy technique to determine sex of psittacine birds. *Proceedings of the American Association of Zoo Veterinarians*, Honolulu, pp. 40–44.

Ingram KA (1978) Laparotomy technique for sex determination of psittacine birds. *Journal of the American Veterinary Medical Association* **176**: 1244–1246.

Ingram KA (1980) Otoscopic technique for sexing birds. In: Kirk RW (ed.) *Current Veterinary Therapy* VII, pp. 656–658. WB Saunders, Philadelphia.

Johnson AL (1986) Reproduction in the female and male. In: Sturkie PD (ed.) *Avian Physiology*, 4th edn, p. 404. Springer Verlag, New York.

Jones RG, Redig PT (2003) Endoscopy guided vasectomy in the immature Japanese quail (*Coturnix coturnix japonica*). *Proceedings of the European Association of Avian Veterinarians*, Tenerife, pp. 117–123.

Jones DM, Samour JH, Knight JA, Ffinch JM (1984) Sex determination of monomorphic birds by fiber-optic endoscopy. *Veterinary Record* **115**: 595–598.

Kollias GV Jr (1988) Avian endoscopy. In: Jacobson ER, Kollias GV Jr (eds) *Contemporary Issues in Small Animal Practice*, pp. 75–104. Churchill Livingstone, New York.

Lawton MPC (1996) Anesthesia. In: Beynon PH, Forbes NA, Harcourt-Brown NH (eds) *Manual of Raptors, Pigeons and Waterfowl*, pp. 79–88. British Small Animal Veterinary Association, Cheltenham.

Le Resche RE (1971) PhD. thesis, Johns Hopkins University, Baltimore.

Lierz M (2004) Endoskopie. In: Pees M (ed.) Leitsymptome bei Papageien und Sittichen, pp. 185–194. Enke Verlag, Stuttgart.

Lierz M, Hafez HM (2005) Endoscopy guided multiple entry surgery in birds. *Proceedings of the European Association of Avian Veterinarians*, Arles, pp. 184–189.

McDonald SE (1982) Surgical sexing of birds by laparoscopy. *California Veterinarian* 5: 16–22.

McDonald SE (1987) Endoscopic examination. In: Burr EW (ed.) *Companion Bird Medicine*, pp. 166–174. Iowa State University Press, Ames, IA.

McDonald SE (1996) Endoscopy. In: Rosskopf WJ Jr, Woerpel RW (eds) *Diseases of Cage and Aviary Birds*, 3rd edn, pp. 699–717. Williams & Wilkins, Baltimore.

Pye GW, Bennett RA, Plunske R et al. (2001a) The effect of endoscopy salpingohysterectomy in juvenile cockatiels (*Nymphicus hollandicus*) on ovulation. *Proceedings of the European Association of Avian Veterinarians*, Munich, pp. 66–69.

Pye GW, Bennett RA, Plunske R, Davidson J (2001b) Endoscopic salpingohysterectomy of juvenile cockatiels (*Nymphicus hollandicus*). *Journal of Avian Medicine and Surgery* 15: 90–94.

Risser AC (1971) A technique for performing laparotomy on small birds. *Condor* 73: 376–379.

Rosskopf WJ Jr, Woerpel RW (1996) Practical anesthesia administration. In: Rosskopf WJ Jr, Woerpel RW (eds) *Diseases of Cage and Aviary Birds*, 3rd edn, pp. 664–671. Williams & Wilkins, Baltimore.

Samour JH (1991) Avian endoscopy. In: Brearley MJ, Cooper JE, Sullivan M (eds) *A Colour Atlas of Small Animal Endoscopy*, pp. 97–109. Wolfe Publishing, London.

Samour JH (1996) Veterinary medicine, falcons and falconry in the Middle East. *Proceedings of the Association of Avian Veterinarians*, Tampa, pp. 233–239.

Samour JH, Stevenson M, Knight JA, Lawrie AJ (1983) Sexing penguins by cloacal examination. *Veterinary Record* 113: 84–85.

Samour JH, Jones DM, Knight JA et al. (1984a) Comparative studies of the use of some injectable anesthetic agents in birds. *Veterinary Record* 115: 6–11.

Samour JH, Markham J, Nieva O (1984b) Sexing ratite birds by cloacal examination. *Veterinary Record* 115: 167–169.

Satterfield WC (1980) Diagnostic laparoscopy in birds. In: Kirk RW (ed.) *Current Veterinary Therapy* VII, pp. 659–661. WB Saunders, Philadelphia.

Satterfield WC, Altman RB (1977) Avian sex determination by endoscopy. *Proceedings of the American Association of Zoo Veterinarians*, Honolulu, pp. 45–48.

Sladen WJL (1978) *International Zoo Yearbook* 18–77.

Taylor M (1989) A morphologic approach to the endoscopic determination of sex in juvenile macaws. *Journal of the Association of Avian Veterinarians* 3: 199–201.

Taylor M (1990) Endoscopy. *Proceedings of the Association of Avian Veterinarians*, Phoenix, pp. 319–324.

Taylor M (1992) *Endoscopy. Laboratory Manual*, pp. 1–10. Association of Avian Veterinarians, Lake Worth, FL.

Taylor M (1994) Endoscopic examination and biopsy techniques. In: Ritchie BW, Harrison GJ, Harrison LR (eds) *Avian Medicine: Principles and Application*, pp. 327–354. Wingers Publishing, Lake Worth, FL.

Wilson GH, Richey L, McBride M et al. (2004) Chemical castration of pigeons via endoscopic intratesticular injection. *Proceedings of the Association of Avian Veterinarians*, New Orleans, pp. 91–93.

Hauser WMP (1977) Game bird breeders. *Aviculturists, Zoologists and Conservationists Gazette* 26: 6–10, 10–11.

Assessment of body condition and lipid content using total body electrical conductivity

Peter J. Hudson

One of the major difficulties in experimental studies of live animals is to obtain an estimate of body condition or body composition noninvasively. Traditionally, estimates have evaluated mass with respect to a measure of body size, usually a skeletal measurement (e.g. tarsus size) or a feather measurement (wing cord). However, such estimates are by necessity relatively coarse and measurements of mass include lipid, muscle mass, fat and gut contents.

There is a range of alternative techniques for estimating relative body condition. One is to make an indentation of the pectoralis muscle on to dental paste and to subsequently obtain an estimate of pectoral volume. A second is to use a piece of wire pushed over the pectoralis to provide a cross sectional representation of the pectoralis muscle and, using correction figures from dead birds, to estimate pectoralis volume. A third is to use an ultrasound device that measures the time taken for an ultrasound wave to travel to a tissue interface and can be used to estimate the thickness of pectoralis muscle.

These techniques have the advantage that they allow comparative and quantitative estimates of body condition for a single individual and can be used regularly over a period of time. However, none of these techniques can be used to make a reasonable estimate of body composition or the relative ratio of lipid content to muscle mass. A wide range of studies require reasonable estimates of lipid storage, since lipids provide a major way of storing energy prior to reproduction, migration or surviving harsh conditions. Previously it was not possible to obtain an accurate estimate of an individual's lipid store without killing the animal and solvent-extracting lipids from the homogenized carcass. Such an approach restricts the possibility of undertaking detailed studies on individuals and estimating changes in lipid content associated with life history strategies. A relatively recent technique is to use total body electrical conductivity (TOBEC, Fig. 3.218), which permits workers to estimate precisely lean body mass, percentage body fat and the total water content of individuals in a comparative way and make quantitative estimates of body condition between individuals and with respect to time.

TOBEC equipment

Current TOBEC equipment for birds is produced by EMSCAN Inc. (Springfield, IL) and is sold in the UK through Biotech Instruments Ltd (Kimpton, Herts). The basic equipment consists of scanning recording equipment associated with one of a series of chambers. Choice of chamber is determined by the diameter of the species under study and ranges from 30 mm, suitable for animals weighing less than 10 g, through to 203 mm, for animals weighing about 1 kg, although animals as large as 8 kg can be measured in this system. All the animal's tissues should fit into the chamber and the body should fill more than half the diameter of the chamber. In growth

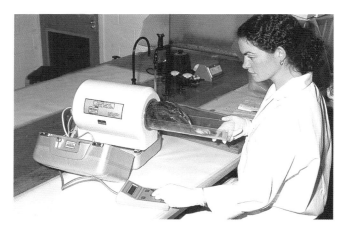

Fig. 3.218 Estimation of body condition and lipid content using total body electrical conductivity (TOBEC).

studies or in studies with a wide variation in body size, two chambers may be necessary. The system is designed to be used both in the field, using a DC battery system and a hand-held recording device, or connected up to a computer in the laboratory.

TOBEC methodology

The basic methodology for the TOBEC system is to place an animal in a measurement chamber, open at each end, surrounded by a solenoid that produces a stable, cylindrical electromagnetic field. Placing the animal in the chamber alters the electromagnetic inductance of the coil, the extent of which is determined by the body's electrolytes, specifically in the hydrated tissues. By measuring the change in the phase relationship between voltage and current when a high-frequency signal is passed through the coil, an estimate of lean tissue mass can be determined, given that body water is a constant proportion of lean tissue and that the body lipids have a relatively poor conductivity (just 5% of lean tissues). By comparing lean and actual body mass a reasonable estimate of lipid content can be obtained.

Animals need to be restrained before being inserted into the chamber, either through anesthesia or by inserting the animal in a suitable and approved holding device. Some workers use soft plastic jackets with Velcro fasteners. The process of inserting the restrained bird into the chamber and obtaining a reading takes about 20 s for each specimen. There are no harmful effects if the bird is caught and measurements are taken at repeated intervals. Care should be taken to achieve repeatable results, since a change in orientation can alter results. With reasonable care, errors should be less than 5%. Some workers find that the sequence at which birds are scanned can alter the results, so repeated measures are recommended whereby a series of birds are scanned at random, and usually five readings should be taken with the bird in and the bird out and obvious outliers in the results ignored. Only part of

the detection chamber is used and a certain homogeneity in the bird's composition is assumed, so birds must be placed centrally and in the same location in the chamber each time. A curved carrier plate is provided with each chamber and these can be used to ensure that bodies are located in the same area of the scanning range. The best location for most bird species is with the mid-sternum position close to the midpoint of the chamber. The index of total body electrical conductivity is estimated as:

TOBEC Chamber reading empty – Bird in chamber reading/Normalization constant (from manufacturer)

During field work, the scanning equipment should not be placed in direct sunlight and reading should be taken only after the chamber has been placed in the shade for 15 min or more. Usually it is best to ensure that the bird is lying well within the central part of the electromagnetic field. Metal tags may also alter the readings, while plastic tags and rings appear not to, but it is wise to check all possible causes of variation. Tags should be scanned separately and the difference of these values taken from the final values given by the machine.

Other conductive material must be kept well away from the chamber, including the operator's hand, and there should be no contact between the bird and the user.

TOBEC calibration

The examining device needs to be calibrated and ideally a series of birds need to be sacrificed and lipids extracted. The estimates of electrical conductivity can be very accurate but properties of the subject that relate conductivity to fat-free mass have a range of characteristics that will influence estimates of fat-free mass. The calibration is basically:

Fat free mass – Conductivity Index Calibration Factor.

If the group under examination is heterogeneous, with variations with respect to age and sex, then reduced error in the result can be achieved by producing a calibration curve for each respective group or adding terms to the above equation and using multiple regression to estimate fat-free mass. Including length within the calibration equation can help to increase the predictive power of the equation, and if dead birds are used body temperature should be included.

With endangered species or species that cannot be sacrificed, calibration may be possible through the use of stable isotopes dilution.

FURTHER READING

Castro G, Wunder BA, Knopf FL (1990) Total body electrical conductivity (TOBEC) to estimate total body fat of free-living birds. *Condor* **92**: 496–499.

Scott I, Grant M, Evans PR (1991) Estimation of fat-free mass of live birds: use of total body electrical conductivity (TOBEC) measurements in studies of single species in the field. *Functional Ecology* **5**: 314–320.

Anesthesia and soft tissue surgery

4

General anesthesia

Martin P. C. Lawton

The routine use of isoflurane in avian practice has almost made anesthesia of birds a predictably safe and uneventful procedure. There is, however, more to anesthesia than masking a bird down with isoflurane. The unique anatomy and physiology of the bird affect the design and use of anesthetic circuits, intubation or placement of an airsac tube, as well as the method of resuscitation should an emergency occur. The aims of anesthesia should be to provide a smooth, reliable induction with adequate restraint, muscle relaxation and analgesia, followed by a fast, but full, uneventful recovery (Lawton, 1996a, 1996b).

Anatomical and physiological considerations

Anatomical considerations

Only the most important characteristics of avian anatomy that have a direct bearing on the management and maintenance of anesthesia will be discussed here. For a more detailed description of avian respiratory anatomy see King and McLelland, 1975 and McLelland, 1990.

Trachea

The avian trachea has complete interlocking rings, which are cartilaginous in some species and ossified in others. This has implications when intubation of birds is undertaken, as cuffed endotracheal tubes, if used, could damage these complete rings (Fitzgerald and Blais, 1993). Unlike mammals, birds can still vocalize even when intubated because of the location of the syrinx at the tracheal bifurcation (Heard, 1997). Some Anseriformes and other species do have diverticulum and bulbous expansions, while others have complicated tracheal loops or even a double trachea (penguins) (Edling, 2003), which can lead to complications with dead space within the trachea.

Airsacs

The class Aves has a unique respiratory system, employing airsacs that act as bellows and reservoirs when breathing (Fig. 4.1). Most birds have nine airsacs, some of which pneumatize bones while some leave the celomic cavity and terminate subcutaneously (Fedde, 1986). As a generalization, there are usually the following airsacs: paired cranial thoracic, caudal thoracic, abdominal and clavicular, and a single cervical. The airsacs are avascular and contribute less than 5% towards respiratory gas exchange (Edling, 2003).

The position of a bird under anesthesia will effect the ability of the airsacs to work normally. In dorsal recumbency, the weight of the abdominal organs will cause a partial collapse of the abdominal and thoracic airsacs. Intermittent positive pressure ventilation (IPPV) can help to overcome the effects on respiration of dorsal positioning.

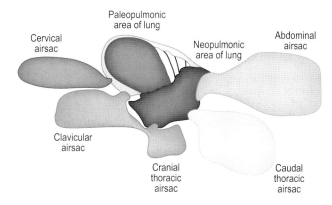

Fig. 4.1 Relationship of airsacs to paleopulmonic and neopulmonic area of lungs.

Lungs

The avian lungs are relatively rigid and do not move appreciably during respiration. The diaphragm is absent and therefore lungs do not collapse when the thoracic (celomic) cavity is entered surgically (or endoscopically). The avian lung is a 'flow-through' system. The entrances between the airsacs and the lungs are either via ostia or sometimes via large tubes, the saccobronchi. The primary bronchus also has an extrapulmonary portion that extends through the lung to the abdominal airsac (Edling, 2003). This arrangement of lungs interconnecting with the airsacs allows the bird to be artificially ventilated either via the trachea or via an abdominal airsac tube (see below).

The lungs are divided into paleopulmonic and neopulmonic areas. During inspiration the air flow is divided between these two areas but gaseous exchange mainly occurs in the paleopulmonic area with only a limited amount occurring in the neopulmonic area. Air that passes through the paleopulmonic area enters the cervical, clavicular or cranial thoracic airsacs, whereas air that goes through the neopulmonic area passes into the caudal thoracic and abdominal airsacs. There has been some debate as to whether inspired air passes over the lung tissue twice (James *et al.*, 1976) or only once (Scheid and Piiper, 1971; Fitzgerald and Blais, 1993). During both inspiration and expiration, although air moves bidirectionally through the neopulmonic area, air will only ever travel unidirectionally (caudal to cranial) through the paleopulmonic area (Fedde, 1986). The unidirectional flow through the paleopulmonic parabronchi is thought to be due to the aerodynamic shape and angle of the bronchi and cranial airsacs creating a flow resistance within the lungs, as no valves have been grossly identified.

Physiological considerations

Trachea

The tracheal length and volume is greater in birds than in mammals of equal body mass. The tracheal dead space is 4.5 times that of mammals. Birds compensate by increasing their tidal volume and decreasing respiratory frequency as compared with a mammal of equal size (Fedde, 1986). This increased tidal volume must be maintained during anesthesia to prevent hypocapnia associated with the increased dead space volume of the trachea and any endotracheal tube used.

Inspiration and expiration

Avian inspiration occurs when the inspiratory muscles increase the body volume by movement of the thoracoabdominal body wall (in particular, the sternum is moved downwards and the ribs move outwards). This increase in the body volume results in a negative pressure build-up within the airsacs, causing air to be 'sucked in' through the nares and mouth, pass through the lungs and into the airsacs. On handling or positioning a bird prior to surgery, any pressure to the ribs and in particular the sternum may affect the ability to breathe, as the necessary body volume changes may not occur.

Expiration occurs when the expiratory muscles cause a reduction in the size of the body volume by compression of the thoracic skeleton (Fig. 4.2) and is not passive, unlike the situation in mammals. The reduction of the body volume causes an increased pressure within the airsacs, forcing gas from the airsacs back into the lungs (Fig. 4.3) and then out via the mouth or nares. The airsacs thus act as bellows. On the relaxation of the respiratory muscles, the sternum is midway between its inspiratory and expiratory position. A deeply anesthetized bird may not generate sufficient muscular contractions to allow adequate 'pumping' of air back through the lungs. Sinn (1994) advised the routine use of positive IPPV (20–40/min at 15 mmHg) to overcome any possibility of hypocapnia and to maintain adequate oxygenation.

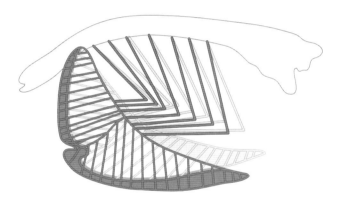

Fig. 4.2 Demonstration of the movement of the keel and ribs during respiration. The blue-shaded area represents expiration while the red shaded area represents inspiration.

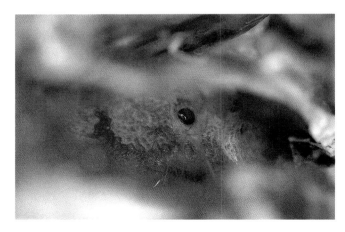

Fig. 4.3 Ostia between the lungs and the caudal thoracic airsac.

Gaseous exchange

Gaseous exchange within the avian lung relies on a cross-current exchange system in which the air within the air capillaries flows at right angles to the flow of blood through the blood capillaries. This cross-current exchange system is more effective than that found in mammalian lungs. The cross-current flow causes a potential increase in the partial pressure of carbon dioxide (P_{CO_2}) expired and an increase in P_{O_2} within the blood. Avian lungs are considered to be 10 times more effective than mammalian lungs (James et al., 1976).

In birds, CO_2 is mainly in the form of hydrogen bicarbonate in the plasma, with only small amounts as dissolved or plasma-bound CO_2. Carbonic anhydrase is responsible for the production of the bicarbonate and the subsequent dissociation of the hydrogen ion. It appears that CO_2 has no direct effect on the oxygen affinity of hemoglobin other than through the metabolic release of hydrogen ions. In the lungs, the hydrogen bicarbonate enters the red blood cells and the resulting metabolism releases the CO_2, which is then breathed out. A small change in the P_{CO_2} leads to a large change in the blood CO_2.

Ventilation triggers

Ventilation during anesthesia is affected by a number of physiological factors that should be considered in an anesthetized patient. As with most Taxa, inhalation of CO_2 stimulates ventilation. There are known to be receptors in the carotid bodies and the intrapulmonary chemoreceptors, as well as CO_2 directly stimulating the nervous system (Fedde, 1986). The carotid bodies are responsible for controlling ventilation when there is a reduction in the P_{O_2} in the arteries, hypoxia or an increase in the P_{CO_2}. Pain will also stimulate respiration. Increases in body temperature will cause a thermal polypnea but not usually hyperventilation. Under anesthesia, subjecting the larynx and trachea to cold gases is known to slow breathing and may even produce apnea. Temperature also has an influence on the O_2 affinity of hemoglobin: an increased temperature in active tissue favors a release of O_2 from the hemoglobin but if the bird cools down too much under anesthesia then the release of oxygen is affected as the binding with hemoglobin is increased.

Hypoglycemia

Birds are very prone to hypoglycemia when anesthetized. It is not recommended that birds be starved prior to gaseous induction, but where possible induction should be performed when the crop (where present) is empty. It is often overlooked that the total time a bird is starved would not just include any period before anesthesia (if any), but also the time up until the bird has fully recovered and is willing to eat. Cooper (1989) stated that small birds should never be deprived of food for longer than 3 h. Starvation may also reduce hepatic detoxification of certain anesthetic agents (Carter-Storm, 1988). Regurgitation is seldom a problem in granivorous psittacine birds, unlike waterfowl or frugivorous birds, in which a period of starvation has previously been recommended (Mandelker, 1987).

Volatile anesthesia

There are a number of anesthetic agents that have historically been used for induction and maintenance of birds. Ether, one of the older volatile anesthetic agents, can be dismissed on the basis that it is unsafe, as the safety margin is below that of more modern anesthetic agents, there is a risk of explosion and it is irritant to the mucosa. Although methoxyflurane has been used in the past with very good results, the lack of availability and the requirement of a dedicated vaporizer, together with the disadvantage of the hangover effect (50% being metabolized), has virtually removed its use from avian practice. The two agents that are likely to be used routinely in a practice situation are halothane and isoflurane, and these are compared in Table 4.1. Rosskopf and Woerpel (1996) consider that, if veterinary surgeons are unwilling to invest in isoflurane and the necessary equipment to use it, they should refer the case for surgery to a practice that is properly equipped. Recent studies (Lennox et al., 2002) have shown that isoflurane has very little effects on natural physiological processes, such as gastrointestinal transit time, and therefore can be used in situations where previous stressful restrain was required (such as for barium meal radiography of the gastrointestinal tract).

Many avian veterinarians are now using the next-generation 'isoflurane'. Sevoflurane is proving even safer than isoflurane and is considered by many to be the anesthetic agent of choice for birds. Sevoflurane has an even lower blood gas partition coefficient than isoflurane (0.69), giving a shorter recovery time compared to isoflurane. It is thought that sevoflurane will increase the chance of success in critical or prolonged procedures (Edling, 2003). However, the cost difference between sevoflurane and isoflurane may make its routine use hard to justify.

Equipment (anesthetic machines, face masks, endotracheal tubes, anesthetic chambers)

Although it is possible to use volatile anesthetic agents in a Boyle's bottle or by the primitive method of placing a soaked cotton wool swab directly into a chamber with a bird, this is not advised. The use of a dedicated

TABLE 4.1 Comparison of isoflurane and halothane		
	Isoflurane	**Halothane**
Safety margin This is the ratio of lethal dose to anesthetizing dose (Dohoo, 1990)	5.7 This safety margin alone makes other agents obsolete (Rosskopf et al., 1992)	3.0 High concentrations of anesthetic agent are 'held' in the airsacs after induction, which may lead to fatalities
Blood gas partition coefficient The higher the value, the greater the solubility in blood and tissue distribution	1.4 at 37°C Very low solubility allows rapid induction and rapid recovery, with less retention in the body tissues compared to halothane	2.3 at 37°C Higher solubility gives more potential for redistribution from the body compartments back into circulation after induction, and a slower recover than isoflurane
Degree of metabolism Any metabolism will slow the speed of elimination from the body, and often metabolites can cause a 'hangover' effect	0.3% Virtually no metabolism allows excretion solely by expiration. 2% isoflurane has been used for prolonged anesthesia and recovery was still rapid, occurring within 6 min and full recovery considered to occur within 21 min (Clutton, 1986)	15–20% Because of increased distribution in body tissues (associated with the higher blood gas partition coefficient) and increased metabolism, there is a slower recovery than with isoflurane. Recovery is delayed if there is any underlying liver disease
Muscular relaxation	Very good	Poor
Analgesia	Good	Poor
Respiratory effects	Little respiratory depression	Marked respiratory depression
Cardiac effects	Possibility of slight myocardial depression, which results in little or no change in the heart rate (Jenkins, 1993)	Moderate myocardial depression. There is catecholamine sensitization
Contraindications	None reported	Hepatic dysfunction, cardiovascular disease or catecholamine release
Overdose	There is usually apnea before cardiac arrest. This allows a good change of prompt artificial ventilation, leading to a full recovery	Apnea and cardiac arrest usually occur simultaneously, making artificial ventilation and a full recovery more difficult than with isoflurane

vaporizer is recommended to allow an exact concentration to be given (irrespective of temperature or air pressure, within certain ranges). Ideally, the anesthetic machine should be on a mobile trolley with shelves for placing the monitoring equipment, such as respiratory and cardiac monitors, together with drugs to deal with an emergency (Fig. 4.4). It is not possible to use the same vaporizer for both halothane and isoflurane because of the differences in these volatile fluids, unless the vaporizer is cleaned and recalibrated prior to each change. An anesthetic machine with a 'Selectatec' fitting will allow easy changing between dedicated vaporizers should this be required, e.g. for different classes.

There are several advantages in the use of IPPV (Fig. 4.5) for any anesthetized bird as this allows control over not only the rate and depth of respiration but also oxygenation and the prevention of hypercapnia.

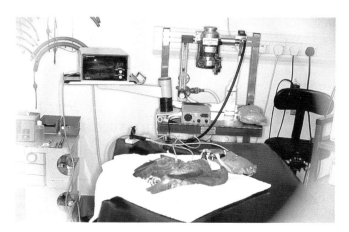

Fig. 4.4 Anesthetic trolley with isoflurane vaporizer, respiratory monitor, cardiac monitor and emergency drug box.

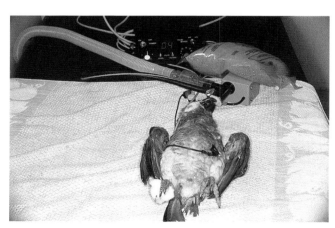

Fig. 4.5 Intermittent positive pressure ventilation of an African gray parrot (*Psittacus erithacus*).

Whether using IPPV, intubation and a suitable circuit or just a face mask, the flow rate of oxygen to the lungs must be kept high in order to prevent hypercapnia. The gaseous flow rate should be a minimum of three times the normal minute volume (i.e. approximately 3 ml/g bodyweight – a 400 g Amazon parrot (*Amazona* sp) needs 1.2 l/min), although I use 2–3 l/min irrespective of size.

Face mask

Isoflurane allows a relatively easy method of induction by face mask (other than for diving birds), reducing many of the complications of handling and injecting and the stresses that are involved with these procedures. Therefore, the most basic anesthetic circuit consists of a vaporizer, a source of carrier gas (usually oxygen) and a face mask. To keep the bird relaxed and prevent flapping, the patient should be adequately restrained, for instance in a towel (Figs 4.6–4.8). Face masks can be purchased or self-made from disposable items such as syringe cases (for small birds, Fig. 4.9) or soft-drink bottles (for macaws

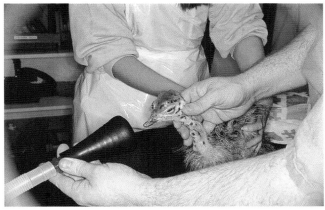

Fig. 4.8 Use of a Hall's mask for induction of an ostrich chick (*Struthio camelus*).

or long-beaked birds, Figs 4.10 and 4.11). The advantages of using disposable face masks are the elimination of the risk of spread of infection between birds and often a more

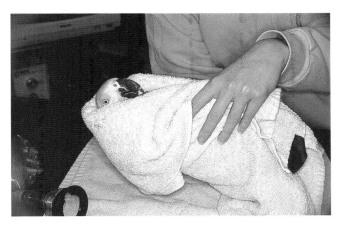

Fig. 4.6 Restraint of African gray parrot in a towel prior to induction via face mask.

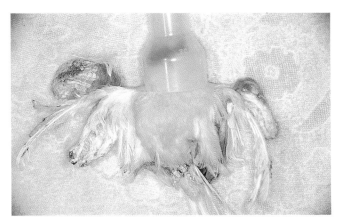

Fig. 4.9 Anesthesia of a canary (*Serinus canaria*) before removal of feather cysts, with a syringe case adapted as a face mask.

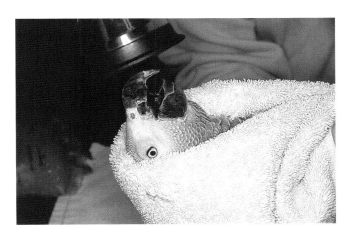

Fig. 4.7 Face mask induction of an African gray parrot with isoflurane anesthesia.

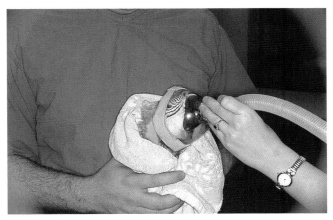

Fig. 4.10 A cut-down soft drink bottle, with the edges protected with sticking plaster, makes an ideal mask for a blue and gold macaw (*Ara ararauna*).

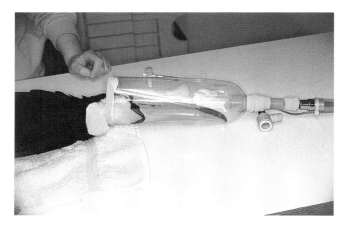

Fig. 4.11 A soft drink bottle makes an extended face mask for long-billed birds such as toucans (*Ramphastos* sp.).

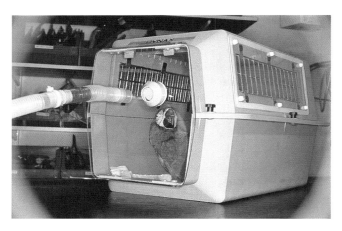

Fig. 4.13 An adapted cage with Perspex makes a suitable anesthetic induction chamber.

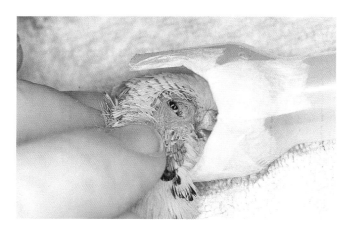

Fig. 4.12 A syringe face mask can be cut to allow access to the eye area while still maintaining anesthesia without intubation.

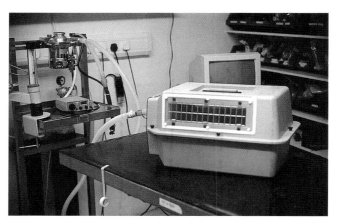

Fig. 4.14 An anesthetic chamber attached to the anesthetic machine and scavenging tubes.

suitable mask for an avian patient than those currently on the market. If a disposable face mask is not used, then it is important that the mask is cleaned well before using it on another patient. A face mask does have disadvantages, especially if examining or operating around the head, although a mask can be adapted for this (Fig. 4.12).

Anesthetic chambers

For birds that are likely to be highly stressed by the handling required for masking down, the use of an anesthetic chamber is advised (Figs 4.13 and 4.14). Birds tend not to be distressed by being in an anesthetic chamber, especially if the volatile anesthetic agent is isoflurane. Anesthetic chambers can be very simple, such as a cage and a bag placed over it into which the volatile anesthetic is introduced, or dedicated purpose-built chambers fitted in an anesthetic machine and with scavenging capacity. The main disadvantages of using an anesthetic chamber are usually cost and the slightly increased length of time before the intubation can be performed when compared with a bird that is masked down.

Endotracheal intubation

Once a patient is induced, although it is possible to maintain anesthesia just with a face mask (Fig. 4.15), endotracheal intubation should be considered except for the shortest procedures. An airway should be provided to allow maintenance of the bird under anesthesia but also for ventilation should apnea occur. Intubation of birds is easy, because of the forward-placed glottis behind the base of the tongue (Figs 4.16 and 4.17). With the mouth held open and, in the case of psittacines, the tongue gently pulled forward, a suitably sized tube can be introduced through the glottis (Fig. 4.18). Even small budgerigars or cockatiels may be intubated using cut-down cannulas or catheters (Fig. 4.19), although these small-diameter tubes may become blocked with respiratory secretions. Because of the great differences in the size of birds, a wide range of tubes also have to be available, which can be purpose-made tubes or pre-made out of cut-down intravenous catheters or urinary cannulas (Figs 4.20 and 4.21). Most catheters and cannulas have lure fittings and can therefore be connected to an anesthetic circuit

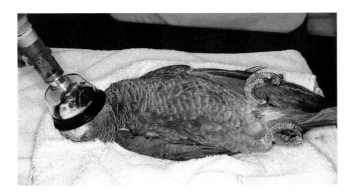

Fig. 4.15 An African gray parrot maintained under anesthesia with just a face mask.

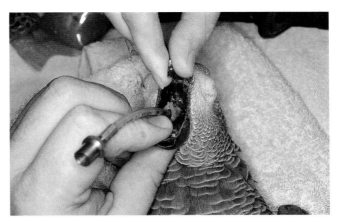

Fig. 4.18 Intubation of an anesthetized African gray with a Bethune 2.5mm endotracheal tube.

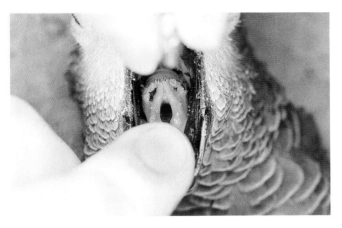

Fig. 4.16 An anesthetized African gray parrot showing glottal opening and base of tongue.

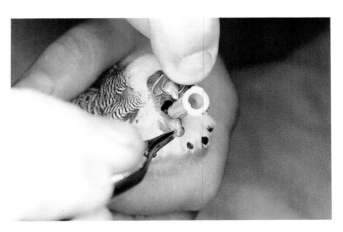

Fig. 4.19 A cut-down intravenous catheter makes an ideal endotracheal tube for a budgerigar (*Melopsittacus undulatus*).

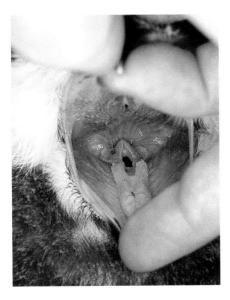

Fig. 4.17 The glottal opening of a European eagle owl (*Bubo bubo*). Compare this with Fig. 4.16.

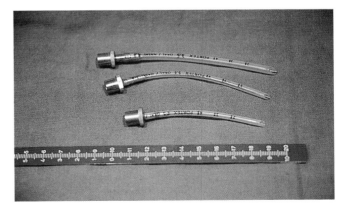

Fig. 4.20 A selection of Bethune endotracheal tubes suitable for birds.

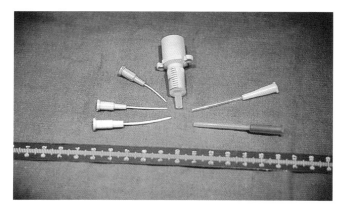

Fig. 4.21 Prepared intravenous cannulas or urinary catheters with a syringe adaptor.

force to open the valves. Intubation will allow ventilation of the bird should this prove necessary, and also allows scavenging of waste gases, an increasing requirement under most countries' legislation. Scavenging of waste gases is difficult, if not impossible, with an open face mask unless a more expensive active scavenging system, such as Fluvac (designed for a face mask), is used.

Airsac intubation

When undertaking surgery around the beak, head or face, a mask or even an endotracheal tube is likely to restrict access. The presence of airsacs and the unique air flow from the abdominal and caudal thoracic airsacs into the lungs means that when a tube is placed into one of the airsacs, anesthetic gases can be introduced (Figs 4.24 and 4.25). The site for the placement of an airsac tube is a matter of preference but is usually similar to the site chosen for endoscopic examination. Traditionally, this is the left side just behind the ribs, although Sinn (1994) has suggested the use of short endotracheal tubes or rubber tubes into the clavicular or caudal thoracic airsacs. The

(Fig. 4.22) by using a cut-down 2 ml syringe fitted on to an endotracheal adaptor (usually 8.5 mm). Once intubated, a bird should be maintained on a Bethune or Ayre's T-piece system (Fig. 4.23). Circle circuits should not be used for the avian patient as it is not able to exert sufficient

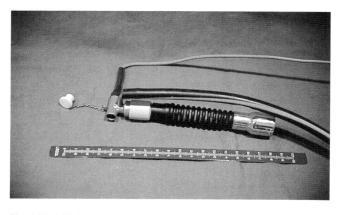

Fig. 4.22 A Bethune anesthetic circuit with scavenging and respiratory monitor probe attached.

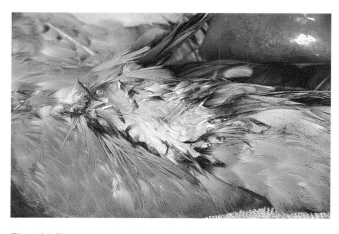

Fig. 4.24 Placement of an airsac tube in a scarlet macaw (*Ara macao*).

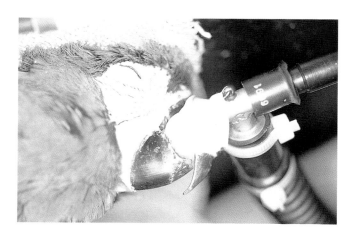

Fig. 4.23 The Bethune circuit attached to a Bethune endotracheal tube. Note the reduction of dead space between the circuit and bird.

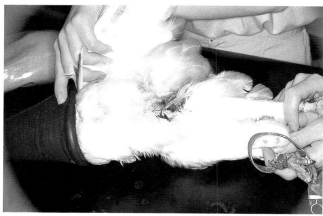

Fig. 4.25 A restrained owl with head in mask breathing 100% oxygen while an airsac tube is placed.

placement of the airsac tube is usually performed after induction by injection, face mask or anesthetic chamber. In cases of severe airway obstruction it is possible to place the tube in a physically restrained conscious bird. The placement of the tube in a conscious bird is quick and appears to cause little discomfort or distress. In emergency situations to reduce the risks that are associated with handling respiratory distress, the bird may be restrained with its head in a mask into which 100% oxygen is being delivered (Lawton, 1996b).

As large a tube as possible (French gauge 14) should be placed attached to the anesthetic circuit. IPPV via the placed tube is required while the bird is under anesthesia, as birds with airsac intubation will usually stop breathing spontaneously as a result of the expulsion of all carbon dioxide from the respiratory system (Korbel *et al.*, 1993). Ventilated birds will not breathe again spontaneously until after perfusion via the airsac is terminated and the blood carbon dioxide levels rise. The tube can be removed postoperatively or left *in situ* in cases of dyspnea (e.g. after surgery to the neck or in cases of aspergillosis plugs of the syrinx).

Injectable anesthesia

If an injectable agent is to be used, the bird should be accurately weighed. Without an accurate weight it is not possible to calculate an accurate dose, and an overdose and even a fatality could occur. Where induction with a volatile anesthetic agent is performed, it is less stressful to weigh the bird after induction but prior to the administration of any other agent. Injectable anesthetic agents are listed in Table 4.2.

Anesthesia monitoring

Despite the considered safety of isoflurane, there is no excuse for complacency over monitoring during anesthesia. The depth of anesthesia may only be correctly controlled if the bird is carefully and continuously monitored. Monitoring of birds should be approached in exactly the same way as monitoring of any mammalian species, although it is considered to be more challenging (Flammer, 1989).

Reflexes

In birds the best reflexes to monitor are the palpebral reflexes, corneal reflexes, cere reflexes, toe pinch reflexes and wing twitch. As the bird becomes more deeply anesthetized, the standard reflexes usually slow and decrease in strength, and will eventually disappear. The toe (Fig. 4.26), cere and wing reflexes disappear as the bird enters a medium plane of anesthesia. The corneal reflex (Fig. 4.27) is usually the last reflex to be abolished and shows that the bird is very deeply anesthetized (Lawton, 1996a). The tone of the jaw should also be assessed: it becomes less tense as the bird enters a medium plane of anesthesia.

Circulatory volume

Birds are thought to be better able to tolerate blood loss than mammals (Heard, 1997), although hemorrhage is still a problem. The amount of blood loss during surgery should be carefully monitored (if necessary by measuring swabs) and fluid therapy or even a blood transfusion should be considered. In an emergency situation pigeon blood can be used for most species, although there are always risks involved in this procedure, not least from viral infections.

The weight of the bird before and after surgery will allow assessment of fluid loss. Although many different figures for fluid requirements exist, Sinn (1994) suggested that the normal daily requirement is approximately 5% of bodyweight in milliliters, while up to 10% of bodyweight in milliliters may be required for a dehydrated bird. If a daily intake of less than 5% is achieved, supplementation should be considered.

Pain

The response of the bird during surgery to painful stimuli will often show as a change in respiration, heart rate or movement. The control of pain both during and after anesthesia is to be recommended. Analgesics (especially when anesthetic agents with poor analgesic properties are used) allow a more stable maintenance of anesthesia and reduce the possibility of surgical shock. Suitable analgesic agents are listed in Table 4.3; see also Local anesthesia and analgesia, below.

Electrocardiogram

Figures 4.28–4.32 illustrate electrocardiogram (ECG) equipment and lead placements. Where possible, the use of a cardiac monitor is recommended, although an esophageal stethoscope can be of use. Cardiac monitors are essential when certain anesthetic agents, such as xylazine, are used, to indicate whether atrioventricular block occurs. The standard lead placements are over the distal lateral tarsometatarsus and the carpal joints of each wing (Burtnick and Degernes, 1993) using atraumatic clamps or silver needles (Figs 4.29 and 4.30). As an aid to the assessment of pain, the heart rate is dramatically effective (Figs 4.31 and 4.32). It is not uncommon for a cockatiel, on feeling pain, to increase its heart rate from 300 beats/min to over 700 beats/min (Lawton, 1996a). The heart rate should never fall below 120 beats/min (Doolen and Jackson, 1991).

TABLE 4.2 Injectable anesthetic agents

Agent	Dose and route	Comments on use	Disadvantages
Alphaxalone/ alphadolone	5–10 mg/kg IV; 36 mg/kg IM, IP	Alphaxalone/alphadolone was considered a relatively good anesthetic agent (Harcourt-Brown, 1978). There is a wide safety margin but only a short length of action (Mandelker, 1987). The large volumes required make IV the preferred route. There are now better alternatives to this agent	Following IV administration there is often a transient apnea (Cooper and Frank, 1973, 1974), which can be alarming. IP or IM routes produce immobilization but poor analgesia (Cooper and Frank, 1973, 1974). There are reports of deaths when used in red-tailed hawks (Cooper and Redig, 1975)
Ketamine	20–50 mg/kg SC, IM, or IV In waterfowl 18 mg/kg, with further 9 mg/kg incremental doses as necessary, was reported as producing good immobilization (Borzio, 1973). Forbes (1991) recommended a sliding dosage: 30 mg/kg for up to 150 g bodyweight, 20 mg/kg for 200–400 g, 10 mg/kg for up to 1 kg but only 5 mg/kg for birds over 2 kg	First reported use in birds in 1972 (Mandelker, 1972). Historically, ketamine was the drug of choice; it is now used less often in avian practice, although it is useful for reducing stress when handling larger species such as swans or other waterfowl Ketamine has been used orally (Garner, 1988) as a means of immobilizing a captive-bred hawk that had flown off and was avoiding recapture. The dose used was 100 mg/kg in a 30 g piece of meat, although it took up to 2 h to have the desired effect. This route may also be used for catching ducks on a pond, free-ranging peacocks etc. Ketamine may give up to 30 min anesthesia, with full recovery taking up to 3 h (Ensley, 1979). The speed of recovery is dose-dependent, which is inversely proportional to the body size (Boever and Wright, 1975). Large waterfowl tend to recover more slowly than other birds because of their decreased metabolism	Ketamine by itself is a good sedative but a poor anesthetic, with poor muscle relaxation and little analgesia, although there is little respiratory or cardiovascular depression (Flammer, 1989). With ketamine, hippus (rhythmic contraction and dilation of the pupil) is seen until the bird becomes deeply anesthetized (Lawton, 1984) There is often wing flapping during recovery, even when used in combination with tranquilizers. This may continue for several minutes (Mandelker, 1987) The kidneys eliminate ketamine. Toxicity may be noted in debilitated or dehydrated birds, and those with renal dysfunction. IV fluids can hasten recovery from ketamine by causing diuresis Doses of 35 mg/kg IV may cause immediate cardiac arrest or prolonged apnea followed by cardiac arrest in a number of raptors, others that survive having convulsions after induction (Redig and Duke, 1976)
Ketamine/ diazepam or midazolam	Ketamine 10–30 mg/kg IV and diazepam 1–1.5 mg/kg IM or 0.2 mg/kg midazolam SC, IM	These are good combinations allowing a smooth induction and recovery when compared to ketamine by itself. The benefit of midazolam is that it can be mixed in the same syringe as ketamine, while diazepam has to be given as a separate injection	Mandelker (1988) considered these as the most effective combinations available but, with the introduction of medetomidine, which can be reversed, this no longer true
Ketamine/ medetomidine	1.5–2 mg/kg ketamine + 60–85 µg/kg medetomidine IM (reversed by atipamezole 250–380 µg/kg IM)	The addition of medetomidine provides sedative and analgesic properties, with good muscle relaxation but no arrhythmias or respiratory depression (Jalanka, 1989). This combination is particularly good for waterfowl	Medetomidine has hypotensive, bradycardic and hypothermic effects
Ketamine/ xylazine	4.4 mg/kg ketamine + 2.2 mg/kg xylazine IV (then reversed by yohimbine 0.1 mg) (atipamezole 250–380 µg/kg IM can be used to reverse the effects of xylazine)	The synergistic action of the combination of xylazine with ketamine produces smooth induction and improved muscle relaxation without difficulties in recovery due to residual ketamine effect (Degernes et al., 1988). Petruzzi et al. (1988) found that 18.5 mg/kg ketamine and 1.5 mg/kg xylazine to be effective in raptors	Unreversed, there is a prolonged recovery and postoperative depression that may result in the bird being unable to perch properly or unable to feed, leading to hypothermia, hypoglycemia, and even death (Lawton, 1984). Lumeij (1993) also reported two deaths postoperatively (24 h and 50 h) in goshawks, which were attributed to severe sinus bradycardia
Propofol	1.33–14 mg/kg IV	Very high safety margin and easily metabolized. A very smooth, rapid induction good muscle relaxation with a short duration of 2–7 min (Heard, 1997)	High cost. Propofol is metabolized far too quickly in birds to be of realistic use by itself as an agent for surgery. The combination of propofol and isoflurane may lead to difficulties in keeping the bird anesthetized. Intravenous propofol is

TABLE 4.2 Injectable anesthetic agents *(continued)*

Agent	Dose and route	Comments on use	Disadvantages
			considered to be more stressful than mask induction with isoflurane (Lawton 1996a, 1996b)
Tiletamine/zolazepam	5–10 mg/kg IM	Tiletamine is a phencyclidine derivative that is more potent than ketamine. This combination provides good immobilization and is considered safe (Kreeger *et al.*, 1993)	Tiletamine causes convulsions unless given with a sedative, thus the manufactured combination
Xylazine	1–20 mg/kg IM or IV (reversed with yohimbine hydrochloride, 0.1–0.2 mg/kg IV or atipamezole 250–380 µg/kg IM)	Seldom used as a sole agent	Xylazine by itself is unreliable, causes bradycardia and AV block and is extremely respiratory depressant (Mandelker, 1987). The bradycardic effects can be reduced if atropine is used. Raptors may show a hypersensitivity to external stimuli, including increased trembling, vocalization and labored respiration, and higher dosages did not increase the depth of sedation (Freed and Baker, 1989)

AV, atrioventricular; IM, intramuscular(ly); IP, intraperitoneal(ly); IV, intravenous(ly); SC, subcutaneous(ly).

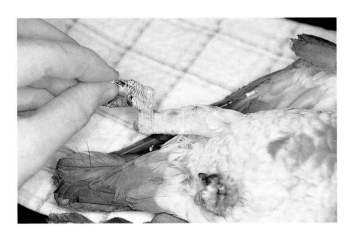

Fig. 4.26 Demonstration of the toe pinch reflex in an African gray parrot.

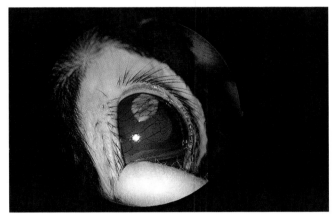

Fig. 4.27 The corneal reflex is one of the last reflexes to be abolished under anesthesia.

TABLE 4.3 Analgesic agents

Agent	Dose rate	Comments
Buprenorphine	0.02 mg/kg IM	Opiate analgesic that can cause some respiratory depression. I consider that this, in combination with carprofen, offers the best analgesia for severe trauma
Butorphanol	3 mg/kg IM	Has been used in parakeets (Bauck, 1990)
Carprofen	5–10 mg/kg IV, IM or PO	A very effective analgesic that can be used in combination with buprenorphine to have a synergistic effect in cases of severe pain. I have used this drug for long-term management of painful conditions without noted side effects
Flunixin–meglumine	1–10 mg/kg IM	Has been used, but carprofen is considered more effective
Ketoprofen	5–10 mg/kg IM	Better then flunixin but not as good as carprofen
Meloxicam	0.5–1 mg/kg PO twice daily	Half-life is shorter in large birds than in small birds (Wilson *et al.*, 2004)

IM, intramuscular(ly); IV, intravenous(ly); PO, oral(ly).

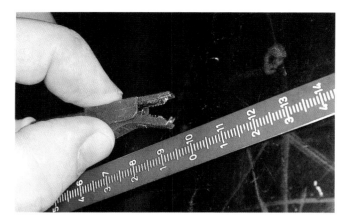

Fig. 4.28 Suitable small ECG clamp, which is relatively atraumatic.

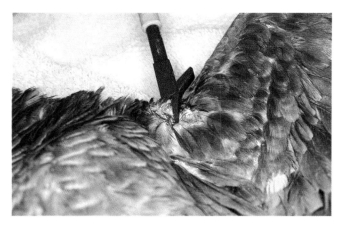

Fig. 4.29 Placement of an ECG clamp on to the wing, at elbow level, in an African gray.

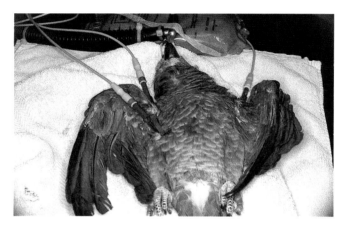

Fig. 4.30 The standard placement of electric leads for ECG monitoring in an African gray: one on each wing and one on the right hind leg.

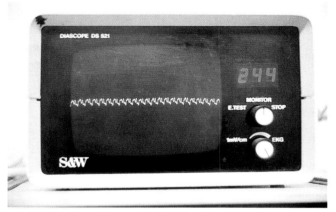

Fig. 4.31 The appearance of the ECG trace from an anesthetized African gray parrot.

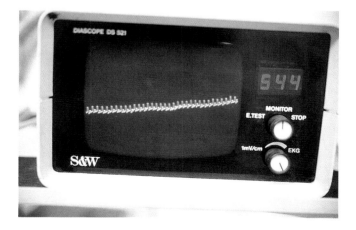

Fig. 4.32 The same ECG trace for an African gray parrot as shown in Fig. 4.31, but after a response to pain. The ECG trace is a very good method of establishing the depth of anesthesia in avian patients.

Doppler flow apparatus can also be used and may give an audible signal of arterial flow as well as monitoring heart rate and rhythm (Heard, 1997). Some manufacturers produce a cloacal probe, or alternatively a pediatric probe may also be used.

Respiration monitor

Electronic monitoring of respiration is considered the best indicator of the depth and stability of anesthesia in the absence of response to pain. The pattern of respiration is also important: it should be stable and continually monitored during anesthesia (Figs 4.33 and 4.34). A sudden change in pattern, especially in the depth of respiration (from shallow to deep), may indicate that the bird's plane of anesthesia is lightening or that the

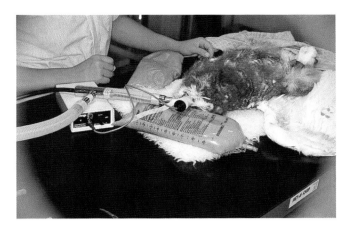

Fig. 4.33 Careful monitoring of an anesthetized owl with respiratory monitor and continuous visual monitoring.

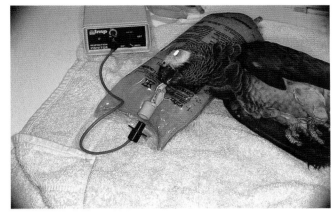

Fig. 4.34 Postoperatively an African gray parrot is disconnected from the anesthetic circuit, but a respiratory monitor probe is placed by the tube to continue monitoring respiration until the bird is fully recovered.

bird is feeling pain. As the bird enters a deeper plane of anesthesia, the rate and depth usually decrease. Depending on the bird's body size, the respiration rate should not fall below 25–50 beats/min (Doolen and Jackson, 1991); below this there is a risk of hypercapnia. The respiratory rate of any anesthetized bird should never fall below its normal resting rate (Coles, 1985).

The majority of respiratory monitors work on thermal changes between inspired and expired gases. This can lead to difficulty in measuring small birds, especially when the flow rates of the cold carrier gases are high. A sensitive cardiac monitor (especially if it has an amplifier) will pick up the movement of the respiratory muscles and allow a further method of assessing the respiration. Pulse oxymeters with a cloacal probe are useful to assess the oxygenation of the blood and also the rate of respiration. The use of IPPV allows the anesthetist to provide a defined suitable rate and depth of respiration, thus removing the requirement of further monitoring. This is particularly useful in a patient with underlying respiratory disease.

Respiration should be carefully monitored (even if just by watching the movement of the sternum) until the bird is fully recovered from the anesthetic. If isoflurane is being used, consideration should be given to holding the bird until it is recovered enough to perch (or to be released), allowing continuous observation. When injectable agents have been used, it may be necessary to strap or wrap the bird to prevent bruising or damage of the head or wings; this is particularly important when ketamine has been used (alone or in combination).

Temperature

Warmth should be provided before induction, during anesthesia and in the recovery period (Fig. 4.35). Sick or anesthetized birds may not be able to maintain their core body temperature adequately (Figs 4.36 and 4.37). Sick

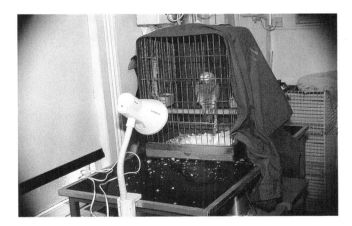

Fig. 4.35 An African gray parrot recovering from anesthesia is placed in a cage with an infrared lamp near to provide extra heat. Care has to be taken not to overheat the bird.

birds attempting to maintain their high core temperature may become hypoglycemic as a result of hypothermia. Hypothermia can cause peripheral vasoconstriction, bradycardia, hypotension and, when severe, ventricular fibrillation (Heard, 1997).

Anesthetizing a bird and placing it on to a cold operating table may result in a rapid fall in body temperature. The core body temperature of birds is usually between 40°C and 44°C (104–111.2°F) (Carter-Storm, 1988), with that of smaller birds being 41°C (105.8°F) (Cooper, 1989). Excessive removal of feathers or preoperative washing or application of surgical spirit at the site of surgery will result in lost insulation and heat loss. Anesthetized birds should be placed on to a towel or insulated Vetbed®; the use of heating pads or lights can also help to reduce heat loss but care must be taken to prevent overheating or burns. Bubble wrap or 'space' sheets can also be used for wrapping most of the bird to prevent unnecessary heat loss. The use of OpSite® (Smith & Nephew, Fig. 4.38) will reduce the need to pluck a bird bald yet maintain

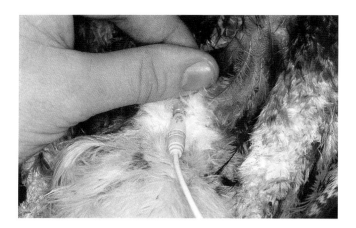

Fig. 4.36 Placement of a temperature probe into the vent of a Harris hawk (*Parabuteo unicinctus*).

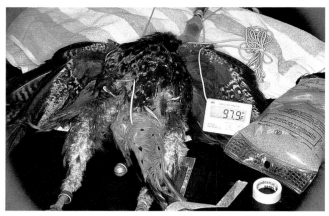

Fig. 4.37 An anesthetized Harris hawk showing the monitoring of core body temperature via a cloacal probe.

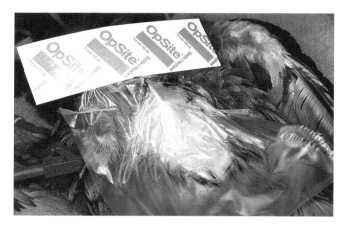

Fig. 4.38 The use of OpSite® surgical drape allows the removal of feathers to be kept to a minimum at the time of surgery. By reducing the quantity of feathers lost, the insulating properties of the plumage are not interfered with in the postoperative period.

procedures. Figs 4.39 and 4.40 illustrate the administration of anesthesia using isoflurane to a gyrfalcon (*Falco rusticolus*).

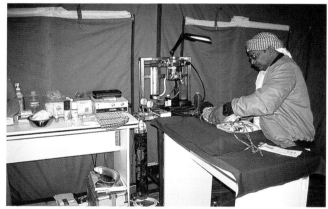

Fig. 4.39 A veterinary technician in the process of anesthetizing a gyrfalcon (*Falco rusticolus*) within a field hospital. (Courtesy of Dr. J. Samour).

an adequately clear surgical site. Cold anesthetic gases will also have a chilling effect on the bird but there is little that can be done to prevent this other than keeping the overall duration of anesthesia time to the shortest possible.

The cloacal temperature should be monitored during anesthesia (Doolen and Jackson, 1991). Likewise, a continuous assessment should be made of the degree of hemorrhage during surgery to prevent surgical shock and resultant hypothermia.

Anesthesia under field conditions

Nowadays modern hunting parties from the Middle East carry fully equipped field hospitals in which falcons can safely be anesthetized for different medical

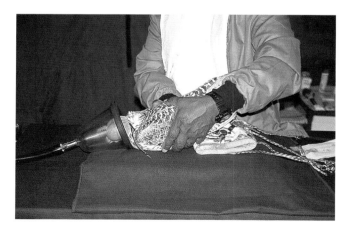

Fig. 4.40 The same falcon as in Fig. 4.39. Note that the hood has been left on the falcon while its head is within the face mask. This facilitates handling and restraint during the induction period. (Courtesy of Dr. J. Samour).

REFERENCES

Bauck L (1990) Analgesics in avian medicine. *Proceedings of the Association of Avian Veterinarians*, Phoenix, pp. 239–244.

Boever WJ, Wright W (1975) Use of ketamine for restraint and anesthesia of birds. *Veterinary Medicine/Small Animal Clinician* **70**: 86.

Borzio F (1973) Ketamine hydrochloride as an anesthetic for wildfowl. *Veterinary Medicine/Small Animal Clinician* **35**: 1364.

Burtnick NL, Degernes LA (1993) Electrocardiography of fifty-nine anesthetized convalescing raptors. In: Redig PT, Cooper JE, Remple JD et al. (eds) *Raptor Biomedicine*, pp. 111–121. University of Minnesota Press, Minneapolis.

Carter-Storm A (1988) Special considerations for general anesthesia of birds. *Clinical Insight* **2**(3):61.

Clutton RE (1986) Prolonged isoflurane anesthesia in the golden eagle. *Zoo Animal Medicine* **17**: 103.

Coles BH (1985) *Avian Medicine and Surgery*, 2nd edn. Blackwell Scientific, Oxford.

Cooper JE (1989) Anaesthesia of exotic species. In: Hilbery ADR, Waterman AE, Brouwer GJ (eds) *Manual of Anaesthesia of Small Animal Practice*, 3rd edn. British Small Animal Veterinary Association, Cheltenham.

Cooper JE, Frank LG (1973) The use of the steroid anesthetic CT 1341 in birds. *Veterinary Record* **92**: 474.

Cooper JE, Frank LG (1974) The use of the steroid anesthetic CT 1341 in birds. *Raptor Research* **8**: 20.

Cooper JE, Redig PT (1975) Unexpected reaction to the use of CT 1341 by red tailed hawks. *Veterinary Record* **97**: 352.

Degernes LA, Kreeger TJ, Redig PT (1988) Ketamine–xylazine anesthesia in red-tailed hawks with antagonism by yohimbine. *Journal of Wildlife Diseases* **24**: 322.

Dohoo SE (1990) Isoflurane as an inhalational anesthetic agent in clinical practice. *Canadian Veterinary Journal* **31**: 847.

Doolen MD, Jackson L (1991) Anesthesia in caged birds. *Iowa State University Veterinarian*, **53**(2): 76.

Edling TM (2003) Inhalation anesthesia, monitoring and anesthetic pain management. *Proceedings of the Association of Avian Veterinarians*, Pittsburgh, pp. 319–329.

Ensley P (1979) Cage bird medicine and husbandry. *Veterinary Clinics of North America: Small Animal Practice* **9**: 391.

Fedde MR (1986) Respiration. In: Sturkie PD (ed.) *Avian Physiology*, 4th edn, pp. 191–220. Springer-Verlag, New York.

Fitzgerald G, Blais D (1993) Inhalation anesthesia in birds of prey. In: Redig PT, Cooper JE, Remple JD et al. (eds) *Raptor Biomedicine*, pp. 128–135. University of Minnesota Press, Minneapolis.

Flammer K (1989) Update on avian anesthesia. In: Kirk RW, Bonagura JD (eds) *Current Veterinary Therapy* X. WB Saunders, Philadelphia.

Forbes NA (1991) Birds of prey. In: Beynon PH, Cooper JE (eds) *Manual of Exotic Pets*. British Small Animal Veterinary Association, Cheltenham.

Freed D, Baker B (1989) Antagonism of xylazine hydrochloride sedation in raptors by yohimbine hydrochloride. *Journal of Wildlife Diseases* **25**: 136.

Garner MM (1988) Use of an oral immobilizing agent to capture a Harris' hawk (*Parabuteo unicinctus*). *Journal of Raptor Research* **22**: 70.

Harcourt-Brown NH (1978) Avian anaesthesia in general practice. *Journal of Small Animal Practice* **19**: 573.

Heard DJ (1997) Anesthesia and analgesia. In: Altman RB, Clubb SL, Dorrestein GM, Quesenberry K (eds) *Avian Medicine and Surgery*, pp. 807–828. WB Saunders, Philadelphia.

Jalanka HH (1989) Chemical restraint and reversal in captive markhors (*Capra falconeri megaceros*): a comparison of two methods. *Journal of Zoo and Wildlife Medicine* **20**: 413.

James AE, Hutchings G, Bush M et al. (1976) How birds breathe: correlation of radiographic with anatomical and pathological studies. *Journal American Radiographic Society* **17**: 77.

Jenkins JR (1993) Post-operative care of the avian patient. *Seminars in Avian and Exotic Pet Medicine* **2**: 97–102.

King AS, McLelland J (1975) *Outline of Avian Anatomy*. Baillière Tindall, London.

Korbel R, Milovanovic A, Erhardt W et al. (1993) Aerosaccular perfusion with isoflurane – an anesthetic procedure for head surgery of birds. *Proceedings of the European Association of Avian Veterinarians*, Utrecht.

Kreeger TJ, Degernes LA, Kreeger JS, Redig PT (1993) Immobilization of raptors with tiletamine and zolazepam (Telazol). In: Redig PT, Cooper JE, Remple JD et al. (eds) *Raptor Biomedicine*, pp. 141–144. University of Minnesota Press, Minneapolis, MI.

Lawton MPC (1984) Avian anaesthesia. *Veterinary Record*, **115**: 71.

Lawton MPC (1996a) Anaesthesia. In: Beynon PH, Forbes NA, Lawton MPC (eds) *Manual of Psittacine Birds*, pp. 49–59. British Small Animal Veterinary Association, Cheltenham.

Lawton MPC (1996b) Anaesthesia. In: Beynon PH, Forbes NA, Harcourt-Brown NH (eds) *Manual of Raptors Pigeons and Waterfowl*, pp. 79–88. British Small Animal Veterinary Association, Cheltenham.

Lennox AM, Crosta L, Buerkle M (2002) The effects of isoflurane anesthesia on gastrointestinal transit time. *Proceedings of the Association of Avian Veterinarians*, Monterey, pp. 53–55.

Lumeij JT (1993) Effects of ketamine-xylazine anesthesia on adrenal function and cardiac induction in goshawks and pigeons. In: Redig PT, Cooper JE, Remple JD et al. (eds) *Raptor Biomedicine*, pp. 145–149. University of Minnesota Press, Minneapolis.

McLelland J (1990) *A Colour Atlas of Avian Anatomy*. Wolfe Publishing, London.

Mandelker L (1972) Ketamine hydrochloride as an anesthetic for parakeets. *Veterinary Medicine/Small Animal Clinician* **68**: 55.

Mandelker L (1987) Anesthesia and surgery. In: Burr EW (ed.) *Companion Bird Medicine*. Iowa State University Press, Ames, IA.

Mandelker L (1988) Avian anesthesia, part II: injectable agents. *Companion Animal Practice* **2**(10): 21.

Petruzzi V, Coda S, Ximenes LA, Naitana P (1988) L'associazione ketamina-xilazina nell' anesthesia generale dei rapaci. Valutazione di alcuni parametri vitali. *Documenti Veterinari* **6**: 59–62.

Redig PT, Duke GE (1976) Intravenously administered ketamine HCl and diazepam for anesthesia of raptors. *Journal of American Veterinary Medical Association*, **169**(9): 886.

Rosskopf WJ Jr, Woerpel RW (1996) Practical anesthesia administration. In: Rosskopf WJ Jr, Woerpel RW (eds) *Diseases of Cage and Aviary Birds*, 3rd edn, pp. 664–672. Williams & Wilkins, Baltimore.

Rosskopf WJ Jr, Woerpel RW, Reed S et al. (1992) Anesthetic agents: anaesthesia administration for pet birds. *Veterinary Practice Staff* **4**(2): 34.

Scheid P, Piiper J (1971) Direct measurement of the pathway of the respired gas in duck lungs. *Respiratory Physiology* **11**: 308.

Sinn LC (1994) Anesthesiology. In: Ritchie BW, Harrison GJ, Harrison LR (eds) *Avian Medicine: Principles and Applications*, pp. 1066–1074. Wingers Publishing, Lake Worth, FL.

Wilson GH, Hernandez-Divers S, Budsberg SC et al. (2004) Pharmacokinetics and use of meloxicam in psittacine birds. *Proceedings of the Association of Avian Veterinarians*, New Orleans, pp. 7–9.

Local anesthesia and analgesia

Judith C. Howlett

Local anesthesia

Local anesthetics have limited application and are not in standard use in avian anesthesia. This is partly due to the fact that birds are thought to be very sensitive to local analgesics. It is easy to overdose, and higher levels of the drug may be toxic. Another consideration is that the bird still has to be physically restrained even if a local anesthetic is successfully employed. The physical restraint can be very stressful for the bird and there may not therefore be any advantage over administering a general anesthetic.

Lignocaine

Dose rate if used as a local anesthetic should be diluted 0.2% or less.

Analgesia

Few studies have been carried out on the effects of analgesics in birds. They are thought to have relatively high pain thresholds. The following agents, which have been developed for use with horses or dogs, have been used in birds without adverse effect (Ritchie and Harrison, 1994). For more recent information the reader is referred to reviews by Paul-Murphy (2006) and Marx (2006).

Analgesic agents

Acetylsalicylic acid

- **Presentation**: Aspirin tablets – acetylsalicylic acid 5 g, 60 g
- **Uses**: May be effective as an analgesic, antipyretic and anti-inflammatory agent in some species
- **Dose rate**: No dosage recommendations are available. Murray (1994) recommends 30 mg/200 g bodyweight without adverse effect.

Buprenorphine hydrochloride

- **Presentation**: Vetergesic – buprenorphine hydrochloride 0.3 mg/ml
- **Pharmaceutical company**: Animalcare Limited (UK)
- **Uses**: Buprenorphine is a potent (opiate) long-acting analgesic and sedative used for relief of postoperative pain in dogs that appears to be effective in controlling pain in avian patients
- **Dose rate**: A dose of 0.1–0.5 mg/kg to provide postoperative analgesia
- **Contraindications**: Should not be used in birds with impaired liver or respiratory function, nor with other opioid type analgesics.

Butorphanol

- **Presentation**:
  - Torbugesic injection – butorphanol tartrate 10 mg/ml
  - Torbutrol injection – butorphanol 0.5 mg/ml
  - Torbutrol tablets – butorphanol 1 mg, 5 mg, 10 mg
- **Pharmaceutical company**: Willows Francis (UK)
- **Uses**: Butorphanol is a synthetic opiate used for antitussive effects and for analgesia and sedation. Used to control abdominal pain; can be used for postsurgical pain

- **Dose rate**: 1–2 mg/kg IM in African gray parrots and 1–3 mg/kg IM in Hispaniolan Amazon parrots (Paul-Murphy et al., 1999; Paul-Murphy and Ludders, 2001)
- **Contraindications**: Should be used with caution in birds with liver disease.

Flunixin-meglumine

- **Presentation**:
  - Finadyne injection – flunixin-meglumine 10 mg/ml
  - Finadyne granules – flunixin-meglumine 250 mg/10 g packet
  - Finadyne tablets – flunixin-meglumine 5 mg, 20 mg
- **Pharmaceutical company**: Schering–Plough Animal Health (UK)
- **Uses**: Flunixin-meglumine is a potent nonsteroidal, non-narcotic with anti-inflammatory, anti-endotoxic and antipyretic properties. May be helpful in some cases of shock and trauma. Antipyretic use in the cases of hyperthermia
- **Dose rate**: 1–10 mg/kg
- **Contraindications**: May cause vomiting and diarrhea in some birds.

Carprofen

- **Presentation**: Zenecarp Inj – carprofen 50 mg/ml
- **Pharmaceutical company**: C-Vet Veterinary Products (UK)
- **Uses**: Carprofen is a nonsteroidal anti-inflammatory drug with analgesic and antipyretic properties
- **Dose rate**: 5–10 mg/kg IM
- **Contraindications**: Should not be used in animals suffering from renal, hepatic or cardiac disease.

Ketoprofen

- **Presentation**: Ketofen 10% Inj – ketoprofen 100 mg/ml; Ketofen 5 mg, 20 mg tablets
- **Pharmaceutical company**: Rhone Mérieux (UK)
- **Uses**: Ketoprofen is a potent, non-narcotic, nonsteroidal anti-inflammatory agent with analgesic and antipyretic properties
- **Dose rate**: 5–10 mg/kg IM
- **Contraindications**: Not to be used in animals with impaired hepatic, renal or cardiac function.

Copper indometacin

- **Presentation**: Vetapharm Avi-gesic – copper indometacin 0.2 mg/ml
- **Pharmaceutical company**: Vetapharm, Wagga Wagga (Australia)
- **Uses**: Copper indometacin is a nonsteroidal anti-inflammatory agent with analgesic properties for birds
- **Dose rates**: 0.2 ml/100 g IM.

Meloxicam

- **Presentation**:
  - Metacam® Oral Suspension 1.5 mg/mL
  - Metacam® Injection 5 mg/mL

- **Pharmaceutical Company:** Boehringer Ingelheim (UK)
- **Uses:** Meloxicam is a COX2 selective NSAID with antipyretic, analgesic and anti-inflammatory properties. Can be used to control postoperative pain, and acute and chronic pain associated with musculoskeletal disorders
- **Dose rate:** Dose rates of 0.2–0.5 mg/kg. Oral suspension can be diluted for use with small species to give accurate dosing
- **Contraindications:** Can cause hepatic, renal and gastrointestinal

REFERENCES

Marx KL (2006) Therapeutic agents. In: Harrison GJ, Lightfoot TL (eds) *Clinical Avian Medicine*. Spix Publishing, Palm Beach, FL.

Murray M (1994) Management of critical avian trauma cases. In: Fudge A, Jenkins JR (eds) *Seminars in Avian and Exotic Animal Pet Medicine: Critical Care*. WB Saunders, Philadelphia.

Paul-Murphy J (2006) Pain management. In: Harrison GJ, Lightfoot TL (eds) Clinical avian medicine. Spix Publishing, Palm Beach, FL, pp. 233–239

Paul-Murphy J, Ludders J (2001) Avian analgesia. *Exotic Animal Practice* **4**: 35–45.

Paul-Murphy J, Brunson DB, Miletic V (1999) A technique for evaluating analgesia in conscious perching birds. *American Journal of Veterinary Research* **60**: 1213–1217.

Ritchie BW, Harrison GJ (1994) Formulary. In: Ritchie BW, Harrison GJ, Harrison LR (eds) *Avian Medicine: Principles and Application*, pp. 457–478. Wingers Publishing, Lake Worth, FL.

FURTHER READING

Hall LW, Clarke KW (1983) Anaesthesia of birds, laboratory animals and wild animals. In: Hall LW, Clarke KW (eds) *Veterinary Anaesthesia*, pp. 355–364. Baillière Tindall, London.

Lawton MPC (1996) Anaesthesia. In: Beynon PH, Forbes NA, Harcourt-Brown NH (eds) *Manual of Raptors, Pigeons and Waterfowl*, pp. 79–88. British Small Animal Veterinary Association, Cheltenham.

National Office of Animal Health (1998–99) NOAH – *Compendium of Data Sheets for Veterinary Products 1995–96*. National Office of Animal Health, Enfield, UK.

Paul-Murphy J, Fialkowski J (1991) Injectable anesthesia and analgesia in Birds. In: Gleed RD, Ludders JW (eds) *Recent Advances in Veterinary Anesthesia and Analgesia*. Companion Animals International Veterinary Information Service (www.vis.org) Ithaca, New York, USA.

Rosskopf WJ Jr, Woerpel RW (1996) Practical anesthesia administration. In: Rosskopf WJ Jr, Woerpel RW (eds) *Diseases of Cage and Aviary Birds*, 3rd edn, pp. 664–671. Williams & Wilkins, Baltimore.

Sinn LC (1994) Anesthesiology. In: Ritchie BW, Harrison GJ, Harrison LR (eds) *Avian Medicine: Principles and Application*, pp. 1066–1088. Wingers Publishing, Lake Worth, FL.

Hypothermia

Judith C. Howlett

Birds have a high basal metabolic rate and a high body temperature and therefore they metabolize drugs very quickly. Birds are physiologically less efficient than mammals at maintaining body temperature and consequently undergo more rapid changes in body temperature during anesthesia. Loss of heat during anesthesia can compromise the outcome of anesthetic survival. Birds will become hypoglycemic in an effort to produce body heat. Even with the supplementation of heat, there will still be a drop in core body temperature. The addition of heat will reduce the rate of heat loss, especially over a prolonged period.

Points to consider in the prevention/reduction of heat loss in avian anesthesia

- Ensure that the bird is kept in a warm environment before any surgical procedure involving anesthesia.
- Birds should be placed on a low-level heat pad and towel, or water circulating heat pads throughout anesthesia, to avoid contact with any cold conducting surface and to help minimize the loss of physiological responses as a result of reduced core body temperature.
- Temperature should be monitored throughout the procedure. It is important to record the cloacal temperature between 3 and 5 min to gain an accurate reading, whether using a traditional or electronic thermometer. The longer the procedure the greater the temperature loss, which can result in cardiac arrhythmia and prolonged recovery time. In severe temperature loss of over 5.6°C (10°F) the bird may not recover. If necessary, additional heat may be given in the form of heat lamps, wrapping in towels, warm IV drips, etc.
- Hypothermia can be induced by excessive removal of feathers for surgery and overliberal use of alcohol during the preparation; this should be kept to a minimum.
- Cool anesthetic gases through the respiratory tract can also affect the body temperature, although this cannot be avoided.
- On recovery the bird should be put back into a warm environment and monitoring should be continued until the bird is fully recovered.

FURTHER READING

Coles BH (1985) Anaesthesia. In: *Avian Medicine and Surgery*, 2nd edn, pp. 125–147. Blackwell Science, Oxford.

Harrison GJ, Lightfoot TL (eds) *Clinical Avian Medicine*. Spix Publishing, Palm Beach, FL.

Lawton MPC (1996) Anaesthesia. In: Beynon PH, Forbes NA, Harcourt-Brown NH (eds) *Manual of Raptors, Pigeons and Waterfowl*, pp. 79–88. British Small Animal Veterinary Association, Cheltenham.

Rosskopf WJ Jr, Woerpel RW (1996) Practical anesthesia administration. In: Rosskopf WJ Jr, Woerpel RW (eds) *Diseases of Cage and Aviary Birds*, 3rd edn, pp. 664–671. Williams & Wilkins, Baltimore.

Sinn LC (1994) Anesthesiology. In: Ritchie BW, Harrison GJ, Harrison LR (eds) *Avian Medicine: Principles and Application*, pp. 1066–1088. Wingers Publishing, Lake Worth, FL.

Anesthetic emergencies

Judith C. Howlett

As with any animal under anesthesia, a bird should be monitored regularly throughout the duration of the anesthetic. Isoflurane is now widely regarded as the safest anesthetic to use with birds. Monitoring of an anesthetic requires the undivided attention of the anesthetist, who may be either the veterinarian or veterinary nurse. The heart rate should be monitored either by auscultation with a stethoscope or electronically and should be recorded regularly. Any changes should be acted upon immediately. Respiration rate should also be counted regularly; an ECG combined with respiration monitor is also an advantage. Regular monitoring can help minimize problems that may occur and alert the anesthetist when they do, so prompt action may be taken.

It is advantageous to have an emergency kit on hand that includes drugs such as Dopram, so that they can be quickly found and administered as necessary.

Anesthetic emergencies

Respiratory depression

- Reduce level of anesthesia or switch off anesthetic gas
- Intubate if bird not already intubated
- Flush with O_2 until bird recovers
- Do not overventilate as this can wash out CO_2 and inhibit chemoreceptors stimulating ventilation
- Prognosis good.

Respiratory arrest

- If it occurs as a response to an injectable anesthetic, give the reversal agent intravenously immediately
- If as a result of inhalational anesthesia, switch off anesthetic gas and flush with O_2 only
- Intubate if bird not already intubated
- Inflate chest with gentle breaths through an endotracheal tube or administer O_2 by positive pressure ventilation if breathing does not resume
- Give Dopram IV or drops on the tongue
- Continue monitoring until the bird has fully recovered
- Prognosis good if using isoflurane.

Cardiac arrest

- Switch off anesthetic gas and use sternal massage
- Continue ventilation as for respiratory arrest
- Give IV or IC epinephrine or norepinephrine
- Poor prognosis.

Hemorrhage

- The blood volume of birds is small; care should be taken to minimize any surgical bleeding as shock may occur and, in severe cases, death
- Fluids should be given to increase the circulating blood volume.

FURTHER READING

Coles BH (1985) Anaesthesia. In: *Avian Medicine and Surgery*, 2nd edn, pp. 125–147. Blackwell Science, Oxford.

Harrison GJ, Lightfoot TL (eds) *Clinical Avian Medicine*. Spix Publishing, Palm Beach, FL.

Lawton MPC (1996) Anaesthesia. In: Beynon PH, Forbes NA, Harcourt-Brown NH (eds) *Manual of Raptors Pigeons and Waterfowl*, pp. 79–88. British Small Animal Veterinary Association, Cheltenham.

Rosskopf WJ Jr, Woerpel RW (1996) Practical anesthesia administration. In: Rosskopf WJ Jr, Woerpel RW (eds) *Diseases of Cage and Aviary Birds*, 3rd edn, pp. 664–671. Williams & Wilkins, Baltimore.

Sinn LC (1994) Anesthesiology. In: Ritchie BW, Harrison GJ, Harrison LR (eds) *Avian Medicine: Principles and Application*, pp. 1066–1088. Wingers Publishing, Lake Worth, FL.

Soft tissue surgery

Neil A. Forbes

Experience required

Any aspiring avian surgeon should first become a competent small animal surgeon. The sympathetic handling of soft tissues is mandatory for successful avian surgery. In view of small body size and increased metabolic rate, avian surgery demands exactness and precision, as any errors are magnified. Surgery on birds of less than 2 kg requires micro surgical techniques and equipment, together with a significant manual dexterity. For avian surgery to be safe and effective, hemorrhage, tissue trauma and anesthetic time, as well as anesthetic and metabolic complications, must all be minimized and good postoperative care (including analgesia) is mandatory.

Preparation

Energy and nutritional status must be assessed and any circulatory or blood deficit corrected. Intraoperative and postoperative hypothermia, analgesia, sepsis and shock must be controlled (see Anesthesia section, above). Presurgical starvation should be sufficient purely to ensure an empty crop (budgerigar 1 h, parrot 3 h, raptor 6–8 h). Crop emptying time varies with species, weight, health and the food ingested. Starvation should not exceed that essential minimum, especially in smaller species, which will rapidly become hypoglycemic (see above). All birds over 100 g are intubated to protect the airway from gastric reflux.

Equipment required

Hypothermia

Heat loss should be minimized and an external source of heat provided.

Skin preparation

Sufficient feathers are removed (never flight feathers) to enable adequate sterile access to the operative site. Adjacent feathers may be retracted with proprietary office adhesive tape. The use of adhesive transparent surgical drapes facilitates patient observation, minimal feather removal and control of heat loss.

Sterile cotton buds

These are invaluable for applying 'point pressure' to control hemorrhage, as well as moving tissues in an atraumatic manner.

Magnification

Some form of magnification is essential for all patients under 1 kg in size. A bifocal surgical lens attached to a rechargeable halogen light source, with a variable focal distance, is ideal; economic alternatives are not ideal but remain practical.

Microsurgical instruments

A small number of high-quality instruments with miniaturized ends but standard handles, preferably counter weighted (to minimize finger fatigue), are required – fine-pointed scissors, needle holders, 2× artery forceps, atraumatic grasping forceps (e.g. Harris ring tip forceps), a retractor (e.g. Alm) – are the essentials. Delicate tissues must be handled in an atraumatic, sympathetic manner. Instruments are delicate and their care is essential. Where possible, handles should be round in outline, so that instrument tip movement can be accomplished by a finger rolling action, rather than the more normal wrist movement, to reduce tissue trauma. Spring-loaded locking instruments will also greatly assist in reducing finger fatigue.

Suture materials

The minimum number of sutures should be used, employing a monofilament material 4-0–6-0, causing minimal tissue reaction. Taper-cut swaged-on needles are indicated in most situations. Required suture strength duration relates to the speed of tissue healing. Tendons, ligaments and fascia heal slowly (50% strength in 50 days) and should be repaired using polydioxanone or nylon. Birds tolerate bandages or dressings poorly. In areas where some additional support is required over a suture line, hydrocolloidal skin dressings (Granuflex®, Convatec®) may be sutured in place. These dressings will promote healing while preventing traction over the wound.

Hemoclips (and applicators)

These are essential for clamping intra-abdominal vessels where ligation is not practical.

Radiosurgery

The correct use of radiosurgery will facilitate incision (monopolar forceps) while avoiding excessive tissue damage, in the absence of hemorrhage. Accurate control of bleeding points (using the bipolar forceps) is possible. Hemorrhage control prevents blood loss and maintains uninterrupted visualization of the surgical field, thus reducing surgical time and facilitating precision of surgery. A unit with a frequency of 3.8–4.0 MHz, and monopolar and bipolar electrodes is required. The smallest possible electrode size is always used, in order to minimize lateral heat and hence collateral tissue damage. The electrode should be in contact with the tissue for the minimum time possible, to minimize tissue damage. Once a cut has been made the operator should not return to the same tissue with a single wire within 7 s, or 15 s if it is a loop electrode. Fully rectified, fully filtered (90% cutting 10% coagulation) current should be used for cutting skin and biopsy collection. Fully rectified (50% cutting and 50% coagulation) current should be used for dissection with hemostasis, while partially rectified (10% cutting, 90% coagulation) current should be used for coagulation.

Surgical lasers

Laser surgery is now more readily available. Tissues may be cut or ablated (vaporized) using contact (least collateral damage – typically 300–600 u) or non-contact (when visualization is improved, although lateral damage tends to be slightly greater) modes. Using either technique, blood vessels of up to 2 mm diameter may be incised in the absence of any hemorrhage. Laser surgery can be used endoscopically. There is no doubt that the application of surgical lasers will have an increasing role in avian surgery during the next few years (Bartels, 2002). The main advantages are the reduction of edema, postoperative swelling, lateral damage and healing times, and less postoperative pain, enabling more extensive procedures (e.g. orchidectomy) to be performed.

Microsurgery

Surgeons must gain familiarization with magnification. Slight instrument movements are exaggerated when magnified; however the surgeon's natural ability to control such movements is improved by magnification. Increased manual control is essential, which necessitates a sitting position with forearm support. Assess all risks and possible complications prior to surgery so that you are not fazed by them as they occur. Never commence surgery unless you are wholly familiar with the anatomy. Ensure that all the equipment that is required for a procedure is available and sterile prior to anesthetic induction. The operating table must be stable (against movement of people or machinery in the vicinity) and staff should be advised not to touch or knock the table during surgery as even slight patient movements result in significant surgical risks.

Surgery of the skin and adnexa

Feather cysts (plumafolliculoma)

These are ingrown feathers causing significant inflammatory swellings. They occur most commonly at the sites of insertion of primary or secondary flight feathers. They may occur subsequent to infection or trauma (including flight feather plucking). Feather cysts are common in canaries and are considered to be hereditary. Under anesthesia cysts may be lanced and cleaned out in the hope that the feather will then grow back normally; such an approach should initially be used for tail and primary flight feathers. Alternatively, the entire cyst, including the dermal papilla, may be surgically removed.

Uropygial (or preen) gland

The uropygial gland may suffer from ductal blockage, gland abscessation or neoplasia. Blockage is often overcome with digital pressure, resulting in a jet of thick, oily secretion. Infection and neoplasia can be difficult to differentiate as both result in a significant inflammatory response. Adenoma, adenocarcinoma and squamous cell carcinoma may occur. A biopsy should always be taken in cases of doubt. Abscesses are treated by curettage, topical and systemic antibiosis. Hemi- or complete preen gland removal is typically indicated in neoplastic cases. Surgical removal must extend to the avascular ventral fibrous connective tissue that attaches firmly to the dorsal surface of the pygostyle and caudal vertebrae. The two sides of the gland are separated by a central septum; in early cases, one side of the gland alone may be removed. The skin overlying the gland should be preserved in order to enable postoperative closure.

Treating soft tissue wounds and injuries

Birds typically have very thin skin, with minimal soft tissue structures (in particular on the extremities). In birds, desiccation and devitalization of subcuticular tissues following loss of skin integrity is common. If skin cannot be closed for first intention healing, then desiccation must be prevented by application of hydrocolloidal or vapor membrane dressings. Tissue damage/necrosis/organic contamination or significant bacterial or fungal infection will preclude first-intention healing (Redig, 1996). In the majority of cases, debridement and irrigation will facilitate primary-intention closure. The commonest site for skin deficit is the cranium (subsequent to trauma while in flight). In these cases single-pedicle or bi-pedicle cervical grafts may be used to move loose skin from the neck up over the deficit. Free skin grafting tends not to be successful. Skin closure may be achieved with vertical or horizontal mattress sutures, in particular if there is potential for wound site tension. Psittacine wounds are generally best protected (e.g. hydrocolloidal sewn on dressings) or covered, although parrots are generally reluctant to accept bandaging.

Neoplasms

Birds, like all species, suffer from a range of cutaneous, subcutaneous and internal neoplasms. Approach to these should be similar to that used in other species. Fine-needle aspiration or biopsy is indicated prior to removal. Species, site and age maybe predictive in relation to tumor type (Forbes et al., 2000).

Lipoma

A benign tumor of fat tissue, lipoma is a common finding in many psittacine species, particularly budgerigars. Lipomas are commonly situated over the bird's breast. Affected birds may present with a ventrally displaced tail. Obesity should be controlled prior to surgery. Birds on seed-based diets should be converted to a lower energy diet. Dietary L-carnitine may facilitate nonsurgical resolution of lipoma (De Voe et al., 2003).

Xanthoma

These are non-neoplastic masses, commonly found on extremities, especially following trauma or hemorrhage. Microscopically, intradermal deposits of cholesterol clefts are evident with an associated inflammation. They often present as yellowish subcutaneous plaques, diffuse thickening or lobulated masses, which on occasions ulcerate. Xanthomas are naturally highly vascularized and invasive. Reduction of the dietary fat content may assist but surgical removal (if possible) at initial presentation is recommended. If, after removal, the skin cannot be closed, the deficit may be covered with tissue glue. If the wing tip is affected, amputation is indicated.

Gastrointestinal tract techniques

Tongue

Psittacines use their tongues and chew on solid, hard, abrasive and fragmentary objects; penetrations, lacerations and foreign bodies in the psittacine tongue do occur. Any recurrent or nonhealing lesion of the tongue should be fully investigated with this in mind. Differential diagnosis includes *Cryptococcus neoformans*, mycobacteria and neoplasia. Tongue pathology may be caused by candidiasis, trichomoniasis or bacterial granuloma. Noninfectious differential diagnoses include hypovitaminosis A (cysts or abscesses), lymphoreticular neoplasia, cystadenoma and squamous cell carcinoma.

Proximal esophagus

Esophageal stricture formation may occur after infections (trichomoniasis, capillariasis, candidiasis), tube feeding trauma, thermal or caustic trauma, foreign body ingestion or iatrogenic surgical trauma. An ingluviostomy tube may be placed to facilitate supportive and medical care. Strictures may be relieved by serial mechanical dilation using esophageal balloon dilators, cuffed endotracheal tubes or passing tubes or cannulae of increasing size over several weeks.

Ingluviotomy

This is indicated for the retrieval of crop, proventricular or ventricular foreign bodies (using magnets encased in plastic tubes, lavage or endoscopy), the placement of an ingluviotomy or proventriculotomy tube, or the collection of biopsies (Fig. 4.41). Crop calculi, ingluvioliths or 'sour crop' are resolved by ingluviotomy. The

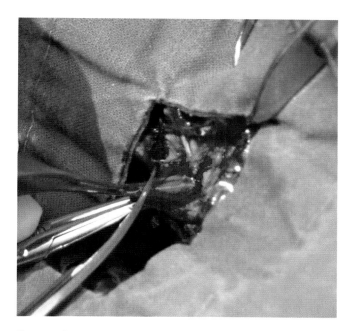

Fig. 4.41 Crop biopsy for the diagnosis of proventricular dilation disease.

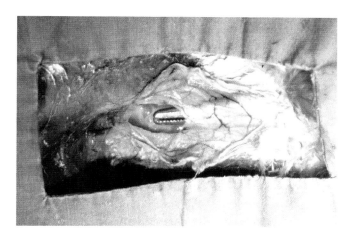

Fig. 4.42 Ingluviotomy incision.

bird is placed in dorsal or lateral recumbency; intubated, with the head elevated above the level of the crop. A probe is placed per os into the crop to delineate the position of the organ. The skin is incised over the left lateral crop wall, close to the thoracic inlet (Fig. 4.42). The crop wall is localized and isolated. An incision site is selected to avoid blood vessels and such that post-operative tube feeding is not compromised. Stay sutures are placed in the crop and an incision one-third to half the length of the skin incision is made. Crop closure is achieved with 4-0–6-0 synthetic monofilament absorbable material, using a continuous double inversion pattern, followed by skin closure.

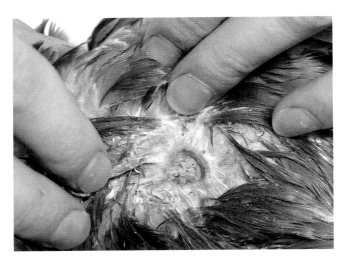

Fig. 4.43 Crop burn in a young African gray parrot (*Psittacus erithacus*).

Crop burns

These arise subsequent to feeding overheated (commonly microwaved) food (Fig. 4.43). Surgical repair should not be attempted for at least 4 days, such that devitalized tissue can be differentiated from healthy tissue. The crop wall and skin will be adherent. These layers are separated, all devitalized tissue is removed and the crop wall and skin are closed as above.

Crop or esophageal lacerations

These may occur following traumatic tube feeding or external trauma (e.g. talon punctures from a raptor). Tears are often not recognized at the time of trauma but instead later when a significant build-up of fetid toxin-producing food material has occurred subcutaneously. Surgical exploration, closure of the crop wound, drainage (pharyngostomy tube placement if required), fluid therapy, analgesia, anti-inflammatory and antibiotic therapy will be required prior to surgical skin closure for some days.

Ingluviostomy tube placement

Tube placement is indicated where the mouth, proximal or distal esophagus or crop requires bypass. The bird is prepared and an ingluviotomy is performed and crop emptied. An appropriately sized rubber or plastic feeding tube is passed via the incision into the esophagus and advanced caudally into the proventriculus. A skin suture is placed around the tube exit point. Tape is placed either side of the feeding tube as it exits the skin incision and is sutured to the skin. The capped feeding end is attached to the bird's back. Regular small meals are administered; the tube is flushed clean after each use. A tube may be left in situ for several weeks.

Celiomic surgery

Celiotomy

Opening of the posterior airsacs is inevitable during celiotomy. This leads to loss of volatile anesthetic agents from the airsac together with increased heat loss. Surgical openings may be packed off or plugged with abdominal organs. Alternatively, parenteral anesthetic agents may be used. During any celiotomy procedure, the bird's head should be raised at 30–40° to prevent any surgical irrigation fluid from entering the lung field.

Left lateral celiotomy

This is the most useful approach and is used for access to the gonads, left kidney, oviduct, ureter, proventriculus and ventriculus. The bird is placed in right lateral recumbency. The uppermost wing should be reflected dorsally while the left leg is restrained in a dorsocaudal direction. The skin web between the abdominal wall and the left leg is incised to facilitate further abduction of the left leg. A skin incision is created from the sixth rib to the level of the pubic bone on the left abdominal wall (Fig. 4.44). The superficial medial femoral artery and vein will be visualized traversing dorsal to ventral across the lateral abdominal wall ventral to the coxofemoral joint. These vessels should be cauterized with the bipolar forceps prior to transection (Fig. 4.45). The musculature (external and internal abdominal oblique and transverse abdominal muscles) should be tented up away from the celomic contents and incised with sharp, fine scissors. The incision is extended from the pubis to the 8th rib. Bipolar forceps are extended from a caudal position around the anterior aspect of the 8th rib to cauterize the intercostal vessels prior to transecting the rib (with large scissors) (Fig. 4.46). The same procedure is repeated with the 7th rib. A retractor

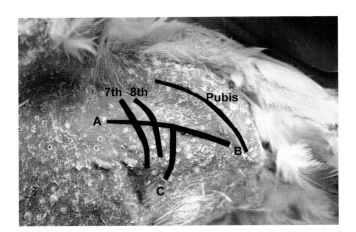

Fig. 4.44 Celiotomy approach, showing landmarks, 7th and 8th rib and pubis, and incision site (A–B) with extension flap (C).

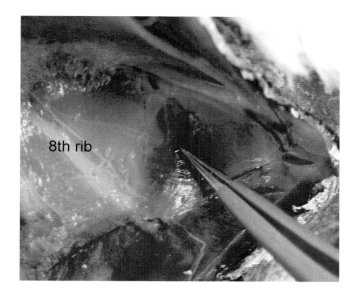

Fig. 4.45 Radiosurgery of medial femoral artery and vein.

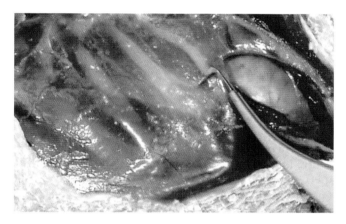

Fig. 4.46 Bipolar radiosurgical cauterization of intercostal vessels.

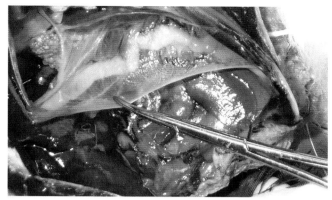

Fig. 4.47 Salpingohysterectomy with ventral oviductal ligament broken down.

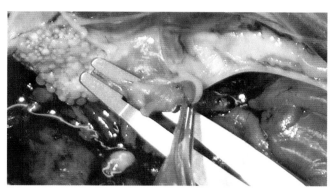

Fig. 4.48 Application of a hemoclip between the infundibulum and the ovary.

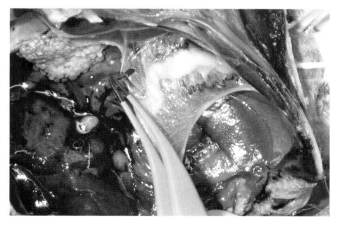

Fig. 4.49 Bipolar cutting and cauterization of the dorsal oviductal ligament.

(e.g. Heiss, Alm or Lonestar) is applied to enable full visualization of the abdominal cavity. On completion of the intercelomic surgery, the incision is closed using 4-0–6-0 absorbable monofilament synthetic material in a continuous or interrupted pattern in two layers. The intercostal muscles are opposed and no attempt is made to rejoin the transected ribs.

Preconditioning

If time permits, surgery may be delayed to facilitate involution of the gonads (medically or by reduced day light), so as to reduce gonad size and blood supply.

Salpingohysterectomy

Removal of the avian ovary is challenging and dangerous (as it is firmly attached to the dorsal abdominal wall). Cessation of egg laying may be achieved by *total* removal of the oviduct and uterus. A review of ovariectomy techniques is discussed by Echols (2002). The oviduct is recognized as a white structure (compared with gut) found ventral to the caudal lobes of the kidney. The ventral suspensory ligament (of the oviduct and uterus) is broken down with blunt dissection (Fig. 4.47). A significant blood vessel enters the infundibulum from the ovary on its medial aspect. The latter should be clamped off with two hemoclips prior to transection (Fig. 4.48). The dorsal suspensory ligament of the uterus

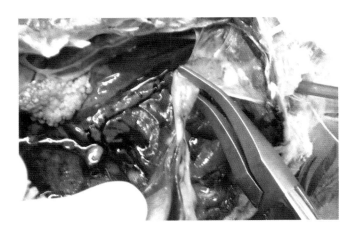

Fig. 4.50 Hemoclip application to the distal oviduct.

should be identified extending from the dorsal abdominal wall to the uterus. In this ligament are a number of blood vessels, which should be coagulated or clipped (Fig. 4.49). The uterus and oviduct are then exteriorized. Moving dorsocaudally towards the cloaca care is taken not to damage the ureters. The placement of a cotton bud per cloaca will assist in delineating where the uterus should be clamped off. The latter is achieved by applying two clips to the uterus and transecting on the uterine side of these (Fig. 4.50). All hemorrhage is controlled prior to closure of the abdominal muscle wall and the skin, each with a simple continuous suture pattern.

Egg-binding (dystokia)

Cesarian section

Where a hen is suffering from egg binding and both the egg and hen are of high financial or conservational value or she is suffering from egg binding that is nonresponsive to medical intervention or per cloacal egg implosion, cesarian section may be considered as an alternative. Typically a midline incision is indicated. The oviduct is incised directly over the egg, avoiding significant blood vessels. After egg removal, the oviduct is inspected and the cause of binding determined and rectified. If correction is impossible, salpingohysterectomy is indicated at a later date. The oviduct is closed with single interrupted or continuous pattern using 1.5 m (4–0) or finer absorbable material.

Uterine torsion

Egg binding may arise from a range of etiologies. If the condition does not respond to medical support, in particular if there is a markedly swollen celom, then torsion of the oviduct may be present (Harcourt-Brown, 1996). A number of eggs in a varying state of decay may be present in the proximal oviduct. Torsion typically occurs subsequent to traumatic breach of the oviductal suspensory ligament through which the oviduct will have passed. Such patients are often in poor condition and

represent poor surgical cases. With the bird stabilized, a ventral midline incision gives access the oviduct. The torsion may be reduced (surgical drainage of the oviduct may be required) and the ruptured suspensory ligament repaired. Alternatively a salpingohysterectomy may be performed.

Orchidectomy

The testicles (like the ovaries) are attached to the dorsal abdominal wall adjacent to the aorta, and connected only by a short testicular artery. The left testicle is identified, the caudal pole is elevated and a hemoclip is placed under the testicle (Fig. 4.51). The testicle is then surgically cut away from the clip, after which a further clip is applied from the caudal direction, between the testicle and the existing clip, so the process is continued until the testicle can be totally removed. If any testicular tissue is left, there is a possibility of regeneration. Access to the right testicle will be more difficult requiring blunt dissection through the airsac wall, or via a fresh incision on the contralateral abdominal wall.

Neutering

Neutering as described above is a high risk procedure while a vasectomy is less risky. Salpingohysterectomy has previously been recommended to prevent breeding. The current view is that, with the reduction of the energy density of the diet (by converting seed and nut eating birds to a pelleted and fresh fruit and vegetable diet), together with the initial use of leuprolide acetate (a GnRH agonist) and the institution of behavioral modification training (to gain dominance over the bird), surgery is rarely indicated.

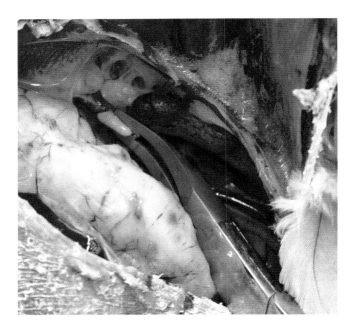

Fig. 4.51 Hemoclip application to left testis from the caudomedial aspect.

Endoscopic testicular biopsy

This is indicated in order to investigate the reason for clear egg production.

Proventriculotomy for access to proventriculus or ventriculus

Proventriculotomy is most commonly indicated for the removal of foreign objects, which are not retrievable per os or ingluvies. Proventricular biopsy is not recommended as the diagnostic method of choice where proventricular dilation disease is suspected, in view of the unacceptable risk of postoperative wound dehiscence with serious complications (McCluggage, 1992). Although the technique has been described, ventriculotomy is generally avoided, in view of the highly muscular walls (the physiological postoperative muscular activity of the ventricular wall), the inability to form an inversion closure and the increased vascularity compared with the proventriculus. Ventricular foreign bodies can be accessed via an incision in the isthmus between the proventriculus and the ventriculus. Access is gained via the left lateral celiotomy approach; sufficient exposure is necessary to visualize the suspensory membranes and to avoid the proventricular vessels along its greater curvature. The ventriculus (gizzard) is identified as a muscular organ with a white tendinous lateral aspect. Blunt dissection is used to break down the ventricular suspensory attachments. Two stay sutures are placed in the tendinous lateral aspect of the ventriculus, and exteriorized if possible (Fig. 4.52). The abdomen should be packed off around the ventriculus, with gauze swabs to minimize the effect of any leakage. The

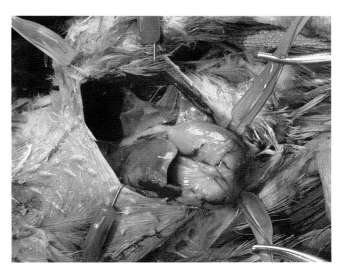

Fig. 4.52 Exteriorization of ventriculus by placement of stay sutures in the ventricular fascia.

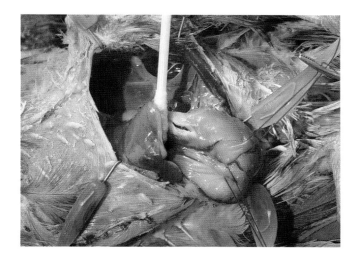

Fig. 4.53 Proventricular–ventricular isthmus showing incision site for access to ventricular lumen.

triangular portion of liver, which covers the isthmus, is identified. Using a sterile cotton bud, the liver is elevated, revealing the optimum incision site into the isthmus (junction between the proventriculus and the ventriculus) (Fig. 4.53). An initial stab incision is made, which is extended with iris scissors. Suction should be available to remove enteric contents in a controlled manner. Enteric contents are removed, after which an endoscope may be passed into the lumen to verify that all foreign objects have been removed. The incision is closed in two continuous layers (opposed then inverted) using 4-0–8-0 synthetic absorbable mono-filament material. After closure the liver is tacked over the incision site. The proventricular wall is deficient in collagen and so sutures tear readily as they are tightened. Sutures should be placed a sufficient distance from the wound edge but not so far that undue pressure is required to close the wound, so as to minimize the risk of tearing. As birds have no mesentery, enterotomy carries a higher risk of postoperative leakage and peritonitis. The liver instead overlies the incision, serving the same role. Ventricular suspensory ligaments are not repaired. Abdominal wall closure is as described above.

Neoplasia of the proventriculus and ventriculus is uncommonly reported in psittacine birds. In the author's experience they are most commonly presented in aged (over 30 years) Amazon parrots (*Amazona* sp.). Carcinoma of the proventriculus occurs more commonly than adenocarcinoma of the ventriculus. Clinical signs may include the passage of undigested seed and regurgitation. The bird may appear sick and weak, often suffering from secondary infections or other complications. Sizable lesions may be seen radiographically and may be confirmed following per os endoscopic biopsy. The gross appearance of proventricular adenocarcinoma is often not striking and is only likely to be differentiated on histopathological examination. By the time of diagnosis, such cases do not normally lend themselves to surgical correction. However such lesions are often amenable to chemotherapy using cisplatin 1 mg/kg every 7 d on three occasions (Fillipich *et al.*, 1999).

Yolk sacculectomy

In neonate chicks, the presence of an infected or unretracted yolk sac necessitates surgical removal. Clinical signs include anorexia, lethargy, constipation, diarrhea, weight loss and abdominal distension. Following induction of anesthesia, the bird is placed in dorsal recumbency. A small incision is delicately created cranial to the umbilicus. This incision is extended around the umbilicus and the umbilical stump is excised. The yolk sac is exteriorized and the duct ligated. Care is taken to avoid rupture or spillage of the yolk sac contents. The abdominal incision is closed in two layers. Survival rates for such surgery in sick psittacine neonates are not good. As yolk sac retention is frequently linked to incubation abnormalities, there may be other simultaneous pathology.

Enterotomy

Enterotomy is an infrequent procedure typically necessitated following trauma to the gastrointestinal tract, iatrogenic surgical damage, intussusception, torsion, adhesions, enteroliths or areas of necrosis. The procedure carries a guarded to grave prognosis. If colon is prolapsed via the cloaca (Fig. 4.54), an intussusception must be present. Such cases require an immediate midline (with or without flap) celiotomy, reduction of the intus-

susception and removal of any devitalized gut. Intussusception may be secondary to linear foreign bodies or subsequent to enteric infections. If the patient is shocked it may be prudent to create a stoma or a loop colostomy, with reattachment several days later (VanDerHeyden, 1993). Midline flap incisions give optimal access. Microsurgical instrumentation and techniques are mandatory. Blood vessel appositional clamps (e.g. Acland clamps) are invaluable to atraumatically achieve intraoperative intestinal occlusion while simultaneously maintaining the tissue sections in apposition during suture placement. Vascular clamps prevent tissue slippage but are only low-pressure to minimize tissue damage. When passing needles through fine tissue, it is important that the needle is encouraged to follow its natural curvature, otherwise an excessive needle hole is created. Finger rolling action on round-bodied needle holders, as opposed to wrist action, minimizes tissue damage.

Intestinal anastomosis

This may be achieved with end-to-end (Fig. 4.55) or side-to-side methods. If the gut is less than 2 mm in diameter then six to eight simple interrupted sutures are used (similar to a blood vessel anastomosis). If the gut is more than 2 mm in diameter a continuous pattern should be used. The advantages of a continuous pattern is that it reduces surgery time, yields improved apposition and so reduces risk of leakage, reduces tissue irritation and

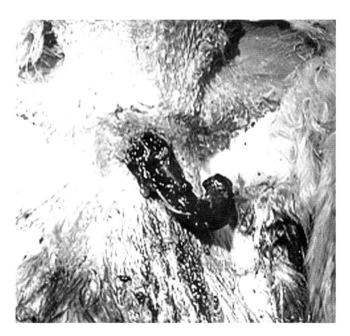

Fig. 4.54 • Colon prolapsed per cloaca.

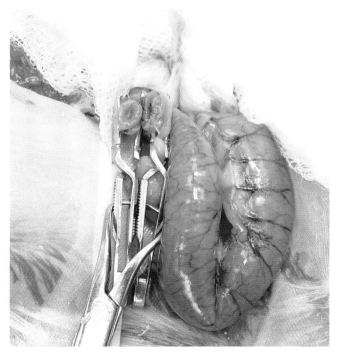

Fig. 4.55 Application of clamps in preparation for end-to-end intestinal anastomosis.

achieves improved endothelialization. Care should be taken not to overtighten a continuous pattern, as this would then cause a purse string and compromise food passage across the repair site.

Sutures are initially placed at 12 pm and 6 pm then sutures are placed in the caudal section of gut before placing sutures in the anterior aspect. If the sections of gut being joined are of unequal size, or where end-to-end anastomosis is technically difficult for other reasons, a side-to-side or side-to-end technique may be used. If using a side-to-side the end sections may be closed with sutures or hemoclips. One section of gut is offered up to the side of the other and the back of the anastomosis is sutured, prior to the aperture being created and then the front being sutured. If necessary, the front repair sutures may be pre-placed.

Ventral midline celiotomy

This approach gives poor visibility of the majority of the celiom. Nevertheless, it will facilitate surgery of the small intestine, pancreatic biopsy, liver biopsy or colopexy and is used in diffuse abdominal disease such as peritonitis, egg binding and cloacal prolapses. The bird is placed in dorsal recumbency, the midline prepared and the legs abducted caudally. The skin of the abdominal wall is tented and an initial incision is made using scissors or the single wire radiosurgical electrode (care is required to prevent iatrogenic visceral damage). The risk is minimized by creating the incision caudally over the cloaca rather than over the small intestine. The incision is extended with fine scissors. This approach can be extended along the costal border cranially and to the pubis caudally to create a flap on one of both sides of the midline to increase access. This approach is particularly useful for access to the caudal uterus and cloaca.

Cloacal conditions

Cloacal conditions are common in pet birds, with varied etiologies such as cloacitis (caused by papilloma, neoplasia), urolith, mycobacteriosis, parasitic, neoplasia, cloacal prolapse associated with oviductal or urethral obstruction, other oviductal disease or behavioral (hypersexuality and lack of dominance) abnormalities (Crib, 1984; Sundberg *et al.*, 1986; VanDerHeyden, 1988; Lumeij, 1994; Best, 1996; Antinoff *et al.*, 1997; Taylor and Murray, 1999).

Organs prolapsed through the cloaca

Apart from partial cloacal prolapses, prolapsed cloacal masses (papilloma (Fig. 4.56), neoplasia or mycobacterial granuloma – see Ch. 5 for differential diagnosis), total prolapses can occur, where the colonic, urethral and

oviductal junctions may be everted. Alternatively, the oviduct or colon may be prolapsed (Fig. 4.57). Differentiation of the tissues involved is important and is achieved by assessing the size of the structures present (Best, 1996). Birds presented with such prolapses are typically extremely shocked. Fluid therapy, analgesia and anti-inflammatory therapy are all mandatory. If a colonic or uterine prolapse is present, inevitably there must be an intussusception. Pushing the offending organ back through the cloacal opening and placing

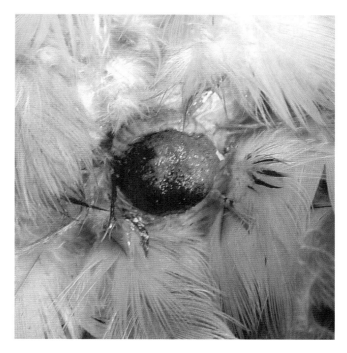

Fig. 4.56 Cloacal papillomas.

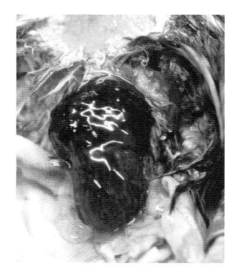

Fig. 4.57 Oviduct prolapse per cloaca.

a purse string suture along will not lead to a satisfactory outcome. Such action must be followed by a celiotomy, and reduction of, or removal of the intussuscepted material.

Cloacolith

These are firm, rough surfaced aggregations of urates. They are uncommon and the pathogenesis is unclear. In the author's experience these occur most frequently in carnivorous birds, especially in birds that have recently undergone extended nesting or brooding behavior, such that they may not have voided feces as frequently as normal. Birds present with repeated straining, often passing scant traces of blood. The condition is readily diagnosed on digital exploration of the cloaca. The bird is anesthetized; the cloacolith may be fragmented with artery forceps and removed piecemeal. Analgesics and antibiosis should be administered. There is often an area of severe inflammation in the ventral wall of the cloaca. The patient should undergo cloacal endoscopic examination 10–14 d after treatment to ensure that there is no reoccurrence.

Liver biopsy

With the patient in dorsal recumbency a 2–3 cm incision through skin and then abdominal musculature is created parallel to and 0.5 cm caudal to the caudal edge of the sternum just lateral to the midline (Fig. 4.58). The liver will be identified beneath the sternum. The liver is visually examined for any apparent lesions. If a specific lesion is present then biopsy at that site is indicated. If no discrete lesion is apparent a wedge biopsy is collected

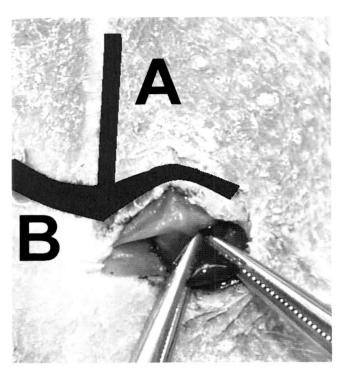

Fig. 4.59 Liver biopsy, 1 cm left lateral to midline, 0.5 cm caudal to sternum.

from the caudal border of both the left and right lobes of the liver. In both situations two pairs of fine artery forceps are used to triangulate and isolate a wedge of liver tissue (1 cm wide and 0.75 cm deep) (Fig. 4.59). The segment of liver is removed and the forceps removed a minute later. Alternatively, a monopolar loupe electrode may be used to harvest a biopsy. In such cases, the power is activated prior to making contact with the tissues, ensuring a sufficient margin between the incision and the tissue to be examined. Cauterized tissue yields poor histopathological results.

Pancreatic biopsy

A number of pancreatic diseases have been reported (Graham and Heyer, 1992; Speer, 1998; Ritzman 2000) but little research has been reported into the clinical significance of amylase and lipase levels (Fudge, 1997), although a fourfold increase in amylase level may be suggestive of pancreatic pathology. Currently, histopathology is the diagnostic tool of choice (Speer, 1998). Clinical signs associated with avian pancreatitis include anorexia, abdominal discomfort (colic), weight loss, polyuria, polydipsia, abdominal distension, polyphagia or pale bulky feces, although many cases are asymptomatic. The bird is anesthetized, intubated and placed in dorsal recumbency. A small (1–2 cm) craniocaudal incision is made in the midabdominal region. Care is taken not to

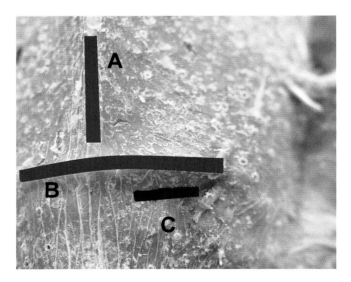

Fig. 4.58 Landmarks for liver biopsy. A, carina of sternum.

damage underlying viscera. The pancreatic lobe in the duodenal loop of the small intestine is readily located and exteriorized. The dorsal and ventral pancreatic loops are separated by the pancreatic artery (which must not be damaged). Although lesions may be apparent in other areas of the pancreas, the distalmost aspect of the organ is harvested. To safely achieve this, the distal edge is lifted and the underlying tissues examined for the presence of the artery, prior to careful biopsy removal. If specific lesions are present, these should be biopsied (if in the ventral or dorsal lobe), but not the splenic lobe – so long as this can be achieved without damaging the arterial supply to the remaining pancreatic tissue. The incision is closed in a routine manner.

Renal biopsy

This is a frequently used technique in the diagnostic work-up of kidney disease. The technique is simple and carries few risks if undertaken endoscopically.

Respiratory surgery

Tracheotomy

This procedure is most commonly indicated in the treatment of syringeal or tracheal aspergilloma or retrieval of a tracheal foreign body. This technique is more commonly necessitated in psittacines compared to raptors as in the former case the distal trachea narrows significantly, which makes endoscopic treatment of such lesions more difficult. Airsac intubation should be performed prior to undertaking tracheal surgery. A hypodermic needle may be usefully placed across the trachea distal to any foreign body to prevent the material passing caudally. The bird is placed in dorsal recumbency, with the head directed towards you. The front of the bird should be elevated at 45° to the tail, so as to facilitate interoperative visualization into the thorax. A skin incision is made adjacent to the thoracic inlet. The crop is identified, bluntly dissected and displaced to the right. The interclavicular airsac is entered and the trachea elevated. The sternotrachealis muscle (attached bilaterally to the ventral aspect of the trachea) is transected. Stay sutures may be placed into the trachea in order to draw it in an anterior direction. In most species it is impossible to completely exteriorize the syrinx. A tracheotomy may now be performed, cutting half of the tracheal circumference, through the ligament between adjacent tracheal cartilages (using a no. 11 scalpel blade). Foreign material may be scraped out using a Volkmann's spoon, and foreign bodies (e.g. seed) may be removed at the tracheotomy site or may be moved craniad using a suitable catheter as a probe, or on occasions with

a forceful blast of air from a hypodermic syringe. The incision is repaired with single interrupted sutures (6/0 Maxon, two or three sutures only) placed to include two rings either side of the incision. If additional access is required, the superficial pectoral muscles may be elevated and an osteotomy of the clavicle performed. On closure the two ends of the clavicle are apposed but not rejoined. The muscle is replaced and sutured into position. The crop is sutured back into place to create an airtight repair over the interclavicular airsac, using a continuous suture pattern and absorbable suture material. The skin is closed in a routine manner.

Trachectomy

In cases where a severe tracheal stenosis occurs, typically following trauma (most commonly associated with recent intubation – especially in macaws) or infection, tracheal resection and removal of the affected tissue can be performed (Fig. 4.60). Depending on the site of the lesion, most species can cope with losing up to five tracheal rings. In such cases, close apposition of cartilages following surgery, using a suture material that elicits minimal tissue reaction (e.g. polydioxanone, Ethicon), is used in order to minimize the risk of intraluminal granuloma formation. Trauma to tracheal tissues during surgery must be minimized. It is preferable to place sutures in the trachea at the time of resection, to facilitate apposition and anastomosis. Two to four sutures are used (depending on patient size) and are all preplaced before any are tied.

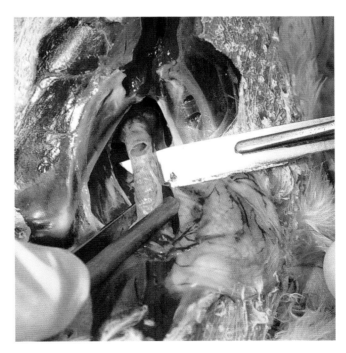

Fig. 4.60 Tracheotomy with reflexion of superficial pectoral muscles and left clavicle resection to increase thoracic inlet access.

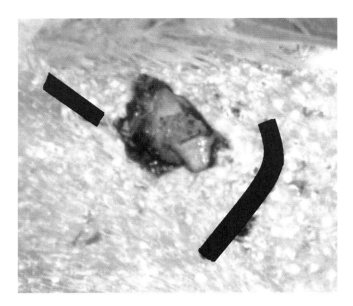

Fig. 4.61 Lung biopsy site under 6th rib.

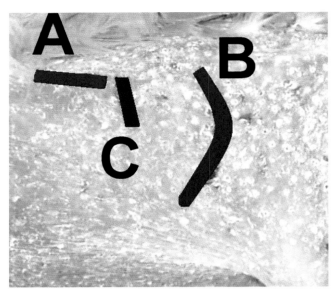

Fig. 4.62 Lung biopsy landmarks – A, scapula; B, 8th rib; C, incision over 6th rib.

Lung biopsy

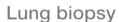

May be collected endoscopically via the air sac or surgically (a method favored by this author). Fine-definition radiographs or CT may usefully assist the surgeon in locating an area of lung tissue with apparent abnormalities from which biopsy is most likely to yield a useful result. The bird is laid in lateral recumbency, the leg extended caudally and the wing abducted dorsally. The fifth (i.e. 5th of eight) rib is located (typically at the caudal extremity of the scapula). A skin incision is made over the rib from the scapula to the level of the uncinate process. The incision is continued down on to the rib (Fig. 4.61). The lung tissue may be visualized on either side of the rib. A section of rib (0.5 cm) overlying the lung is removed and a biopsy is harvested using iris scissors from beneath the position of the rib (Fig. 4.62). The skin alone is closed afterwards.

Devoicing birds

This procedure is considered to be a mutilation by the Royal College of Veterinary Surgeons and quite rightly is illegal in the UK. Even in countries where it is not prohibited, it is a risky procedure with an uncertain short- and long-term outcome, i.e. many birds continue to vocalize despite surgical devoicing.

Postsurgical care

Postsurgical care greatly affects the outcome of the procedure. Prevention of self-trauma, a rapid recovery, sufficient analgesia, fluid, thermal and nutritional support as well as the minimization of stress are all vital.

REFERENCES

Antinoff N, Hoefer HL, Rosenthal KL, Bartick TE (1997) Smooth muscle neoplasia of suspected oviductal origin in the cloaca of a blue fronted Amazon parrot (*Amazona aestiva*). *Journal of Avian Medicine and Surgery* **11**: 268–272.

Bartels KE (ed.) (2002) Lasers in medicine and surgery. *Veterinary Clinics of North America – Small Animal Practice* 32: xiii–xv.

Best R (1996) Breeding problems. In: Beynon PH, Forbes NA, Harcourt-Brown NH (eds) *Manual of Raptors, Pigeons and Waterfowl*, pp. 208–215. British Small Animal Veterinary Association, Cheltenham.

Cribb PH (1984) Cloacal papilloma in an Amazon parrot. *Proceedings of the Association of Avian Veterinarians*, Denver, pp. 35–37.

De Voe RS, Trogdon M, Flammer K (2003) Diet modification and L-carnitine supplementation in lipomatous budgerigars. *Proceedings of the Association of Avian Veterinarians*, Denver, pp. 161–163.

Echols SM (2002) Surgery of the avian reproductive tract. *Seminars in Avian and Exotic Pet Medicine* **11**: 177–195.

Fillipich LJ, Bucher AM, Charles BG (1999) The pharmacokinetics of cisplatin in sulfur-crested cockatoos (*Cacatua galerita*). *Proceedings of the Association of Avian Veterinarians*, Denver, pp. 229–233.

Forbes NA, Cooper JE, Higgins RJ (2000) Neoplasms of birds of prey. In: Lumeij JT, Remple JD, Redig PT *et al.* (eds) *Raptor Biomedicine III*, pp. 127–146. Zoological Education Network, Lake Worth, FL.

Fudge AM (1997) Avian clinical pathology – hematology and chemistry. In: Altman RB, Clubb SL, Dorrestein G, Quesenberry K (eds) *Avian Medicine and Surgery*, pp. 151. WB Saunders, Philadelphia.

Graham DL, Heyer GW (1992) Diseases of the exocrine pancreas in pet, exotic and wild birds: a pathologist's perspective. *Proceedings of the Association of Avian Veterinarians*, Denver, pp. 190–193.

Harcourt-Brown NH (1996) Torsion and displacement of the oviduct as a cause of egg-binding in four psittacine birds. *Journal of Avian Medicine and Surgery* 10: 262–267.

Lumeij JT (1994) Gastroenterology. In: Ritchie BW, Harrison GJ, Harrison LR (eds) *Avian Medicine: principles and application*, pp. 482–521. Wingers Publishing, Lake Worth, FL.

McCluggage D (1992) Proventriculotomy: a study of selected cases. *Proceedings of the Association of Avian Veterinarians*, Denver, pp. 195–200.

Redig PT (1996) Avian emergencies. In: Beynon PH, Forbes NA, Harcourt-Brown NH (eds) *Manual of Raptors, Pigeons and Waterfowl*, pp. 30–41. British Small Animal Veterinary Association, Cheltenham.

Ritzman TK (2000) Pancreatic hypoplasia in eclectus parrot (*Eclectus roratus polychloros*). *Proceedings of the Association of Avian Veterinarians*, Denver, pp. 83–87.

Speer BL (1998) A clinical look at the avian pancreas in health and disease. *Proceedings of the Association of Avian Veterinarians*, Denver, pp. 57–64.

Sundberg JP, Junge RE, O'Banion MK *et al.* (1986) Cloacal papillomatosis in psittacines. *American Journal of Veterinary Research* **47**: 928–932.

Taylor M, Murray M (1999) A diagnostic approach to the avian cloaca. *Proceedings of the Association of Avian Veterinarians*, Denver, pp. 301–304.

VanDerHeyden N (1988) Psittacine papillomas. *Proceedings of the Association of Avian Veterinarians*, Lake Worth, pp. 23–25.

VanDerHeyden N (1993) Jejunostomy and jejuno-cloacal anastomosis in macaws. *Proceedings of the Association of Avian Veterinarians*, Denver, pp. 35–37.

5 Medical procedures

Medicament administration

Jesus Naldo

Medication may be administered to birds by any of the following major routes: parenteral, oral, nebulization and topical. Each one has its own advantages and disadvantages, which should be considered before a particular route is chosen (Table 5.1).

Parenteral administration

This implies administration of medicaments by needle or similar piece of equipment. The parenteral route is the method of choice in treating seriously ill birds that require immediate, direct and aggressive therapy (Figs 5.1–5.10). An exact dose can be administered with minimal stress and blood levels can be rapidly achieved. The main routes of administration that are used in birds are intramuscular (IM), intravenous (IV), subcutaneous (SC), intraperitoneal (IP), intrasinal (IS), intraosseous (IO), intratracheal (IT) and intranasal (IN). A variety of agents can be administered to birds by injection. There are certain general considerations that must be borne in mind, regardless of the route used or the medication applied. These are as follows.

TABLE 5.1 Different routes of injection and recommended sites

Route of administration	Site(s) of injection
Intramuscular	Pectoral muscle
	Quadriceps muscle
Intravenous	Basilic vein
	Right jugular vein
	Medial metatarsal vein
Subcutaneous	Inguinal web
	Interscapular area
	Axillary region
Intraperitoneal	Peritoneal cavity
Intranasal	Nares
Intrasinal	Infraorbital sinuses
Intraosseous	Proximal tibiotarsus
	Distal ulna
Intratracheal	Oropharynx
	Tracheal cartilage rings

- *The choice of needle (size and length) is important.* A needle causes tissue damage and, while this may appear to be slight, it can be very significant, especially in small birds. In general terms, a needle of as narrow a gauge and as short a length as is consistent with efficient administration of the drug is desirable. However, it should be noted that a thin needle may prove unsatisfactory for thick, viscous compounds and that too short a needle may make it impossible to place a depot of a drug (and this may be irritant) deep into the musculature.
- *The site chosen must take into consideration the particular circumstances.* For example, irritant injections will cause muscle degeneration. Therefore, one must assume that there may be some impairment of flight, if the pectoral muscles are used, or walking/running if leg muscles are used. A useful guide is to inject such compounds into the muscle mass, which is less likely to cause the bird inconvenience or adverse effect. Thus, terrestrial birds such as quail, which prefer to walk rather than fly, should generally have injections into their pectoral muscles, whereas a falcon, which depends very much upon its powers of flight, may be injected more safely in the leg muscles.
- *The volume of the injected medication must be considered.* As a general guideline the maximum volumes that can be given by intramuscular injection per site are as follows: macaw and cockatoo, 1 ml; Amazon or African gray parrot, 0.5 ml; cockatiel and small conure, 0.2 ml; budgerigar, canary and finch, 0.1 ml (Rupley, 1997). A volume up to 1.5 ml per site can be administered in birds weighing more than 1500 g. Use several injection sites if larger volumes are to be administered. Multiple injections in the same side of the breast or the use of irritating drugs may result in muscle necrosis or atrophy.
- *Subcutaneous injections* are preferable when large volumes are injected. However, part of the medication may leak out and irritating drugs may cause skin necrosis and ulceration.
- *Intravenous injections* should be given only during emergencies and single-dose drug administration. Rapid therapeutic levels are achieved when this route is used; however, hematomas are common.

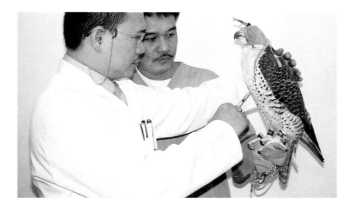

Fig. 5.1 Intramuscular injection into the pectoral muscle of a peregrine falcon (*Falco peregrinus*).

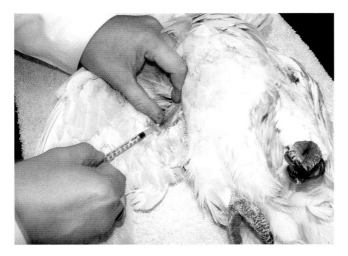

Fig. 5.3 Venipuncture of the basilic vein of a salmon-crested cockatoo (*Cacatua moluccencis*) under isoflurane anesthesia. The same site is used for administering intravenous medications.

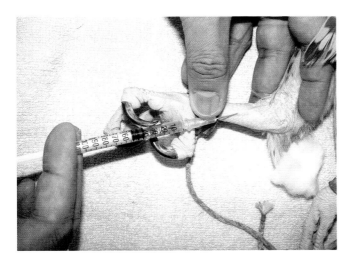

Fig. 5.5 Intravenous injection into the medial metatarsal vein of a lanner falcon (*Falco biarmicus*).

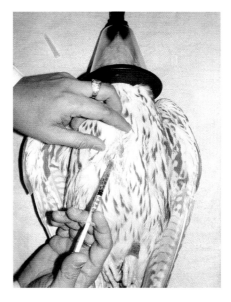

Fig. 5.2 Intramuscular injection into the pectoral muscle of a saker falcon (*Falco cherrug*) under isoflurane anesthesia.

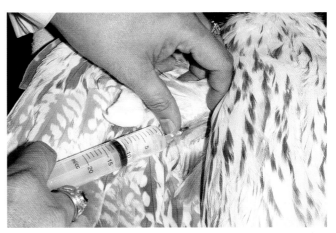

Fig. 5.4 Intravenous fluid administration into the basilic vein of a saker falcon under isoflurane anesthesia.

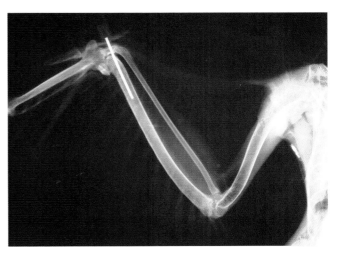

Fig. 5.6 Intraosseous administration into the distal ulna of a saker/gyr hybrid falcon (*Falco cherrug–Falco rusticolus*).

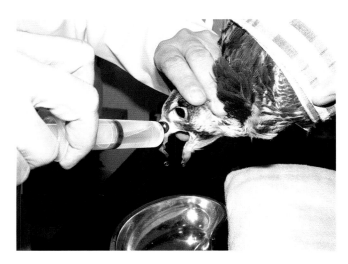

Fig. 5.7 Nasal flushing in a peregrine falcon.

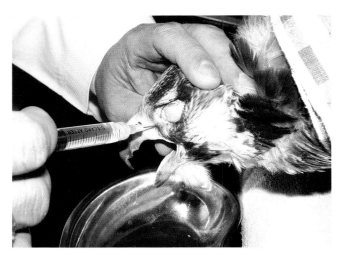

Fig. 5.8 Sinus flushing in a peregrine falcon.

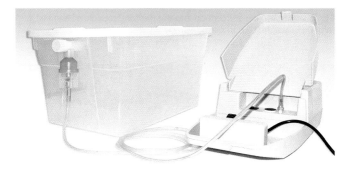

Fig. 5.9 Air compressor, nebulizer and nebulizing chamber used for small birds.

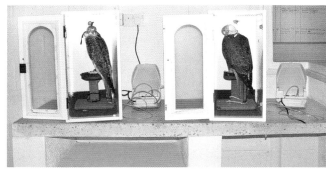

Fig. 5.10 Nebulizing chambers and air compressors used for falcons and other large birds.

Intraosseous injections can be used for nonirritating medications and for repeated drug administration.

● *Intratracheal injection* is used to deliver drugs to the lungs and airways of birds (Jenkins, 1997). It is an effective route for administering amphotericin B to birds with aspergillosis. Volumes up to 2 ml/kg of water-soluble medication may be administered safely using a small-diameter metal feeding needle. The medication is injected into the trachea with some force, then the bird is released and allowed to recover.

● *Infraorbital sinus injection* is useful for flushing and administering medication to birds with sinusitis. It can also be used to dislodge exudates and foreign bodies from the sinuses or to obtain samples for cytology, culture and sensitivity testing. Sterile water and an antibiotic or antifungal solution may be used for treatment of sinusitis. Do not use irritating solutions for sinus flushing (Rupley, 1997).

● A *nasal flush* may be used for both therapeutic and diagnostic purposes in infraorbital sinus infections. Antibiotics and antifungals recommended for nebulization can be used in a lower dose.

The amounts of fluids for nasal flushing are 1–3 ml for a budgerigar and up to 10–15 ml for a large macaw or cockatoo (Jenkins, 1997; Rupley, 1997). I have used a volume up to 40 ml on each naris to dislodge large amounts of rhinoliths and debris in falcons.

Oral administration

The administration of drugs or other compounds by the oral route has much to commend it, especially in terms of ease of administration. Oral administration can include 1) incorporation of the compound in the food or water or 2) administration by crop or stomach tube. The practicalities of the latter will be discussed below but some general points about oral administration will first be given.

● Administration in food or water, while apparently simple, can present problems. Some birds rarely, if ever, drink and thus administration in drinking water may prove futile. Birds that are unwell may not feed or may take in very little food, and thus compounds/drugs in the food may not be ingested, let alone

TABLE 5.2 Oral administration: advantages and disadvantages		
Route of administration	**Advantages**	**Disadvantages**
Directly by mouth – capsules/tablets	Can be administered by the owner Provides a definite drug volume administered to individual bird	Can be stressful for both the patient and the person giving the medication Limited to tame and relatively docile birds Absorption into the gut can be unpredictable Time-consuming in large number of birds
Fluids and suspensions via crop or stomach tube	Very useful for gastrointestinal-tract-associated conditions Allows accurate dosing Fast arrival time into the gut Good absorption	Can be stressful, because of repeated handling Risk of regurgitation and aspiration Time-consuming in large number of birds
Medicated feed	Handling of birds not required. No stress Birds will self-medicate several times daily Food consumption is more consistent than water consumption Very practical in large number of birds Useful for prevention, follow-up treatment or treatment of gastrointestinal-tract-associated conditions Reliable gut concentrations or blood levels	Unsatisfactory in anorectic birds Food intake may be affected by the taste Unpredictable interaction between drug and food Depending on the type of drug used, there may be insufficient absorption to reach therapeutic blood levels (see also water intake, below)
Medicated drinking water	Handling of birds not required. No stress Birds will self-medicate several times daily Probably the only possible route when medicating large flocks or wild birds Reduces bacterial contamination in drinking water Helps to control the multiplication of bacteria in the oropharynx	Intake and absorption of antibiotics administered in drinking water are unreliable, especially in species adapted to arid conditions that drink very little Some drugs are not stable or soluble in water Therapeutic blood levels are rarely achieved Inadequate intake of antibiotics may lead to drug-resistant bacteria

absorbed. Even if a bird is drinking and eating, it may not take in adequate medication because it is aware of the appearance or the taste of the compound in the food.

- Even if the compound is ingested, apparently in adequate amounts, absorption from the gastrointestinal tract may be insufficient to produce adequate blood levels of that agent (this is not applicable to drugs that are intended only for action within the intestinal tract). The absorption may be inadequate under any circumstances or may be reduced because the crop, stomach or intestines are full of food. Even the efficacy of drugs intended for use within the intestine may be reduced if there are large quantities of ingesta present.

It will be appreciated, therefore, that oral administration of drugs, while very tempting, and sometimes very useful, is not without its drawbacks (Table 5.2). Before embarking on this course of action, the veterinary surgeon should check the points above and reassure him/herself that the therapy is likely to prove effective. When drugs are put in the food, this can be done in a number of ways. Birds that are being fed a proprietary mash or pelleted diet can have the compound included either at source (the manufacturer) or mixed at a later stage by the owner or veterinary surgeon. In the case of birds that eat fruit, it may be possible to inject the compound into a particularly favored item. Birds that eat meat or whole animals can have certain agents secreted within the meat or the body of the prey.

When it comes to administration in drinking water, assuming that the bird is of a species that regularly drinks, the question of appearance and palatability comes to the fore. Some drugs impart coloration to the water and this may discourage a bird from drinking or reduce its intake. Likewise, the taste of a drug may reduce palatability. The effect of color can be minimized by providing the bird with water in a dark brown or similarly colored container for a few days before medication starts. Palatability is less easy to solve but, in some cases, the addition of sugar or another sweet substance to the water may help to disguise the taste of the medication.

It will be clear from the preceding paragraph that oral administration is not a panacea. In times past, a standard treatment for sick cage birds in many veterinary practices was 'oxytetracycline in the drinking water'. Over the years many authors have drawn attention to the unreliability of such an approach and the modern avian veterinarian is well aware that s/he must be more enterprising if drugs are to be effective.

Nebulization

Used for local administration to the upper respiratory tract, nebulization allows drug penetration into the airsacs, which can be the site of several important infections, including aspergillosis, mycoplasmosis and *Escherichia coli* infection. An ideal nebulizer unit should produce particles smaller than $3\,\pi$m in diameter in order to reach the airsacs and lungs. The parabronchi of birds

TABLE 5.3 Nebulization therapy: advantages and disadvantages

Advantages	Disadvantages
Effective treatment can be achieved with less stress involved, even in repeated medication Drugs can be delivered directly to the site of infection, including those that are relatively toxic when given parenterally Humidifies the inspired air	Can lead to environmental contamination No drug levels in the blood or lower respiratory tract Should usually be combined with systemic therapy

vary in size from 0.5–2 mm and the air capillaries vary from 3–10 πm in diameter (King and McLelland, 1984). Nebulization is likely to penetrate a limited portion of the lower respiratory tract; however, clinical improvement is often observed. Table 5.3 outlines the advantages and disadvantages of this treatment.

The nebulization equipment consists of the following:

- Air compressor
- Oxygen
- Nebulizer
- Enclosed chamber.

Some antibiotics and antifungal medications commonly nebulized are listed in Table 5.4. A broad-spectrum antibiotic should be used to initiate nebulization before culture and sensitivity results are known. The selection of antibiotic can be altered based on sensitivity testing.

Patients should be nebulized for 10–30 min 2–4 times daily, in conjunction with systemic therapy (Rupley, 1997).

A novel disinfectant from South Africa, F10 is an aldehyde-free, quaternary ammonia with biguanidine compounds that offers complete spectrum virucidal, bactericidal, fungicidal and sporicidal activity (Verwoerd, 2001). F10 diluted 1:250 has been used to nebulize psittacines, bustards and raptors with aspergillosis or bacterial airsacculitis (Bailey and Sullivan, 2001; Chitty, 2002; Forbes, 2001; Stanford, 2001; Verwoerd, 2001). It has been used in African gray parrots in combination with oral terbinafine (Chitty, 2002) and in raptors in combination with itraconazole (Forbes, 2001; Stanford, 2001). Several factors that make F10 an ideal agent to nebulize include: it is well tolerated by patients, safe to humans and is used for disinfection in food manufacture in South Africa. It is nonirritant to tissues and noncorrosive to metal or plastic (Verwoerd, 2001). Birds with clinical signs of respiratory disease are nebulized with F10 as part of the initial stabilization prior to diagnostic investigation (Chitty, 2002; Stanford, 2001).

Topical administration

Topical drug administration gives the advantage of direct application to the site of the insult, with advantages and disadvantages as outlined in Table 5.5.

TABLE 5.4 Some common nebulizing agents

Medication	Dosage	Administration time and frequency	References
Acetylcysteine 20%	200 mg/9 ml sterile water 200 mg/8 ml sterile water and 1 ml amikacin or gentamicin	15 min b.i.d.	Rupiper et al. 2000
Amikacin sulfate	50 mg/10 ml saline	15 min b.i.d.	Forbes 1996, Rupiper et al., 2000, Rupley 1997
Aminophylline	25 mg/10 ml saline	15 min b.i.d.	Rupiper et al., 2000
Amphotericin B	10 mg/10 ml saline 100 mg/15 ml saline	15 min b.i.d. 15–20 min q.i.d.	Rupiper et al., 2000, Rupley 1997 Forbes 1996
Carbenicillin	200 mg/10 ml saline	15 min b.i.d.	Rupiper et al., 2000, Rupley 1997
Cefotaxime	100 mg/10 ml saline	10–30 min b.i.d.–q.i.d.	Rupley 1997
Chloramphenicol	100 mg/10 ml saline 200 mg/15 ml saline	15 min b.i.d. 15 min q.i.d.	Rupiper et al., 2000 Forbes 1996
Clotrimazole	1% solution	30–60 min	Rupiper et al., 2000
Doxycycline	200 mg/15 ml saline	15–20 min q.i.d.	Forbes 1996
Enrofloxacin	100 mg/10 ml saline	15–20 min q.i.d.	Forbes 1996
Erythromycin	50 mg/10 ml saline 100 mg/10 ml saline 200 mg/10 ml saline	15 min t.i.d. 15 min t.i.d. 15–20 min q.i.d.	Rupiper et al., 2000 Rupley 1997 Forbes 1996
Gentamicin	50 mg/10 ml saline 50 mg/8 ml sterile water and 1 ml 20% acetylcysteine	15 min t.i.d. 15 min t.i.d.	Forbes 1996, Rupley 1997 Rupiper et al., 2000
Piperacillin	100 mg/10 ml saline	10–30 min b.i.d.–q.i.d.	Rupley 1997
Spectinomycin	200 mg/15 ml saline	15–20 min q.i.d.	Forbes 1996
Sulfadimethoxine	200 mg/15 ml saline	15–20 min q.i.d.	Forbes 1996
Terbinafine hydrochloride	500 mg and 1 ml acetylcysteine 20% in 500 ml distilled water	20 min t.i.d.	Dahlhausen et al., 2000
Tylosin	100 mg/10 ml saline or 1 g powder/50 ml DMSO or distilled water	10–60 min b.i.d.	Forbes 1996, Rupiper et al., 2000, Rupley 1997
F10 disinfectant*	10 ml of a 1:250 dilution	20–30 min b.i.d.–t.i.d.	Bailey and Sullivan 2001, Chitty 2002, Forbes 2001, Stanford 2001, Verwoerd 2001

* Health and Hygiene (Pty) Ltd, PO Box 347, Sunninghill 2157, South Africa; www.healthandhygiene.net

TABLE 5.5 Topical therapy: advantages and disadvantages

Topical medicaments	Advantages	Disadvantages
Ophthalmic ointments	Remain in the eyes and exert their therapeutic action longer than eye drops or solutions. Can be squeezed directly into the nostrils of birds to treat sinusitis	Excessive amount of ointment contaminating skin of eyelids may cause irritation and self-mutilation
Creams and ointments	Useful for localized infections, such as dermatitis or skin trauma, that do not warrant systemic injections	Can cause clogging of the feathers. May lead to self-mutilation. May cause toxicosis if ingested when the bird preens. Steroid-containing creams can cause polydipsia if used excessively
Ear and eye drops	Useful in treating rhinitis by instillation of the external nares. Preferable to ointments as this will limit damage to feathers	Short duration of therapeutic action
Aerosol antibiotic/anthelmintic sprays	Does not cause clogging of the feathers	The color of the spray stains the feathers making them look unpleasant
Powders	Useful for the treatment of ectoparasites	
Antibiotic ointment/DMSO impregnated gauze swab	Useful in treating localized soft tissue swelling on the foot	
Antibiotic-impregnated polymethyl methacrylate (AIPMMA) beads	Useful in treating bumblefoot and other infected, ischemic wounds. Higher local concentrations of antibiotic can be achieved without relying on vascular supply and tissue integrity	

The use of antibiotic-impregnated polymethyl methacrylate (AIPMMA) beads, following surgical debridement, offers an effective method for the delivery of antibiotics to an infected, ischemic site (Klemm, 1993). This technique has been used in birds for the treatment of osteomyelitis, cellulitis (Wheler *et al.*, 1996) and bumblefoot (Remple and Forbes, 2000). Some antibiotics that can be incorporated in AIPPMA beads include piperacillin, rifampin, amoxicillin, clindamycin, enrofloxacin and gentamicin (Remple and Forbes, 2000).

REFERENCES

Bailey TA, Sullivan T (2001) Aerosol therapy in birds using a novel disinfectant. *Exotic DVM* **3**(4):17.

Chitty J (2002) A novel disinfectant in psittacine respiratory disease. *Proceedings of the Association of Avian Veterinarians*, Monterey, pp. 25–27.

Dahlhausen B, Lindstrom JG, Radabaugh S (2000) The use of terbinafine hydrochloride in the treatment of avian fungal disease. *Proceedings of the Association of Avian Veterinarians*, Portland, pp. 35–39.

Forbes NA (1996) Respiratory problems. In: Beynon PH, Forbes NA, Lawton MPC (eds) *Manual of Psittacine Birds*, pp. 147–157. British Small Animal Veterinary Association, Cheltenham.

Forbes NA (2001) Aspergillosis in raptors. *International Falconer* **9**:44–47.

Jenkins JR (1997) Hospital techniques and supportive care. In: Altman RB, Clubb SL, Dorrestein GM, Quesenberry K (eds) *Avian Medicine and Surgery*, pp. 232–252. WB Saunders, Philadelphia.

King AS, McLelland J (1984) *Birds: Their Structure and Function*, 2nd edn. Baillière Tindall, London.

Klemm KW (1993) Antibiotic bead chains. *Clinical Orthopaedics and Related Research* **295**: 63–76.

Remple JD, Forbes NA (2000) Antibiotic-impregnated polymethyl methacrylate beads in the treatment of bumblefoot in raptors. In: Lumeij JT, Remple JD, Redig PT *et al.* (eds) *Raptor Biomedicine III*, pp. 255–263. Zoological Education Network, Lake Worth, FL.

Rupiper DJ, Carpenter JW, Mashima TY (2000) Formulary. In: Olsen GH, Orosz SE (eds) *Manual of Avian Medicine*, pp. 553–589. CV Mosby, St Louis.

Rupley AE (1997) *Manual of Avian Practice*. WB Saunders, Philadelphia.

Stanford M (2001) Use of F10 in psittacines. *Exotic DVM* **3**(4):18.

Verwoerd D (2001) Aerosol use of a novel disinfectant as part of an integrated approach to preventing and treating aspergillosis in falcons in the UAE. *Falco* **17**:15–18.

Wheler CL, Machin KL, Lew LJ (1996) Use of antibiotic-impregnated polymethacrylate beads in the treatment of chronic osteomyelitis and cellulitis in a juvenile bald eagle (*Haliaeetus leucocephalus*). *Proceedings of the Association of Avian Veterinarians*, Tampa, pp. 187–194.

FURTHER READING

Dorrestein GM (1996) Principles of therapy. In: Beynon PH, Forbes NA, Harcourt-Brown NH (eds) *Manual of Raptors, Pigeons and Waterfowl*, pp. 47–54. British Small Animal Veterinary Association, Cheltenham.

Dorrestein GM (2000) Nursing the sick bird. In: Tully TN, Lawton MPC, Dorrestein GM (eds) *Avian Medicine*, pp. 74–111. Butterworth-Heinemann, Oxford.

Flammer K (1994) Antimicrobial therapy. In: Ritchie BW, Harrison GJ, Harrison LR (eds) *Avian Medicine: Principles and Application*, pp. 434–456. Wingers Publishing, Lake Worth, FL.

Forbes NA, Lawton MPC (1996). Examination, basic investigation and principles of therapy. In: Beynon PH, Forbes NA, Lawton MPC (eds) *Manual of Psittacine Birds*, pp. 27–37. British Small Animal Veterinary Association, Cheltenham.

Rosskopf WJ, Woerpel RW (1996). Practical avian therapeutics with dosages of commonly used drugs. In: Rosskopf WJ Jr, Woerpel RW (eds) *Diseases of Cage and Aviary Birds*, 3rd edn, pp. 255–259. Williams & Wilkins, Baltimore.

Enema

Jaime Samour

An enema is a routine medical procedure commonly used in mammalian medicine to relieve constipation.

This condition is very seldom encountered in the avian patient because of differences in the physiology of the digestive system. However, birds affected with severe dehydration and some chronic diseases may suffer from impaction of the lower gastrointestinal tract, especially in raptors, or from uroliths resulting in impaction of the cloaca. An enema, or more appropriately cloacal lavage, is indicated in these cases. Esophageal tubes commonly used for small mammals are ideal for this purpose. In smaller birds, urethral catheters are more appropriate. A lavage solution is prepared using 100 ml of warm water at 37°C (98.6°F), 5 ml vegetable oil or liquid paraffin and 1 ml liquid detergent. The tube or catheter is lubricated with oil or liquid paraffin and inserted gently into the cloaca. The lavage solution can then be injected using a syringe (Figs 5.11 and 5.12).

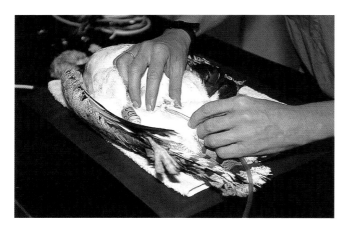

Fig. 5.11 An esophageal tube is ideal for the administration of enemas into medium-sized birds. The tube is lubricated and inserted gently into the cloaca. A houbara bustard (*Chlamydotis undulata*) is shown receiving an enema as a collateral treatment to capture paresia. (Courtesy of Dr. T. A. Bailey).

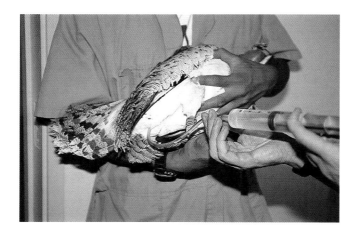

Fig. 5.12 The lavage solution containing warm water, liquid paraffin and liquid detergent is injected through the tube using a large syringe. Note that the bird is being held by a second operator. It is strongly recommended that this operation is carried out over a basin. (Courtesy of Dr. T. A. Bailey).

Fluid therapy

Thomas A. Bailey

Fluid therapy aims to replace fluids lost by a disease process or by restriction of intake (Blood and Studdert, 1988) and, as such, it is a necessary part of the treatment of most injured or debilitated birds, which are assumed to be presented in a state of dehydration (Harrison, 1986).

Total body water, extracellular water and blood volume in adult birds constitute approximately 60%, 18–24% and 4.4–14.3% of the bodyweight respectively (Jones and Pollock, 2000). The daily maintenance fluid requirements are unknown. However, the daily maintenance fluid requirements for raptors and psittacine birds have been estimated at 50 ml/kg/d, or approximately 5% of the bodyweight (Redig, 1984). In the absence of data to the contrary, this estimate is probably appropriate for many species of bird, although it is known that water consumption may vary from 5% to 30% of bodyweight in many free-ranging species. The amount of water needed is generally inversely related to body size and can also vary according to age, reproductive status, dietary intake and the type of food consumed (National Research Council, 1994). For example, young, growing birds will often drink comparatively larger volumes of water than adult birds and dehydration is often more severe in chicks than in adults because of the higher total body water in chicks. The variance in water intake in the domestic fowl (*Gallus domesticus*) is illustrated in Table 5.6.

The hydration status can be estimated from the clinical signs and history. The appearance of the eyes, corneal hydration, ocular pressure and dryness of the oral mucous membranes provide useful information on whether a bird is dehydrated. Skinfold elasticity on the dorsal aspect of the metatarsus and the turgescence, filling time and luminal volume of the brachial vein and artery after digital compression are all good indicators of hydration status (Abou-Madi and Kollias, 1992; Jones and Pollock, 2000):

- Moderate dehydration (>5%) – filling time of the ulnar vein greater than 1–2 s and brief tenting of skin
- Severe dehydration (>10%) – sunken eyes, tacky mucous membranes, skin and eyelid tenting
- Extreme dehydration (15%) – all the above signs plus weakness, increased heart rate, poor pulse quality and collapse.

TABLE 5.6 Variance in water intake in the domestic fowl	
Stage	**Requirement (% bodyweight per day)**
Adult	5.5
Growing	18–20
Laying hen	13.6

Source: Quesenberry and Hillyer, 1995.

TABLE 5.7 Laboratory findings in birds with dehydration	
Increased packed cell volume	Increases by 15–30% (>55% in adults)
Increased total protein	Increases by 20–40% with dehydration
Increased plasma urea	6.5–15.3 × normal

Source: Lumeij 1987; Martin and Kollias 1989.

As with mammals, anemia or hypoproteinemia can affect the accuracy of a packed cell volume (PCV) or solids in detecting dehydration (Table 5.7). In addition, there are age-related changes in the hematology and blood chemistry of juvenile birds, so changes in juvenile birds should be interpreted by comparing PCV, total protein and plasma urea with normal birds of the same age class.

Although the fluid requirements of many species are unknown, the daily maintenance fluid requirements for raptors and psittacine birds have been estimated at 50 ml/kg/d, or approximately 5% of the bodyweight (Redig, 1993). An estimation of the fluid deficit of a bird can be calculated based on bodyweight:

Estimated dehydration (%) × bodyweight (g) = fluid deficit (ml).

Half the total fluid deficit is given over the first 12–24 h along with the daily maintenance fluid requirement. The remaining 50% is divided over the following 48 h with the daily maintenance fluids. An example is provided below. Heidenreich (1995) advises that the maximum amount of fluids that can be administered at one time to a healthy bird is 90 ml/kg/h which amounts to a drip rate of 1.5 ml/kg/min.

Fluid therapy: clinical application

A 900 g houbara bustard presented with trichomonosis of the oropharyngeal cavity. The bird was anorectic and, from the history and clinical findings, was estimated to be approximately 10% dehydrated.

- Total estimated fluid deficit 0.1 (10%) × 900 (g) = 90 ml
- Daily maintenance fluid requirements at 50 ml/kg = 50×0.9 = 45 ml:
  - Fluids required for first 12–24 h = 45 + 0.5×(90) = 90 ml
  - Fluids required for the next 24–48 h = 45 + 0.5×(90) = 90 ml.

Supplemental fluids can be given orally, subcutaneously (Fig. 5.13), intravenously (Fig. 5.14) or by intraosseous cannula (Fig. 5.15). The advantages and disadvantages of each method are presented in Table 5.8.

Further information on the IO cannula technique is presented in Box 5.1. Dextrose 5% saline, lactated Ringer's saline and commercial products such as decarbonated cola-based soft drinks, Pedialyte® (Abbott Laboratories, USA) and Lectade® (Pfizer, UK), have been used successfully for oral rehydration. Although mildly dehydrated birds can be managed conservatively using oral or subcutaneous fluids, the intravenous or intraosseous route is recommended in other cases. A full list of agents used in fluid therapy is presented

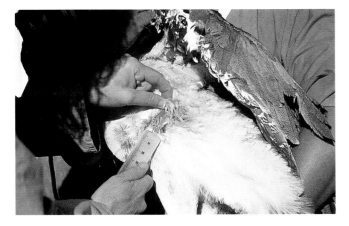

Fig. 5.13 Subcutaneous fluids can be administered in the lateral flank, axilla or intrascapular region in cases of mild dehydration.

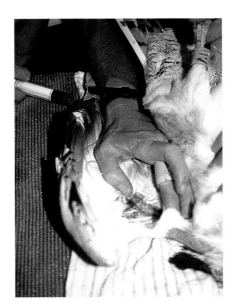

Fig. 5.14 Intravenous fluids and drugs can be given slowly through a butterfly catheter in the right jugular vein.

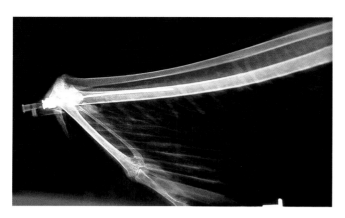

Fig. 5.15 Radiograph showing an intraosseous cannula in the distal ulna of a kori bustard (*Ardeotis kori*).

in Appendix VIII. The selection of intravenous fluids is outlined below:

Crystalloids are considered to be the initial fluid of choice in avian shock or dehydration. 30 min after fluid administration to a bird, only a quarter of the total fluids remain in the vascular compartment (Dorrestein, 2000). Thus the circulatory benefits obtained from fluid therapy are transient and therapy must be repeated. Having a small incubator in the examination or treatment room is useful so that fluids can be warmed to 38–39°C prior to administration. Using warm fluids is particularly important with neonates. Redig (1996) recommends using rapid bolus intravenous injection at a rate of 10 ml/kg/min through a 25-gauge needle or catheter for the first 24–48 h of replacement therapy. A slow IV bolus injection of 10–25 ml/kg of crystalloid fluids can also

safely be given over a 5 min period every 8–12 h. As most of the commonly encountered conditions displace the avian patient toward a state of metabolic acidosis, lactated Ringer's saline is recommended (Redig, 1993). The lactate is metabolized to bicarbonate by the liver. Bicarbonate supplementation may be necessary in severely acidotic states. If it is not possible to measure blood bicarbonate, a dose of 1 mmol/kg can be given every 15–30 min to a maximum of 4 mmol/kg/d (Hernandez and Aguilar, 1994). In cases of severe tissue injury, extreme catabolism and renal failure, calcium gluconate can be administered slowly as a cardioprotectant, while glucose can be given to facilitate the movement of potassium across cell membranes (Dorrestein, 2000).

Hypertonic saline (7.5%) can be used as a resuscitative therapy to restore circulatory function. It causes rapid plasma expansion and its use should be followed by administration of isotonic fluids. Hypertonic saline is indicated in cases of hemorrhagic shock and pulmonary edema and contraindicated in dehydration and head trauma (Dorrestein, 2000). In dog and cat medicine a convenient method for administering hypertonic saline with a colloid is to dilute 23.4% NaCl with 6% hetastarch or 6% Dextran 70 to make a 7.5% solution and infuse at a rate of 4 ml/kg (Day and Bateman, 2006).

Colloids are high-molecular-weight polysaccharides, with a particle size similar to that of albumin, that are restricted to the plasma compartment. They are indicated as a plasma volume substitute in cases of hypovolemic shock caused by hemorrhage, burns, water and electrolyte loss from persistent vomiting or diarrhea. The effect is similar to the administration of hypertonic saline, although the duration (24 h) is longer than that of hypertonic

TABLE 5.8 Types of fluid therapy: advantages and disadvantages

Route	Advantages and disadvantages
Oral fluids	Only effective with mild dehydration
	5% dextrose may be better than lactated Ringer's solution
	Contraindicated with gastrointestinal tract stasis
	Contraindicated with lateral recumbency
	Contraindicated with seizures and head trauma
	Ineffective for shock
Subcutaneous fluids	Primarily used for mild dehydration
	Less effective for shock therapy because of peripheral vasoconstriction
	Effective for providing maintenance fluids
	Given in lateral flank or inguinal regions
	Divide dose among several sites at 5–10 ml/kg/site
	Avoid giving around base of neck because of communications with the cervicocephalic airsac system
Intravenous or intraosseous fluids	Rapidly expand circulatory volume
	Rapidly perfuse kidney
	Indicated in shock
	Indicated with severe dehydration
	Right jugular vein – one-time use
	Medial metatarsal vein – one-time use
	Ulnar intraosseous cannula – multiple use
	Tibial intraosseous cannula – one-time use
	Injection of a large volume of fluid into the ulnar or metatarsal vein is difficult and can result in hematoma formation

Box 5.1 Intraosseous fluids: further information

An intraosseous cannula can be used to administer
- Fluids
- Blood
- Antimicrobials
- Parenteral nutrition
- Colloids
- Glucose.

Advantages of intraosseous cannulas
- Useful in extremely debilitated cases in which the veins are too collapsed
- Ease of placement and maintenance
- Tolerance
- Reduced patient restraint
- Less stress compared with repeated venipunctures.

Intraosseous cannulas can be placed in any bone with a rich marrow cavity:
- Distal ulna in medium-sized to large birds that require days of therapy
- Proximal tibia for short-term therapy.

Note: it has been shown in pigeons that 50% of fluids administered into the ulna enter the systemic circulation within 30 s.

- Heat
- Multivitamins
- Iron dextran
- Antibiotics, if required.

REFERENCES

Abou-Madi N, Kollias GV (1992) Avian fluid therapy In: Kirk RW, Bonagura JD (eds) *Current Veterinary Therapy IX*, pp. 1154–1159. WB Saunders, Philadelphia.

Blood DC, Studdert VP (1988) *Baillière's Comprehensive Veterinary Dictionary*. Baillière Tindall, London.

Day TK, Bateman S (2006) Shock syndromes. In: DiBartola S (ed.) *Fluid, Electrolyte and Acid-base Disorders in Small Animal Practice*, pp. 540–564. Saunders, St Louis.

Dorrestein GM (2000) Nursing the sick bird. In: Tully TN, Lawton MPC, Dorrestein GM (eds) *Avian Medicine*, pp. 74–111. Butterworth-Heinemann, Oxford.

Harrison GJ (1986) What to do until a diagnosis is made. In: Harrison GJ, Harrison LR (eds) *Avian Medicine: Principles and Application*, pp. 356–362. WB Saunders, Philadelphia.

Heidenreich M (1995) *Birds of Prey. Medicine and Management*, pp. 125–128. Blackwell Science, Oxford.

Hernandez M, Aguilar RF (1994) Steroid and fluid therapy for treatment of shock in the critical avian patient. *Seminars in Avian and Exotic Pet Medicine* 3: 190–199.

Jones MP, Pollock CG (2000) Supportive care and shock. In: Olsen GH, Orosz SE (eds) *Manual of Avian Medicine*, pp. 17–47. Mosby Publishing, St Louis.

Lumeij JT (1987) Plasma urea, creatinine and uric acid concentration in response to dehydration in racing pigeons. *Avian Pathology* 16: 377–382.

Martin HD, Kollias GV (1989) Evaluation of water deprivation and fluid therapy in pigeons. *Journal of Zoo and Wildlife Medicine* 20: 173–177.

Mathews KA (2006) Monitoring fluid therapy and complications of fluid therapy. In: DiBartola S (ed.) *Fluid, Electrolyte and Acid-base Disorders in Small Animal Practice*, pp. 377–391. Saunders, St Louis.

National Research Council (1994) *Nutrient Requirements of Poultry*, 9th edn. National Academy Press, Washington, DC.

Quesenberry KE, Hillyer EV (1994) Supportive care and emergency therapy. In: Ritchie BW, Harrison GJ, Harrison LR (eds) *Avian Medicine: Principles and Application*, pp. 382–416. Wingers Publishing, Lake Worth, FL.

Redig PT (1984) Fluid therapy and acid–base balance in the critically ill avian patient. *Proceedings of the Association of Avian Veterinarians*, Boulder, pp. 59–74.

Redig PT (1993) Fluid therapy and acid-base balance in the critically ill avian patient. In: Redig PT (ed.) *Medical Management of Birds of Prey. A Collection of Notes on Selected Topics*, pp. 49–60. Raptor Center, University of Minnesota, St Paul, MN.

Redig PT (1996) Avian emergencies. In: Beynon PH, Forbes NA, Harcourt-Brown NH (eds) *Manual of Raptors, Pigeons and Waterfowl*, pp. 30–41. British Small Animal Veterinary Association, Cheltenham.

saline. Redig (1984) reported a dramatic improvement in avian species in shock given 10–20 ml/kg of 6% dextran. Adverse effects in mammals include hypervolemia and anaphylaxis. In no case should the volume of dextran injected exceed one-third of the plasma volume. If this proportion is exceeded, dextran has a heparin-like action and severe hemorrhage may result (Jones and Pollock, 2000). Colloids are contraindicated in sepsis, volume overload, capillary leak syndromes and coagulopathies (Mathews, 2006). Oxyglobin (Biopure) is an ultrapurified, glutaraldehyde polymerized bovine hemoglobin in modified lactated Ringer's solution. In dogs Oxyglobin provides oxygen-carrying support, improving the clinical signs of anemia for at least 24 h, independent of the underlying conditions. It has been used successfully in many avian species with severe anemia.

Homologous blood transfusions have been shown to be beneficial for birds with chronic anemia (PCV <20%) (Dorrestein, 2000) and are feasible in situations where there are plenty of donor birds of the same species available.

The progress of cases can be monitored using packed cell volume or total protein. Additional therapy to be considered when administering fluids includes:

Tube feeding and nutritional support

Thomas A. Bailey

Nutritional support is crucial for the successful recovery of avian patients that are not eating voluntarily. Enteral feeding uses the digestive tract, while parenteral feeding bypasses the digestive tract by supplying nutrients directly into the vascular system. Enteral nutritional support is generally provided to birds using a tube passed into the crop, or directly into the distal esophagus in birds that do not have a crop.

Equipment needed for tube feeding includes:

- Plastic feeding catheters of various diameters
- Catheter-tipped syringes
- Oral beak specula.

Tube feeding must be avoided in dehydrated patients and in birds that have gastrointestinal disorders, including vomiting, crop stasis and ileus (Harrison, 1986; Quesenberry and Hillyer, 1994).

A sterile feeding tube should be used for each bird to prevent the spread of disease. Parenteral medications should be given before tube feeding, because if they are given afterwards many birds will regurgitate. Oral medications can be given with the feeding mixture.

Tube feeding is far easier with the help of an assistant (Fig. 5.16) but can be done in small to medium-sized birds by one person. The following description applies to a medium-sized bird, such as a houbara bustard, but can be adapted for other species. The bird's neck is straightened vertically with the head grasped around the mandibles. The tube is passed into the oral cavity and down the esophagus on the right side of the neck. Tube placement can be seen by moistening the feathers on the right lateral neck region or by palpation of the tube in the proximal neck. The neck should be kept fully extended during feeding to discourage regurgitation. In birds with a crop the tube is directed into the crop, while in birds without a crop, such as bustards, the tube may be passed into the middle or distal esophagus. In birds without a crop, it is important not to force the end of the tube further than the distal esophagus – this can cause iatrogenic trauma to the proventriculus and/or the gizzard, which can result in perforation of the alimentary tract and death. After feeding the tube is carefully removed to prevent reflux and the assistant continues to hold the bustard with the neck in extension until the bird is released into its enclosure. If reflux of the food occurs during tube feeding, the bird should be released immediately and allowed to clear the oral cavity on its own.

Most hospitalized birds are fed between one and four times a day according to their clinical condition and calorific needs. The frequency of feeding depends on the temperament and clinical status of the bird. When dealing with unfamiliar species it is wise to use low volumes initially in order to gauge the quantity of fluids that the bird can cope with.

The following therapeutic agents can be added to liquid diets (Coles, 1997; Dorrestein, 2000):

- Methylcellulose can help to slow the gastrointestinal transit time and absorb enterotoxins
- Lactulose has a mild laxative effect and also absorbs enterotoxins.

Tube feeding is contraindicated for birds with ileus and impaction. Esophagostomy and duodenostomy are also used in the nutritional supportive of hospitalized avian species (Dorrestein, 2000).

Nutritional requirements

The size, weight, reproductive status and season all affect the daily caloric needs of birds. The basal metabolic rate (BMR) is the minimum amount of energy necessary for daily maintenance. An estimate of the BMR for birds can be made based on metabolic scaling using the following equation (Quesenberry et al., 1991):

$$\mathrm{BMR} = K(W_{kg}^{0.75}),$$

where $K = 129$ in passerine birds and 78 in nonpasserine birds.

The K factor is a theoretical constant for kilocalories used during 24 h for various species of bird, mammal and reptile. The maintenance energy requirement (MER) is the BMR plus additional energy needed for physical activity, digestion and absorption. The MER for hospitalized animals is approximately 25% above the BMR. In passerine birds, MER varies from 1.3–7.2 times the BMR. With growth, stress and disease, animals are in a hypermetabolic state, with daily energy needs that surpass maintenance. The amount of increased demand depends on the type of injury or stress and varies between one and three times the daily maintenance requirement. Table 5.9 lists the adjustments to maintenance for stress. Although not exact, metabolic scaling can be used to estimate the approximate daily caloric needs of birds.

Enteral nutritional formulas

Commercial enteral nutritional formulas marketed for humans are widely available. Some of these diets are available in liquid formulations and others as powder

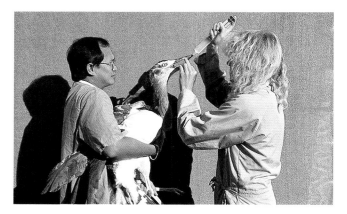

Fig. 5.16 Force-feeding an adult kori bustard (*Ardeotis kori*) affected with capture paresia. A syringe and a stomach tube commercially available to feed neonatal lambs are ideal for the purpose.

TABLE 5.9 Adjustments to maintenance for stress, as a multiple of MER

Factor	MER ×
Starvation	0.5–0.7
Elective surgery	1.0–1.2
Mild trauma	1.0–1.2
Severe trauma	1.1–2.0
Growth	1.5–3.0
Sepsis	1.2–1.5
Burns	1.2–2.0
Head injuries	1.0–2.0

Source: from Quesenberry and Hillyer, 1994.

Box 5.2 Example of metabolic scaling to estimate approximate daily caloric needs of a bustard

A houbara bustard weighing 1200 g is presented for septicemia secondary to bacterial enteritis. Estimating MER as $1.5 \times$ BMR, the daily caloric needs can be estimated as:

- BMR = 78 $(1.2^{0.75})$ or 89 kcal/d
- 1.5×89 kcal/d = 134 kcal/d approximate MER
- 1.2×134 kcal/d = 161 kcal/d increase for sepsis.

If the energy content of the feeding formula is known, the daily caloric needs are divided by the calories per milliliter of formula to calculate the total volume of formula needed per day. For example using a formula that is 1.0 kcal/ml, the total volume of formula needed per day for the houbara is:

- 161 kcal/d $\times 1.0$ kcal/ml = 161 ml needed daily.

formulations that can be mixed with water. The diets vary in caloric density, protein, fat, carbohydrate content and osmolarity. Table 5.10 lists some of the enteral products that are used.

Knowing the exact caloric density per millimeter is convenient for calculating daily maintenance requirements. Once opened, liquid enteral formulas can be refrigerated for 2–3 d. Powdered products can curdle if an inadequate amount of water is used for mixing. Before feeding, the formulas can be heated gently, for example in a syringe under a hot running tap. Powdered products are often mixed with oral fluids, such as Pedialyte® (Abbott Laboratories, USA) and Duphalyte® (Duphar Ltd, UK). It is important to ensure that birds that are given enteral nutrition are adequately hydrated, because many products are hyperosmolar and will contribute to dehydration if fluid requirements are not met (Quesenberry *et al.*, 1991).

Following the weight on a daily basis is the best evaluation of enteral feeding. An example of a clinical application of enteral nutrition is given in Box 5.2.

It is important to encourage hospitalized birds to feed by themselves as quickly as possible. This can be done by offering favorite fresh food items. We offer mealworms, crickets, other invertebrates (such as beetles) and small pink mice to bustards at the National Avian Research Center, United Arab Emirates.

REFERENCES

Coles BH (1997) *Avian Medicine and Surgery*, 2nd edn, pp. 240–279. Blackwell Science, Oxford.

Dorrestein GM (2000) Nursing the sick bird. In: Tully TN, Lawton MPC, Dorrestein GM (eds) *Avian Medicine*, pp. 74–111. Butterworth-Heinemann, Oxford.

Harrison GJ (1986) What to do until a diagnosis is made. In: Harrison GJ, Harrison LR (eds) *Avian Medicine: Principles and Application*, pp. 356–362. WB Saunders, Philadelphia.

Quesenberry KE, Maudlin G, Hillyer EV (1991) Review of methods of nutritional support in hospitalized birds. *Proceedings of the European Association of Avian Veterinarians*, Vienna, pp. 243–254.

Quesenberry KE, Hillyer EV (1994) Supportive care and emergency therapy. In: Ritchie BW, Harrison GJ, Harrison LR (eds) *Avian Medicine: Principles and Application*, pp. 382–416. Wingers Publishing, Lake Worth, FL.

TABLE 5.10 Commercial enteral products: nutrients per 100 kcal energy

Products	Protein (g)	Fat (g)	Carbohydrate (g)	Caloric density (Kcal/ml)
LIQUIDS				
Ensure	4.2	3.36	13.36	1.0
PediaSure	3.0	4.98	10.96	1.0
GELS/SOLIDS				
Hill's a/d diet	8.3	5.2	3.0	1.27
Nutri-plus gel	0.25	5.9	8.3	5.9
POWDERS				
Cerelac	3.7	2.15	16.5	4.19
Complan	4.65	3.22	13.16	4.3
Sustagen	6.13	0.95	16.95	3.8

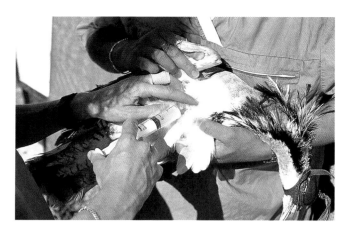

Fig. 5.17 Fluid administration to a severely dehydrated houbara bustard (*Chlamydotis undulata*). The administration of fluids is necessary to maintain the electrolyte balance in birds in cases of severe dehydration due to starvation, diarrhea or hemorrhage. The bird had spent 48 h in a transport box before it was confiscated.

Metabolic drug scaling

Thomas A. Bailey

Medication and vaccination of nondomestic birds is often accomplished by extrapolating dosage regimens from other species, if such data exist, but the effectiveness and safety of this method is not always considered to be satisfactory (Dorrestein, 1991). Anatomical and physiological differences are considered to account for some of the difficulties of extrapolating drug dosages for birds from dosages prescribed for mammals (Dorrestein, 1991). As knowledge of drug disposition and metabolism expands it is becoming clear that large differences exist in dosage, administration interval and organ distribution, not only between birds and mammals but between different avian species (Dorrestein, 1993; Baggot, 1995). Ideally, drug administration should be based on knowledge of the pharmacokinetics of that drug in the species to which it is being administered. Although some pharmacokinetic studies have been carried out in birds, for the majority of the drugs used in every day clinical practice no studies have been performed. Even in the future, it is unrealistic to expect pharmacokinetic data derived from studies in birds to be available for more than a handful of drugs, so it will often be necessary to make estimates of appropriate drug doses and dose frequencies.

Allometric scaling provides a method for examining the structural and functional consequences of changes in size or scale among otherwise similar organisms (Schmidt-Nielson, 1984). It has been found that many physiological variables can be related to bodyweight (W) by mathematical relationships; for example, rates of production and consumption vary with $W^{0.5}$ and the time-spans of biological processes vary with W^1 (Kirkwood, 1983). The use of allometric principles to scale physiological parameters between animals of various sizes is now well established and is widely used in estimating the energy requirements and thus food needs of captive and free-living wildlife (Kirkwood and Bennett, 1992; Kirkwood, 1996). The uptake, distribution and elimination of drugs that are administered to animals similarly involve physiological processes that can be scaled allometrically (Sedgwick, 1993). Thus, when using novel drugs for which no other avian dose is known it is possible to use allometric equations to assist in calculating doses. The reader is recommended to consult the literature to gain a deeper insight into the theories, applications and pitfalls of using metabolic scaling to extrapolate doses between different species (Kirkwood and Bennett, 1992; Pokras *et al.*, 1993; Sedgwick, 1993).

Although allometric equations can appear to be intimidating, it is important to be able to use them to extrapolate drug doses from one species to another. Once one is familiar with the worksheet approach described by Sedgwick (1993), it is relatively straightforward to write the calculations in one of the commonly used spreadsheet or database programs and doses can then be rapidly calculated in the clinic. Such information can provide a starting point for a dose for an unfamiliar medicine and is better than the alternative of guessing! Although the size range of birds is not as vast as other groups of animals, when we consider the size difference in the Otididae between a newly hatched red-crested bustard chick (*Eupodotis ruficrista*) weighing 30 g and a large adult kori bustard (*Ardeotis kori*) of 15 kg we are still dealing with a 500-fold difference. I feel that insufficient attention has been paid to selecting doses to treat chicks and juvenile birds a small fraction of the weight of adult birds and we really should pay greater attention to using metabolic scaling to guide us in the calculation of size-appropriate doses and dose intervals. I have drawn heavily on the papers by Sedgwick (1993) and Pokras *et al.* (1993) in the following two examples.

The specific minimum energy cost (SMEC) for any animal can be calculated as follows:

$$\text{SMEC} = K\,(W_{kg}^{\,0.75} / W_{kg}) = K\,(W_{kg}^{\,-0.25}).$$

where K = energy constant (Table 5.11).

The SMEC dose for a drug is calculated by dividing the dose rate (mg/kg) of the control animal by the control's SMEC (Boxes 5.3 and 5.4). Treatment frequency is the number of times that a drug dose is administered to a patient in a day (24 h) when a treatment regimen is a multiple one. The SMEC frequency is the treatments frequency of a control animal divided by the SMEC (Boxes 5.3 and 5.4). Two worksheet examples are provided. The first shows how to extrapolate an established treatment regimen for azithromycin from humans (control species) in which the dose rate has been established following

TABLE 5.11 Hainsworth's energy groups (Sedgwick, 1993)

Group	Constant (K)	Mean core temperature (°C)
Passerine bird	129	42
Nonpasserine bird	78	40
Placental mammal	70	37

Box 5.3 Example 1: SMEC dose and SMEC frequency scaling worksheet extrapolating standard dosage regimens for azithromycin from humans to three different age and size classes of bustard

Control species SMEC calculations:

The dose rate for azithromycin in a human (bodyweight 70 kg) is 500 mg (7 mg/kg) q24 h.

Control species: human (Weight W_{kg} 70 kg)

Dose rate is 500 mg (7 mg/kg) every 24 h

$SMEC = K (W_{kg}^{-0.75} / W_{kg}) = K (W_{kg}^{-0.25}) = 24.2$

SMEC dose is the dose rate divided by SMEC = 7/24.2 = 0.3

SMEC dose = 0.3

Frequency (number of treatment intervals per 24 h) = 24/24 = 1

SMEC frequency is the frequency divided by SMEC = 1/24.2 = 0.04

SMEC frequency = 0.04.

Species, age and weight	Buff-crested bustard chick (0.05 kg)	Adult male houbara bustard (1.5 kg)	Adult male kori bustard (15 kg)
SMEC	$78(0.05^{-0.25}) = 165$	$78(1.5^{-0.25}) = 70.5$	$78(15^{-0.25}) = 40$
Dose rate calculations	165×0.3 = 49.5	70.5×0.3 = 21.2	40×0.3 = 12
Dose frequency calculations	165×0.04 = 6.6	70.5×0.04 = 2.8	40×0.04 = 1.6
Regimen	50 mg every 4 h	21 mg every 8 h	12 mg every 12 h

Box 5.4 Example 2: SMEC dose and SMEC frequency scaling worksheet extrapolating standard dosage regimens for enrofloxacin established for adult houbara bustards to three different age and size classes of bustard

Control species SMEC calculations:

The dose rate for enrofloxacin in an adult houbara bustard (bodyweight 1.5 kg) is 10 mg/kg q12 h (Bailey *et al.*, 1998).

Control species: houbara bustard (Weight W_{kg} 1.5 kg)

Dose rate is 10 mg/kg every 12 h

$SMEC = K (W_{kg}^{-0.75} / W_{kg}) = K (W_{kg}^{-0.25}) = 70.5$

SMEC dose is the dose rate divided by SMEC = 10/70.5 = 0.15

SMEC dose = 0.15

Frequency (number of treatment intervals per 24 h) = 24/12 = 2

SMEC frequency is the frequency divided by SMEC = 2/70.5 = 0.03

SMEC frequency = 0.03

Species, age and weight	Buff-crested bustard chick (0.05 kg)	Adult female buff-crested bustard (0.5 kg)	Adult male kori bustard (15 kg)
SMEC	$78(0.05^{-0.25}) = 165$	$78(0.5^{-0.25}) = 93$	$78(15^{-0.25}) = 40$
Dose rate calculations	165×0.15 = 25	93×0.15 = 14	40×0.15 = 6
Dose frequency calculations	165×0.03 = 4.9	93×0.03 = 2.8	40×0.03 = 1.2
Regimen	25 mg every 6 h	14 mg every 8 h	6 mg every 24 h

pharmacological trials for different size and age classes of bustard. The second shows how to extrapolate an established treatment regimen for enrofloxacin from adult houbara bustards (control species) in which the dose rate has been established following pharmacological trials (Bailey *et al.*, 1998) to different size and age classes of bustard. The best data for selection of a control animal from which to extrapolate treatment regimens come from pharmacokinetic studies performed in the control species. Clearly of the two examples, we would have more confidence in the values of enrofloxacin for our three different types of bustard, that were extrapolated from pharmacokinetic investigations in houbara bustards (Bailey *et al.*, 1998), rather than the values for azithromycin that were extrapolated from humans to bustards. Azithromycin is used at a dose of 43 mg/kg q24 h in psittacines (Rupiper *et al.*, 2000), not so wildly different from the results of the allometric calculations. Even with the limitations of allometric scaling, I think that the results of these examples help to demonstrate that drug doses should be interpreted with caution and show that a drug dose used safely in adult birds may have a different effect in a chick.

REFERENCES

Baggot JD (1995) Pharmacokinetics: disposition and fate of drugs in the body. In: Adams HR (ed.) *Veterinary Pharmacology and Therapeutics*, 7th edn, pp. 18–52. Iowa State University Press, Ames, IA.

Bailey TA, Sheen, RS, Silvanose C *et al.* (1998) Clinical pharmacology and pharmacokinetics of enrofloxacin after intravenous, intramuscular and oral administration in houbara bustard (*Chlamydotis undulata macqueenii*). *Journal of Veterinary Pharmacology and Therapeutics* 21: 288–297.

Dorrestein GM (1991) The pharmacokinetics of avian therapeutics. *Veterinary Clinics of North America: Small Animal Practice* 21: 1241–1263.

Dorrestein GM (1993) Antimicrobial drug use in pet birds. In: Prescott JF, Baggot JD (eds) *Antimicrobial Therapy in Veterinary Medicine*, pp. 490–506. Iowa State University Press, Ames, IA.

Kirkwood JK (1983) Influence of body size in animals on health and disease. *Veterinary Record* 113: 287–290.

Kirkwood J (1996) Nutrition of captive and free-living wild animals. In: Kelly NC, Wills JM (eds) *Manual of Companion Animal Feeding*, pp. 235–241. British Small Animal Veterinary Association, Cheltenham.

Kirkwood JK, Bennett PM (1992) Approaches and limitations to the prediction of energy requirements in wild animal husbandry and veterinary care. *Proceedings of the Nutrition Society* 51: 117–124.

Pokras MA, Karas AM, Kirkwood JK, Sedgwick CJ (1993) An introduction to allometric scaling and its uses in raptor medicine. In: Redig PT, Cooper JE, Remple JD, Hunter DB (eds) *Raptor Biomedicine*, pp. 211–224. University of Minnesota Press, Minneapolis.

Rupiper DJ, Carpenter JW, Mashima TY (2000) Formulary. In: Olsen GH, Orosz SE (eds) *Manual of Avian Medicine*, pp. 553–589. Mosby, St Louis.

Schmidt-Nielson K (1984) *Scaling: Why is Animal Size so Important?* Cambridge University Press, New York.

Sedgwick CJ (1993) Allometric scaling and emergency care: the importance of body size. In: Fowler ME (ed.) *Zoo and Wildlife Medicine: Current Therapy 3*, pp. 34–37. WB Saunders, Philadelphia.

Claw/talon and beak trimming

Jaime Samour

Overgrown claws and talons are frequently found in captive birds from several orders but in particular from the Psittaciformes, Passeriformes and Falconiformes (Figs 5.18 and 5.19). This condition is usually caused by insufficient wear associated with the use of perches too small in diameter and perching surfaces that are too soft. The claws and talons of birds are composed of a hard, keratinized casing covering the dorsal and lateral aspects, while the ventral surface is formed of a softer structure. Claws and talons are trimmed using nail clippers, a

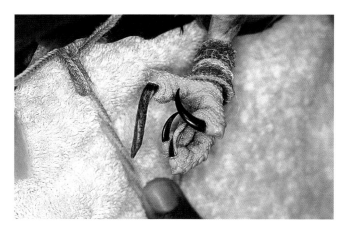

Fig. 5.18 Overgrown talons in a saker falcon (*Falco cherrug*). The use of inadequate perches, in particular during the molting season, is most often responsible for this condition.

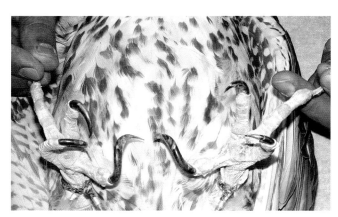

Fig. 5.19 Overgrown and deformed talons in a saker falcon. Regular trimming and reshaping would prevent such deformities.

utility knife with a curved blade, a set of small metal files or fine-grain nail files, as appropriate (Figs 5.20–5.23). In small birds, the overgrown nail is cut using small nail clippers, commonly used for children. The nails are then reshaped using metal files, for larger birds, or fine-grain nail files for smaller species. To trim the talons of larger birds, in particular birds of prey, it is preferable to use the guillotine-type nail clippers commonly used for dogs. The talons are reshaped using a utility knife and by using a combination of flat and round metal files. A hand-held Dremel hand drill with grinder attachments could also be used to reshape strong talons. During the trimming process, hemorrhages may occur if the nails or talons are cut too short. Usually it is only necessary to trim the tips, 3 mm in smaller species and up to 5–8 mm in larger birds. Hemorrhages of the nails and talons can be stopped using a silver nitrate pencil, thermocautery or electrocautery.

Very often, the clinician is confronted with a detached or broken claw or talon. A protective cover can be made using multiple layers of cyanoacrylate glue, antibiotic powder and talcum powder (Molnar and Ptacek, 2001). Alternatively, cyanoacrylate glue and fine sodium bicarbonate powder can also be used to the same effect.

The beaks of cage and aviary birds and birds of prey are also prone to overgrowth due to lack of wear (Figs 5.24 and 5.25). Deformities of the beak, in particular in Psittaciformes, are also frequently found and are usually associated with the continuous use of the beak for hanging, climbing and moving around the cage. Other medical conditions associated with beak deformities include neoplasia, nutritional deficiencies, knemidocoptic mite infestation and traumatic injuries.

The beak can be trimmed using similar instruments as for nail trimming. Nail clippers are very useful in most species. After trimming, the beak can be reshaped using

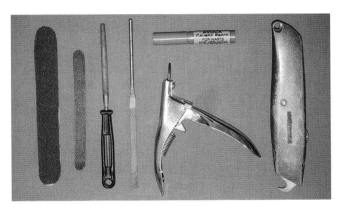

Fig. 5.20 Materials and equipment commonly used for coping the talons of captive birds of prey.

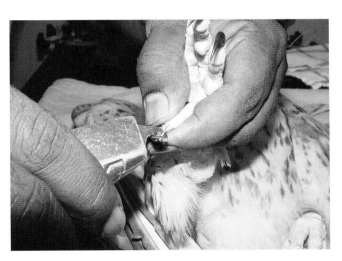

Fig. 5.22 A utility knife (commonly used to cut carpets) fitted with a curved blade is a very useful tool to reshape the talons of falcons.

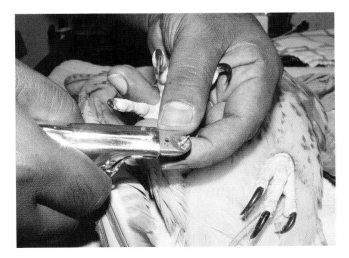

Fig. 5.21 Guillotine type nail cutters are ideal for trimming the talons of falcons and the nails of other birds.

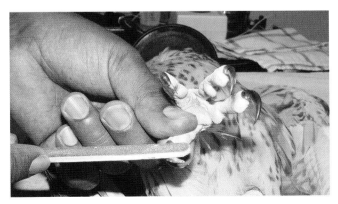

Fig. 5.23 Fine-grain nail files give the final touch in the process of talon trimming and reshaping. The application of mineral oil or paraffin at the end of the procedure is always indicated.

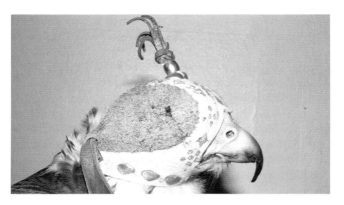

Fig. 5.24 A saker falcon (*Falco cherrug*) with an extremely long beak. It is not uncommon for beaks in such birds to break during feeding.

nail files in small species or a combination of flat and round metal files for larger birds. In birds with a strong and solid beak, such as macaws and cockatoos, the use of a Dremel hand drill with a suitable attachment for sanding down maybe more appropriate.

The lateral aspects of the beak are prone to cracks and splits (Figs 5.27 and 5.28). Periodic filing is sometimes necessary in order to avoid more serious problems, including fractures. It is strongly recommended that the tip of the beak of captive birds of prey used for falconry is clipped at the start of the molting season. Coping is the ancient falconry term meaning the trimming and reshaping of talons and beaks in Falconiformes.

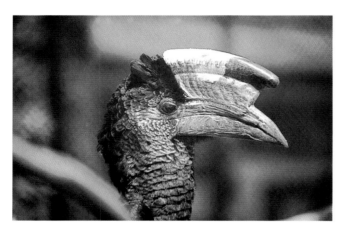

Fig. 5.25 In captivity, hornbills are prone to suffer from cracks, splinting and fractures of the beak. Many of these conditions are related to suboptimal housing, management, nutrition and in many cases disease.

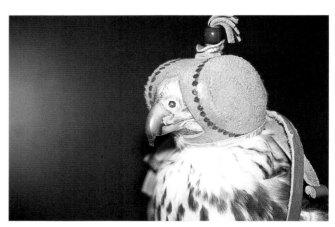

Fig. 5.27 A large crack with diffuse splinting on the lateral aspect of the beak of a saker falcon.

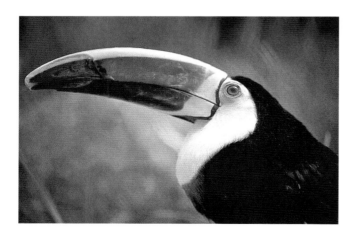

Fig. 5.26 Captive toucans are also prone to suffer from beak abnormalities including splinting and fractures.

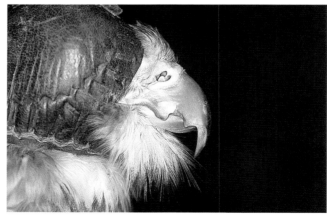

Fig. 5.28 A similar case on a saker falcon showing a normal tomial tooth and a crack with mild splinting further up on the beak.

Several techniques to repair cracks, fissures and fractures of the beak have been described in the literature (Rosskopf and Woerpel, 1996; Altman, 1997; Clipsham, 1997). The techniques include the repair of the beak using pins, stainless steel wire and the use of acrylic and epoxy resins (Figs 5.29 and 5.30).

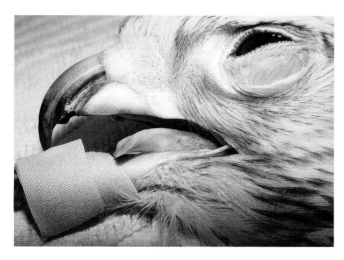

Fig. 5.29 A saker falcon was presented displaying a deep unilateral groove on one side of the beak. Note the absence of a well-defined tomial tooth.

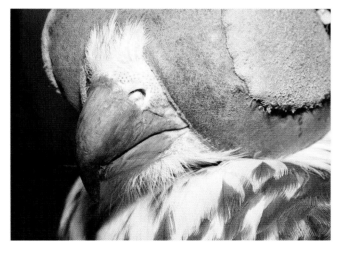

Fig. 5.30 The same falcon after beak repair. The groove was prepared by filing the edges to create a suitable bed for the back filling. Dental acrylic was used in this case to fill up the deficit and acrylic paints were used to match the color of the beak. Beak repair can also be carried out using multiple layers of cyanoacrylate glue and fine sodium bicarbonate powder.

REFERENCES

Altman RB (1997) Beak repair, acrylics. In: Altman RB, Clubb SL, Dorrestein GM, Quesenberry K (eds) *Avian Medicine and Surgery*, pp. 787–799. WB Saunders, Philadelphia.

Clipsham R (1997) Beak repair, rhamphorthotics. In: Altman RB, Clubb SL, Dorrestein GM, Quesenberry K (eds) *Avian Medicine and Surgery*, pp. 773–786. WB Saunders, Philadelphia.

Molnar L, Ptacek M (2001) Traumatic injuries of beak and talon of captive raptors. *Proceedings of the European Association of Avian Veterinarians*, Munich, pp. 246–247.

Rosskopf WJ, Woerpel RW (1996) Beak repair and surgery. In: Rosskopf WJ Jr, Woerpel RW (eds) *Disease of Cage and Aviary Birds*, 3rd edn, pp. 718–721. Williams & Wilkins, Baltimore.

Feather repair

Jaime Samour

The integrity of the primary feathers or remiges and tail feathers or rectrices is of the utmost importance for flight performance in species destined for release back into the wild or for birds of prey used in the ancient sport of falconry. Invariably, feathers tend to suffer bends or fractures during captivity in rescue and rehabilitation centers due to poor aviary or holding cage design or in crash landings or fighting with quarry during training or hunting or due to inadequate transport and handling practices.

Feather repair or imping, a medieval falconry term, is the art of repairing bent or fractured feathers. Modern imping techniques involve total or partial feather replacement or splinting. For a total and partial feather replacement, it is necessary to procure a feather that is of the same species, side (e.g. wing feather), size, sex, age and color. Rescue and rehabilitation centers, falconry enthusiasts and medical facilities devoted to raptors medicine usually maintain a collection of molted feathers and feathers obtained from carcasses. It is recommended to carry out feather examination and feather repair procedures under general inhalant anesthesia.

Materials and instruments used for imping

- Scissors, small, sharp, fine-pointed, 130 mm and 160 mm long
- Guillotine nail cutter, medium and large (e.g. cat and dog size)
- Imping needles, made from steel hairpins, long 50 mm × 1.5 mm, medium 40 mm × 1.5 mm, short 30 mm × 1.5 mm, fine 25 mm × 1 mm
- Hair clips (aluminum), 90 mm long
- Nail files, coarse and fine
- Cyanoacrylate glue, tube, 2 g
- Epoxy glue, fast setting (5 min), twin tubes, 4.2 g
- Sodium bicarbonate, powder, fine
- Pliers, curved, fine-tipped, 130 mm long

- Wire cutters, 200 mm long
- Flat metal file, 150 mm long, fitted with a plastic handle
- Barbecue skewers, bamboo pegs, different diameters (barbecue skewers are ideal)
- Knitting needles aluminum pegs, no. 14 (2 mm), 13 (2.2 mm), 12 (2.5 mm), 11 (3 mm), 10 (3.2 mm) and 9 (3.7 mm)
- Utility knife, fine pointed interchangeable blades
- Cardboard cards, thin, square 5 cm × 5 cm.

Bent feather repair

The treatment to correct bent feathers varies according to the severity of the damage. Usually in mild cases, bent feathers can be straightened up by applying steam, for a couple of minutes, from a boiling kettle. In more severe cases, it is necessary to apply hot water directly on to the affected area and straighten up the shaft of the feather by digital manipulation. Moderate or severe bending might occur at different levels of the shaft. Bent feathers are repaired using the splinting technique (Figs 5.31–5.38). The bend is straightened on its dorsoventral or laterolateral axis with a pair of fine-tipped, curved electrician pliers. The ventral aspect of the feather shaft is then split 12–15 mm in either direction from the bend. A small amount of cotton wool is placed in the newly created groove and secured firmly with cyanoacrylate glue. The glue when combined with the cotton wool creates a strong inner reinforcement mesh. The ventral surface of the feather shaft around the bend is roughened with a fine nail file. A thin layer of cyanoacrylate glue is smeared on to the site approximately 10 mm on either side of the bend.

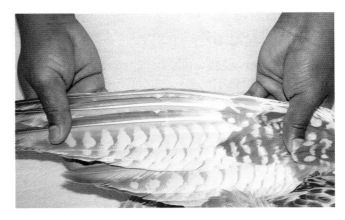

Fig. 5.32 Ventral view of the right wing of an adult female saker falcon (*Falco cherrug*) showing the first three feathers (Arab falconry classification) with partial fractures resulting in severe bends at the mid shaft. This type of fracture commonly occurs when the falcon strikes the perch or the ground during a fight with its quarry.

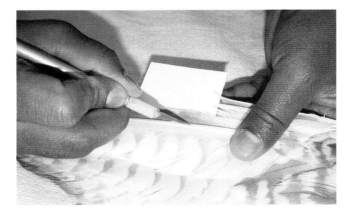

Fig. 5.33 The first step consists in making a longitudinal incision over the fracture extending about 10 mm in either direction of the fracture. The incision should include only the upper layer of the feather shaft.

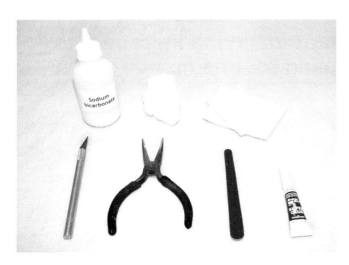

Fig. 5.31 Materials and instruments used by the author for feather repair.

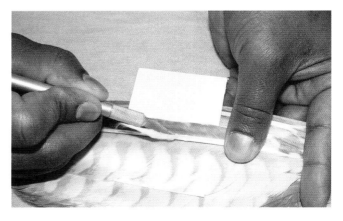

Fig. 5.34 The bend is straightened up on its dorsoventral and laterolateral aspects using a pair of fine-tipped curved pliers. An elongated wad of cotton wool is snugly inserted into the feather shaft using the blunt side of a utility knife.

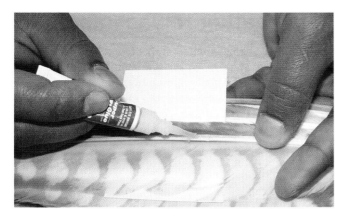

Fig. 5.35 A small amount of methacrylate glue is placed directly on the incision, impregnating the wad of cotton wool. Pressure is then applied laterally over the incision using a pair of fine-tipped curved pliers until the glue sets. When dried the glue-impregnated cotton wool provides a strong inner reinforcement to the damaged feather shaft.

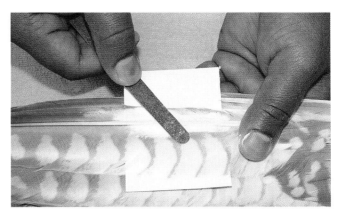

Fig. 5.37 The upper surface of the newly created layer is filed using a fine nail file. The procedure can be repeated two or three times in order to create a thicker layer should this prove necessary.

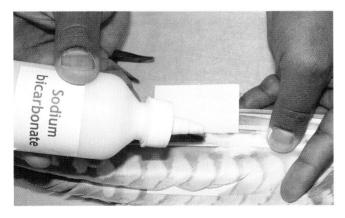

Fig. 5.36 The surface of the feather shaft around the incision is roughened using a fine nail file. A thin layer of methacrylate glue is applied over the area. A small amount of sodium bicarbonate is sprinkled directly on to the glued surface. The powder binds with the glue, creating a strong cement-like layer over the bend.

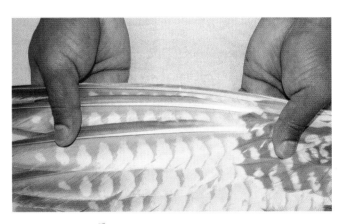

Fig. 5.38 The feathers are now repaired with a strong reinforcement splint formed over the original fracture. The external splint is translucent, making the need of coloring unnecessary.

A small amount of sodium bicarbonate is sprinkled directly on to the freshly glued surface. The sodium bicarbonate binds with the glue creating a strong cement-like layer over the bend. The procedure can be repeated two or three times to create a thicker layer if this proves necessary. The surface and the edges of the newly created layer are filed with a fine nail file. The external splint is translucent, making the need for coloring unnecessary.

Partial feather replacement

Partial feather replacement is indicated if the fracture has occurred at the mid-shaft or at the distal end of the feather. If the fracture is complete and the feather

fragment is missing, a similar fragment must be procured from a donor feather. Conversely, if the fragment is still available, this can then be reattached. In both cases, the ends of the fragments are smoothed out with fine-pointed scissors and a fine nail file in order to make a near perfect joint. A previously prepared imping needle, made from a steel hair fastener, of suitable length and diameter is carefully inserted in both fragments to make a narrow channel. A fine-diameter drill bit can also be used for the same purpose. The needle is then fixed to the fragment with a small amount of cyanoacrylate glue. The fragment is attached to the rest of the feather and checked for correct alignment. Additional glue is then applied to the free end of the needle of the fragment, which is then attached to the rest of the feather (Figs 5.39 and 5.40). Pressure should be applied

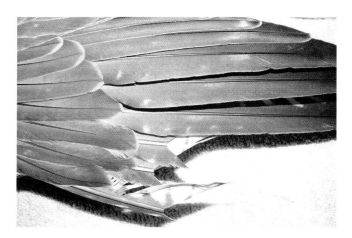

Fig. 5.39 This falcon suffered fractures of the first three primary (Arab falconry) feathers, with loss of the distal fragments. Similar fragments must be procured from donor feathers in order to maintain bilateral symmetry and to ensure adequate flying performance.

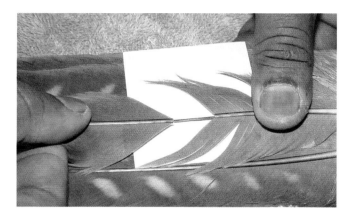

Fig. 5.40 A peregrine falcon (*Falco peregrinus*) suffered a fracture of a deck feather, with loss of the distal fragment. The fragment was fixed using a previously prepared imping needle manufactured from a steel hair fastener.

over the imping site with fine-tipped electrician's pliers for approximately 30 s to allow the glue to set. The dorsal and ventral aspects of the fracture line are then filed with a fine nail file. In partial replacement, it is strongly recommended that a ventral external splint, fabricated from multiple layers of cyanoacrylate glue and sodium bicarbonate, is applied in addition to the method described above to produce a more satisfactory and efficient result. The dorsal aspect of the imping site can be colored, if necessary, with a marker pen. The main disadvantage of this method is that the feather tends to rebreak near either tip of the rigid imping needle when subjected to stress.

Total feather replacement

Total feather replacement is indicated when the feather is fractured at the proximal section of the feather shaft (Figs 5.41–5.50). After examination and determining the number of feathers for replacement, the area should be prepared. First, the covert feathers are deflected backward and held in place using 1″ masking tape to

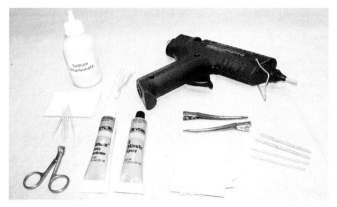

Fig. 5.41 Materials, instruments and equipment used by the author for total feather replacement.

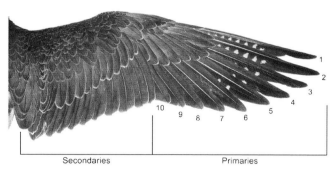

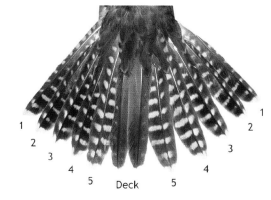

Fig. 5.42 Arab falconry classification of wings and tail feathers.

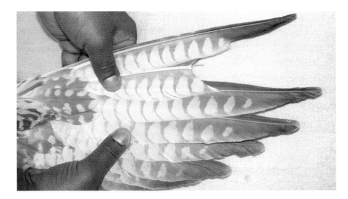

Fig. 5.43 Ventral view of the left wing of an adult female saker falcon showing a fracture of the second feather (Arab falconry classification), with loss of the distal one-third segment.

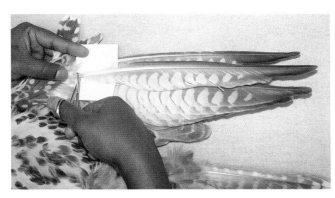

Fig. 5.44 A suitable feather is procured, taking into consideration the species, sex, age and size of the individual and the color and markings of the feather. The feather is measured and cut making sure bilateral symmetry is maintained.

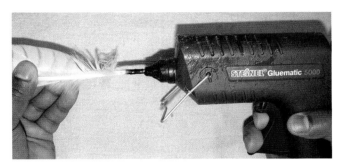

Fig. 5.45 A small amount of hot glue is applied directly into the feather shaft of the newly selected feather. An aluminum imping needle of suitable diameter is promptly inserted into the shaft, as the glue tends to sets in seconds.

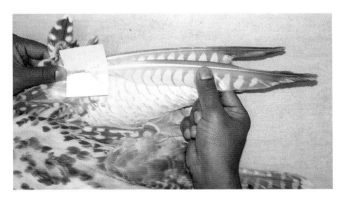

Fig. 5.46 The feather is then inserted into the shaft to double-check the length and correct angle.

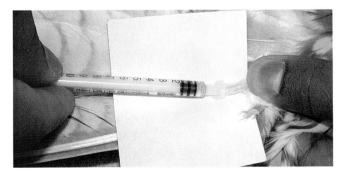

Fig. 5.47 Rapid-setting epoxy glue is then prepared and inserted into the shaft using a tuberculin syringe. Note that a small card has been placed underneath the working site in order to avoid smearing glue on the adjacent feathers.

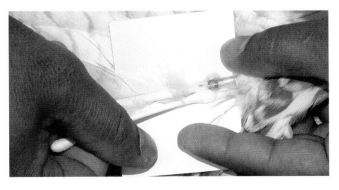

Fig. 5.48 The new feather is then placed into the shaft and any surplus of epoxy glue is wiped off using cotton buds.

expose the base of the shaft. The fractured feather is cut approximately 15–25 mm from the skin with a nail cutter. The new feather is placed in position to assess the length, making sure that bilateral symmetry is maintained with the opposite wing, when replacing a wing feather or the opposite side, if replacing a tail feather. If the feather from the opposite side is missing, the veterinarian or technician should follow the feathering pattern of the wing or tail characteristic of the species. For instance, in a peregrine falcon, primary 10 (no. 1 in Arab falconry) is approximately 5–8 mm shorter than primary 9 (no. 2 in Arab falconry) (Fig. 5.42).

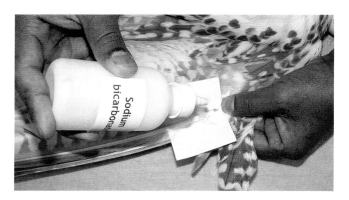

Fig. 5.49 A small amount of sodium bicarbonate is sprinkled on to the working site to bind with any glue residue.

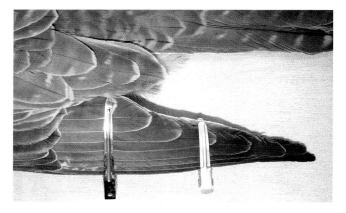

Fig. 5.50 Hair clips are placed to ensure that the feathers remain in the correct position while the glue sets.

imping site should be cleaned using cotton buds and a small amount of sodium bicarbonate is then applied to complete the cleaning process. The wing or the tail should then be closed in the natural anatomical position and all the feathers held in place with hair clips until the glue is set.

It is of paramount importance to ensure that bamboo pegs made from barbecue skewers are immersed in water prior to use, as dried old bamboo pegs are very brittle. Bamboo pegs can also be made from freshly cut green bamboo stems. Conversely, lightweight aluminum pegs can be used for the same purpose. These can be manufactured from knitting needles commonly found in tailor's and handicraft shops and are available in different diameters. These are the pegs I prefer to use. Such pegs offer several advantages. First, knitting needles are cheap and readily available on the market; second, pegs made from these needles can be cut and shaped using common hardware tools, e.g. strong wire cutters and flat files; third, and most importantly, the pegs can be bent to ensure adequate alignment. A useful and comprehensive review of the different techniques used for feather repair and feather replacement was recently published (Remple, 2003). A novel technique concerning feather cysts and repair under the skin is methodically described.

Figs 5.51–5.53 illustrate a related technique for fitting telemetry equipment to the tail feathers of a falcon in order to locate it while free flying.

This general ornithological knowledge is essential to carrying out feather replacement adequately. The feather is cut, and a bamboo peg about 80–100 mm long is prepared by sharpening both ends to approximate the diameter of the shaft of the new feather and the empty shaft of the wing. The wooden peg is first glued into the shaft of the new feather with fast-setting epoxy. Additional glue is then injected with a 1 ml tuberculin syringe into the shaft, making sure the feather is properly aligned. Fractures at the proximal end of growing feathers (e.g. 'green' or 'blood' feathers) are corrected by firstly applying a plug made of cotton wool for a few days and waiting until the feather follicle has stopped bleeding. Small crocodile forceps, commonly used to retrieve foreign objects from the ear, are suitable for removing the cotton plug. When the bleeding has stopped and the feather shaft is judged to be fully grown, a new feather is attached using the technique described above. A small piece of cardboard should be placed under the imping site to prevent the glue from smearing on to adjacent feathers. Any glue residue around the

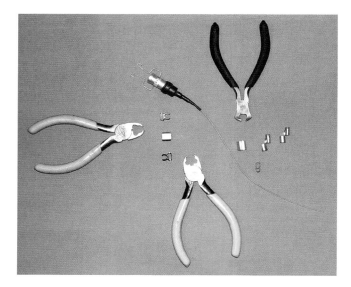

Fig. 5.51 Radio transmitters and the use of telemetry equipment are nowadays widely used in the sport of falconry. A tail kit integrates a small, battery-operated radio transmitter fitted with a long aerial and mounted on a stainless steel clip, and a tail feather clamp.
The photograph shows different types of feather clamps and fixing tools, together with a radio transmitter.

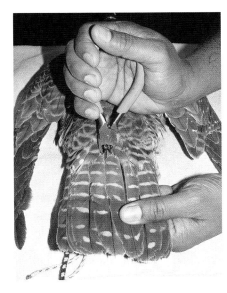

Fig. 5.52 Fixing a Marshal® tail feather clamp to a peregrine falcon using a dedicated Marshal® fixing tool. The clamp is fixed on to a central deck feather. Some operators prefer to add a small amount of epoxy glue to ensure an adequate grip.

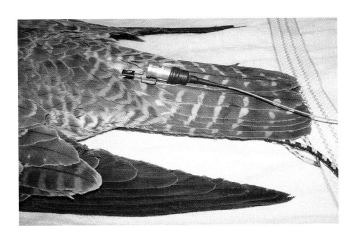

Fig. 5.53 The radio transmitter has been fixed on the tail of the falcon. The use of telemetry equipment allows the falconer to locate the falcon if it flies away during a training session or while on a hunting trip.

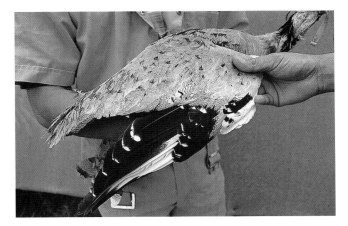

Fig. 5.54 Wing clipping is a very simple avicultural procedure carried out to prevent birds from flying. The main disadvantage of this procedure is that the flight is impaired for only a relatively short period. The wing of the bird is fully extended in preparation for the procedure. (Courtesy of Dr. T. A. Bailey).

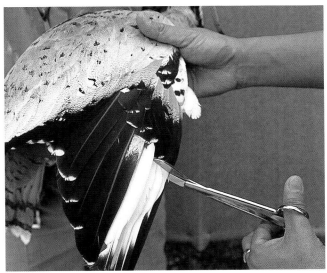

Fig. 5.55 Wing clipping is carried out by simply cutting short the primary feathers of one wing only, using a pair of strong scissors or bandage shears. (Courtesy of Dr. T. A. Bailey).

REFERENCE

Remple JD (2003) Feather tricks: practical pearls for the avian practitioner. *Proceedings of the European Association of Avian Veterinarians*, Tenerife, pp. 185–190.

Wing clipping and pinioning

Jaime Samour

Wing clipping and pinioning are techniques designed to prevent birds from flying. This is indicated when birds such as waterfowl, cranes, storks and flamingoes are housed in open paddocks, or highly nervous terrestrial species are kept in large aviaries. Wing clipping is carried out by simply cutting short the primary feathers of one wing only using a pair of strong scissors (Figs 5.54 and 5.55). It is recommended that the first and second feathers are left intact, since these will give the closed wing a more natural appearance. Excessive trimming should be avoided at all times (Fig. 5.56), since the object of wing trimming is to stop the bird from maintaining a strong and sustainable flight and not to stop the bird flying at all. Excessive trimming could result in accidents if the bird is unable to escape from cage companions or to move freely

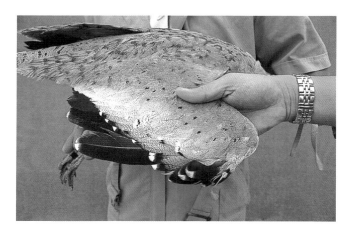

Fig. 5.56 In this case, all the primary feathers were cut. However, it is recommended that the first and second feathers are left intact, since these will give the closed wing a more natural appearance. (Courtesy of Dr. T. A. Bailey).

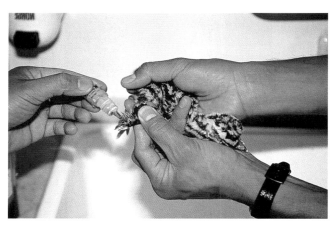

Fig. 5.57 Pinioning is a relatively easy procedure to undertake in young birds. The technique is based on the amputation of the wing tip just below the carpal joint using a pair of scissors. Anesthesia is not necessary. Hemorrhage can be arrested by using silver nitrate pencils or commercially available surgical glue. (Courtesy of Dr. T. A. Bailey).

within the enclosure. Wing trimming should be carried out only when the feathers are fully grown, since the cutting of 'green' or 'blood' feathers will result in profuse bleeding. The main disadvantage of this procedure is that the flight is impaired only for a relatively short period. Birds need to be caught within a 2–3-month period to undergo the same procedure again.

There are several more permanent techniques to deflight birds, including patagiectomy, tenotomy and tenectomy of the extensor tendons, neurectomy, fusing the carpal joint by cerclage and pinioning (Fig. 5.57). Most of these techniques (tenotomy, tenectomy) are not reliable and birds are able to fly within a short time. Other techniques, such as patagiectomy, fusing of the carpal joint and neurectomy are expensive and time-consuming. Therefore, pinioning is the method most widely used in bird gardens and zoological collections worldwide.

Ideally, pinioning should be conducted when the birds are around 1 week old. The process at this age is relatively simple and is conducted using only a pair of scissors. The wing of the bird is cut at the proximal end of the metacarpal bone, although this is sometimes difficult to assess at such a young age. Usually the sectioned stump does not bleed, but it is highly recommended that a commercially available surgical glue is available to apply to the wound in case of hemorrhage.

In adult birds, pinioning is a much larger surgical procedure. The surgery should be performed under full anesthesia. The area around the metacarpal joint is prepared for surgery and a circular incision is made on the skin, around 2–5 cm from the joint depending on the size of the bird. It is recommended that the larger blood vessels are ligated before severing the muscle and tendons. The bones are then cut using an orthopedic saw. The skin is stitched using a purse string suture or simple interrupted stitches. A dressing and a bandage are then applied to the tip of the wing. An alternative to this method consists of amputating the wing tip by disarticulation of the carpal joint instead of severing the wing tip just below the joint. The alula is left in place to provide a more natural appearance.

Lewandowski and Sikarskie (1996) described a different pinioning technique. The area around the metacarpal joint was first infiltrated with a local anesthetic and then a castration rubber band was applied just above the incision site. The skin and underlying tissues, including the bones, were cut using a double-action bone cutter. A dressing and a bandage were then applied to the stump. Sutures were not considered necessary. More recently, a technique to deflight pigeons and cockatiels was described. The birds were placed in sternal recumbency and a surgical incision was made over the shoulder. After debriding the muscles, the tendon of the supracoracoideus muscle was bluntly dissected and a small section, of approximately 4–5 mm, was removed. The muscle fascia and the skin were sutured. After the procedure, none of the birds had normal dorsal extension of the wing, but they could fly if placed outdoors. The authors concluded that neither unilateral nor bilateral tenectomy of the supracoracoideus muscle was an effective method to deflight pigeons and cockatiels (Degernes and Feduccia, 2001).

REFERENCES

Lewandowski AH, Sikarskie JG (1996) Pinioning. A quick and simple technique. *1st International Conference of Zoo and Avian Medicine*, pp. 414–415.

Degernes LA, Feduccia A (2001) Tenectomy of the supracoracoideus muscle to deflight pigeons (*Columba livia*) and cockatiels (*Nymphicus hollandicus*). *Journal of Avian Medicine and Surgery* **15**: 10–16.

Bandages and dressings

Judith C. Howlett

The application of a bandage is a skill in which veterinarians and veterinary technicians should become proficient. A bandage should be comfortable for the patient, look professional and serve the purpose for which it is designed. Several principles must be followed to avoid complications. Bandages should be sufficiently padded, applied evenly and snugly and in three layers, and placed to avoid the newly formed granulation tissue or epithelium. There are many different bandages and dressings available from simple to sophisticated, some of which are listed below (Figs 5.58–5.63).

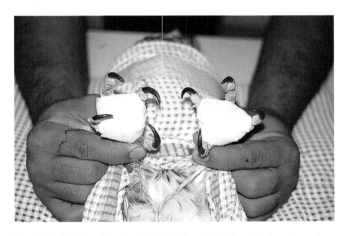

Fig. 5.58 'Ball bandage' on the feet of a saker falcon (*Falco cherrug*) recently operated on for bumblefoot. (Courtesy of Dr. J. Samour).

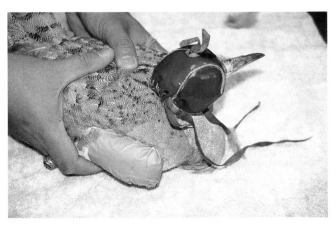

Fig. 5.59 Dressing and bandage applied to the wing of a houbara bustard (*Chlamydotis undulata*) after pinioning was carried out.

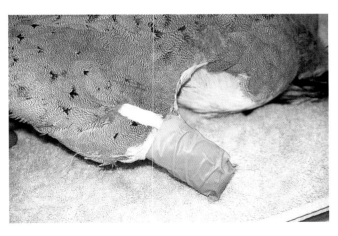

Fig. 5.60 The same bird as in Fig. 5.59 showing the correct way of 'anchoring' the bandage to the wing in order to stop it from slipping. The author currently uses a cohesive bandage, such as Vetrap® instead of Sleek ®, as the preferred choice for the tertiary layer.

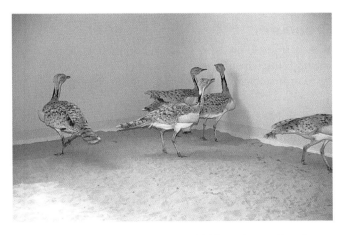

Fig. 5.61 A group of houbara bustards with bilateral protective wing bandages. Such bandages are fitted on the wings of newly arrived birds to prevent injuries during the adaptation period. The birds in the photograph were housed at the quarantine facility of the National Avian Research Center, United Arab Emirates.

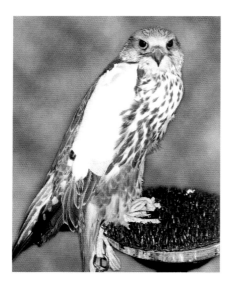

Fig. 5.62 Figure-8 bandage on the wing of a saker falcon (*Falco cherrug*) applied immediately after surgery to stabilize a fracture of the ulna. Careful management of this type of bandage is necessary in order to avoid damage to the patagial membrane.

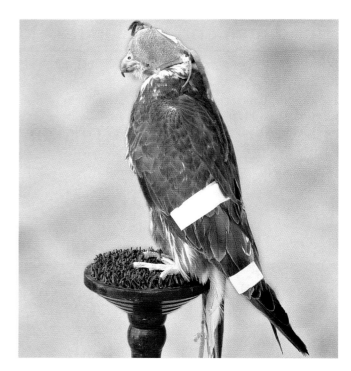

Fig. 5.63 A simple bandage applied to the wing of a saker falcon after surgery to immobilize a fractured radius. In this case, a single intramedullary pin was fixed together with the bandage. This bandage consists of two rings made of 1″ masking tape in order to hold the primary feathers in place and to stop the falcon from opening the wing. This is the bandage of choice used on the wings of falcons after surgery at our hospital to reduce and immobilize fractures of the ulna and/or the radius.

Functions of dressings and bandages

Protection

- To protect wounds following surgery and prevent desiccation
- To provide thermal insulation
- To prevent interference with wounds from beak and claw
- To protect wounds from pathogenic organisms.

Pressure

- As a first aid measure to avert hemorrhage and edema and reduce dead space
- To reduce swelling following trauma or surgery.

Support

- As a first aid measure to minimize further damage from a simple fracture
- To immobilize the affected part and therefore relieve pain following surgery or trauma
- To maintain intravenous and intraosseous catheters.

Absorption, moist environment, holding in place

- Dressings absorb exudate and help debride the wound surface

- Dressings help to maintain a moist environment to encourage granulation and re-epithelialization as quickly as possible
- Correct bandaging keeps a dressing in place.

Comfort

- To provide comfort for the patient.

Other characteristics of an ideal dressing

- Low-adherence or nonadherent
- Requiring infrequent changing
- Free from particulate contaminants
- Safe to use (nontoxic, nonsensitizing, nonallergenic)
- Comfortable and moldable
- Good absorption characteristics (exuding wounds)
- Impermeable to microorganisms
- Sterile
- Available in a suitable range of sizes/forms
- Cost-effective.

Process of selection

The correct dressing for wound management depends not only on the type of wound but also on the stage of the healing process. When selecting a dressing good knowledge of wound healing processes is essential in addition to an awareness of the properties of the dressing available. Successful wound management requires these two factors to be considered together. Many of the principles and techniques of wound management and bandaging in mammals apply to birds, although of course anatomical differences have to be considered. Wound dressing materials for humans are being continually developed with increased knowledge of wound healing processes. The new dressings keep wounds moist and prevent scab formation, which significantly increases the rate of re-epithelialization. Adaptation of these products in avian medicine has significantly improved wound management and healing.

After initial assessment of wound type and appropriate stabilization (if necessary) of the bird it is essential to carry out wound lavage to wash away both visible and microscopic debris before applying any dressings. In human medicine, normal saline or even plain water is the preferred fluid for wound irrigation, as it is not toxic to the tissues. Use of antibiotics in wound flushing is controversial and strong solutions of antiseptics such as chlorhexidine can be toxic to healing tissues, an anachronism to be avoided. Some dressings are marketed specifically as wound-cleaning agents. Studies have shown that wound cleaning does not actually remove bacteria: it merely redistributes them. Following wound lavage, debridement of nonviable tissue can be performed.

Honey, an ancient remedy for the treatment of infected wounds, has recently been 'rediscovered' by the medical profession. Following 10 years' research in Australian, New Zealand and UK hospitals in 2006, Medihoney™ launched two new honey-based wound care products. There are a number of published reports describing the effectiveness of honey in reducing infection from wounds, with no adverse effects, and there is also some evidence to suggest that honey may actively promote healing.

It is good practice to use a standardized wound assessment tool to ensure that valid reliable and consistent information is documented.

Wound assessment

Wound assessment should include:

- Location of wound
- Cause of wound
- Form
- Etiology

- Tissue type:
  1. Necrotic (usually black, covered with devitalized epidermis)
  2. Sloughy (contains a layer of viscous fluid with dead cells – yellow in color)
  3. Clinically infected/malodorous (yellow/green in color)
  4. Granulating (highly vascular granulation tissue – red in appearance)
  5. Epithelializing (shows evidence of pink wound margin)
- Size
- Exudate.

Management objectives of wound treatment

- *Dry necrotic wound*. Debride and provide a moist wound environment
- *Sloughy wound*. Cleanse, debride, absorb, fill in dead space and provide a moist wound environment
- *Highly exuding wound*. Control large amounts of exudate to help prevent maceration while maintaining a moist wound environment
- *Cavity wound*. Protect, hydrate and fill in dead space
- *Granulating/epithelializing wound*. Protect, fill in dead space and provide a moist wound environment
- *Skin tear*. Protect, fixate, absorb and provide a moist wound environment
- *Surgical*. Protect, absorb and provide a moist wound environment.

The three main layers of bandaging and dressings are shown in Table 5.12.

- *Primary or dressing layer* – the dressing that is in contact with the wound. It should be sterile, stay in place against the wound with patient movement and provide a moist wound climate and assist debridement, encourage granulation and re-epithelialization
- *Secondary layer* – for absorption of fluids and wound exudates, padding the wound from trauma, support or immobilize a limb and giving protection to underlying fractures
- *Tertiary layer* – serving to hold other layers in place, provides pressure and keeps inner layers protected from the environment.

Care of bandages

- Bandages should be protected from dirt and wet
- Good observation is necessary to check for movement of the bandage or dressings and the presence of any sores, unpleasant odors, discharges and discoloration

- The bird should be prevented from interfering with the bandage; in psittacines it may be necessary to use an Elizabethan collar or similar neck restraining device

- Most dressings are suitable to be left in situ for 3–7 days and should be left undisturbed to maintain constant temperature, humidity and reduce bacterial access. If wounds are infected or the dressing becomes contaminated it is then essential to change them.

TABLE 5.12 Materials for dressings

Dressing – make and manufacturer	Description and application
PRIMARY LAYER	
Adhesive dressings Fine mesh and open weave pads and gauze swabs	Wet to dry bandaging. Warm saline-soaked gauze swabs with daily changes can be used in the first 3–4 d in open, severely contaminated wounds to encourage debridement and removal of necrotic tissue. These can be followed by hydroactive dressings Disadvantages of wet to dry dressings are that the moist environment may encourage the growth of bacteria and that regular dressing change may disrupt the healing process. With the advent of hydrogels and hydrocolloids they are now obsolete
Antimicrobial dressings Actisorb® plus (Johnson & Johnson) Actisorb® Silver 220 (Johnson & Johnson) Acticoat™ with Silcryst™ (Smith & Nephew) Inadine® (Johnson & Johnson)	Suitable for discharging purulent and contaminated wounds Contains activated charcoal and silver, which inhibits bacterial growth. The dressing creates a favorable environment for effective wound healing by adsorbing and killing microorganisms that contaminate and infect wounds. Activated charcoal also binds bacterial endotoxins Acticoat™ with Silcryst™ nanocrystals works in a similar way to Actisorb® Silver 220 A topical antimicrobial wound dressing impregnated with an ointment containing 10% povidone–iodine (PVP-I). The povidone molecule provides sustained release of iodine
Calcium alginate dressings Sorbsan (Pharma-Plast Ltd, Steriseal Division) Sorbsan Plus (Pharma-Plast Ltd) 3M™ Tegagen™ Alginate Dressing (3M Health Care Ltd) Kaltostat® (ConvaTec Ltd) Kaltogel® (ConvaTec Ltd) AlgiSite™ M (Smith & Nephew) Melgisorb® (Mölnlycke)	Highly absorbent biodegradable alginate dressings are derived from seaweed and are applied to cleanse a variety of secreting lesions; high absorption is achieved via a strong hydrophilic gel that limits wound secretions and minimizes bacterial contamination. Alginate fibers trapped in a wound are readily biodegraded. These cavity dressings are presented in a variety of forms – rope, ribbon filler – depending on product. Area of use: sloughy wounds, cavity wounds, not suitable for dry necrotic wounds or infected wounds. Most require a secondary dressing
Collagen dressings Collamend dressings and particles (Genitrex Animal Health and Nutrition)	Contains collagen and can be used with hydrogels and MVP dressings. Suitable for use with degloved wounds, burns and lacerations. Particles make excellent contact with wound surface, can absorb 60 times their own weight in fluid; help remove exudate and infectious materials from wound; act as an enzymatic debriding agent. Dressings are porous collagen membranes that can be used on any wound type at any stage of healing. Produces fluid containing growth factors. Interacts with the wound bed to form an optimal environment for wound healing. Provides a matrix for cell epithelialization
Honey Medihoney™ Antibacterial Wound Gel Medihoney™ Antibacterial Medical Honey	Antibacterial Wound Gel and Antibacterial Medical Honey are both packaged in single-use tubes. The gel has a high viscosity and is recommended for use with ulcers, surgical sites and burns. Deep wounds, sinuses and necrotic and surgical wounds are best treated with the honey
Hydrocellular (Foam) dressings Allevyn™ (Smith & Nephew) Allevyn™ Cavity Wound Dressing (Smith & Nephew) Tielle® (Johnson & Johnson) Lyofoam (Seton Healthcare Group) Mepilex® (Mölnlycke)	These products consist of hydrophobic polyurethane foam or polyurethane foam film with or without adhesive borders. The side of the dressing that comes in contact with the skin has been heat-treated to collapse the cells of the foam and thus enable it to absorb liquid by capillarity. The dressings are freely permeable to gases and water vapor but resist the penetration of aqueous solutions and wound exudate. When used the dressing absorbs blood or other tissue fluids and the aqueous component is lost through evaporation via the back of the dressing. The dressing maintains a moist, warm environment at the surface of the wound, which is conducive to the formation of granulation tissue and

TABLE 5.12 Materials for dressings *(continued)*

Dressing – make and manufacturer	Description and application
	re-epithelialization. Most foams are suitable for light to medium exuding wounds. They can be held in place with tape or a bandage: a secondary dressing is not usually required. Not recommended for dry or superficial wounds
Hydrocolloid or hydroactive dressings Granuflex® (ConvaTec) DuoDerm® (ConvaTec) DuoDerm® ExtraThin (ConvaTec) Comfeel Hydrocolloid Dressing (Coloplast) 3M™ Tegasorb™ Hydrocolloid Dressing (3M Health Care Ltd) 3M™ Tegasorb™ Thin Hydrocolloid Dressing (3M) RepliCare™ Ultra (Smith & Nephew)	Semi-flexible opaque membranes most are impermeable to moisture vapor and act as a physical barrier on a necrotic wound and help it become rehydrated. The necrotic tissue eventually separates leaving behind yellow partially liquefied material known as slough. The dressings adhere to the normal skin but not to wounds and form a gelatinous mass over the wound that creates a good atmosphere for healing. Hydrocolloids promote the formation of granulation tissue and provide pain relief by covering nerve endings with gel and exudate. These dressings have been successfully used in a variety of avian species and are particularly useful for extensive wounds with an excessive exudate production. Also for wounds that are slow to heal and those in need of debridement. DuoDerm Extra Thin has been successfully used on chronic scalp traumas and held in place with dabs of Vetbond (3M) tissue glue. DuoDerm extra thin has limited absorbency and used in treatment of lightly exuding wounds. It can also be used as a secondary dressing over hydrogels and alginates. DuoDerm can be changed on a weekly basis once healing processes are underway. In their intact state most hydrocolloid dressings are impermeable to water vapor but as the gelling process takes place the dressing becomes progressively more permeable. Hydrocolloids are not suitable for infected wounds
Hydrogels IntraSite™ Gel (Smith & Nephew) Granugel (ConvaTec) Nu-Gel® (Johnson & Johnson) Purilon Hydrogel (Coloplast) Vetalintex Wound Hydrogel (Robinson Animal Healthcare)	Hydrogels' basic structure consists of 2–3% gel-forming polymer such as sodium carboxymethylcellulose, modified starch or sodium alginate, 20% propylene glycol and 80% water. Gel is placed on the wound and covered with a suitable secondary layer (e.g. MVP or thin hydrocolloid dressings) that prevents loss of moisture from the gel or absorption by the outer layer. Water is donated by the gel to the dead tissue and it becomes rehydrated and thus more easily removed. Hydrogels are suitable for use on dry, 'sloughy' or necrotic wounds and lightly exuding wounds. They are suitable for all stages of wound healing except infected or heavily exuding wounds
Low-adherence dressings Melolin™ (Smith & Nephew) Mepitel® (Mölnlycke Health Care) Mepore® (Mölnlycke) Mesorb® (Mölnlycke) N-A Ultra® (Johnson & Johnson Medical) Release® (Johnson & Johnson) Tricotex (Smith & Nephew)	Low-adherence dressings are the current-day alternative to traditional dry dressings such as cotton wool, gauze and lint. N-A Ultra is claimed to be truly nonadherent; the other dressings are considered low-adherence. Most are suitable on dry or lightly exuding wounds. Mepitel, Mesorb and Mepore can be used on medium to heavily exuding wounds, although a secondary dressing may be required to absorb excess exudate
Polysaccharide dressings Debrisan® beads Debrisan® Paste (Pharmacia & Upjohn Ltd)	Consist of pale dextranomer 0.1–0.3 mm diameter beads. When introduced into an exuding wound 1 g of beads will absorb up to 4 g of exudate. When applied to relatively small sloughy wounds the beads absorb fluid and progressively move bacteria and cellular debris away from the wound surface. Not for use on dry or lightly exuding wounds
Iodosorb™ (Smith & Nephew)	Consists of hydrophilic beads of cadexomer (a modified starch hydrogel, which is biodegradable) impregnated with elemental iodine. Suitable for infected exuding cavities. Dressings need to be changed regularly if wound heavily exuding, indicated by loss of color of the iodine
Iodoflex ™ (Smith & Nephew)	Consists of a sterile cadexomer iodine paste sandwiched in protective gauze and changed when there is a loss of color
Polyurethane matrix dressing Cutinova™ Hydro (Smith & Nephew) Hydro-Selective™ Dressing	Cutinova Hydro is a recently introduced dressing developed as a successor to the hydrocolloids. It has been designed to offer the benefits of a hydrocolloid with none of the drawbacks. Its special structure offers a unique mode of action, absorbing water from wound fluid but leaving essential wound healing agents behind in the wound. Cutinova Hydro therefore combines all the proven benefits of clean, moist wound healing with the ability to leave growth factors, essential agents in wound healing and other natural proteins on the wound bed

Continued overleaf

TABLE 5.12 Materials for dressings (continued)

Dressing – make and manufacturer	Description and application
Tulle (nonmedicated) dressings Jelonet™ (Smith & Nephew) Paratulle (Seton)	Can be used for clean superficial wounds. Tulles contain different weights of paraffin per unit area. Paraffin reduces the adherence of the dressing to the wound but requires frequent changes to stop it drying out and being incorporated into granulation tissue. A secondary dressing is always required
Tulle (medicated) dressings Fucidin Intertulle (Leo Laboratories Ltd) Bactigras™ (Smith & Nephew) Serotulle (Seton) Clorhexitulle (Roussel) Sofra-Tulle (Roussel)	Medicated tulle dressings are often used inappropriately for infected superficial wounds. Bactigras, Clorhexitulle and Serotulle are similar, containing 0.5% chlorhexidine. These dressings are suitable if the use of an antiseptic product is deemed necessary. The use of Fucidin Intertulle and Sofra-Tulle is declining in healthcare as both products contain topical antibiotics and lanolin, which carries the risk of skin sensitization
Vapor-permeable adhesive film (MVP) dressings Bioclusive® (Johnson & Johnson) OpSite™ Flexigrid™ (Smith & Nephew) 3M™ Tegaderm™ Transparent Film Dressing (3M Health Care Ltd) Tegaderm™ Plus (3M) Mefilm® (Mölnlycke)	MVP dressings are slim, flexible, transparent polyurethane membranes with an adhesive backing. They are permeable to oxygen but not to water or bacteria, allowing accumulation of fluid exudate under the dressing. The maintenance of an aerobic environment under the dressing prevents scab formation and promotes more rapid epithelialization, while preventing wound desiccation, as well as reducing pain associated with lack of moisture and raw nerve endings These, as well as hydrocolloid membranes, are indicated for a variety of avian wounds, but MVP dressings are more suited to areas that are difficult to bandage (e.g. head wounds) because of the superior adhesive quality and flexibility of the material. Dressings are changed every 2–3 d initially, more frequently if there is excessive exudate production resulting in leakage of fluid from under the dressing. Tegaderm Plus is coated with a layer of acrylic adhesive that contains 2% available iodine in the form of an iodophor; when in contact with the skin it slowly releases the iodine
Secondary layer **Padding** Absorbent cotton Softband Orthoband	Plenty of padding should be used, especially on pressure points and areas easily traumatized (e.g. wing tips)
Bandaging White open weave bandage	A cotton bandage, which has now been superseded by conforming bandage
Conforming bandage Crinx® (Smith & Nephew) Bioband (Leatherite PTY Ltd, Australia) Vet-Band™ (Millpledge Veterinary) Vetband® (Smith & Nephew)	Can be applied firmly over the initial dressing and padding and as the name suggests conforms to the area being bandaged Several layers may be applied. Bioband is an antimicrobial impregnated bandage that prevents the growth of Gram-positive and Gram-negative bacteria and reduces the risk of the bandage becoming a source of external contamination
Tertiary layer **Elastic adhesive bandage** Elastoplast (Smith & Nephew) Treatplast (Animalcare) Veterinary Flexoplast (Robinson)	Usually applied as the external layer to give extra support and hold the other bandage in place. Care should be taken not to wrap it too tightly or to attach it to too many feathers or skin
Cohesive bandage 3M Vetrap Bandaging Tape (3M Health Care Ltd) Coflex (Valley Vet Supply) Coban (3M) Wrapz™ (Millpledge Veterinary) Co-Form™ (Millpledge Veterinary) Easifix®	Consist of water-vapor-permeable, nonwoven polyester fabric containing longitudinal strands of polyester elastane. The fabric is coated with a self-adherent substance that gives the bandage the ability to stick to itself and not to the skin. Care is needed in its application, however, because of the loss of the potential for movement between turns of the bandage to equalize the pressure on local areas. High tension carries the risk of creating a tourniquet effect

Removal of dressings

- Bandages should be removed using round-ended scissors or bandage shears; care needs to be taken not to cut the skin or interfere with the healing process of the wound
- The actual dressing removal will depend on type used; flushing with saline may be necessary
- Contaminated dressings should be suitably disposed of and the scissors used in the procedure should be washed and sterilized
- Hands should be washed with an antiseptic solution before reapplying a new dressing.

The range of dressings available is diverse and, depending upon their structure and composition, dressings may be used to absorb exudate, combat infection, relieve pain, promote autolytic debridement, and provide and maintain a moist environment at the wound surface to promote granulation tissue and the process of epithelialization. Some dressings simply absorb exudate and may therefore be suitable for use with a variety of different wounds. Others have a very clearly defined specialist function and therefore have a more limited range of indications. Wound healing is a dynamic process; no one dressing is suitable for all wound types and few are suitable for the treatment of a single wound during all the stages of the healing process. Good wound management requires a flexible approach in the selection of dressings and understanding of the healing processes. Without taking this knowledge into consideration the process becomes rather capricious and potentially ineffective.

FURTHER READING

Cousquer G (2005) Wound management in the avian wildlife casualty. *World Wide Wounds*. Available online at: http://www.worldwidewounds.org

Degernes LA (1994) Trauma medicine. In: Ritchie BW, Harrison GJ, Harrison LR (eds) *Avian Medicine: Principles and Application*, pp. 417–422. Wingers Publishing, Lake Worth, FL.

Fowler A (2005) *How to Manage Open Wounds in Wildlife*. National Wildlife Rehabilitation Conference. Available online at: http://www.nwrc.com.au/forms/anne_fowler_1.pdf

Merck Veterinary Manual (2006) Emergency medicine and critical care: wound management. Available online at http://www.merckvetmanual.com/

Molan PC (2001) Honey as a topical antibacterial agent for the treatment of infected wounds. *World Wide Wounds*. Available online at: http://www.worldwidewounds.org

Morgan DA (1999) Wound management products on the Drug Tariff. *Pharmaceutical Journal* **263**: 820–825. Available online at: http://www.pjonline.com/Editorial/19991120/education/wounddressings.html

Redig PT (1996) Avian emergencies. In: Beynon PH, Forbes NA, Harcourt-Brown NH (eds) *Manual of Raptors, Pigeons and Waterfowl*, pp. 30–41. British Small Animal Veterinary Association, Cheltenham.

Stewart J (2002) Next generation products for wound management. *World Wide Wounds*. Available online at: http://www.worldwidewounds.org

Thomas S (1997) A structured approach to the selection of dressings. *World Wide Wounds*. Available online at: http://www.worldwidewounds.org

USEFUL WEB SITES

3M Health Care Ltd: http://cms.3m.com/cms/GB/en/2–163/ilkluFY/view.jhtml

Coloplast: http://www.coloplast.co.uk/

ConvaTec Ltd: http://www.convatec.com/UK/

Genitrix Animal Health Ltd: http://www.genitrix.co.uk/products/collamend.htm

Johnson & Johnson: http://www.jnj.com/home.htm

Medihoney: http://www.medihoney.com/

Mölnlycke Health Care: http://www.molnlycke.com/index.asp?id=3142&lang=2

Robinson Animal Healthcare: http://www.robinsoncare.com/AnimalDressings.htm

Smith & Nephew Medical Ltd: http://wound.smith-nephew.com/uk/Home.asp

Veterinary Wound Management Society: http://www.vwms.org/

World Wide Wounds: www.worldwidewounds.org

Protective foot casting

Jaime Samour

Protective foot casts are indicated to reduce pressure-related trauma to the newly created wound in the postoperative care of pododermatitis or bumblefoot (Figs 5.64–5.68). Halliwell (1981) first proposed the application of a thermoplastic tape (Hexcelite®) to immobilize the limbs of birds of prey. Remple and Remple (1987) described a casting method using the same thermoplastic tape as an adjunctive therapy to bumblefoot surgery in falcons. After surgery, a dressing and a bandage are applied to the distal tarsometatarsus and the foot using an elastic nonadhesive bandage (Vetrap®, 3M). Lighter, individual bandages are also placed around the first phalanx of each toe. The cast consists of one piece of thermoplastic tape wrapped

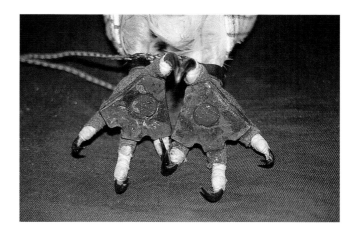

Fig. 5.64 Ventral view of the bandaged feet of a falcon after undergoing bumblefoot surgery. The protective castings are provided with a window at the center of the cast in order to avoid direct trauma to the surgical wound.

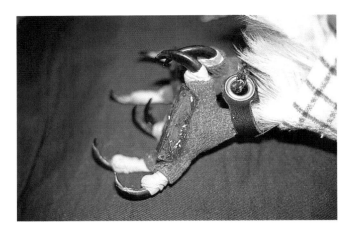

Fig. 5.65 Lateral view of the protective cast.

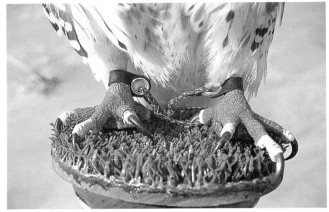

Fig. 5.66 The protective foot cast allows the falcon to stand comfortably on its perch.

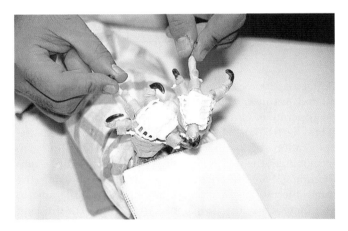

Fig. 5.67 Protective foot cast manufactured with a thermoplastic tape. The cast consists of one piece of the tape wrapped around the tarsometatarsus and extending forward to the first phalanx of each toe. A second piece of the tape is used to make a bridge under the foot, leaving a gap under the plantar surface.

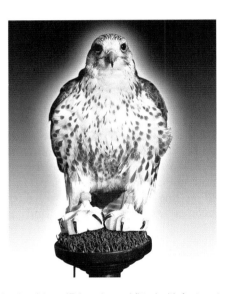

Fig. 5.68 A saker falcon (*Falco cherrug*) fitted with foot casts made of high-grade polystyrene foam. The foot casts can also be constructed from the soft rubber commonly used to manufacture beach sandals.

around the tarsometatarsus and extending forward to the first phalanx of each toe. Narrow strips of nonadhesive tape are used to fix each toe to the cast. A double-thickness piece of the thermoplastic tape is used to make a bridge under the foot, leaving a gap under the plantar surface of the foot. This piece is then secured on both sides of the tarsometatarsus. Before application, the thermoplastic tape should be immersed in hot water to make it pliable and easy to manipulate.

Remple (1993) proposed a new foot casting method for the post-surgical management of bumblefoot. Preformed 'shoes' or plantar casts were made using a commercially available styrene plastic polymer commonly used for car body repairs (Bondo). Casts of different sizes and shapes were prepared using precast molds. A large hollowed area is left at the center of the cast to ensure adequate protection of the newly operated site. After surgery the

foot and the toes, up to the first phalanx, are bandaged using an elastic nonadhesive tape (Vetrap). The cast is then glued on to the bandage.

Riddle and Hoolihan (1993) designed a form-fitting composite-casting method for the legs and wings of birds. This casting method was mainly used in the postoperative care of falcons operated on for bumblefoot. After surgery, the first phalanx of each toe was bandaged using an elastic nonadhesive bandage. A small amount of fast-setting epoxy glue was applied on to the ventral surface of each toe. Then a small ball was made of cotton wool and wrapped in the same nonadhesive tape to form a cylinder. This was then fixed on to the plantar area of the foot at the point of the base of the first phalanx of each toe. The cylinder was secured to the foot using the same nonadhesive tape. Fresh epoxy glue was coated on to the cylinder and was secured to the foot using the same nonadhesive tape. Fresh epoxy glue was coated on to the whole bandage and the cylinder. The sections of the bandage around the tarsometatarsus and the distal end of the toes were left without glue so as to allow a soft buffer layer between cast and skin. The bottom section of the cylinder was cut to provide a window to the plantar area of the foot and to allow periodic inspection and re-dressing of the wound.

Harcourt-Brown (1996) described the use of an adherent hydrocolloidal dressing in combination with a plastic casting material in the postoperative care of bumblefoot. More recently, Remple (2005) proposed the use of a silicone composite dental material to produce a form-fitting and flexible protective cast to aid healing in the postoperative care of bumblefoot. This technique produces a much softer shoe than any of the techniques previously described (Remple and Remple, 1987; Remple, 1993; Riddle and Hoolihan, 1993; Harcourt-Brown, 1996). I favor the use of protective shoes manufactured from a thick soft rubber commonly used to make beach sandals. These can be manufactured in different sizes and stored. Other surgeons prefer to use padded rings (doughnut-shaped) fitted to the feet of the bird using nonadhesive elastic bandages (N. Forbes, personal communication). The use of protective casts in the postoperative management of bumblefoot is not only limited to raptors. Recently, the use of protective shoes manufactured from neoprene was described in penguins (Reidarson et al., 1999). The shoes included a high heel to prevent slippage on icy surfaces and were fastened to the foot of the birds using Velcro straps. A similar technique can probably be used in the postoperative care of bumblefoot in other species, such as flamingoes, waders and shore birds and large waterfowl.

REFERENCES

Halliwell WH (1981) New thermoplastic casting material and its application to birds of prey. In: Cooper JE, Greenwood AG (eds) Recent Advances in the Study of Raptor Diseases, pp. 123–129. Chiron Publications, Keighley.

Harcourt-Brown NH (1996) Foot and leg problems. In: Beynon PH, Forbes NA, Harcourt-Brown NH (eds) Manual of Raptors, Pigeons and Waterfowl, pp. 147–168. British Small Animal Veterinary Association, Cheltenham.

Remple JD, Remple CJ (1987) Foot casting as adjunctive therapy to surgical management of bumblefoot in raptorial species. Journal of the American Animal Hospital Association 23: 633–639.

Remple JD (1993) Raptor bumblefoot: a new treatment technique. In: Redig PT, Cooper JE, Remple JD et al. (eds) Raptor Biomedicine, pp. 154–160. University of Minnesota Press, Minneapolis.

Remple JD (2005) Use of a composite silicone dental impression material to create a form-fitting, flexible, support cushion to facilitate wound healing in bumblefoot. Proceedings of the European Association of Avian Veterinarians, Arles, pp. 467–469.

Reidarson TH, McBain J, Burch L (1999) A novel approach to the treatment of bumblefoot in penguins. Journal of Avian Medicine and Surgery, 13(2): 124–127.

Riddle KE, Hoolihan J (1993) Form-fitting, composite-casting method for avian appendages. In: Redig PT, Cooper JE, Remple JD et al. (eds) Raptor Biomedicine, pp. 161–164. University of Minnesota Press, Minneapolis.

External splinting

Jaime Samour

External splinting devices are commonly used in avian medicine to immobilize injured or fractured limbs in the avian patient. There are various commercially available materials that can be used for this purpose, but many practitioners prefer to manufacture their own immobilizing devices made from materials ordinarily used in veterinary practice.

The ideal types of material for external splinting include commercially available orthopedic thermoplastic tape, aluminum padded finger splints and suitable padding material. The use of thermoplastic tape as the primary material for external splinting is highly recommended since it can be molded to a near-perfect fit over the limb. Aluminum finger splints can also be used as a primary material for external splinting in the case of bone fractures (e.g. tarsometatarsals).

One of the most common sites in birds requiring external splinting is over the radius and ulna. Coles (1985) described a method to immobilize fractures on this site. The method involves suturing a cut section of orthopedic tape padded underneath with a suitable padding material (e.g. polyurethane foam). The sutures are placed through the orthopedic tape and the padding material and they are firmly secured around the base of the secondary feathers of the wing.

A very useful external splint to immobilize fractures on the carpometacarpal bone and digits of wing tip injuries was described by Coles (1985). The method involves 'wrapping' the wing tip using a cut away section of an X-ray film. The two sections of the X-ray film are held in place by sutures applied through the film, the skin and between the shaft of the primary feathers.

Schroeder–Thomas splints have also been used to immobilize fractured legs in different avian species (Redig, 1986). These can be made using 1–2 mm steel wire or aluminum rods. This splint is particularly useful in immobilizing fractured legs of species with short, strong legs such as birds of prey and psittacines. The round section around the femoral area should be well padded in order to avoid abrasion of the skin. The splint should be bent slightly around the joints to accommodate the leg in a normal standing position. The leg is then firmly secured to the splint using nonadhesive tape.

Fractures of the tibiotarsal and tarsometatarsal bones are very common in small birds. Altman (1982) proposed the use of two sections of zinc oxide tape facing each other and placed on either side of the affected area. The tape is firmly secured by compressing the two sections, very close to the limb, using artery forceps. The splint can be removed later using a suitable solvent.

Product reference list

- Hexcelite®, Hexcel Corporation, Dublin, CA, USA.
- Veterinary Thermoplastic®, Imex Veterinary Inc., 1227 Market Street, Longview, TX 75604, USA.
- Sam Splint®, Moore Medical Corp., PO Box 2620, New Britain, CT 06050–2620, USA.

REFERENCES

Altman RB (1982) Disorders of the skeletal system. In: Petrak ML (ed.) *Diseases of Cage and Aviary Birds*, p. 260. Lea & Febiger, Philadelphia.

Coles BH (1985) *Avian Medicine and Surgery*. Blackwell Science, Oxford.

Redig PT (1986) Modification of the Schroeder–Thomas splint for birds. In: Harrison GJ, Harrison LR (eds) *Clinical Avian Medicine and Surgery*, p. 391. WB Saunders, Philadelphia.

Elizabethan collars

Jaime Samour

Elizabethan collars are very useful devices commonly used to stop birds from feather picking, self-mutilation or disturbing bandages and newly operated sites. The aim is to create a physical barrier between the sharp beak and the affected area. Elizabethan collars are commercially available in different sizes and are commonly made from clear vinyl or acrylic. These can also be made of any lightweight, rigid, but flexible material, such as cut away sections of radiographic films. Several modified versions of the traditional Elizabethan collar have been introduced into the market. A tubular shaped neck restraining device is available providing a more comfortable fit around the neck than the traditional disc shaped device. More recently, a spherical neck restraining appliance was introduced into the market. This is a spherical plastic collar that comes in two interlocking sections and is available in different diameters. This collar provides a comfortable fit around the neck and it can be fixed and removed by pet owners.

Product reference list

- Avian Spherical Collar®, GHN Inc., 9299 Mooring Circle, Fort Myers, FL 33912–4919, USA; http://www.aviancollar.com
- Veterinary Specialty Products Inc., PO Box 9311, Mission, KS 66201, USA; http://www.vet-products.com
- Hexcelite®, Hexcel Corporation, Dublin, CA, USA.
- Veterinary Thermoplastic®, Imex Veterinary Inc., 1227 Market Street, Longview, TX 75604, USA.
- Sam Splint®, Moore Medical Corp., PO Box 2620, New Britain, CT 06050–2620, USA.

Trauma-related medical conditions

6

Neck dislocation and fracture

Jesus Naldo

Neck dislocation or fracture is the loss of continuity of the cervical section of the vertebral column. Neck fractures are debatable subjects, as clinicians suggest fractures are not possible in birds because of the compact anatomical structure of the avian cervical vertebrae. Injuries that may result in dislocation or fracture of the cervical vertebral column are traumatic in origin and are usually associated with birds crashing into the fence or the roof of their enclosure. In our practice, both neck fractures and dislocations have been diagnosed (Figs 6.1–6.5). In most cases, affected birds were found dead beside the fence or wall of their aviary. External examination usually revealed bruising on the skin of the neck and swelling of the subcutaneous tissue due to hematoma. Bruising on the head is sometimes an accompanying finding. Initial diagnosis of dislocation or fracture was made through physical examination of the cervical vertebral column. Cervical dislocations and fractures were later confirmed through radiographic and post-mortem examinations.

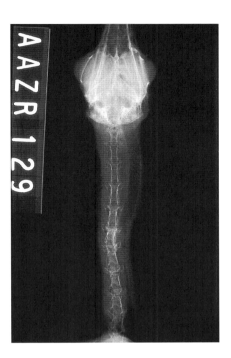

Fig. 6.2 Ventrodorsal radiograph of an adult houbara bustard (*Chlamydotis undulata*) with dislocation of the middle portion of the cervical vertebral column.

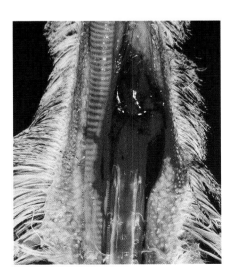

Fig. 6.1 Kori bustard (*Ardeotis kori*), adult. Traumatic cervical dislocation with severe hemorrhage.

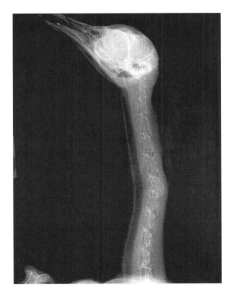

Fig. 6.3 Lateral radiograph of the same bird as in Fig. 6.2.

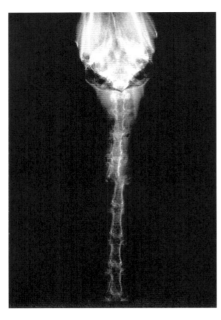

Fig. 6.4 Houbara bustard, adult. Dislocation between the 4th and 5th cervical vertebrae.

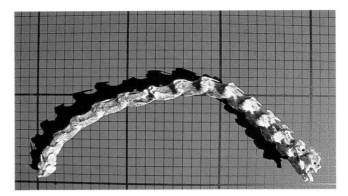

Fig. 6.5 Houbara bustard, adult. Fracture on the lateral aspect of the vertebral body together with the proximal articular process of the 7th cervical vertebra.

Eye and eyelid injuries

Stephen J. Kellner

The anatomy of the avian globe differs greatly from that of the mammalian eye. These differences become relevant when dealing with surgical procedures. The globe is very large, relative to the size of the bird, mainly because of the volume of the posterior segment. Three basic shapes are distinguished, the tubular form in owls, the globose form in diurnal raptors and the flat form in the majority of birds. The shape of the eye is maintained by cartilage in the sclera of the posterior segment and by scleral ossicles in the sclera of the intermediate segment. The pupil is circular and its movements occur mainly in response to accommodation and voluntary control and not to light. The avian lens is soft and pliable. The lens sutures in birds form point sutures unlike the Y-shaped suture lines in mammals. The accommodative apparatus in birds is in direct contact with the lens and enables refractive changes of 80–90 diopters. The retina is avascular and lacks a tapetum. The optic disc is not usually visible because of the overlying pecten. Both rods and cones are present in the retina. Unlike mammals, birds have four types of cone. In addition to the blue, green and red portion of the mammal-visible spectrum, birds have a fourth cone type for detecting ultraviolet wavelengths.

The skin over the whole of the skull in most bird species is not very elastic and is adherent to the bone. Any wound more than a few days old, including lacerations of the eyelids, will have contracted, with resultant fibrosis. The lower lid of birds is the more mobile, containing a fibroelastic tarsal plate, and special care should be taken to restore the lower eyelid. Even very small wounds should be treated surgically without delay. Debridement should be minimal. Most lesions can be dealt with under local anesthesia with 0.5% proxymetacaine hydrochloride with a single layer closure using 6-0 monofilament nonabsorbable suture material. Eyelid lesions due to trauma should be differentiated from lesions due to poxvirus infection. Scarring of the lids may be mistaken for eyelid agenesis or coloboma of the lids, and lid swellings due to trauma should be differentiated from blepharitis and hyperkeratosis in vitamin A deficiency.

The nictitating membrane in birds is well developed, very thin and nearly transparent. Damage to the nictitans prevents spreading of the precorneal tear film, protective blinking and cleaning of the corneal surface, and may have severe consequences. The membrana nictitans is fairly often traumatized in birds of prey. Raptors with corneal problems with slow or no healing tendency should be examined for lesions of the third eyelids. Such lesions are surgically corrected with 10-0 nonabsorbable or 8-0 absorbable sutures under general anesthesia. Foreign bodies, such as grass seeds or parts of feathers, may be lodged between lower eyelid and nictitating membrane. Removal under local anesthesia is straightforward.

The eye globe is very large in birds, with a large posterior segment and a small anterior segment and cornea. Various shapes of avian globe are recognized, maintained by scleral ossicles in middle parts and hyaline cartilage in the sclera of the posterior segment. Corneal injuries and keratitis occur in raptors after accidental collisions, and in other birds during transport. Corneal ulcerations may develop and infections should be ruled out (Figs 6.6 and 6.7). Severe and painful corneal conditions benefit from temporary tarsorrhaphy. Again, this can be performed under local anesthesia with

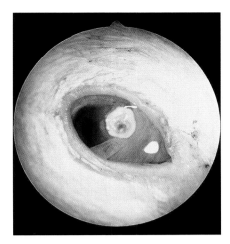

Fig. 6.6 Descemetocele as sequel to a corneal injury in a duck.

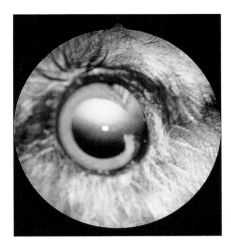

Fig. 6.8 Tear in the iris after collision accident in an owl.

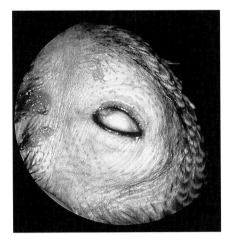

Fig. 6.7 Fungal keratitis that developed after prolonged treatment of corneal erosion with antibiotics in a parrot.

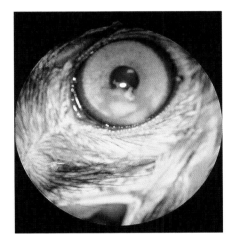

Fig. 6.9 Sterile hypopyon in the anterior chamber of a red kite (*Milvus milvus*) after uveitis.

a soaked cotton tip applied to the skin for half a minute and three or four nonabsorbable 6-0 split-thickness sutures. Unlike the situation in mammals, performing a nictitating membrane flap is not advisable, because of the very delicate nature of the nictitans and the powerful pyramidalis muscle controlling the third eyelid.

Tears in the iris and uveitis are seen commonly after trauma, especially in raptors (Figs 6.8–6.10). Hyphema and vitreous hemorrhage may be extensive and fractures of the scleral ossicles can be found occasionally, leading to phthisis bulbi eventually. Secondary cataract must be expected with extensive damage of the iridial tissue but small tears usually heal uneventfully under local corticosteroid and antibiotic treatment. As the iris muscles are striated, therapeutic or diagnostic mydriasis cannot be achieved with atropine. The application of vecuronium bromide (4 mg/ml, one drop 15 min apart) enables proper ophthalmoscopic examination of lens, vitreous

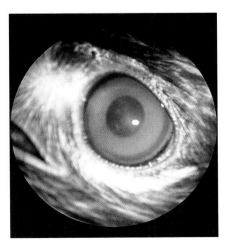

Fig. 6.10 Acute uveitis in a buzzard (*Buteo buteo*) after collision accident.

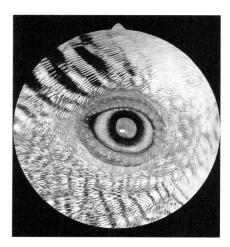

Fig. 6.11 Secondary cataract in a budgerigar (*Melopsittacus undulatus*).

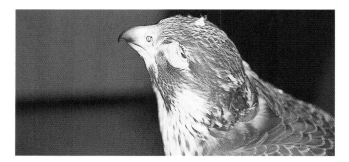

Fig. 6.12 A peregrine falcon (*Falco peregrinus*) with 'sealed' eyelids. 'Sealing' is traditionally carried out by falcon trappers in the East to tame recently caught free-living falcons. Hoods are not normally used since wild-caught falcons can easily remove them. A stitch is placed on the proximal edge of the lower eyelids using a standard stitching needle and a fine cotton thread. The two threads are secured with a knot on the top of the head to 'seal' the eyes. This procedure very often leads to lacerations of the eyelids and cornea and related infections. (Courtesy of Dr. J. Samour).

and fundus. Because of the possibility of severe side effects, the use of vecuronium is no longer advocated for a standard ophthalmic examination. Secondary cataract (Fig. 6.11) should be differentiated from congenital cataract associated with microphthalmos (especially in raptors), inherited cataract (canaries) and cataract associated with old age. Extracapsular cataract extraction is performed in birds but the restoration of full or adequate visual power is not possible in every case. Electroretinography is recommended before cataract removal to evaluate retinal function. Lens luxation is usually seen in very severely traumatized eyes and lentectomy is therefore not routinely performed. Vitreous hemorrhage, retinal detachment and tearing can be seen after accidents or gunshot wounds. Treatment of inflammatory processes with corticosteroids and prevention of further trauma in temporarily blind birds with cage rest and single confinement should be initiated immediately (Figs 6.12 and 6.13). Treatment of trauma to the posterior segment of the eye is usually conservative and conditions such as vitreous hemorrhage may take weeks to dissolve.

A severely damaged eye may require enucleation. Two surgical techniques are available. In both procedures hemostasis is vital, small sutures should be used (6-0–8-0) and care should be taken to avoid excess traction on the globe, which can result in fissures in the orbital septum and in optic chiasm damage and thus contralateral blindness. The transaural approach involves removal of the intact globe and is especially suitable for owls and if the globe is needed for histopathology. After plucking the feathers an incision is made between the lateral canthus and the anterior auricular margin down to the sclera. Skin is dissected to expose the posterior globe and conjunctiva is prepared free. Careful digital pressure is applied to move the globe medially and the optic nerve and extraocular muscles are severed. Hemorrhage is controlled by packing the orbit with hemostyptic pads or foam. Conjunctiva, membrana nictitans and a 2mm strip

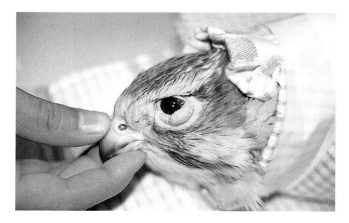

Fig. 6.13 A saker falcon (*Falco cherrug*) displaying extensive pox lesions on the lower eyelid. Falcons in the Middle East are usually affected by avian pox during hunting trips to neighboring countries such as Pakistan. (Courtesy of Dr. J. Samour).

of lid margin are removed and the lids are closed with absorbable sutures.

The globe collapsing enucleation involves the removal of parts of the scleral ossicles of the intermediate segment of the eye to allow access to the retrobulbar structures. After plucking the feathers, the incision line is from the lateral canthus extended dorsal to the anterior auricular margin. The cornea is then incised at the dorsal limbus over 180° and conjunctiva dissected over 360°. A piece of sclera and its ossicle is excised laterally with scissors inserted between the lateral uvea and sclera. The globe can thus be collapsed inwards and the posterior segment is now accessible for removal of the posterior parts. After removal of the conjunctiva, membrana nictitans and lid margin, wound closure is performed with absorbable sutures. Wild birds with reduced vision cannot be safely released into their normal habitat and, while some birds may adapt to life in captivity, this may be especially difficult in birds of prey.

FURTHER READING

Hendrix DVH, Sims MH (2004) Electroretinography in the Hispaniolan Amazon parrot (*Amazona ventralis*). *Journal of Avian Medicine and Surgery* **18**: 89–94.

Kern TJ (1997) Disorders of the special senses. In: Altman RB, Clubb SL, Dorrestein GM, Quesenberry K (eds) *Avian Medicine and Surgery*, pp. 563–589. WB Saunders, Philadelphia.

Kern TJ, Paul-Murphy JR, Murphy CJ *et al.* (1996) Disorders of the third eyelid in birds: 17 cases. *Journal of Avian Medicine and Surgery* **10**: 12–18.

Lavach JD (1996) Diseases of the avian eye. In: Rosskopf WJ Jr, Woerpel RW (eds) *Diseases of Cage and Aviary Birds*, 3rd edn, pp. 380–386. Williams & Wilkins, Baltimore.

Williams D (1994) Ophthalmology. In: Ritchie BW, Harrison GJ, Harrison LR (eds) *Avian Medicine: Principles and Application*, pp. 673–694. Wingers Publishing, Lake Worth, FL.

Keel injuries

Jaime Samour

Keel injuries are described as the loss of continuity of the skin and, very often, the adjacent pectoral muscles around the carina or prominence of the ventral median section of the keel bone (Figs 6.14–6.16). Severe injuries could also lead to lacerations and splinting of the carina.

Deep ulcerative wounds around the keel region are very commonly diagnosed in psittacines (Hochleithner and Hochleithner, 1996) and are normally associated with self-mutilation. This type of lesion is produced by the sharp beak during intensive feather plucking on the pectoral area. This behavioral problem may degenerate and lead to ulcerative wounds on the skin and underlying tissues. Keel lesions can also be associated with inadequate feather clipping in many species, but large psittacines in particular. Normally, only the primary feathers of one wing should be clipped. However, it is a common practice among novice pet owners or aviculturalists to clip the

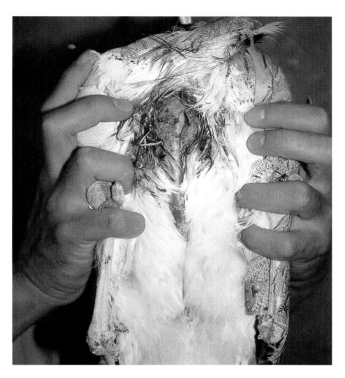

Fig. 6.15 Chronic open wound with associated fibrosis and infection on the keel region of a houbara bustard (*Chlamydotis undulata*). The lesion was caused by repeatedly crashing against the fence of the enclosure.

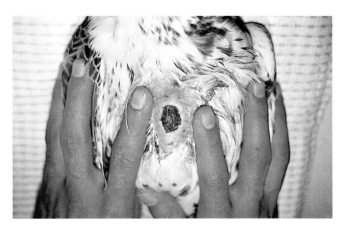

Fig. 6.16 A dry ulcerative lesion on the keel of a saker falcon. This lesion was the result of unnoticed and repeated 'crash landings'. Note the granulating ring around the lesion. Injuries of this type are repaired by debriding in a semicircular pattern around the lesion and by partial resection of the keel bone. The recommended suture technique is the application of interrupted mattress stitches and the use of short segments of plastic tubing to avoid tension over the edges of the wound. Alternatively, gauze swab or dressings could be incorporated into the suture to serve the same purpose.

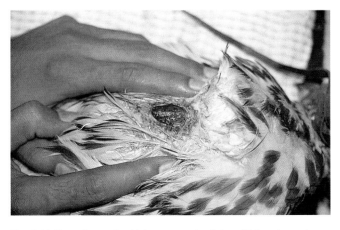

Fig. 6.14 Recent open keel injury on a saker falcon (*Falco cherrug*) after a 'crash landing'. The bird suffered a severe cut on the skin and underlying tissues when it hit rocky ground.

primary feathers of both wings. This normally results in birds crashing continuously to the floor of cages and aviaries, leading to severe injuries.

In other species, such as bustards, storks and cranes, keel injuries are associated with repeated crashing against fences of open paddocks or the walls of aviaries and enclosures. Birds of prey used in the sport of falconry are very often involved in 'crash-landings'. During training exercises, a falcon or a hawk may fail to grasp the lure offered very close to the ground or miss catching a prey during a hunting trip and crash on the floor.

Hochleithner and Hochleithner (1996) recently described a surgical technique for the correction of ulcerative lesions of the keel in psittacines. This technique is not only suitable to repair keel injuries in psittacines but can also be used to correct similar lesions in other species. The technique involves the surgical removal of the necrotic tissue followed by blunt dissection of the pectoral muscles adjacent to the keel and partial resection of the bone. The muscles are sutured using interrupted horizontal mattress sutures and the skin is also sutured with similar stitches secured to a gauze swab to minimize tension over the edges of the wound.

REFERENCE

Hochleithner M, Hochleithner C (1996) Surgical treatment of ulcerative lesions caused by automutilation of the sternum in psittacine birds. *Journal of Avian Medicine and Surgery* **10**: 84–88.

Wing tip injuries

Jaime Samour

Wing tip injuries are also a common occurrence in many bird species and are normally associated with trauma. There are different types of lesion on the wing tip of birds and they can be classified under the following categories: wounds and ulcers, luxations and fractures, bursitis, and edema and dry gangrene syndrome.

Wounds and ulcers

These are normally caused by birds crashing into the fences or walls of their enclosures. Wounds on the wing tips are normally vertical, covering the frontal aspect of the carpal joint. Repeated injury to the same site may lead to ulcerative wounds, fibrosis and, in extreme cases, ankylosis of the joint. The primary treatment consists of debriding the fibrous tissue, if present, and the application of sutures. A dressing and a bandage are essential, not only for wound healing but also to protect the wing tip from further injury. An important aspect to remember is to anchor the bandage to the feathers, since bandages on the wing tip tend to slip off. It is also essential to correct the main cause of the injuries by minimizing disturbance and padding the walls of cages and enclosures.

Luxations and fractures

Luxations and fractures of the carpal joint are often the result of severe trauma (Figs 6.17–6.19). Luxations of the carpal joint are best treated using external fixation devices. Chronic luxations are very often difficult to correct and usually result in partial or total ankylosis. Martin *et al.* (1993) reviewed eight cases of elbow luxation in birds of prey. More recently, Ackermann and Redig (1997) published a very useful paper on the surgical repair of elbow luxation in raptors. Fractures of the carpometacarpus are common in many species of bird. This type of fracture is very often

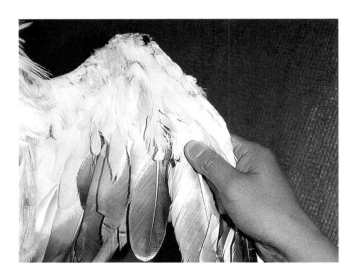

Fig. 6.17 Carpal joint injury showing ulceration and associated mild fibrosis in a houbara bustard (*Chlamydotis undulata*).

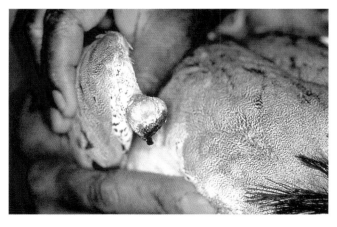

Fig. 6.18 Chronic carpal joint injury in a houbara bustard. Note the tumor-like growth on the ventral aspect of the joint due to proliferative fibrosis. These types of lesions are also caused by repeated trauma to the wing tip by crashing against the wall or fences of enclosures.

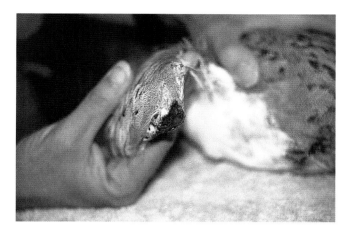

Fig. 6.19 Acute carpal joint injury in a Houbara bustard. The wound is open and bleeding severely. Such injuries are susceptible to myiasis in tropical countries and should be sutured and a dressing and bandage applied.

associated with injuries to the wing tip when juvenile birds begin experimenting with the newly feathered wings. This is a common occurrence that goes largely undiagnosed in large terrestrial species such as cranes, storks and bustards (J. Naldo, personal communication). Fractures of this level are best corrected by reduction and immobilization using an external splint, as suggested by Coles (1985), or a suitable bandage (Degernes, 1994; McCluggage, 1996, 1997).

Bursitis

Inflammation of the synovial capsule of the carpal joint is often diagnosed in tethered birds of prey (Fig. 6.20) (Cooper, 1978; Simpson, 1996). 'Blain' is the old term used by falconers to describe this condition. Bursitis of the carpal joint is the result of repeated injury to the ventral aspect of the wing against the floor when attempting to escape from the approaching handler. The treatment

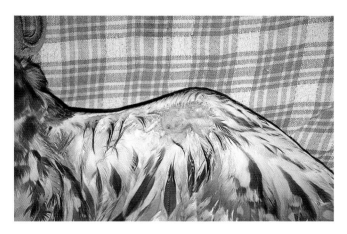

Fig. 6.20 'Blain' or bursitis of the carpal joint in a saker falcon (*Falco cherrug*). Lesions of this type are caused by repeated injury to the ventral aspect of the wing.

of bursitis includes antibiotic and corticosteroid therapy, poultices and dressings combined with suitable bandages.

Edema and dry gangrene syndrome

This syndrome is characterized by edema, transudate around the base of the distal primary feathers and avascular-necrosis-related clinical signs. This type of lesion has been most commonly diagnosed in birds of prey. The exact etiology is unknown but cold weather is probably responsible, since the syndrome is usually diagnosed in temperate countries during the winter and early spring. Birds of prey kept tethered to perches, and therefore less active, are more commonly affected compared with other birds kept in free-flying aviaries (Forbes, 1991; Simpson, 1996).

Treatment can be attempted by trying to restore adequate blood circulation and the administration of antibiotics and corticosteroids. Prognosis is usually reserved, as many affected birds slough and lose the distal wing tip (Forbes, 1991; Simpson, 1996).

REFERENCES

Ackermann J, Redig P (1997) Surgical repair of elbow luxation in raptors. *Journal of Avian Medicine and Surgery* **11**: 247–254.

Coles BH (1985) *Avian Medicine and Surgery*. Blackwell Science, Oxford.

Cooper JE (1978) *Veterinary Aspects of Captive Birds of Prey*. Standfast Press, Saul, Gloucestershire.

Degernes LA (1994) Trauma medicine. In: Ritchie BW, Harrison GJ, Harrison LR (eds) *Avian Medicine: Principles and Application*, pp. 417–433. Wingers Publishing, Lake Worth, FL.

Forbes NA (1991) Wing tip edema and dry gangrene in birds. *Veterinary Record* **129**(3): 58.

Martin HD, Bruecker KA, Herrick DD *et al.* (1993) Elbow luxations in raptors: a review of eight cases. In: Redig PT, Cooper JE, Remple JD, Hunter DB (eds) *Raptor Biomedicine*, pp. 199–206. University of Minnesota Press, Minneapolis.

McCluggage DM (1996) Bandaging and collaring. In: Rosskopf WJ Jr, Woerpel RW (eds) *Diseases of Cage and Aviary Birds*, 3rd edn, pp. 672–674. Williams & Wilkins, Baltimore.

McCluggage DM (1997) Bandaging. In: Altman RB, Clubb SL, Dorrestein GM, Quesenberry K (eds) *Avian Medicine and Surgery*, pp. 829–836. WB Saunders, Philadelphia.

Simpson GN (1996) Wing problems. In: Beynon PH, Forbes NA, Harcourt-Brown NH (eds) *Manual of Raptors, Pigeons and Waterfowl*, pp. 169–179. British Small Animal Veterinary Association, Cheltenham.

Bumblefoot

Nigel H. Harcourt-Brown

Bumblefoot is a disease process mainly confined to birds that are overweight, inactive and have access to poor perches; it may affect chronically ill birds too. It is nearly always seen in captive birds, mainly falcons but not usually hawks, also in owls, waterfowl, cockatiels and occasionally other species. The disease has been reviewed by Harcourt-Brown (1994, 1996, 2000) and more recently by Cooper (2002). Mueller *et al.* (2000) found that inactivity and lack of exercise played a role in the occurrence of bumblefoot. The incidence in wild-caught falcons halved if they were trained twice daily rather than once daily. Wild-caught birds housed in free-flight aviaries during molting also showed a lower incidence of bumblefoot than those tethered and perched on blocks. Lierz (2003) reported an incidence of bumblefoot of 10.1% in 4193 falcons used for falconry in the United Arab Emirates. Peak incidences occurred in the 2 months after capture and after the hunting season finished and training was stopped. Saker and gyrfalcons were more often affected than peregrine falcons. Lierz showed that at the end of the hunting season a sudden cessation of daily exercise caused more cases of bumblefoot than a gradual decrease in exercise over 6 weeks.

The following account of bumblefoot is based on falcons but can be sensibly applied to cases in other species.

A predictable chain of events occurs in overweight, underexercised birds; this has been classified into either three stages (Cooper, 1978) or five stages (Oaks, 1993; Remple, 1993). The changes are dynamic, so divisions tend to be arbitrary; they are usually caused in the first instance by poor circulation of blood to the foot (Figs 6.21–6.23). Because of poor perfusion, the bird's feet become less able to respond to infection, as a sequel to pressure necrosis or due to puncture wounds; poor perfusion also hinders healing.

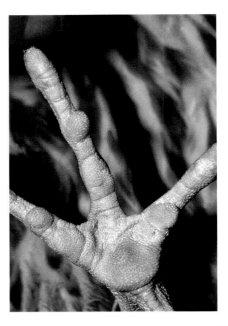

Fig. 6.22 The integument coloration of the immature saker falcon (*Falco cherrug*) is usually blue, but this bird has also had early bumblefoot: the digital and metatarsal pads have flattened, the reticulate scales have become flattened and smooth and there is a reactive hyperemia in these areas.

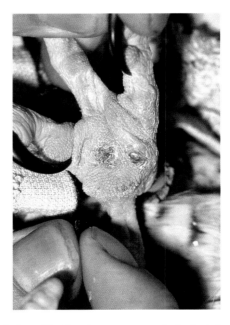

Fig. 6.23 Early proliferative changes are seen in the foot of a peregrine falcon and are greatest at points of maximum weight-bearing. Although the skin has lost its suppleness and there is thickening of the digital pads, as well as the obvious changes on the metatarsal pad, subcutaneous infection has not yet occurred.

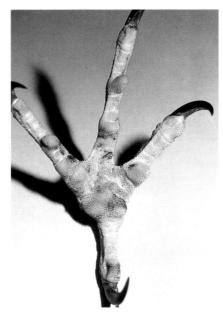

Fig. 6.21 The plantar aspect of the foot of a normal peregrine falcon (*Falco peregrinus*). The reticulate scales of the digital and metatarsal pads have a well-defined papilliferous appearance and the integument is a homogenous yellow color.

Treatment is based on removal of diseased tissue and especially purulent material; killing the infection; providing conditions to allow increased blood supply to the affected areas; and returning the plantar aspect of the foot to as near normal as possible. A combination of medication, surgery and husbandry changes is often necessary to achieve this (Figs 6.24–6.33). After treatment, a foot that has no scar tissue and has a relatively normal shape to its plantar aspect is far more likely to remain healthy than a foot that is a misshapen mass of scar tissue.

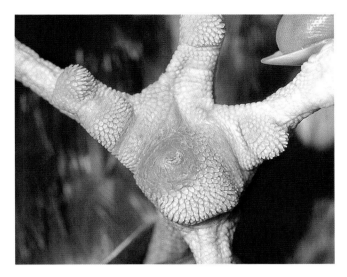

Fig. 6.24 A single proliferative lesion has thickened, forming a 'corn'. Separation has occurred between the surrounding thinned epidermis and the hyperkeratinized corn, and has allowed infection through the integument. An abscess is forming in the plantar surface of the foot.

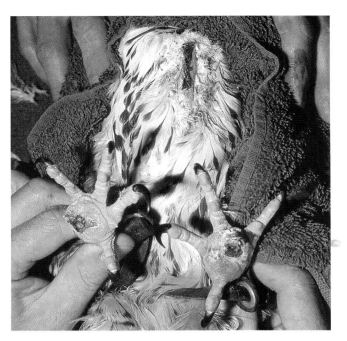

Fig. 6.25 In cases where the above changes are not noticed, commonly when the bird is placed in a large aviary to go through its annual molt, the bird can have advanced changes when brought for treatment. This bird has been lying in sternal recumbency for some time prior to presentation; the feet have become very swollen and contain pus. The sternal injury was also treated in a similar manner to that suggested for Fig. 6.16.

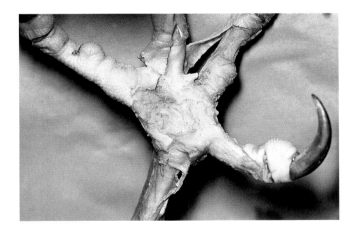

Fig. 6.26 The etiology of bumblefoot is indivisibly linked to poor circulation of blood to the feet causing a failure of devitalized tissue to respond to infection and also to heal. A latex cast of the vascular supply to the foot of a peregrine falcon with bumblefoot shows the lack of the vascular response to inflammation. Treatment must be centered on techniques that increase the blood supply to the affected area of the foot.

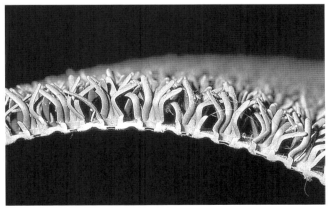

Fig. 6.27 Astroturf (easily available as doormats at the local hardware or DIY store) provides a constantly yielding surface that also distributes the weight of the bird through different points of contact when perching. All perching surfaces should be covered with Astroturf, especially during treatment of bumblefoot or any other condition causing single leg lameness (e.g. a fracture of one leg).

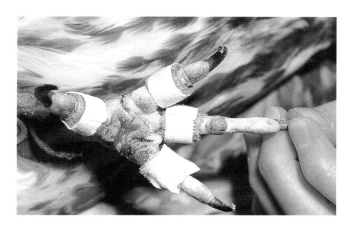

Fig. 6.28 A female saker falcon with bumblefoot has had the purulent material and infected scar tissue removed. A purse string suture has been applied to reduce the deficit. The toes have been bandaged in preparation for a foot cast using several layers of a soft, conforming bandage and a single layer of zinc oxide tape.

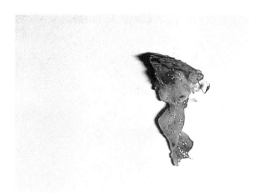

Fig. 6.29 A complete plug of purulent tissue and surrounding deeper infection has been removed from the saker falcon in Fig. 6.24.

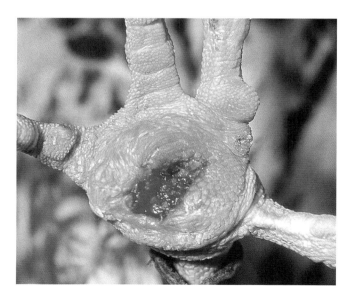

Fig. 6.30 An adult saker falcon was presented with two scabbed and swollen feet. Changes had been present for many months. The base of the foot was distorted with scar tissue. The scab has been removed in this view.

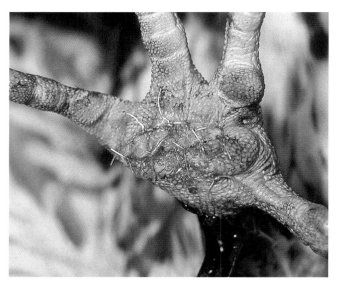

Fig. 6.31 Surgical removal of all abnormal tissue shown in Fig. 6.30 allowed reconstruction of a more normal plantar aspect of the foot. Skin sutures were placed to obliterate dead space and to oppose skin edges.

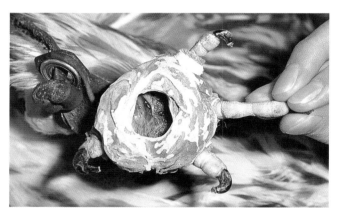

Fig. 6.32 The foot was prepared for a foot cast, after the manner of Riddle and Hoolihan (1993). Bandages are used to cushion the toes, to prevent pressure problems in this site, and the plantar surface of the foot has a temporary bandage placed over it to ensure that the surgical site is not in contact with the cast. When formed, the cast may be bandaged or glued to the toe bandages. Bandaging is preferred if the foot is being redressed regularly.

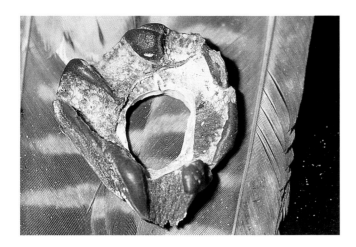

Fig. 6.33 The casting material used was car body filler (Repair Metal for Good, Henkel Home Improvements). A circle of 'recycled' stainless steel orthopedic pin should be used as a reinforcing rod within the cast. A grinder is used to shape the interior of the cast to ensure that the weight of the bird is taken on the bandages around toes. This cast is durable and can be reused.

However, birds that have suffered from bumblefoot are more likely to be affected again, especially if they are kept in the same manner.

Severely swollen feet should be examined radiographically.

All cases of bumblefoot in falcons, regardless of their stage of development, should have the following changes in their husbandry (Harcourt-Brown, 1996):

- A good diet plus vitamin and mineral supplement
- Cover all perching surfaces with Astroturf or similar product: concrete, wood, or perches with rope wound around them are all unsatisfactory. Birds kept permanently in aviaries should have perches of different sizes, preferably suspended so that they 'give' when the bird alights. Broad perches and favorite perching/roosting sites must be covered with Astroturf
- If the bird is housed indoors, new, dry wood shavings should be used to cover the floor, especially if the bird is lying down rather than perching. A layer about 7–10 cm (3–4 ") deep should be put down on a permanently dry floor; wet floors lead to mold forming and the bird is at risk of acquiring aspergillosis. If the bird is housed out of doors, new grass is the surface of choice. Move the bird off gravel, concrete, etc.
- Reduce the weight of the bird to its flying weight
- Aviary birds should be jessed and manned as soon as possible. This allows more direct management of the condition
- Increase exercise: even flying three times a day on a creance will help the resolution of bumblefoot; flying free is even better.

In some cases there may be swelling but no pus formation; antibiotic and anti-inflammatory treatment should be given until the swelling has gone (7–10 d course). In other cases, with a large scab and no infection, sodium fusidate ointment (Fucidin ointment, Leo Laboratories) should be applied to the scab and surrounding skin twice daily until the scab lifts and can be removed. Ointment containing corticosteroids should not be used. Dry, flaky feet may need dressing with hand cream.

Many more advanced cases of bumblefoot are infected with a *Staphylococcus* sp. (Figs 6.34 and 6.35). Lincomycin, clindamycin and marbofloxacin are very useful drugs in these cases; the majority of staphylococcal infections are sensitive to these antibiotics. Lincomycin

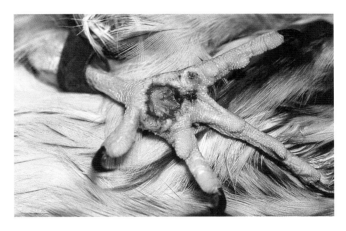

Fig. 6.34 A merlin (*Falco columbarius*) was presented with bilateral, sudden-onset, severe bumblefoot. The scab was removed, a swab taken, and the bird placed on lincomycin; its feet were dressed and placed in a padded bandage. A pure culture of *Staphylococcus aureus* was grown, which was sensitive to lincomycin.

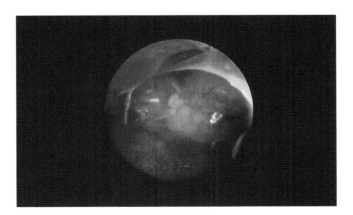

Fig. 6.35 In spite of appropriate treatment the merlin in Fig. 6.34 failed to respond. Endoscopy revealed changes indicative of fatty liver and kidney syndrome. The prognosis was therefore very grave and the bird was euthanized. This is an endoscopic view through the oblique septum revealing a pallid enlarged cranial division of the left kidney, overlain by the ovary.

and marbofloxacin are injectable and easy to give as a tablet, in food (lincomycin: 50 mg/kg twice daily by mouth; marbofloxacin: 10 mg/kg once daily by mouth). Clindamycin comes in capsules, which are difficult to divide. These antibiotics are well absorbed from the gut and reach the tendon sheaths, joints, bone and other infected tissues. Preoperative antibiotics are useful as they remove infection, reducing swelling and inflammation prior to surgery. Cefalexin, amoxicillin, clavulanic-acid-potentiated amoxicillin and ampicillin are not useful. Figs 6.36 and 6.37 illustrate other advanced cases of bumblefoot with contrasting causes. If the bird could be in pain, antibiotic treatment should be combined with analgesia. Meloxicam and carprofen are both useful drugs that can be given orally (carprofen 1–2 mg/kg

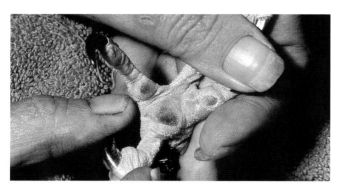

Fig. 6.36 A well intentioned veterinary surgeon amputated the severely traumatized leg of a peregrine falcon. This photograph of the remaining, previously normal foot was taken 10 d after the amputation. Chronic single-leg disability or amputation always results in euthanasia of captive birds due to bumblefoot, even in species that are not usually affected by the condition.

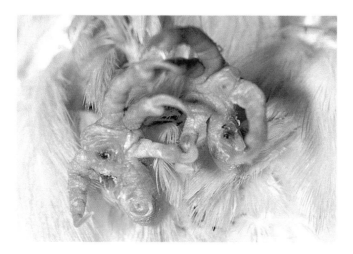

Fig. 6.37 A chronic case of bumblefoot in a cockatiel (*Nymphicus hollandicus*) due to complete lack of flying exercise, obesity and long-term malnutrition (seed diet only). Many cases of bumblefoot can be improved in this species if there is good owner compliance; if the owner is not helpful and committed the bird will die. Requirements include a lower calorie diet with vitamin and mineral supplementation – small size all-in-one diets are ideal; perches covered with rubber cushioned carpet underlay; no sandpaper on the floor of the cage; and regular daily periods out of the cage for walking and if possible flying exercise.

b.i.d.; meloxicam 0.1–0.2 mg/kg s.i.d.) and by injection (carprofen 1 mg/kg SC). They make the bird feel more comfortable and reduce swelling but should not be used in place of antibiotics. Nonsteroidal anti-inflammatory drugs should always be given postoperatively.

Lack of response to antibiotic therapy, or aggressive infection, makes bacteriology vital. Cultures must be made from the deeper and more active areas of infection. Some cases will be infected by Gram-negative bacteria (e.g. *Pseudomonas* spp.) and others by yeasts or fungi. Clindamycin, enrofloxacin, marbofloxacin, trimethoprim–sulfonamide, ketoconazole and itraconazole can all be used. Oral administration of medication is preferred as some cases may require several weeks or even months of therapy. Serious infections worsen the prognosis. Remple and Forbes (2000) showed that antibiotic-impregnated polymethylmethacrylate beads could be introduced during surgery into chronically infected areas, allowing the antibiotic to leach out slowly into the surrounding tissues, where it reaches significant levels. As the effect is local, it is possible to use a relatively toxic antibiotic such as gentamicin with safety.

In birds' feet, pus is always caseous unless mixed with joint or tendon sheath fluid. Surgery is necessary to remove the pus and scar tissue. A preoperative antibiotic should be used for 5 d and the recommended routine changes should be made to the husbandry. The bird should be anesthetized and placed in dorsal recumbency. The feet should be prepared for surgery by cleaning and applying a chlorhexidine in alcohol skin scrub; this sterilizes and penetrates better than any other regimen. Scar tissue in the skin and subcutaneous tissues and all purulent material must be removed by dissection. Pus often forms abscesses in the skin web between the digits and around the distal tarsometatarsus; removal leaves a pocket of dead space. Antibiotic-impregnated beads inserted into these pockets prevent the abscess from reoccurring. Infected tendon sheaths or joint capsule require pus removal and irrigation; any breach or incision should be repaired once the infection is removed. The aim of surgery after removal of infection is to return the plantar aspect of the foot to normal. If possible, the skin should be sutured to allow first intention healing. Monofilament sutures are best: polydioxanone, nylon, or Supramid (Braun). If the foot is very infected and deformed, a purse-string suture can be used to reduce the wound but allow daily cleaning and antiseptic dressings. This encourages healing by second intention and is accomplished through the hole in the foot cast (Fig. 6.32). A second operation may be needed to reconstruct the metatarsal pad. In either case, foot casting postoperatively is very helpful to the healing process as it allows blood to circulate to the healing tissues (see section on protective foot casting in Ch.5).

Some severe cases of bumblefoot have progressed to one or more of the following states: gross and pervading infection with pus in the flexor tendon sheaths leading to distortion of the digits and occasionally septic arthritis of the phalangeal joints; septic arthritis of the metatarsophalangeal joint(s); rupture of the flexor tendons, usually at the metatarsophalangeal joint; and osteomyelitis of the sesamoid bone ventral to the origin of digit II. These conditions all carry a poor prognosis but it is possible to salvage some of these birds (Harcourt-Brown, 1994). However the treatment will be expensive and time-consuming for the owner, as well as painful and stressful for the bird; euthanasia must be considered as an option.

REFERENCES

Cooper JE (1978) *Veterinary Aspects of Captive Birds of Prey*, Standfast Press, Saul, Gloucestershire.

Cooper JE (2002) Foot conditions. In: *Birds of Prey: Health and Disease*, pp. 121–131. Blackwell Science, Oxford.

Harcourt-Brown NH (1994) Diseases of the pelvic limb of birds of prey. FRCVS Thesis, Royal College of Veterinary Surgeons, London.

Harcourt-Brown NH (1996) Foot and leg problems. In: Beynon PH, Forbes NA, Harcourt-Brown NH (eds) *Manual of Raptors, Pigeons and Waterfowl*, pp. 163–167. British Small Animal Veterinary Association, Cheltenham.

Harcourt-Brown NH (2000) *Birds of Prey: Anatomy, Radiology, and Clinical Conditions of the Pelvic Limb.* CD-ROM, Zoological Education Network, Lake Worth, FL.

Lierz M (2003) Aspects of the pathogenesis of bumblefoot in falcons. *Proceedings of the Association of Avian Veterinarians*, Tenerife, pp. 178–184.

Mueller MG, Wernery U, Koesters J (2000) Bumblefoot and lack of exercise among wild and captive-bred falcons tested in the United Arab Emirates. *Avian Diseases* **44**: 676–680.

Oaks JL (1993) Immune and inflammatory responses in falcon staphylococcal pododermatitis. In: Redig PT, Cooper JE, Remple JD et al. (eds) *Raptor Biomedicine*, pp. 72–87. University of Minnesota Press, Minneapolis.

Remple JD (1993) Raptor bumblefoot: a new treatment technique. In: Redig PT, Cooper JE, Remple JD et al. (eds) *Raptor Biomedicine*, pp. 154–160. University of Minnesota Press, Minneapolis.

Remple JD, Forbes NA (2000) Antibiotic impregnated polymethylacrylate beads in the treatment of bumblefoot in falcons. In: Lumeij JT, Remple JD, Redig PT et al. (eds) *Raptor Biomedicine III*, pp. 255–266. Zoological Education Network, Lake Worth, FL.

Riddle KE, Hoolihan JA (1993) Form-fitting, composite-casting method for avian appendages. In: Redig PT, Cooper JE, Remple JD et al. (eds) *Raptor Biomedicine*, pp. 161–164. University of Minnesota Press, Minneapolis.

Fractures

Patrick Redig, Luis Cruz

The objectives in avian fracture management are to stabilize the fracture, allow or promote load sharing and allow limited use during healing. Reduction of morbidity from appliance installation leads to reduction in overall patient morbidity and promotes rapid recovery. Retention of bone length and angular and rotational alignment of the limb is also sought, but exact anatomical reduction of bone fragments may be unnecessary in many instances.

The characteristics of orthopedic appliances that achieve these objectives include rigidity, versatility, efficacy, malleability and lightness of weight. There are several design and functional objectives that a fixation device must be able to meet.

- The device must stabilize the forces that apply tension, torsion, shearing and bending moments to bone. In the case of oblique and comminuted fractures, protection against collapse is also essential
- The device needs to allow weight bearing and range of motion activity without damage to the limb or adjacent body parts
- The device needs to promote load sharing to the extent the fracture will allow it. Oblique fractures have no inherent ability for load sharing, hence the fixation must be strong enough to bear the entire load applied to the bone. As healing progresses, the fixator may be partially dismantled in a process referred to as dynamic destabilization, thereby shifting load sharing to the healing bone and increasing the healing rate
- With good fixation and good overall vascular condition at a fracture site, healing can often be achieved in 18–25 d, which is well within the lifespan of a fixation device. However, most fractures require more time, and the integrity of the fixator must be maintained for the duration. Loosening of pins is not an inevitable consequence and can be avoided by proper placement and the use of positive-profile threaded pins.

The avian skeleton and fracture management

The fixator is one half of the equation in fracture repair; the patient is the other. The avian skeleton is fundamentally and significantly different from the mammalian skeleton and presents unique challenges to fracture fixation. The bone cortices are thin and brittle but very strong. Their strength is derived from their monocoque (i.e. eggshell-like) anatomy. A defect in the wall greatly reduces their strength. There is also less holding power for fixation hardware. It is essential that fixation pins obtain solid purchase in two cortices. There is a paucity of soft tissue over many of the long bones. Thus, comminuted bone fragments may be displaced and are prone to lose their vascular supply. Additionally, the skin is very thin and bone fragments exteriorize easily. Bone so exposed is most often not viable and sequesters in 2–3 weeks if not removed. There is a dearth of cancellous bone in the avian skeleton and, to date, established methods for bone grafting have not been proven clinically. Lastly, with regard to pelvic limb fractures, given the bipedal locomotion of birds, a unilateral fracture puts tremendous strain on the contralateral leg that must be managed. Successful fracture management in birds requires not only application of good fixation but also the management of many of these other challenges that are unique to birds.

Materials

The materials and devices used chiefly in avian fracture repair are intramedullary pins, both Steinmann pins and K-wires (Kirschner wires less than 1.6 mm (0.062") diameter), external skeletal fixators (ESFs) using conventional bars and clamps or a polymer connecting bar (methacrylate or epoxy), and carbon fiber rods. Bone plating has received scant attention in avian species for a variety of reasons, including morbidity associated with placement, the need for follow-up surgery to remove plates in the case of wild birds destined for release, and lack of demonstrated efficacy (Christen et al., 2005). A list of products mentioned in the following pages appears at the end of the section.

For ESF devices, partially threaded, positive-profile thread pins[a] designed specifically for birds and small exotics are commercially available. These offer a greater holding power in the thin cortices. These pins also have a roughened surface on the end opposite the threading that is designed to engage the matrix of acrylic bonding materials. Negative-profile pins may be used as secondary anchor pins in a complex construct but they should not be used in a high-stress application as they are likely to break at the junction of the threads with the pin. Special 'center-threaded' pins with positive-profile threads for type II fixators are also available in larger sizes. They are useful in birds weighing more than 4–5 kg.

Resinous materials such as methacrylate and epoxies are one category of material used to connect the pins of an ESF. Among acrylics, dental acrylic[b] or horse hoof repair products[c,d] are suitable. The acrylic can be molded over the pins after curing to a dough stage or loaded in a syringe during the liquid stage of curing and injected into a molding material such as a Penrose drain or plastic drinking straw. Epoxies are less suitable because of their more viscous and sticky character in the uncured state and their softness and flexibility after curing. Plumber's epoxy is supplied as a hand-moldable dough that makes it more user-friendly, but it is less rigid upon curing than acrylics. Epoxies do have the advantage that, as adhesives, they bond tightly to the ESF pins, while the acrylics form only a mechanical lock.

The other class of material used for external fixator bars are casting tapes[e,f,g] that have heat-sensitive resins impregnated in their synthetic material matrix. These tapes are unbreakable and have substantial holding power. Some of them (e.g. Hexcelite) have a mildly adhesive character so that they adhere to the ESF pins. They are odorless and moldable to fit any configuration of pin placement. Thermoplastics require immersion in hot water to activate the resin and may be reheated at a later time, for instance with a heat gun or hot water compress, so that adjustments can be made to the fixator. Their bonding to steel pins can be improved by coating the latter with a layer of cyanoacrylate adhesive[h] just prior to applying the tape (R. Hess, personal communication).

While there are several different methods for repairing various avian fractures described in the literature, a construct known as the external skeletal fixator–intramedullary pin tie-in fixator (TIF, also called a hybrid fixator), and variations thereof, has yielded exceptional results in a variety of fractures involving most long bones (Redig, 2000). It consists of an intramedullary pin that fills approximately three-quarters of the bone marrow cavity and two external skeletal fixator pins placed at the proximal and distal ends of the affected bone (Fig. 6.38a-c). The intramedullary pin is bent at 90° at its exit point and rotated into the same plane as the ESF pins. A piece of thin-walled latex tubing (e.g. Penrose drain) is placed on to the pins as a mold. The mold is filled with horse hoof repair acrylic injected through a syringe, thus binding all of the pins together. This technique was developed to provide longitudinal and rotational stability for humeral fractures without resorting to additional external coaptation such as a figure-of-eight bandage in the postoperative period and has been extended to other long bones. Coaptation by figure-of-eight bandaging is used as an adjunct to fixation for wing fractures in some instances.

This section is organized according to the layout of the bones in the appendicular skeleton, commencing with the pectoral limb. Surgical approaches, fixation techniques and pre- and postoperative radiographs of actual cases are used to present a broad, but detailed overview.

Methods of fixation for the humerus

General considerations

The humerus can be divided into three zones for evaluation of fractures and selection of fixation devices. The *proximal zone* extends from the subcondylar region near the shoulder joint to the distal extension of the pectoral crest. The *diaphyseal zone* extends from the distal end of the pectoral crest to the apex of the distal diaphyseal curvature and the *distal zone* involves the curved portion of the distal humerus.

A method for fixation of proximal zone humeral fractures: tension band – tie-in

Fractures that occur in the proximal zone are most often transverse. A complicating factor for fixation is the curvature of this segment of bone. Additionally, it is often difficult to gain sufficient purchase on the proximal fragment with an intramedullary pin as would be used in a conventional TIF and there is insufficient bone to accept an ESF pin proximal to the fracture site. An alternative

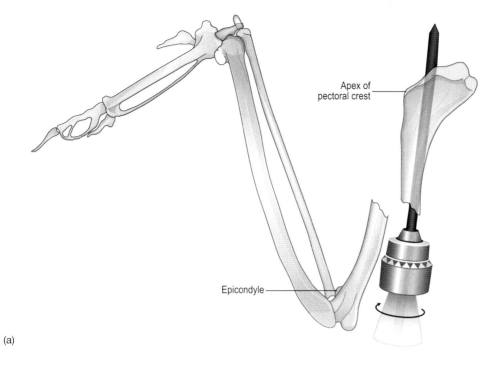

(a)

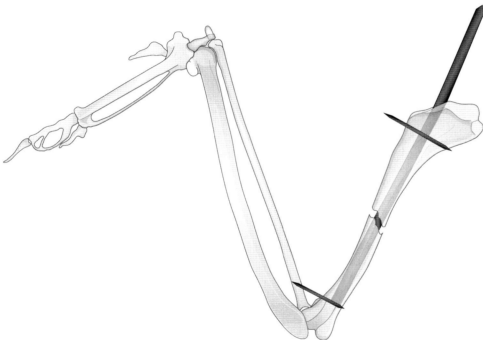

(b)

Fig. 6.38 (a–c) See overleaf for caption.

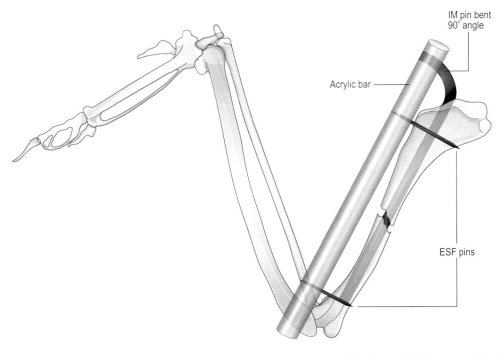

(c)

Fig. 6.38 (a) Placement of an intramedullary (IM) pin by retrograde insertion into the proximal fragment of the humerus. (b) Fracture reduction and normograde driving of the IM pin into the distal humeral fragment and the placement of the external skeletal fixator (ESF) pins at proximal and distal locations. (c) The completed tie-in fixator (TIF). Note 90° bend in IM pin and inclusion of it along with both ESF pins into a cylindrical acrylic connecting bar.

is a variation of the TIF using a tension band (Fig. 6.39). The method resembles one used for repair of proximal humeral fractures in humans. It involves exposure of the proximal humerus from the dorsal aspect (Fig. 6.39d) and placement of two small-diameter K-wires in cross-pin fashion at the fracture site in the proximal fragment. These pins are driven retrograde so as to exit on either side of the pectoral crest (Fig. 6.39e). The fracture is reduced and the pins are driven into the distal fragment, putting pressure on the sides of the bone as a result. A cerclage wire (the only place where cerclage wire will be recommended) is passed through a hole drilled transversely in the distal fragment about one bone diameter distal to the fracture site and another drilled through the blade of the pectoral crest just behind the exit point of the K-wires (Fig. 6.39f). Periosteal elevation of the deltoid muscle and the pectoral muscle from the humerus is required in order to accomplish this. Once the wire is placed, it is tightened in a figure-of-eight pattern, thereby completing a tension band. The K-wires are left projecting at the head of the humerus for future retrieval. (In smaller birds – less than 300 g – it is sufficient to simply place the K-wires.) The muscle is sutured back to the pectoral crest and skin is closed over the top. For additional support, two ESF pins may be placed in the

distal fragment. In that case, the K-wires protruding from the proximal fragment are bent at 90° and a methacrylate bar is used to connect all elements together in a tie-in. The wing is bandaged to the body for about 1 week.

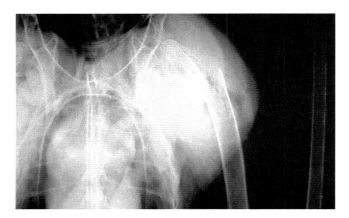

(a)

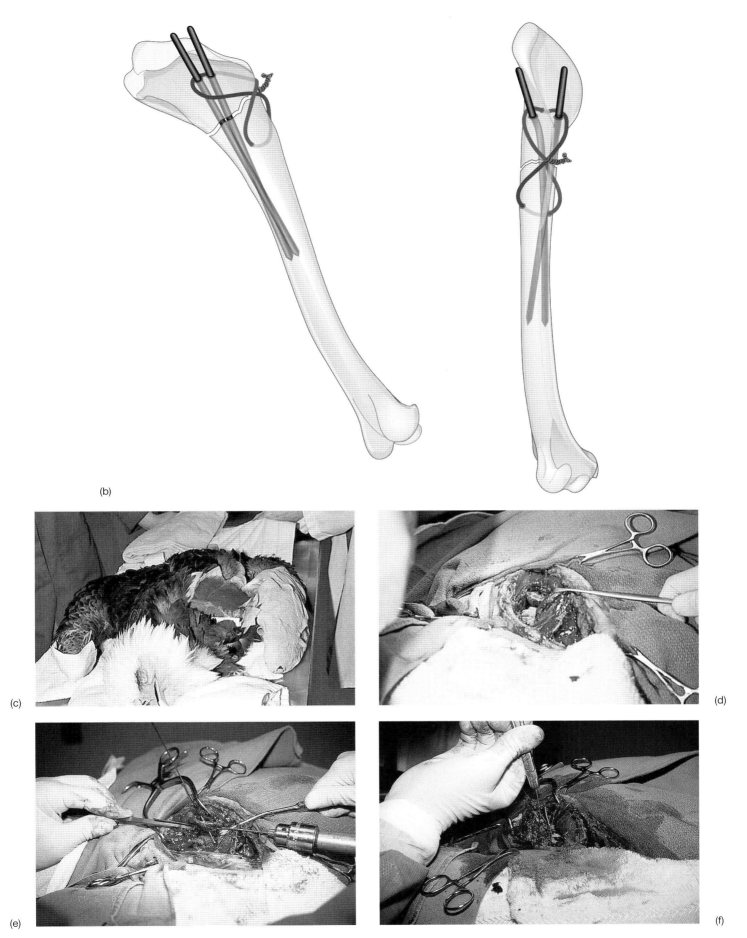

Fig. 6.39 (a–i) See overleaf for caption.

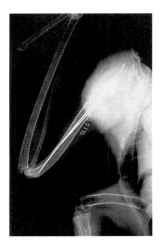

(g)

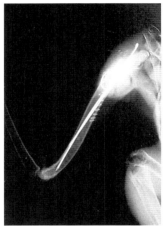

(h)

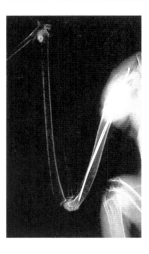

(i)

Fig. 6.39 Treatment of a fracture of the proximal humerus. (a) Preoperative radiograph of a fracture in the proximal segment of the humerus of a bald eagle (*Haliaeetus leucocephalus*). In this case, the transverse fracture was accompanied by a partial avulsion of the pectoral crest. (b) Illustration of the tension band method of fixation for a. Following surgical exposure of the proximal fragment, two 1.6 mm (0.062″) diameter Kirschner wires were driven retrograde in cross-pin fashion from sites dorsal and ventral to the pectoral crest in the proximal fragment, the fracture was reduced and the pins were driven normograde into the distal fragment. Transverse holes were drilled in the distal fragment one bone diameter distal to the fracture site and another through the blade of the pectoral crest. Cerclage wire was passed in figure-of-eight fashion through the holes and behind the K-wires. (c) Preparation of the operative site for a dorsal approach to the humerus. Feathers were plucked from a site craniad to the shoulder to just distal to the midshaft of the humerus. (d) Exposure of the fracture site. The belly of the deltoid muscle was split longitudinally and reflected, leaving its attachment to the diaphysis of the humerus intact while allowing exposure to the blade of the pectoral crest. Ventral to the crest, the major pectoral muscle was elevated. (e) Placement of K-wires. Two 1.6 mm (0.062″) Kirschner wires were retrograded into the proximal fragment, crossing in the intramedullary space and exiting on either side of the pectoral crest. Following this, the fracture was reduced and the pins were driven into the distal fragment. (f) Placement and tightening of the cerclage wire in figure-of-eight fashion. The large tightened wire is the figure-of-eight cerclage. The smaller wire being tightened is one of several used to reattach an avulsed portion of the pectoral crest. (g) Postoperative radiograph. Normal anatomical realignment has been achieved, preserving the curvature of the proximal humerus. (h) Radiograph, 23 d postoperatively. Alignment and approximation of fragment satisfactory, callus forming well. Passive range of motion physical therapy was started on postoperative day 2. (i) Radiograph, 31 d postoperatively. Healing was complete. One K-wire was removed, the other was not retrievable. The cerclage wire was a permanent implant.

Application of the TIF to midshaft diaphyseal fractures of the humerus: the archetypical TIF

Diaphyseal fractures of the humerus are repaired readily unless there is excessive comminution or extensive exteriorization of bone fragments. Most diaphyseal fractures are oblique, with the proximal fragment tending to project through the dorsal surface of the wing and the distal fragment either projecting through the skin on the ventral surface or pulled up against the radius and ulna because of the contraction of the carpal extensor muscles. The radial nerve crosses from caudal to cranial in the midshaft and must be preserved during the dorsal surgical approach. Manipulation of this nerve is a constant feature of managing diaphyseal fractures. The triceps tendon courses distally on the caudal aspect of the bone, wrapping around the distal condyle and attaching to the olecranon. The triceps muscle is very strong and the bending moment it applies to the humerus is a force that must be counteracted by the fixation. The general steps involved in the placement of the TIF on a mid-diaphyseal humeral fracture are illustrated in Figure 6.38a–c and demonstrated in the series of in-surgery images and radiographs in Figure 6.40.

A method of fixation for distal and subcondylar humeral fractures: the cross-pin TIF

The cross-pin method of repairing distal fractures is a variation of the 'tie-in' procedure; however, the placement of the K-wires is technically different from

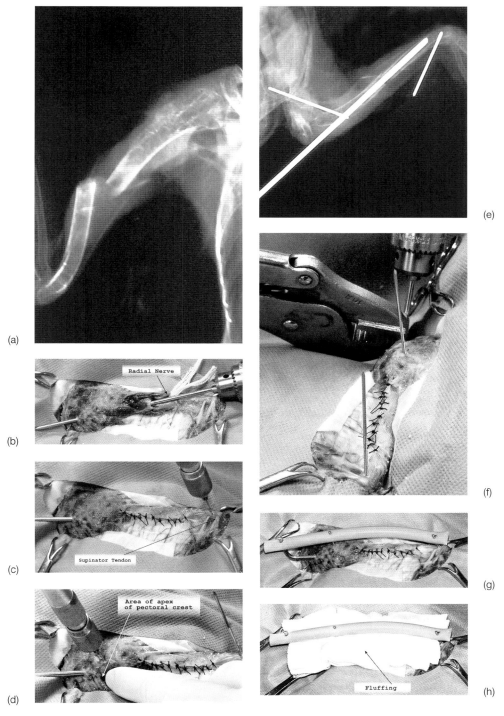

Fig. 6.40 (a–k) See overleaf for caption.

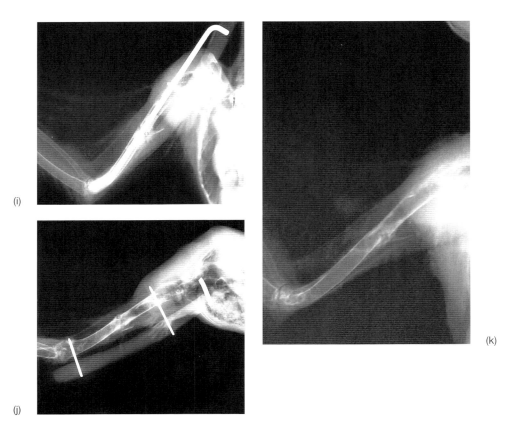

(i)

(j)

(k)

Fig. 6.40 Fixation of a mid-diaphyseal humeral fracture using a tie-in fixator. (a) Preoperative radiograph. This case consisted of a closed, transverse, midshaft diaphyseal fracture in a short-eared owl (*Asio otus*). (b) Introduction of the intramedullary (IM) pin. The pin was inserted in retrograde fashion into the proximal fragment at the fracture site. Note the retraction of the radial nerve with a gauze loop. (c) Placement of the external skeletal fixator (ESF) pins. Positive-profile threaded pins (Imex Veterinary Inc., Texas, USA) were used. The first was placed in the diaphysis proximal to the condyles at the level of the epicondyle to which the tendon of origin of the supinator and common digital extensor attaches (see also Fig. 6.38b). (d) The second ESF pin was placed in the diaphysis of the proximal humerus at a point adjacent to the apex of the curvature of the pectoral crest (Fig. 6.38b), a point that can be palpated for reference. To protect the soft tissues from damage by the pin threads, a tissue tunnel was created with a hemostat and the surrounding muscles were retracted. (e) Intraoperative image taken at the point where the IM pin has been placed in the proximal and distal fragments and the two 1.15 mm (0.045″) diameter. ESF acrylic interface pins (Imex Veterinary, Longview, TX) have been installed. (f) Bending of the IM pin. In order to tie the IM to the ESF, the end of the IM pin was bent 90°. It is imperative to stabilize the pin with locking pliers to prevent transfer of bending forces to the bone. (g) Fixator bar attachment. Application of the fixator bar is accomplished by forcing a piece of thin-walled rubber tubing (e.g. Penrose drain – 10 mm (3/8″) diameter) over the pins. It is then filled with an acrylic horse-hoof repair material injected through the nozzle of an irrigating syringe. After the acrylic has cured, excess material is trimmed away. (h) 'Fluffing', sterile 2×2 gauze pads, was placed between the fixator and the skin to absorb exuded fluids and reduce postoperative swelling and movement of soft tissues. It was changed 18–24 h postoperatively. Note use of acrylic for the fixator bar in this instance. (i) Postoperative radiograph after completion of TIF. We chose to use only proximal and distal ESF pins in this case, to reduce morbidity in the vicinity of the highly traumatized soft tissues adjacent to the fracture site (compare with Fig. 6.48). (j) Radiograph, 21 d postoperatively. The IM pin has been removed but the ESF pins and connecting bar were left in place for an additional week. (k) Radiograph after removal of fixator; healing was complete in 30 d.

the placement of a conventional intramedullary pin. Part of the stability achieved is due to lateral pressure of the pins on the walls of the pneumatic cavity of the bone.

Two K-wires are placed in retrograde fashion, exiting the condyle opposite the side of the marrow cavity from which they are introduced and at a 20–30° angle to the long axis of the bone. They should be retrograded until the ends are flush with or just slightly beyond the edge of the fracture site (Fig. 6.41a). The fracture is reduced and the pins are driven into the proximal fragment,

1–2 cm at a time, alternately, until seated in the proximal fragment (Fig. 6.41b). The most common mistake at this point is to insert one pin too far in advance of the other. External fixation pins are inserted as described above. A conventional stainless steel bar (3.2 mm (1/8″) diameter) for a small-animal-sized KE device and the corresponding clamps are used to connect the fixation pins and at least one of the IM cross-pins together in a tie-in (Fig. 6.41b). Radiographs taken from a case illustrating this kind of fracture management are shown in Figures 6.41c and 6.41d.

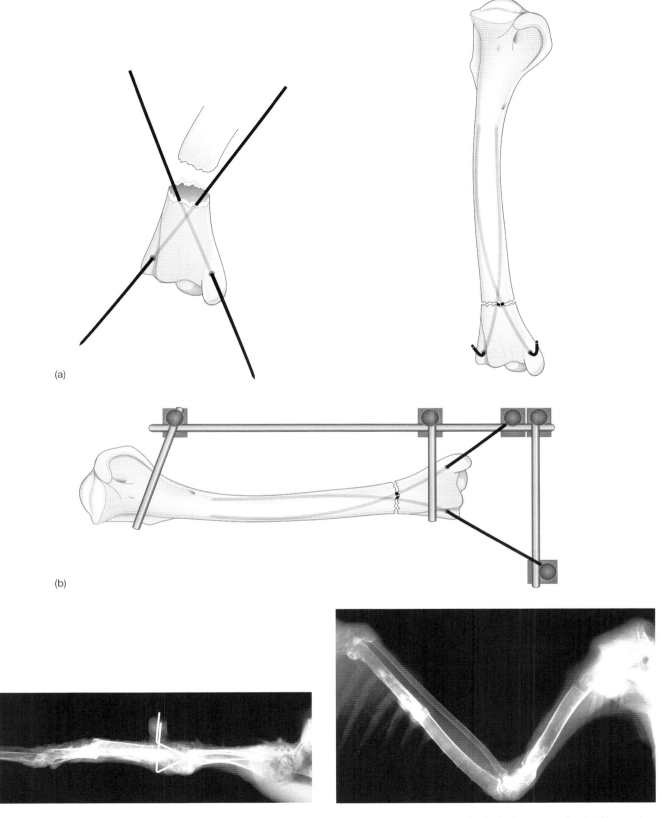

Fig. 6.41 Cross-pin TIF method for distal humeral and femoral fractures. (a) Placement of small-diameter pins in the fragments of a distal humeral fracture where there is otherwise insufficient bone to gain purchase on the distal fragment with a conventional intramedullary pin. (b) The cross-pin TIF as it would be applied to a distal humeral fracture. (c) In this postoperative radiograph of a great horned owl, the relationship of the cross-pins to the condyles and the fracture site is shown, as well as the manner of incorporating these pins into a TIF. (d) Radiograph, 4 weeks postoperatively and after removal of the fixator; the completely healed fracture is shown.

Methods of fixation for diaphyseal forearm fractures

General considerations

Most forearm fractures may be repaired with the TIF applied to the ulna and stabilization of the radius with an intramedullary pin to avoid synostosis (a bony bridge between the radius and ulna). Less complex methods such as figure-of-eight bandaging (Fig. 6.42) may be used if assured restoration of flight capacity is not a required outcome.

Important aspects of pin placement for various fixators

The method and location of the placement of IM pins in the radius and ulna is critical in minimizing joint morbidity. The radius can be repaired by retrograde placement of the IM pin with exit of the pin occurring at the distal end. The anatomy of the carpal joint allows this without undue morbidity. The ulna must be pinned in normograde fashion with the pin being inserted in the proximal end just distal to the point of attachment of the triceps tendon (Fig. 6.43a). Retrograde placement of the IM pin in the ulna is

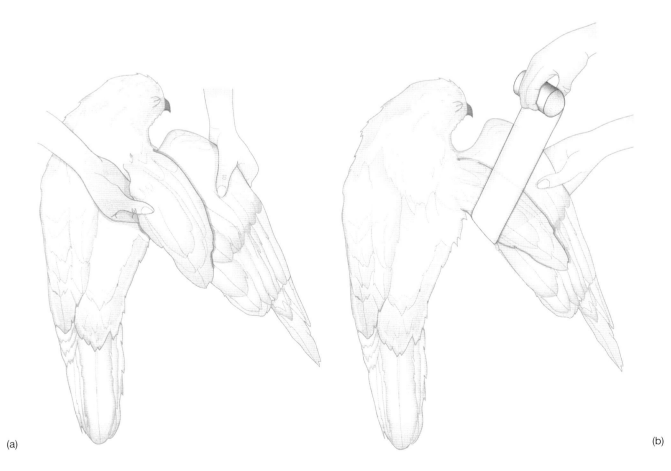

(a)   (b)

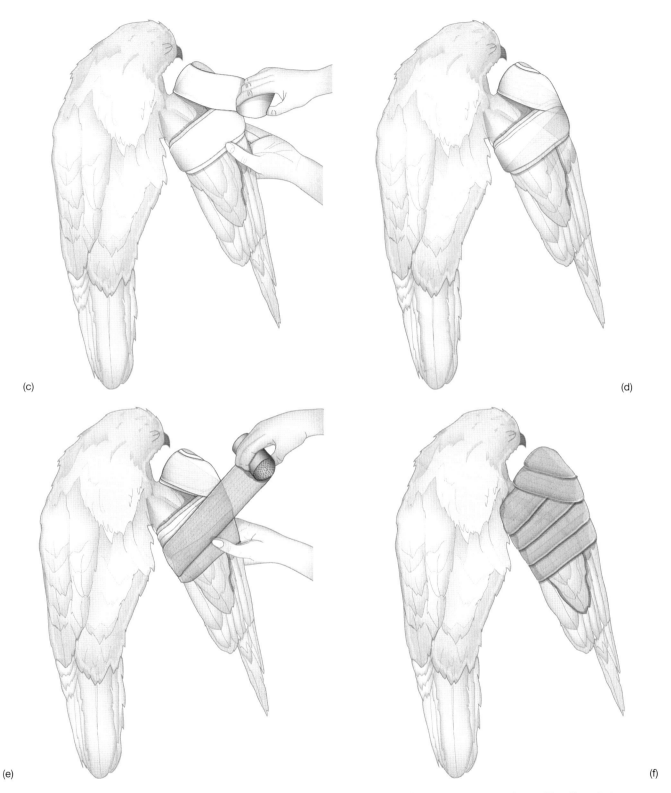

(c)

(d)

(e)

(f)

Fig. 6.42 The figure-of-eight bandage is most easily applied with the patient under anesthesia and in sternal recumbency. The affected wing is partially extended and the tertiary coverts are identified and included under the bandage (a). Conforming gauze (e.g. Johnson & Johnson Kling gauze) is used for the first layer of the bandage. The free end of the gauze is held in place with the fingers of one hand on the ventral side of the wing at the leading edge (b) and brought from underneath the wing behind the tertiary coverts and over the dorsal surface. Four rounds of gauze are applied in this fashion, with attention being given to keeping the gauze evenly distributed between the elbow and the axilla. After this, the wrap is extended by bringing the gauze around the leading edge of the wing, anterior to the humerus (c) and continue in a figure-of-eight manner until a bulky, but not tight, wrap has been applied (d). An overwrap of nonadherent stretch bandage (e.g. 3M Vetrap) is applied over the gauze. This should begin at the elbow in the same manner as the conforming gauze wrap (e) and extend cranially, completing a figure-of-eight as shown in (f). When completed the bandage should stabilize the elbow and carpal joints without overflexing the carpus. The leading edge of the primary feathers should lie parallel to the secondary feathers.

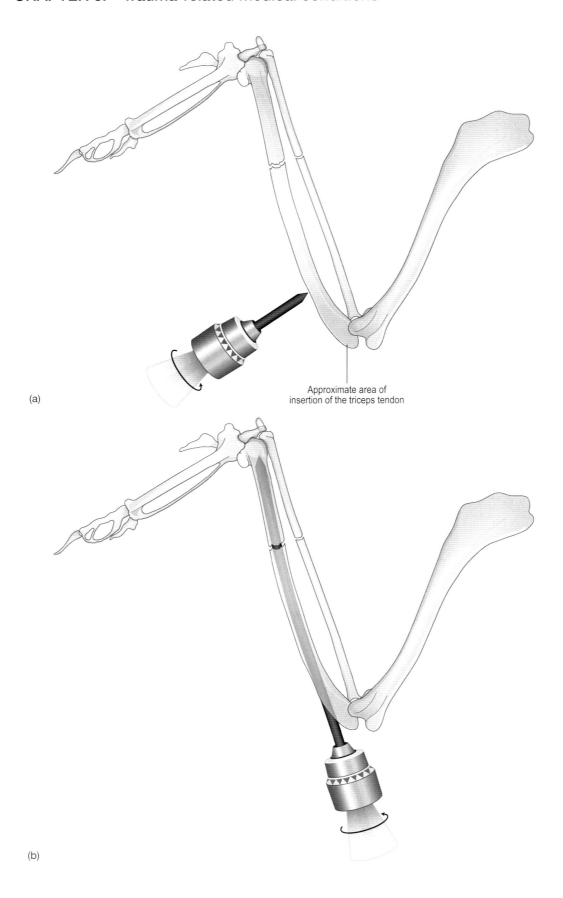

(a)

Approximate area of
insertion of the triceps tendon

(b)

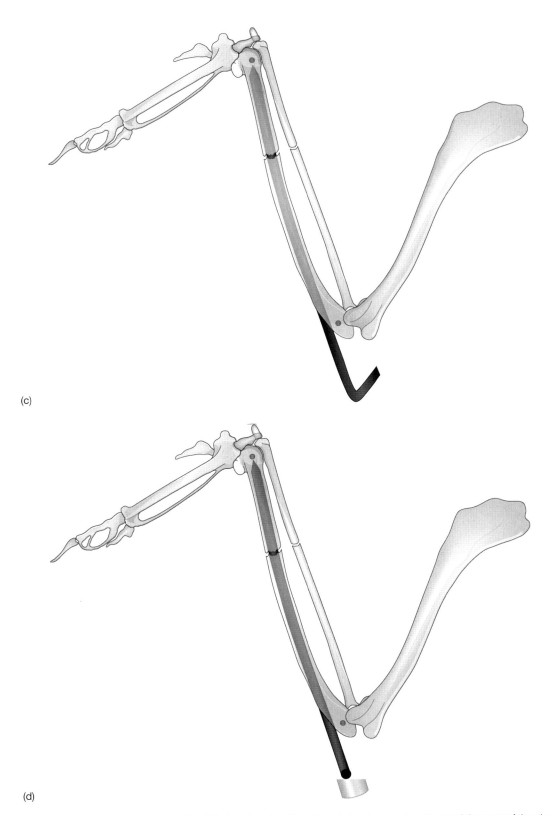

(c)

(d)

Fig. 6.43 Illustrations for normograde placement of an IM pin in the ulna. The ulnar pin is introduced on the caudal aspect of the ulna between the feather follicles of the last (most proximal) secondary feathers and nearly perpendicular to the long axis of the bone (a). An elongated hole is cut in the cortex of the bone and the angle of the pin with the bone is reduced so that, as the pin penetrates the ulnar cortex, the two are longitudinally aligned. The pin is now driven normograde through the reduced fracture and seated in the distal end of the bone (b). Care must be taken to not penetrate the distal end of the ulna. Conversion of the pin in the ulna to a tie-in fixator by the addition of ESF pins, bending the IM pin 90° (c) and applying a connecting bar yields final results (d).

contraindicated as the pin exits the ulna at the olecranon and will damage the joint, the triceps tendon, or both. In addition, a pin exiting at the olecranon will cause joint damage from movement associated with controlled physical therapy in the postoperative period. Specific recommendations for fixation of various types and locations of forearm fractures are detailed below.

Proximal to midshaft ulnar fractures, radius intact or fractured

If the radius is intact and the ulnar fracture is stable (e.g. well-aligned transverse fractures) a suitable treatment option is simple coaptation with a figure-of-eight bandage[i,j] (Fig. 6.42). Be certain that the ulna is aligned in both ventrodorsal and caudal-cranial radiographic planes when using this option.

If the radius is fractured, an intramedullary pin in the radius with no fixation applied to the ulna (Fig. 6.44), especially if the latter is comminuted, or a type I ESF on the ulna (Fig. 6.45) are viable options (a TIF is not usable owing to the extremely short length of proximal ulna in these cases). The radial pin may be placed by introduction at the fracture site of the radius and retrograded toward the metacarpus, or, with good technique, it may be drilled into the distal end of the radius and normograded into the proximal fragment after fracture reduction. In some instances where the ulnar fracture has a very proximal location, only one ESF pin in a type I fixator can be placed in the proximal fragment, but at least this will provide longitudinal and rotational stability of this bone segment.

Coaptation with a figure-of-eight bandage or taping the wing to the body for 7–10 d is advantageous. Physical therapy can be undertaken within the first week by temporarily removing the bandage while the patient is anesthetized.

Midshaft and distal ulnar fractures, radius intact or fractured

Several options for radius and ulna repair are detailed below and fixation choice depends on the characteristics of the injury and the desired outcome. Figures 6.43a–d illustrate the basic steps in application of an acrylic bar-TIF to the ulna.

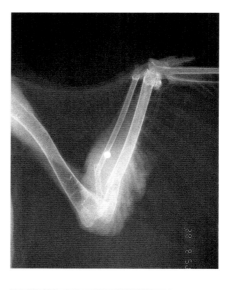

(a)

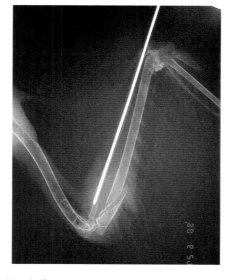

(b)

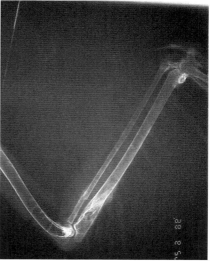

(c)

Fig. 6.44 This red-tailed hawk (*Buteo jamaicensis*) was admitted with a high-energy, comminuted fracture of the proximal radius and ulna (a) that was repaired by retrograde placement of an IM pin in the radius only (b) to preserve remaining soft tissue in the vicinity of the ulnar fracture. The wing was coaptively supported with a figure-of-eight bandage and a satisfactory union was realized in 33 d (c).

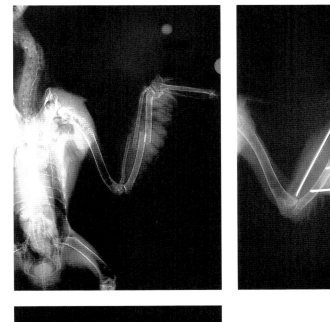

(a)

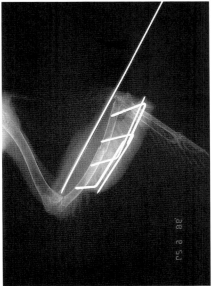

(b)

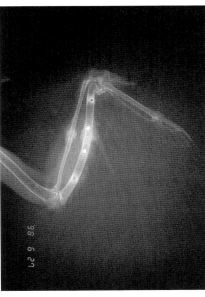

(c)

Fig. 6.45 Radiographs of fixation with an ESF on the ulna and an IM pin in the radius. This Cooper's hawk (*Accipiter cooperi*) was admitted with fractures of the radius and ulna (a). An intramedullary pin was inserted in the radius in retrograde fashion, exiting at the carpus. A type I ESF was applied to the ulna with an acrylic connector bar (b). Healing progressed normally and the fixation was removed in 28 d (c). Pinning the ulna with an IM pin would have been an acceptable alternative in this case.

- For ulnar fractures in which the radius is intact and return to flight is not required necessarily, a figure-of-eight coaptation bandage is adequate. If flight is required, better chances for success will be had with fixation in the form of an IM pin, a type I ESF, or a tie-in fixator (preferred – see below)
- For simple fractures of either or both the radius and ulna, intramedullary pins may be applied as depicted in Figure 6.46. This method provides longitudinal alignment and stabilization, but requires a figure-of-eight bandage for 10–14 d postoperatively. Normograde insertion of the IM pin into the ulna should be used (Fig. 6.43a,b)
- A type I ESF applied to the ulna is recommended if the fracture is comminuted (Fig. 6.47). Note the use of three ESF pins on either side of the fracture in order to provide adequate stability

- A TIF (Fig. 6.48) is the best option in any ulnar fracture in the distal two-thirds of the bone where return to flight is the desired outcome and fracture/soft tissue condition permits its application. The TIF is applied as depicted in Figure 6.43. Small ESF pins may be placed along the diaphysis of the ulna in birds with very long forearms (eagles, cranes) for additional stability. In Figure 6.48b, note the use of a two pin ESF with a conventional Kirshner–Ehmer bar and clamps as a temporary fixator. This can be applied quickly during the admission examination and will prevent bone ends from exteriorizing and improve circulation while the opportune time to do the definitive fixation is awaited. Fracture repair may be delayed in this manner for up to a week; the wing with a temporary fixator applied is taped to the body in the meantime.

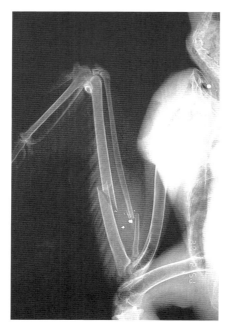

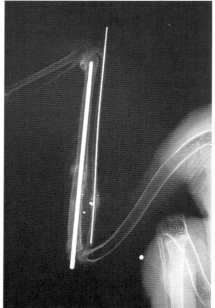

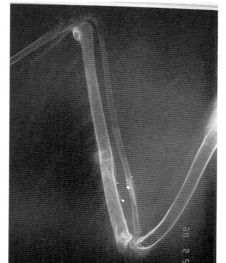

Fig. 6.46 Where both bones are fractured, IM pins, one each in the radius and the ulna, yield satisfactory results. The radial pin is placed first by retrograding it in the distal fragment, exiting at the metacarpus. This golden eagle (*Aquila chrysaetos*) was admitted with a low-energy projectile injury to the radius and ulna (a) with minimal accompanying soft tissue injury. Intramedullary pins were inserted in the radius and ulna, the former in retrograde fashion exiting at the carpus, the latter in normograde fashion (b). Healing of both fractures was complete in 70 d (c).

Special cases of the forearm: Radius fractured proximally or distally, ulna intact

Management options include 1) no fixation, and coaptation – recommended only for very proximal radial fractures; and 2) an intramedullary pin typically installed by retrograde placement, exiting at the distal end of the radius for diaphyseal and distal fractures.

Proximal radial fractures occur commonly in falcons and occasionally in other raptors, presumably from overhead wire strikes. They may or may not be accompanied by varying degrees of elbow luxation (Fig. 6.49). In most cases the proximal fragment is too short for pinning. Coaptation, applied for 3–4 weeks with intermittent physical therapy beginning after the second week, is most commonly used. If the ulna is luxated from the humerus, imbrication of the edges

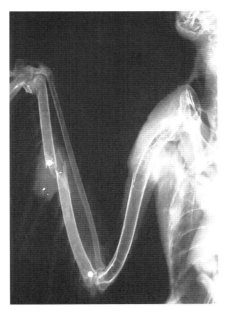

(a)

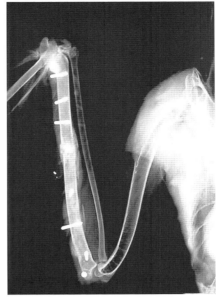

(b)

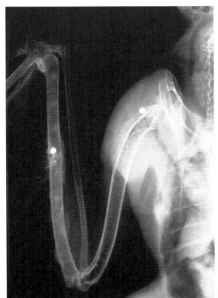

(c)

Fig. 6.47 This red-tailed hawk was presented with a midshaft fracture of the ulna in which there was displacement of the fragments and a high risk of synostosis with the radius if reduction and stabilization were not undertaken. (b) Radiograph, 2 weeks postoperatively, showing the implantation of a type I external skeletal fixator. Owing to the soft tissue damage present at the fracture site, this type of fixation was chosen instead of a TIF. In order to assure rigidity and longevity of the fixator, three positive profile threaded pins were used, placed perpendicularly to the bone, on either side of the fracture. (c) Radiograph, 5 weeks postoperatively and after removal of the fixator. Healing of the fracture with a minimum of external callus can be seen.

of the triceps tendon and the common digital extensor tendon will aid in stabilization of the joint. Undesired outcomes include arthritis at the elbow and non-union.

Radial fractures in the distal three-quarters of the bone are best managed by intramedullary pinning (Fig. 6.50). The radius is a very mobile bone and even when the ulna is intact and the wing is stabilized with a figure-of-eight bandage the radius tends to move, hence the requirement for immobilization. There is a high probability of the formation of a synostosis, a bony bridge between the two bones, especially with more distally located fractures, if the radius is not stabilized.

Methods of fixation for the major metacarpal

General considerations

Fractures of the major metacarpal bone are challenging to manage. The majority of metacarpal fractures are high-energy fractures. The energy of the fracturing agent, be it a fence wire, powerline or projectile, is concentrated over a very small area that has little soft tissue protection. The small amount of soft tissue

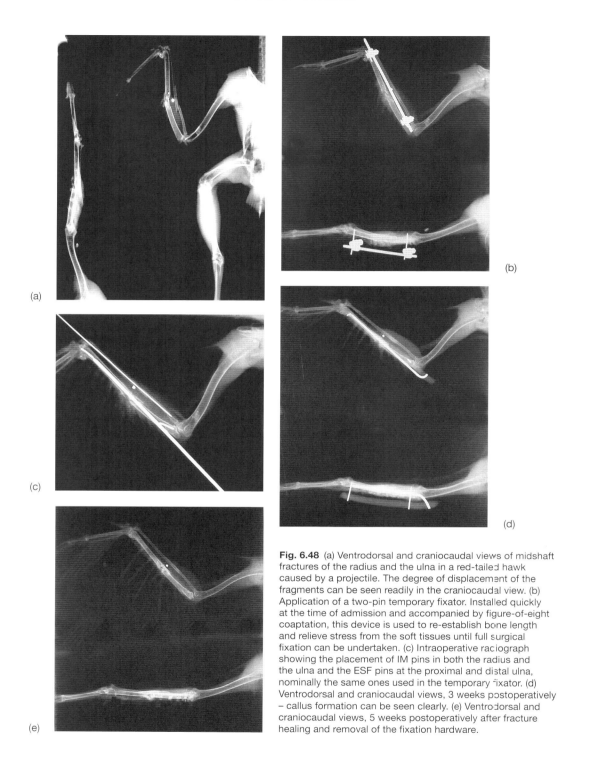

Fig. 6.48 (a) Ventrodorsal and craniocaudal views of midshaft fractures of the radius and the ulna in a red-tailed hawk caused by a projectile. The degree of displacement of the fragments can be seen readily in the craniocaudal view. (b) Application of a two-pin temporary fixator. Installed quickly at the time of admission and accompanied by figure-of-eight coaptation, this device is used to re-establish bone length and relieve stress from the soft tissues until full surgical fixation can be undertaken. (c) Intraoperative radiograph showing the placement of IM pins in both the radius and the ulna and the ESF pins at the proximal and distal ulna, nominally the same ones used in the temporary fixator. (d) Ventrodorsal and craniocaudal views, 3 weeks postoperatively – callus formation can be seen clearly. (e) Ventrodorsal and craniocaudal views, 5 weeks postoperatively after fracture healing and removal of the fixation hardware.

present absorbs a good portion of that energy and is severely damaged in the process. Metacarpal fractures typically present as open and/or comminuted. The minor metacarpal bone is capable of providing internal support and load-sharing if it is not fractured, thereby improving the prognosis. However, the success rate with any type of management is lower than that seen with other long bone fractures except the tarsometatarsus.

Treatment options range from coaptation using a reinforced splint (curved-edge splint) and figure-of-eight bandage to type I ESFs. Metacarpal fractures are highly unstable and re-establishment of load-sharing is not possible, hence the fixator or coaptation device must bear the entire load during healing. The TIF has been less successful than other fixation modes.

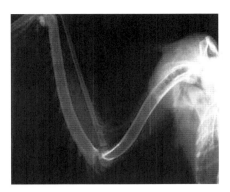

(a)

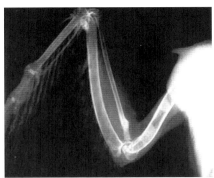

(b)

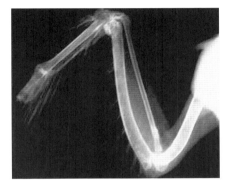

(c)

Fig. 6.49 Proximal radial fractures (within 2–3 bone diameters of elbow). (a) Admission. (b) 3 weeks. (c) 5 weeks. This peregrine falcon was admitted with a low-energy, closed, transverse fracture of the proximal radius. The ulna was intact and the elements of the elbow joint were luxated. In this location the radius was protected and contained by soft tissue. This fracture was adequately managed with coaptation – a figure-of-eight bandage, however, the outcome was accompanied by joint degeneration.

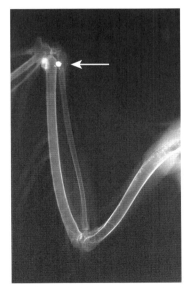

(a)

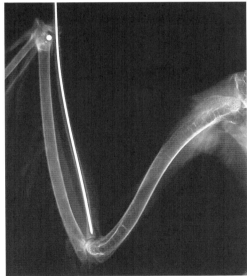

(b)

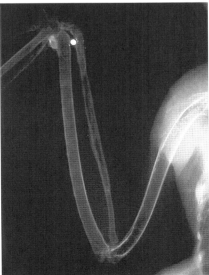

(c)

Fig 6.50 Distal radial fracture in a bald eagle (*Haliaeetus leucocephalus*) caused by a projectile. (a) The arrow indicates the site of the fracture. (b) Postoperative ventrodorsal view after an IM pin has been placed. In this instance, the pin was introduced in the distal end of the radius at the metacarpus and driven normograde through the distal fragment and into the proximal. (c) 5 weeks postoperatively, after the fracture had healed and the fixation removed. The site of the fracture is indicated by the arrow.

Coaptation is suitable for the low-energy, transverse, reducible fracture, especially if the minor metacarpal is intact. Because the wing must be bound in a splint for upwards of 3 weeks, the potential for immobilization-related morbidity is substantial. Splints made from moldable material (e.g. Sam Splint^k or veterinary thermo-plastic (VTP)^f molded into a 'curved edge splint' has been a satisfactory means of coaptively stabilizing metacarpal fractures (Figs 6.51 and 6.52). Conventional external fixation is another choice for highly comminuted metacarpal fractures with extensive soft tissue damage, as reduction, alignment and stabilization can be

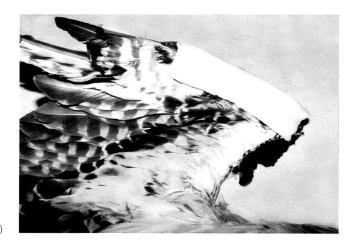

(a)

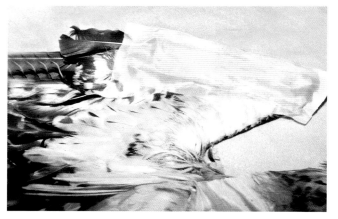

(b)

Fig. 6.51 Curved edge splint made from moldable material for an osprey (*Pandion haliaetus*). Veterinary thermoplastic (VTP®, Imex) is a heat-activated casting tape. (a) A strip of material was cut sufficiently long to span the distance from the proximal end of the radioulnar-carpometacarpal joint to well beyond the joint with the second phalanx and wide enough to span the width of the metacarpal bone. (b) A right-angled bend was made in the material as shown (VTP® is immersed in hot water for molding). It was placed on the ventral side of the wing with the bent edge wrapping the cranial edge. Several overlapping pieces of adhesive tape placed dorsally and ventrally, pressing opposing adhesive surfaces together where possible, were used to affix the splint directly to the wing. The wing was then wrapped in a conventional figure-of-eight bandage with gauze padding added to the dorsal surface to gently press the bone elements into the splint as the figure-of-eight is applied.

accomplished with minimal manipulation of the soft tissue. The least desirable choice is an intramedullary pin, as one incurs the liability of morbidity associated with implanting the pin but does not achieve stability without further coapting the limb. Tie-in fixators have not been consistently effective. Delaying application of fixation by 5–7 d post-injury to allow soft tissues some time to recover before insulting them again with hardware placement has led to improved healing success with metacarpal fractures. This is particularly true in falcons, where metacarpal fractures are most often accompanied by moderate to severe edema. This must be reduced before repair of the fracture is attempted. This is accomplished by twice daily hot-packing the wing for 5–10 min, application of dimethylsulfoxide (DMSO) over the area once or twice, and administering peripheral vasodilating drugs (e.g. isoxuprine^l). In the meantime, the wing is kept bandaged in a figure-of-eight and taped to the body. No other bone in the avian skeleton requires more attention to careful assessment and selection of a proper fixation device to maximize the healing potential of a fracture.

Specific management recommendations

Midshaft comminuted or distal major metacarpal fractures may be repaired with coaptation with a single-sided curved-edge splint (Figs 6.51–6.52) or with a type I ESF, as illustrated in Figure 6.53.

The tie-in method for fractures of the femur

General considerations

With abundant soft tissue protection afforded by heavy muscle, the femur responds favorably to most attempts at fixation. The approach to fixation resembles that of the humerus and the ESF-IM pin tie-in works well. For insertion of the IM pin, the femur is approached from the lateral aspect. The bird is laid with the contralateral side down. The affected leg is abducted and the distal portion of the ipsilateral wing is placed underneath the leg, between the medial aspect of the leg and the body wall. The incision is made at about the 4 o'clock position on the femoral shaft as viewed from the distal end on, extending from the condyles at the distal end to the proximal end. Blunt dissection is used to separate the quadriceps femoris muscle from the ventral flexor muscle group. The femoral artery, vein and nerve lie deep and ventral to the femur; they will be visualized but do not present a serious hazard during repair of the bone.

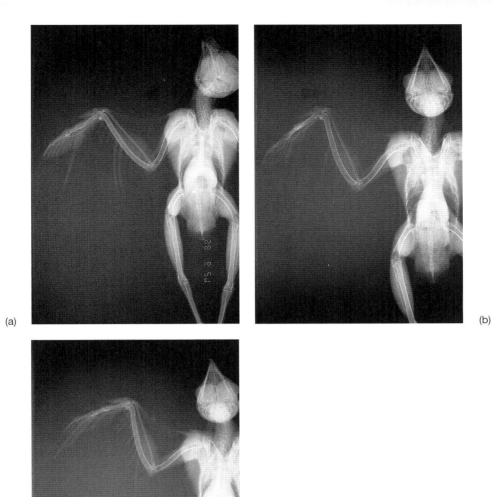

(a)

(b)

(c)

Fig. 6.52 This American kestrel (*Falco sparverius*) was admitted with a closed, midshaft major metacarpal fracture accompanied by severe soft tissue contusion (a). A curved edge splint (made from a foam-clad aluminum splint material – Sam Splint®) was applied and the fracture was healing slowly at 24 d. (b). Complete union was realized in 60 d (c).

Fractures of the femur

Femoral fractures can be managed in a manner closely analogous to the humerus. The application of a TIF is illustrated diagrammatically in Figure 6.54. For diaphyseal fractures, the intramedullary pin for the TIF is typically introduced at the fracture site and retrograded proximally. The distal ESF pin is placed from lateral to medial in the condyles. The proximal ESF pin is placed from lateral to medial by palpating the dorsal rim of the acetabulum and selecting a point on the femur 2–4 mm distad. A smaller pin than that used distally is typically selected as it must share the marrow cavity with the IM pin. As the medial side of the femur cannot be palpated, determination of proper drilling depth for the pin must be done by 'feel'. Characteristically, resistance to the rotation of the pin chuck can be felt when the trocar of the pin is drilling through bone cortex. Accordingly, one feels resistance when passing through the first cortex, lack of resistance as the pin is threaded through the pneumatic cavity, and increased resistance again when the trocar strikes the opposite cortex. Gentle downward pressure is applied to the pin while threading continues. Two to three full rotations of the chuck, after an increase in resistance, is sufficient to seat the pin in the opposite cortex. Angular deflections of the pin chuck should now result in the entire bone fragment moving in concert. If gross movement of the bone is not detected, it means that only one cortex has been engaged. After placement of the ESF pins, the exteriorized portion of the IM pin is bent at 90° and the elements are bonded together with a bar and clamps or with an acrylic bar.

Fractures of the proximal femur may be repaired using a tension band wiring system using two K-wires and cerclage wire (Harcourt-Brown, 1996). Distal fractures may be repaired using a cross-pin method similar to the distal humerus (see above). Again, tying the one or both of the cross-pins to an ESF will provide excellent stabilization. An example of femoral fracture management in a bald eagle with a TIF is depicted in Figure 6.55.

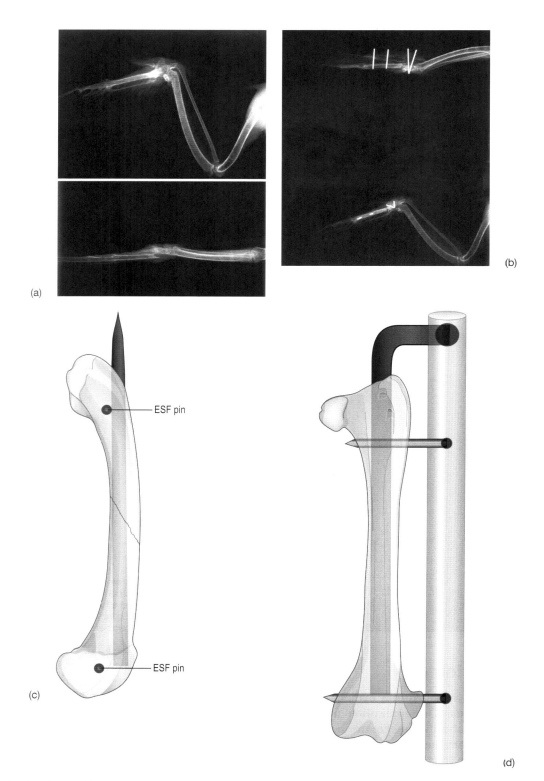

(a)

(b)

(c)

ESF pin

ESF pin

(d)

Fig. 6.53 Application of a type I fixator to a proximal major metacarpal fracture in a peregrine falcon (*Falco peregrinus*). (a) Note the vertical displacement of the fragments seen in the craniocaudal view. (b) Intraoperatively, the ESF pins were used to manipulate the fragments into alignment that was verified radiographically prior to application of the acrylic bar. (c, d) A temporary jig made from a conventional Kirschner–Ehmer bar and clamp device was used to hold the fragments in alignment while the acrylic bar was applied and cured. The fracture healed in 6 weeks and all fixation elements were removed.

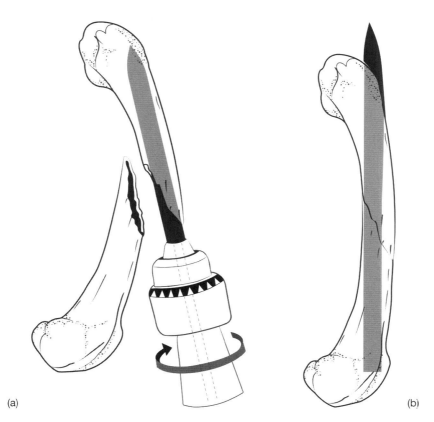

(a)   (b)

Fig. 6.54 Application of a type I fixator to a femoral fracture. (a) After exposure and gentle elevation of the proximal fragment, the IM pin, selected to fill approximately 70% of the marrow cavity, is inserted at the fracture site. (b) The fracture is reduced and the pin is driven and seated in the distal fragment. Locations for placing the two K-wires are indicated by an X. The most distal pin is placed first, and is driven through the condyles. Since it does not share the bone marrow space with the IM pin, it can be a stout pin (e.g. 1.6 mm (0.062″)) in a 1 kg patient.

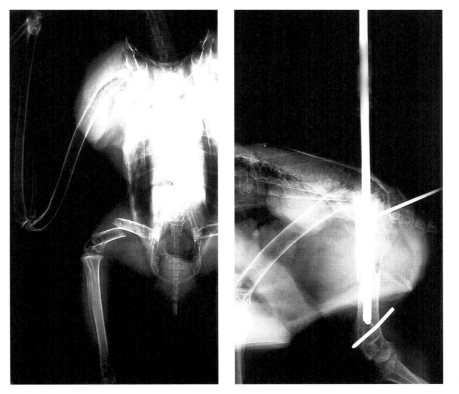

(a)   (b)

Fig. 6.55 (a-c) See overleaf for caption.

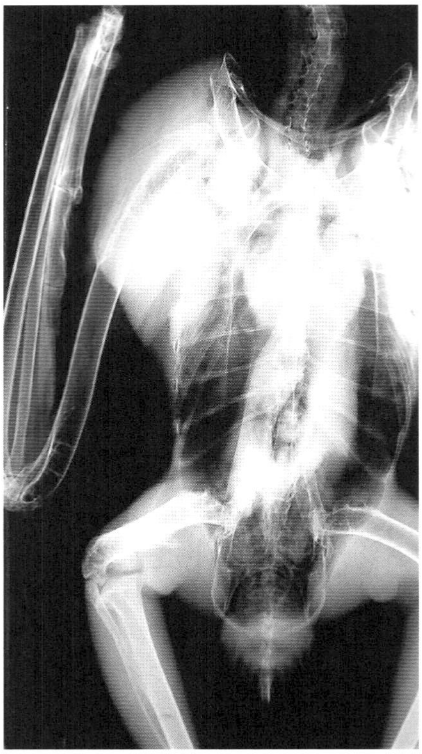

Fig. 6.55 Bald eagle (*Haliaeetus leucocephalus*) with a midshaft femoral fracture. (a) Admission radiograph. (b) Intraoperative radiograph taken to check placement of IM and ESF pins. (c) Radiograph taken at 5 weeks postoperatively, after fracture healing and removal of all hardware.

(c)

Methods of fixation for fractures of the tibiotarsus

General considerations

The tibiotarsus is a very straight bone with a narrow marrow cavity and one that tapers from proximal to distal. The proximal two-thirds are well protected by soft tissue and the primary loads borne during normal use are compressive. The bone is roughly triangular in shape in the proximal half with the base of the triangle lying in a medial to caudal–medial orientation. Satisfactory orthopedic management of fractures of this limb mandates rotational alignment of the stifle and hock joints and lateral to medial alignment of the fragments; anterior to posterior alignment is less critical. In order to preserve integrity of the contralateral foot, immediate postoperative weight bearing is desirable, although injury to soft tissue often results in impaired use even though the fixation is capable of load bearing. Fractures in the proximal one-third are most often transverse, thus offering opportunities for load sharing. A TIF has proved very effective in managing fractures of this bone. Both ends of the tibiotarsus are protected by adjacent leg bones and associated joints; hence penetration of the proximal and distal ends is a morbidity factor when the intramedullary

pin is inserted. Careful placement of the IM pin mitigates this potential problem.

Fractures of the tibiotarsus

Among raptors kept for falconry purposes, fractures of the tibiotarsus in the proximal one-third arising from bating accidents are seen frequently (Harcourt-Brown, 1996). These are typically low-energy, transverse fractures. Wild casualty birds most often have complicated and comminuted, high-energy fractures involving the tibiotarsus. Owing to the large muscle masses, especially in the proximal region, tibiotarsal fractures are seldom open and prognosis is good. Two caveats exist for wild casualty birds: 1) nerve damage often accompanies their fractures of the tibiotarsus, leading to slow return to use of the lower limb, and 2) spinal injury often accompanies these fractures but may be hard to detect at admission because of the analgia in the broken limb. Failure to properly assess this condition may lead to an unnecessary and unproductive fixation procedure. An additional caveat with any tibiotarsal fracture is to avoid using only an IM pin, as this cannot provide adequate rotational stability.

While a type II ESF has been advocated by many surgeons and yielded satisfactory results (Redig 1986a; Hess, 1994, Harcourt-Brown, 1996; Bennett 1997), we have found that an adaptation of the TIF produces exceptional results, again making it the method of choice in all but those cases involving severe comminution, in which a type II external skeletal fixator may be an appropriate choice, or for very distal fractures, where cross-pinning is recommended (Harcourt-Brown, 1996).

For application of the TIF to the tibiotarsus, the IM pin is introduced to the tibial table on the medial aspect of the femorotibial joint and passed normograde into the proximal fragment (Fig. 6.56). The pin is placed

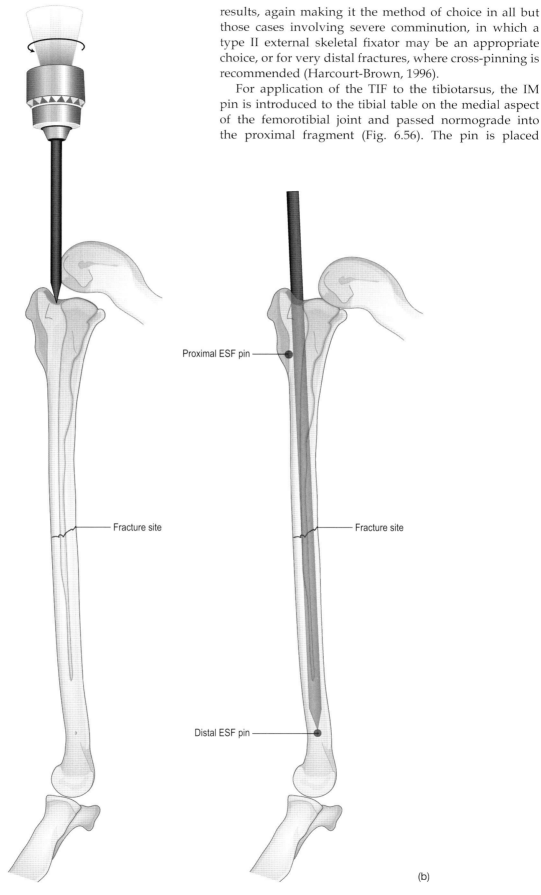

Fracture site

Proximal ESF pin

Fracture site

Distal ESF pin

(a)

(b)

Fig. 6.56 (a–d) See overleaf for caption.

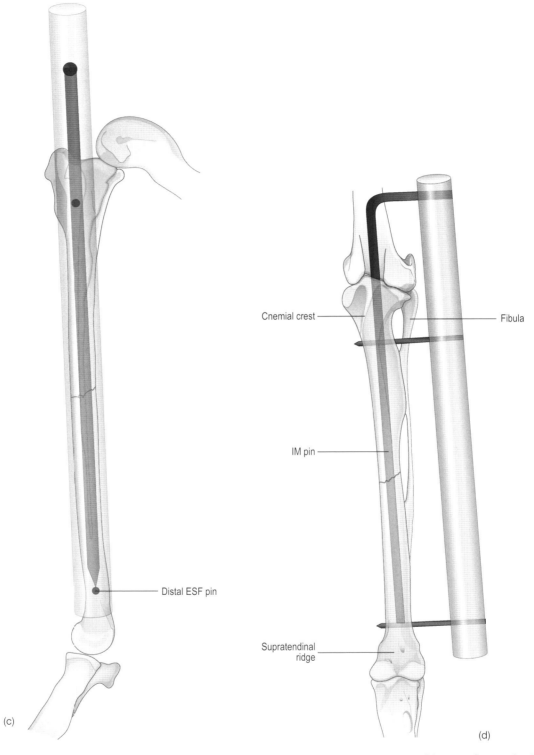

Fig. 6.56 Application of a type I fixator to the tibiotarsus. (a) Lateral view of the introduction of an IM pin into the tibiotarsus. See text for details of insertion of the pin. (b) Relative placement of the IM pin and the proximal and distal ESF pins. (c) The TIF as viewed from the lateral side of the tibiotarsus. (d) Craniocaudal view of the TIF applied to the tibiotarsal bone. Note that the distal ESF pin is inserted proximal to the supratendinal ridge and that the connector bar is on the lateral side of the leg.

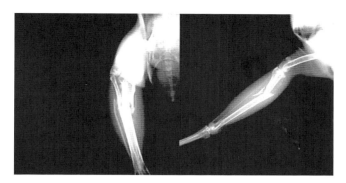

(a)

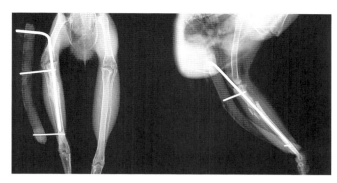

(b)

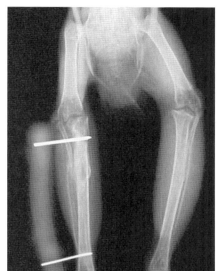

(c)

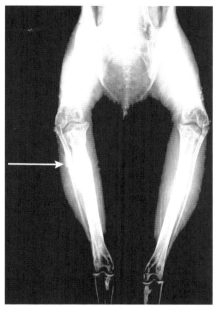

(d)

Fig. 6.57 Proximal fracture of the tibiotarsus and fibula in a barred owl (Strix varia). (a) Radiograph at the time of admission. (b) Craniocaudal and lateral postoperative radiographs after the repair of the tibiotarsal fracture with a TIF. (c) Radiograph, 3 weeks postoperatively. Healing is progressing well and the IM pin has been removed. The elements of the ESF were left in place for continuing support of the fracture. They were removed 5 weeks postoperatively. (d) Radiograph, 5 weeks postoperatively; all fixation has been removed and the fracture is well healed (arrow).

through the skin along the medial edge of the patellar tendon nearly parallel to the joint surface. The trocar of the pin is worked underneath the tendon, pushing the latter laterally. The pin is aligned with the long axis of the tibiotarsal proximal fragment and advanced distally. The fracture is reduced and the pin is advanced into the distal fragment. When selecting the IM pin, use the marrow cavity diameter as measured at the distal end as this bone tapers substantially in the distal portion (Harcourt-Brown, 1996). Threaded ESF pins are placed transversely distally and proximally. The distal pin must be placed 1–2 bone diameters proximal to the hock joint in order to avoid injury to vessels and tendons at the end of the bone and should not be driven distal to the supratendinal ridge (Fig. 6.56d). The proximal pin should be introduced on the craniolateral aspect just distal to the tibial plateau and craniad to the fibula. It should be directed caudomedially to avoid the neurovascular bundles on the medial side

of the proximal tibiotarsus (Harcourt-Brown, 2000). The IM pin is again bent at 90° and directed laterally so that it can be joined to the ESF pins with an acrylic bar or conventional fixator clamps and a bar (Fig. 6.56d).

Postoperatively, one should expect little or no weight bearing on the affected leg for 3–5 d because of transitory neuroparalysis arising either from the injury itself or the surgical procedure; 'knuckling over' is common. It is important to wrap the digits of the affected limb with protective materials (e.g. Vetrap®) to prevent abrasion of the dorsal surfaces. Concurrently, the asymmetric weight bearing predisposes bumblefoot formation in the contralateral foot, so it too should be given protective bandaging (Fig. 6.57 shows radiographs of a healing sequence). Proximal fractures of the tibiotarsus in which the proximal fragment is too short to accept a TIF may be managed with a transarticular fracture as depicted in Figure 6.58.

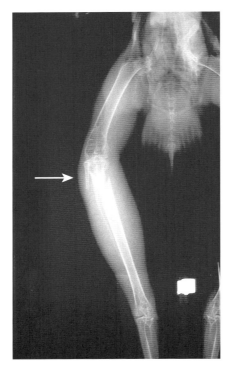

(a)

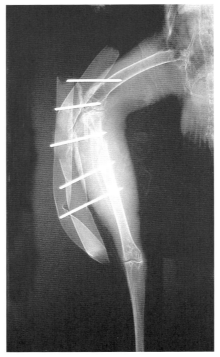

(b)

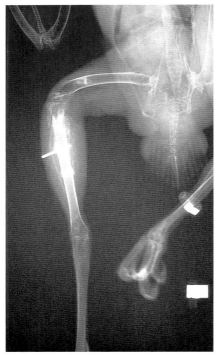

(c)

Fig. 6.58 Method of transarticular fixation for proximal tibiotarsal fractures. (a) This Cooper's hawk fractured its proximal tibiotarsus in a struggle with a cock pheasant. (b) The proximal fragment was too short to be stabilized adequately with a conventional type II fixator. Accordingly, a type I transarticular fixator was applied, consisting of 0.045″ diameter positive-profile acrylic interface threaded pins, with two pins distal to the fracture, one pin in the short proximal tibiotarsal fragment, and two in the femur. A piece of 3/8″ (9.6 mm) diameter Penrose drain was pressed over the pins and the leg was positioned with the stifle joint flexed as in a normal perching configuration. The tubing was filled with horse hoof repair acrylic. The fracture site was accessed from the medial side and the alignment of the bones after reduction was visually observed while the fixator bar was applied and the acrylic cured. Where the tubing became constricted following the acute angle at the stifle, some of the tubing was removed after the acrylic cured and the concave surface of the flexure was reinforced with additional acrylic material. (c) The fracture was slow to heal but union was achieved in 27 d. One pin had broken below the skin line and was left in place. 4 months was required for return to full function.

Methods of stabilization and fixation for tarsometatarsal fractures

Like the metacarpus, the tarsometatarsus has a paucity of soft tissue coverage and therefore many of the same management problems. Anatomically, it is quite different in that it has no marrow cavity in the proximal one-third in hawks and owls, while in falcons a marrow cavity runs the full length (Harcourt-Brown, 2000). In cross-section, it is a U-shaped bone formed embryonically from the fusion of elements of the metatarsal and tarsal bones. The flexor tendons run in a channel on the caudal aspect; veins are present on the lateral and medial aspects and arterial blood supply along with nerves are found on the cranial aspect. Also, the bone is protected by articular surfaces at both ends. These factors combine to render intramedullary pinning a poor fixation choice. Additionally, when a bird is perching at rest, the bone is positioned at an angle to the perching surface so load bearing applies bending forces as well as rotational forces to the bone.

Fixation choices

In birds weighing up to 150 g with closed and otherwise uncomplicated fractures, an effective means of stabilization has been coaptation in the form of a tape splint combined with taping the hock in flexion so the tarsometatarsus is splinted by the tibiotarsus (Figs 6.59 and 6.60). A cast of a thermoplastic material can be used, particularly in a closed fracture in which no wound management

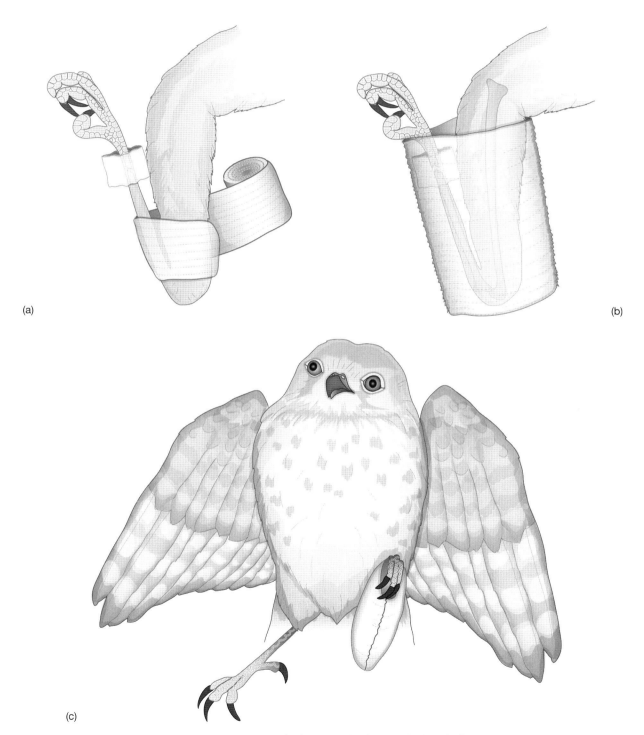

(a)

(b)

(c)

Fig. 6.59 Tarsometatarsal fractures: (a) coaptation by tape splint (b,c) combined with taping the hock in flexion.

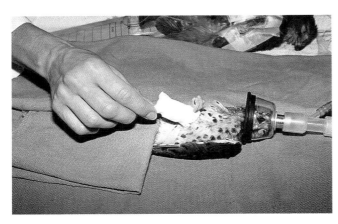
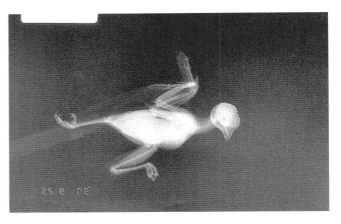

Fig. 6.60 This American kestrel was presented with a closed mid-shaft tarsometatarsal fracture. (a) The fracture was stabilized with an Altman tape splint and the leg was splinted to the tibiotarsus using conforming gauze and Vetrap® applied directly to the leg. (b) The fracture healed uneventfully in 18 d.

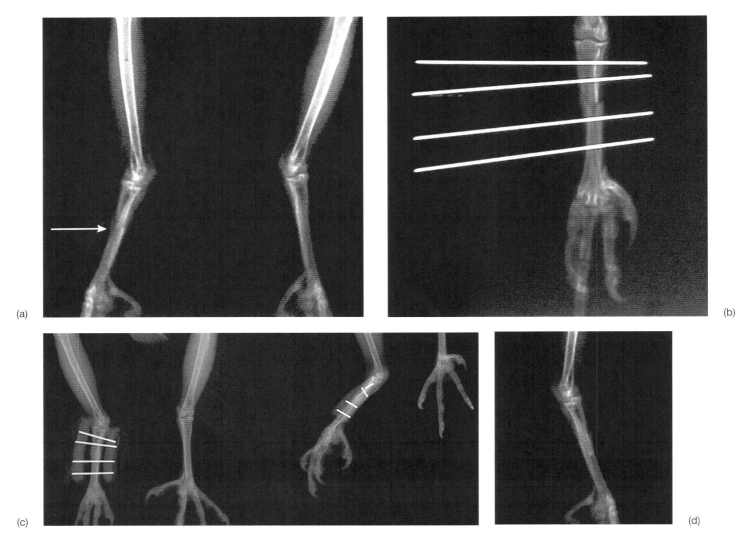

Fig. 6.61 This prairie falcon (*Falco mexicanus*) was presented with an open, transverse fracture of the tarsometatarsus (a). (b, c) In order to facilitate access to the wound for regular management, a type II fixator was applied. (d) Healing was complete in 35 d.

procedures are required. Schroeder–Thomas splints are yet another alternative for birds weighing less than about 1–1.5 kg (Redig, 1986b).

Fixator application in the form of a type II ESF is applicable in a wide variety of situations and is the method of choice in any situation where there is comminution or there are open wounds that require management (Fig. 6.61). Care must be taken not to pass the pins through the flexor channel on the caudal aspect of the bone. Because of the bending loads applied to this bone, it is useful to place three pins on either side of the fracture site, if possible, rather than only two.

Postoperative management of fracture repair patients

Postoperatively, patients are inspected within 24 h of surgery. In uncomplicated cases, bandaging material is removed and the surgical site is cleaned. A thin layer of a triple antibiotic ointment (e.g. neomycin, bacitracin, polymyxin B) is applied over the suture line and pin tracts and a light absorbent bandage is reapplied. Complicated,

open fractures will require daily wound treatment until granulation is well under way. Bactericidal cefalosporin antibiotics will have been given perioperatively (e.g. cefatoxime – Claforan^m) and patients are maintained on oral enrofloxacin (Baytril$^{®n}$) or clavulanated amoxicillin (Clavamox$^{®o}$) for up to 5 d postoperatively. In patients with open, contaminated fractures and infected bones, clindamycin (Antirobe$^{®p}$) is used instead. Radiographs are taken at days 10–14 and 20–24 postoperatively and at biweekly intervals thereafter, if needed. Up to 10 d postoperatively, adjustments in alignment can be made. By 21 d, uncomplicated fractures will be well on their way to complete healing and partial dismantling – dynamic destabilization – (Egger, 1993) of the fixator may take place. Some fractures will be healed already. If healing is not progressing well, evidence of sequestra will be seen radiographically at around 3 weeks. Sequestra should be surgically removed when their extent is clear and reassessment of the patient and the repair process should be made accordingly. In uncomplicated cases, all fixation should be removed by 6 weeks. Bone strength is usually substantial at this point and the patient can be allowed full use of the limb.

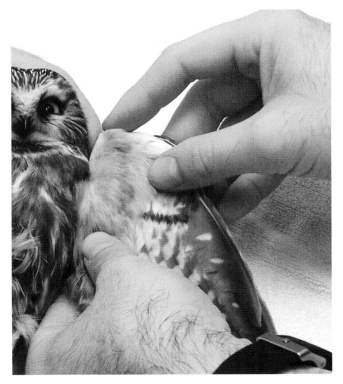

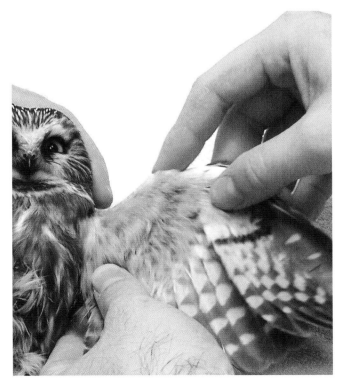

(a)

(b)

Fig. 6.62 (a-c) See overleaf for caption.

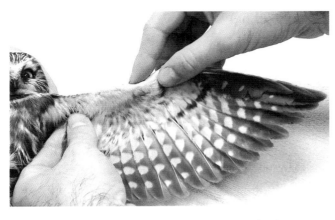

Fig. 6.62a–c Passive range of motion physical therapy for the prevention of patagial contraction being conducted on a saw-whet owl (*Aegolius funereus*). These sessions are conducted under anesthesia in the immediate postoperative period and awake after the first week; each session, lasts about 5 m in and consists of repetitive extensions and flexions, and extend-and-hold manipulations.

Physical therapy for managing wing fractures

Physical therapy in the form of passive range of motion (PROM) exercise is begun 1–2 d postoperatively for humeral fractures and at around 10 d for other wing fractures. The patient is typically anesthetized for this. PROM is done for 5 min sessions twice weekly for the first 1–2 weeks, after which no further gains are likely to be achieved. Stretch and hold exercises are alternated with range of motion movements to the extent the limb will allow at any given time (Fig. 6.62). Care is taken not to overextend the limb during these exercises.

Management of the patagium

Severe contraction of the patagium often accompanies humeral fractures that have been coaptively supported with a figure-of-eight bandage and/or not provided with range-of-motion physical therapy postoperatively. The bone may heal satisfactorily but there can be severe restriction on wing extension after the fracture is healed (Fig. 6.63). There are two ways of preventing this problem. The first is to apply adequate fixation to the fracture that allows full range of motion postoperatively without the need for additional immobilization by bandaging (e.g. a tie-in fixator). The second is to institute passive physical therapy and patagial massage within the first postoperative week and maintain this throughout the healing period. This is performed under isoflurane anesthesia and consists of an approximately 5 min session performed every 2 d. The exercises consist of range-of-motion movements and stretch and hold manipulations (Fig. 6.62). Particular attention needs to be paid to focal areas of thickening along the leading edge of the wing (ligamentum propatagialis). Kneading and stretching of this ligament will minimize or remove these. By instituting this procedure beginning on the second postoperative day, contraction problems of the patagium and reduction in wing extension can be avoided.

Lacerations of the patagium may be managed either by suturing or by secondary-intention healing. However, the elastic fibers of the patagium do not hold sutures and the area of the wound should be protected from movement during healing. A suitable method for providing this protection consists of using a manila cardboard (file folder) stent that is cut to a shape and size approximately 20% larger than the area of the wound. After wound dressing material has been applied to the wound, this cardboard is placed over the wound. Sutures are placed through the patagium and through

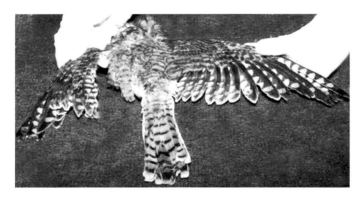

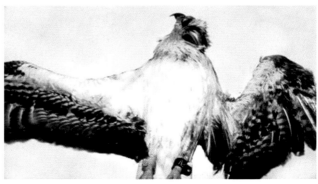

Fig. 6.63 Severe patagial contraction can occur during the healing of a humeral fracture if: (a) a figure-of-eight bandage is used to provide coaptive support (species: kestrel), and (b) no postoperative physical therapy is given (species: osprey).

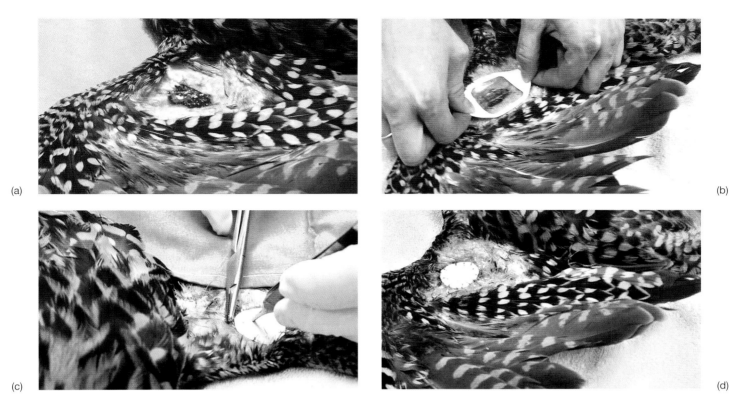

(a)

(b)

(c)

(d)

Fig. 6.64 Management of a patagial wound using a cardboard stent. (a) Nonperforating wound on ventral side of patagium (hybrid falcon). (b) Application of wound dressing material over wound. (c) Suturing a cardboard stent over the treated and dressed wound. (d) Completed stent in place. The wing should be bound to the body and subjected to passive range-of-motion exercise approximately twice weekly.

the cardboard, working around the perimeter of the latter (Fig. 6.64). Because of the loosening of the sutures in the patagium, this stent is replaced at weekly intervals or more often as needed, until the wound is healed.

Luxations

Luxations of the elbow

Moderate success has been obtained in the surgical repair of caudal-dorsal luxations of the elbow (Ackerman and Redig, 1997). Such intervention must take place early in the postinjury period (i.e. at 2–3 d) to be successful. A curved incision is made over the lateral surface of the wing that includes the distal end of the humerus and the proximal portion of the antebrachium. The tendon of origin of the supinator muscle, if still intact, is transected to provide exposure of the joint. The end of the ulna is levered into place by inserting a flat periosteal elevator in between the proximal ulna and the dorsal humeral condyle and levering the ulna distally until it aligns with the humeral condyle. Application of traction to the distal ulna is helpful in this maneuver. The cut ends of the tendon of the supinator are sutured. A pseudocollateral ligament is made by suturing the edge of the triceps tendon to the common digital extensor tendon with the surgeon's preferred choice of suture material. After closure, the elbow is stabilized with a transarticular external skeletal fixator for 7–10 d. Physical therapy is instituted following removal of the fixator and the wing is kept immobilized in between bouts with coaptation.

Minor luxations of the elbow can be managed more effectively compared to simple coaptation by incising the skin over the elbow and suturing the edge of the triceps tendon to the common digital extensor. This procedure is highly recommended on a pre-emptive basis for patients with proximal radial fractures (Fig. 6.48) as these often have a degree of ulnar subluxation associated with them that is not apparent upon physical examination or by radiology.

Luxations of the stifle

Stifle luxations may be repaired by a transarticular external skeletal fixator involving the implantation of threaded ESF pins in the femur and tibiotarsus that are then connected by an acrylic bar molded to fit the contour of the stifle fixed in a partially flexed perching position (Fig. 6.58). If the acrylic is molded within a latex tube (Penrose drain), the flexion at the stifle will create a constriction and a thinned area in the acrylic bar. This is remedied by placing a reinforcing dollop of acrylic material in the acute angle after removing the latex tubing from the surface of the fixator bar.

Another method of stifle stabilization involves placing intramedullary pins in both the femur and the tibiotarsus (Bowles and Zantop, 2002). The pins project from their respective bones at the stifle and are bonded together with a dollop of acrylic material. Luxations of the shoulder elements and the femur are typically managed with cage rest and, in the case of the shoulder, coaptive bandaging of the wing to the body for a period of 10–14 d.

ACKNOWLEDGMENTS

The authors wish to express their sincere thanks to veterinary residents at the Raptor Center, including Dr. David Howard, Dr. Elizabeth Stone, Dr. Janette Ackermann, Dr. Jalila Abu, Dr. Juli Ponder, Dr. Hugo Lopez and Dr. Miguel Saggese, who have been instrumental in the long progression of the development and testing of these methods, along with the veterinary technical staff of TRC, including Lori Arent MS, Toni Guarnera CVT and Jane Goggin, who expend countless hours and great skill and care in the postoperative management of orthopedic patients. Very special thanks go to Dr. Chikako Akaki, who produced the original illustrations for this text, photographed the radiographs and kept all the various components in order during several developmental revisions. Additionally, revisions of existing illustrations, along with new ones for this edition, were provided by Giovanny Rojas, a professional advertising/graphic designer who volunteered his expertise. Thanks also to Drs Larry Wallace and Denny Aron for taking a special interest in tutoring me in principles of orthopedics and their many suggestions for applying them to avian fracture management. Finally, thanks to Animal Care Products, 3M Co., St Paul, MN for their generous donation of rare earth radiographic screens and film that allows comprehensive radiographic documentation of fracture assessment and healing, and to Imex Veterinary Inc., Texas, for manufacturing and providing the acrylic fixator half-pins used in the development and clinical testing of these methods. Portions of this material have been published previously in the *Proceedings of the Association of Avian Veterinarians*.

REFERENCES

Ackerman J, Redig PT (1997) Surgical repair of elbow luxations in raptors. *Journal of Avian Medicine and Surgery* **11**: 247–254.

Bennett RA (1997) Orthopedic surgery. In: Altman RB, Clubb SL, Dorrestein GM, Quesenberry K (eds) *Avian Medicine and Surgery*, pp. 733–766. WB Saunders, Philadelphia.

Bowles HL, Zantop DW (2002) A novel surgical technique for luxation repair of the femorotibial joint in a Monk Parakeet (*Myiopsitta monachus*). *Journal of Avian Medicine and Surgery* **16**: 34–38.

Christen C, Fischer I, von Rechenberg B *et al.* (2005) Evaluation of a maxillofacial miniplate compact 1.0 for stabilization of the ulna in experimentally induced ulnar and radial fractures in pigeons (*Columba livia*). *Journal of Avian Medicine and Surgery* **19**(3): 185–190.

Egger EL (1993) External skeletal fixation – general principles. In: Slatter DH (ed.) *Textbook of Small Animal Surgery*, 2nd edn, pp. 1641–1656. WB Saunders, Philadelphia.

Harcourt-Brown NH (1996) Foot and leg problems. In: Beynon PH, Forbes NA, Harcourt-Brown NH (eds) *Manual of Raptors, Pigeons and Waterfowl*, pp. 147–168. Iowa State University Press, Ames, IA.

Harcourt-Brown NH (2000) Tendon repair in the pelvic limb of birds of prey. In: Lumeij JT, Remple JD, Redig PT *et al.* (eds) *Raptor Biomedicine III*, pp. 201–238. Zoological Education Network, Lake Worth, FL.

Hess R (1994) Orthopedic techniques for the pelvic limb. In: Fudge AM, Redig PT (eds) *Seminars in Avian and Exotic Pet Medicine*, pp. 63–72. WB Saunders, Philadelphia.

Redig PT (1986a) Non-surgical management of avian fractures. In: Harrison GJ, Harrison LR (eds) *Clinical Avian Medicine and Surgery*. WB Saunders, Philadelphia.

Redig PT (1986b) Evaluation and non-surgical management of avian fractures. In: Harrison, GJ, Harrison, LR (eds) *Clinical Avian Medicine and Surgery*, pp. 380–394. WB Saunders, Philadelphia.

Redig PT (2000) The use of a hybrid fixator (intramedullary pin-external skeletal fixator) for stabilization of long bone fractures in raptors – a review of 26 cases. In: Lumeij JT, Remple JD, Redig PT *et al.* (eds) *Raptor Biomedicine III*, pp. 239–254. Zoological Education Network, Lake Worth, FL.

FURTHER READING

Bennett RA, Kuzma AB (1992) Fracture management in birds. *Journal of Zoo and Wildlife Medicine* **23**: 5–38.

Brown RE, Klemm RD (1990) Surgical anatomy of the propatagium. *Proceedings of the Association of Avian Veterinarians*, pp. 176–181.

Degernes LA, Roe SC, Abrams CF Jr (1998) Holding power of different pin designs and pin insertion methods in avian cortical bone. *Veterinary Surgery* **27**: 301–306.

Howard DJ, Redig PT (1994) Orthopedics of the wing. In: Fudge AM, Redig PT (eds) *Seminars in Avian and Exotic Pet Medicine*, pp. 51–62. WB Saunders, Philadelphia.

Piermattei DL, Flo GL (1997) *Brinker, Piermattei and Flo's Handbook of Small Animal Orthopedics and Fracture Repair*, 3rd edn, p. 743. WB Saunders, Philadelphia.

Rochat MC, Hoover JP, Digesualdo CL (2005) Repair of a tibiotarsal varus malunion in a bald eagle (*Haliaeetus leucocephalus*) with a type 1A hybrid external skeletal fixator. *Journal of Avian Medicine and Surgery* **19**: 121–129.

Simpson GN (1996) Wing problems. In: Beynon PH, Forbes NA, Harcourt-Brown NH (eds) *Manual of Raptors, Pigeons and Waterfowl*, pp. 169–179. British Small Animal Association, Cheltenham.

PRODUCT REFERENCE LIST

[a] Acrylic Half-pins®, Imex Veterinary Inc., 1227 Market Street, Longview, TX 75604, USA.

[b] Caulk® Dental Acrylic, Dentsply International Inc., York, PA 17405, USA.

[c] Technovit®, Jorgensen Laboratories, Inc., 1450 North Van Buren Ave., Loveland, CO 80538, USA.

[d] Hoof Wall Restorative Material, Equithane, 600 East Hueneme Road, Oxnard, CA 93033–8600, USA.

[e] Hexcelite®, Hexcel Corporation, Dublin, CA, USA.

[f] Veterinary Thermoplastic®, Imex Veterinary Inc., 1227 Market Street, Longview, TX 75604, USA.

[g] Bolite®, Jorgensen Laboratories, Inc., 1450 North Van Buren Ave., Loveland, CO 80538, USA.

[h] Vetbond®, 3M Animal Care Products, St Paul, MN 55144–1000, USA.

[i] Kling Gauze®, Johnson & Johnson Products, Inc., New Brunswick, NJ 08903, USA.

[j] Vetrap®, 3M Animal Care Products, St Paul, MN 55144–1000, USA.

[k] Sam Splint®, Moore Medical Corp., PO Box 2620, New Britain, CT 06050–2620, USA.

l Isoxsuprine, Geneva Pharmaceuticals, Inc., 2655 West Midway Blvd, Bloomfield, CO 80038-0446, USA.

m Claforan®, Aventis Pharmaceuticals, 399 Interpace Parkway, Parsippany, NJ 07054, USA.

n Baytril®, Bayer Corporation, Pharmaceutical Division, 400 Morgan Lane, West Haven, CT 06516, USA.

o Clavamox®, Pfizer, Inc., 235 East 42nd St New York, NY 10017–5155, USA.

p Antirobe®, Pharmacia & Upjohn, 100 Route 206, North Peapack, NJ 07477, USA.

Wounds

Thomas A. Bailey

A wound is a bodily injury caused by physical means, with disruption of the normal continuity of structures (Blood and Studdert, 1988; Figs 6.65–6.76). Wounds are classified as:

- *Open*: when the injury causes a break in the covering of the body surface (e.g. skin or mucous membrane). These injuries can be seen and blood loss estimated. The main types of open wound are described in Box 6.1
- *Closed*: when the injury does not penetrate the thickness of the skin to cause a break in the body covering. This category includes anything from minor bruising to serious damage to internal organs (e.g. rupture of the liver). Because these wounds cannot be seen, blood loss is difficult to evaluate. The main types of closed wound are described in Box 6.2.

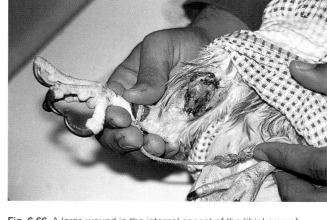

Fig. 6.66 A large wound in the internal aspect of the tibial area of a leg in a saker falcon (*Falco cherrug*). Fights between falcons are not uncommon, in particular when they try to steal the food of eating companions. (Courtesy of Dr. J. Samour).

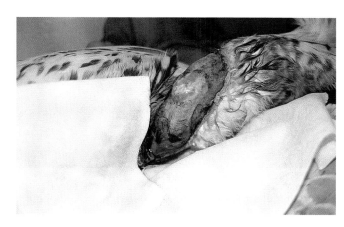

Fig. 6.67 A similar wound to that in Fig. 6.66, but on the cranial area of the femorotibial region of a leg in a saker falcon. (Courtesy of Dr. J. Samour).

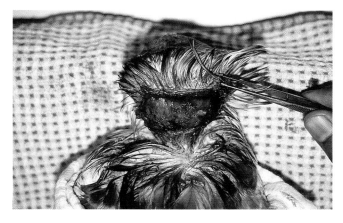

Fig. 6.65 A lanner falcon (*Falco biarmicus*) with a large transversal wound across the occipital area of the head. The wound was produced during an encounter with a larger falcon within a hunting vehicle. The borders of the incision were slightly swollen because of proliferation of granulating tissue. (Courtesy of Dr. J. Samour).

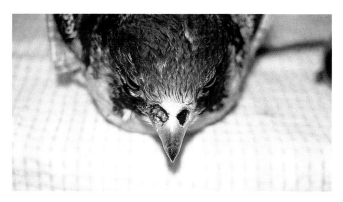

Fig. 6.68 A red-hot nail was driven across the nares of this peregrine falcon (*Falco peregrinus*) with the subsequent loss of tissue. The lesion was artificially caused by a Middle Eastern veterinarian trying to treat the bird for a common rhinitis. 'Branding' lesions are still commonly seen in falcons, domestic animals and even people across the Middle East. The bird was euthanized on humane grounds. (Courtesy of Dr. J. Samour).

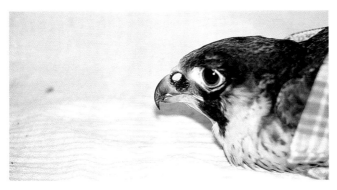

Fig. 6.69 The same falcon as in Fig. 6.68 seen from the lateral view. (Courtesy of Dr. J. Samour).

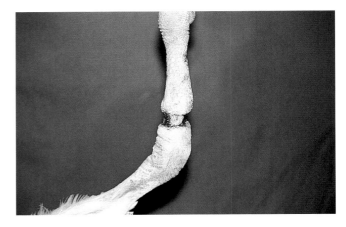

Fig. 6.72 Ring constriction lesion on the leg of a kori bustard (*Ardeotis kori*) caused by the use of a small metal band. (Courtesy of Dr. J. Samour).

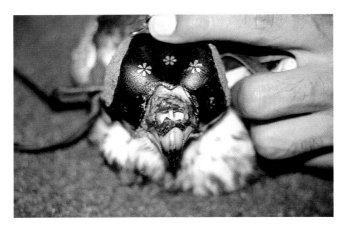

Fig. 6.70 This saker falcon was 'branded' on the cere by its owner trying to treat a large proliferative lesion of avian pox. The whole nasal bridge became necrotic and fell off. The bird was euthanized on humane grounds. (Courtesy of Dr. J. Samour).

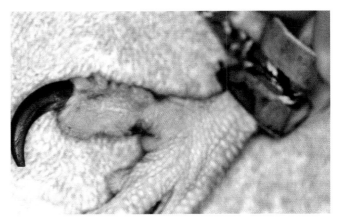

Fig. 6.73 A similar constriction lesion as in Fig. 6.72, caused by a jess entangled around the base of the hind toe of a saker falcon. Comparable lesions are caused by cotton wool strands, commonly used for nesting material, or string from food bags, entangled around the toes of cage birds. (Courtesy of Dr. J. Samour).

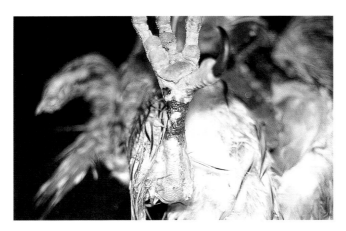

Fig. 6.71 Saker falcon displaying extensive abrasion on the tarsal-metatarsal region of the leg due to the use of small and unsuitable falconry jesses. Similar lesions are observed in wild-caught birds of prey trapped using wire traps. (Courtesy of Dr. J. Samour).

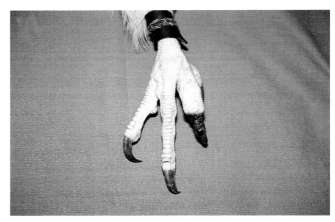

Fig. 6.74 Avascular distal necrosis of a toe in a saker falcon due to extensive scabs produced by avian pox. (Courtesy of Dr. J. Samour).

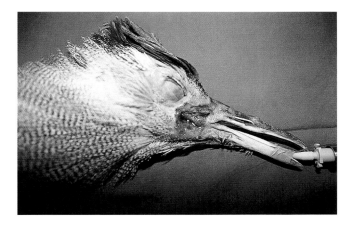

Fig. 6.75 Lacerated wound on the lateral aspect of the face of a kori bustard. The wound occurred during a fight with a companion. Aggression during the breeding season is a very common occurrence among members of this species.

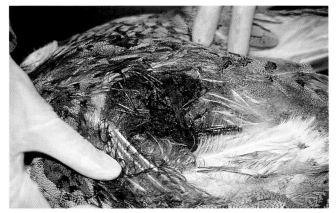

Fig. 6.76 Extensive and severe abrasion under the wing of a houbara bustard (*Chlamydotis undulata*) produced by an exceedingly tight harness made of Teflon ribbons (note the dark band across lesion). The harness in question was placed on the bird as part of a satellite telemetry study. (Courtesy of Dr. J. Samour).

Box 6.1 Open wounds: the main types

Incised
Caused by a sharp instrument so that the skin edges are cut and clearly defined. These wounds can penetrate deeply to damage underlying structures.

Lacerated
Caused by road accidents, tearing or fighting. These wounds are irregular in shape, with jagged uneven edges, and there may be loss of skin. There is a risk of infection from ingrained dirt and bacterial contamination. If areas of skin and underlying tissues are torn away from a lacerated wound, as a loose flap, this is known as an avulsed wound.

Puncture
Caused by blows from sharp pointed instruments such as nails, thorns, fishhooks and talons of birds of prey or teeth in bite wounds. Although the wound is small it may penetrate deeply. Infection is common.

Contused
A contused wound is one in which there is bruising.

Abrasion
Caused by rubbing off the top layer of skin (epidermis) to expose the dermis.

Box 6.2 Closed wounds: the main types

Contusion (bruise)
Caused by a blow with a blunt instrument, which causes rupture of blood vessels in the skin and soft tissues beneath.

Hematoma
If blood loss under the skin is greater than in a contusion, a rounded, fluid-filled swelling called a hematoma is formed. This is commonly seen following poor venipuncture technique of the brachial vein.

Healing of wounds

Wounds heal by one of two methods: 1) first-intention healing or 2) granulation. First-intention healing occurs when the edges of the wound are not widely separated and are held together by blood clots. Blood vessels grow into the clots and promote healing through the production of scar tissue, which ties the wound edges together. First-intention healing can only take place in incised wounds where the edges are close together, which can be achieved by suturing or bandaging while healing takes place (see section on bandages and dressings in Ch. 5.) Granulation healing occurs when the wound edges are widely separated, and is a slower process. Granulation tissue is moist, bright red and formed by clusters of cells on the exposed tissue of the wound. Granulation fills the gap between the wound edges and when it is level with the skin surface new epithelial cells spread across the top to complete the healing process. Granulation tissue usually heals lacerated, avulsed and infected wounds and the repair process can take many weeks.

Treatment of wounds

Treatment of open wounds comprises the following steps:

- Control hemorrhage: the primary objective is to locate the origin of the hemorrhage and to provide rapid hemostasis
- Remove cause of injury
- Remove contaminating foreign bodies: dirt, grit and feathers are commonly found in wounds. Irrigation of the wound with warm sterile saline will remove most contaminants
- If bacterial infection is suspected cultures for bacterial isolation should be taken after the surface contaminants have been removed
- Remove feathers around the wound: it is better to cut feathers in the vicinity of the wound
- Remove necrotic tissue – this should be surgically debrided
- Cleanse the wound using a suitable antiseptic solution such as chlorhexidine or diluted F10
- Apply dressing to the wound (see section on bandages and dressings in Ch. 5)
- Place a surgical drain in a contaminated wound
- Insert polymath
- Treat shock: especially fluid therapy should commence at an early stage (see fluid therapy section in Ch. 5).

Rebandaging and debriding twice a day can prepare infected or old wounds for closure in a few days. Treatment of closed wounds such as contusions and hematomas consists of firm bandaging to limit swelling. The treatment of common traumatic wounds/injuries in avian species is summarized in Box 6.3. Dorsal cervical single pedicle advancement flaps have been used in three different bird species with cranial skin defects. Healing was successful in all three cases (Gentz and Linn, 2000). Useful reviews of wound management in raptors (Burke *et al.*, 2002) and the use of skin flaps and grafts for wound management in raptors has been recently reported (Stroud *et al.*, 2003). The use of xenogeneic grafts in the repair of skin defects in birds has been described (Hernandez-Divers and Hernandez-Divers, 2003). These grafts are manufactured using porcine small-intestinal submucosa. The authors concluded that the wounds treated healed in 6 weeks with less intensive care than was required for healing by second intention.

Wounds that are large, have extensive tissue damage and are either contaminated or infected should be managed as open wounds. This type of wound should be allowed to heal by contraction and epithelialization. The correct use of bandages and medication helps to provide an optimal environment for wound healing. Traumatic wounds may be left open for drainage and healing.

Myiasis caused by blowflies is a frequent complication of avian wounds, particularly in tropical climates and in birds housed in open paddocks or outdoor aviaries. Although it is usually a complication after traumatic injuries, it can also occur in patients hospitalized with bandage wounds. The treatment of myiasis comprises removal of the larvae, irrigation and flushing with diluted antiseptic solution or hydrogen peroxide. Parenteral injection with ivermectin or spraying the affected area with 0.0005% ivermectin (Malley and Whitbread, 1996) is recommended. Products containing coumaphos (e.g. Negasunt, Bayer) should be used sparingly around the affected area to discourage reinfection but should not be applied directly to the wound itself.

Other traumatic injuries, not strictly classified as wounds, include: ring constriction, burns, avascular distal necrosis, self-mutilation and frostbite.

Box 6.3 Treatment of common traumatic wound injuries in avian species

Blood feather damage
Remove damaged feather from affected follicle but beware of causing damage to the germinal epithelium. Seal open shaft with surgical glue or use gentle pressure to stop blood loss.

Beak or nail injuries
Treat with a cauterizing agent such as a silver nitrate stick or an electrosurgical electrode. Severely torn nails may require amputation. Molnar and Ptacek (2001) described the repair of talon injuries in raptors using cyanoacrylate glue, talcum powder and antibiotic mixture to make a 'talon cap' over the distal process of the digit. A similar technique has been used to protect torn talons and beak injuries in falcons using cyanoacrylate glue and sodium bicarbonate (J. Samour, personal communication).

Oropharynx injuries
May need to anesthetize the bird and suture the wound directly or use electrocautery. Topical epinephrine may be useful.

Teeth or claw related injuries
Irrigation, cleaning and drainage. Bacteria, especially *Pasteurella* spp., commonly infect these wounds and can cause a fatal septicemia.

Wing tip trauma
These are usually abrasions and are best cleaned and bandaged. However, surgical resolution may be indicated for fresh incised or lacerated wounds (see Wing tip injuries, above).

Head wounds
Usually caused by trauma and can result in extensive loss of the skin on the scalp. The use of hydrocolloid or hydroactive dressings will speed up healing. These may need to be sutured in place.

Keel injuries
Usually require surgical resolution. Because they are usually caused by impact trauma they require a protective device to prevent further injury (see Keel injuries, above).

Infected joints
Infectious causes of lameness in cursorial birds can result from tenosynovitis, arthritis and osteomyelitis. Infection of joints, commonly the tibiotarsal-tarsometatarsal joint, can result after a traumatic wound or from hematogenous spread. Treatment protocols for septic arthritis should be aggressive. Joint lavage, antibiotic therapy, nonsteroidal anti-inflammatory drugs, analgesics, antibiotic-impregnated polymethacrylate beads, topical DMSO and intra-articular injection of antibiotics have been used. The methods for making these antibiotic beads are discussed by Remple and Forbes (2000).

REFERENCES

Blood DC, Studdert VP (1998) *Baillière's Comprehensive Dictionary*. Baillière Tindall, London.

Burke HF, Swaim SF, Amalsadvala T (2002) Review of wound management in raptors. *Journal of Avian Medicine and Surgery* **16**: 180–191.

Gentz EJ, Linn KA (2000) Use of a dorsal cervical single pedicle advancement flap in three birds with cranial skin defects. *Journal of Avian Medicine and Surgery* **14**: 31–36.

Hernandez-Divers SJ, Hernandez-Divers SM (2003) Xenogeneic grafts using porcine small intestinal submucosa in the repair of skin defects in 4 birds. *Journal of Avian Medicine and Surgery* **17**: 224–234.

Malley AD, Whitbread TJ (1996) The integument. In: Beynon PH, Forbes NA, Harcourt-Brown NH (eds) *Manual of Raptors, Pigeons and Waterfowl*, pp. 129–140. British Small Animal Veterinary Association, Cheltenham.

Molnar L, Ptacek M (2001) Traumatic injuries of beak and talons of captive raptors. *Proceedings of the European Association of Avian Veterinarians*, Munich, pp. 246–247.

Remple JD, Forbes NA (2000) Antibiotic impregnated polymethylacrylate beads in the treatment of bumblefoot in falcons. In: Lumeij JT, Remple JD, Redig PT *et al.* (eds) *Raptor Biomedicine III*, pp. 255–266. Zoological Education Network, Lake Worth, FL.

Stroud PK, Amalsadvala T, Swaim SF (2003) The use of skin flaps and grafts for wound management in raptors. *Journal of Avian Medicine and Surgery* **17**: 78–85.

FURTHER READING

Harrison GJ, Woerpel RW, Rosskopf WJ, Karpinski LG (1986) Symptomatic therapy and emergency medicine. In: Harrison GJ, Harrison LR (eds) *Avian Medicine: Principles and Application*, pp. 362–375. WB Saunders, Philadelphia.

Hiscock S (1989) First aid. In: Lane DR, Cooper BC (eds) *Jones's Animal Nursing*, 2nd edn, pp. 22–96. Butterworth-Heinemann, Oxford.

Redig PT (1996) Avian emergencies. In: Beynon PH, Forbes NA, Harcourt-Brown NH (eds) *Manual of Raptors, Pigeons and Waterfowl*, pp. 30–41. British Small Animal Veterinary Association, Cheltenham.

Management-related diseases

7

Metabolic bone disease

James Kirkwood

The use of terminology describing disorders of the growth, mineralization, maturation and maintenance of bone is inconsistent in the literature. The term metabolic bone disease covers a variety of clinical entities including those outlined below (Fowler, 1986) and in Figures 7.1–7.4.

- *Osteoporosis*: a depletion of osteoid, the organic matrix of bone. In this condition, which can be caused by prolonged cachexia, disuse of bones or senility, the mineralization of remaining osteoid is normal
- *Osteomalacia*: a softening and weakening of bones due to decreased mineralization of osteoid. This is a common consequence of calcium deficiency. There may be increased osteoid deposition at points of stress, in response to weakening of the bone

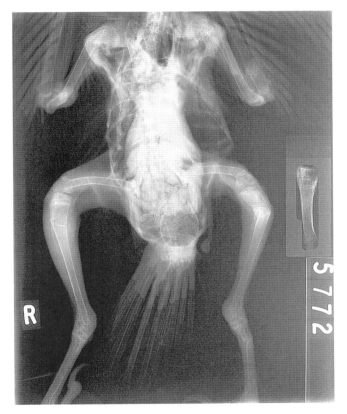

Fig. 7.1 Radiograph of nestling raven (*Corvus corax*), approximately 3 weeks after hatching, with severe nutritional bone disease. This bird was reared in captivity. There are multiple skeletal distortions associated with pathological fractures due to very poor mineralization of bones. This is due to calcium deficiency and develops rapidly in carnivorous birds fed on meat without bone.

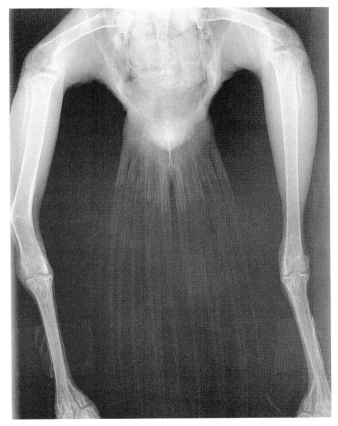

Fig. 7.2 Radiograph of mature raven with deformity of the right tibiotarsus. This bird was reared in captivity. It is thought likely that this deformity arose through pathological fracture during growth.

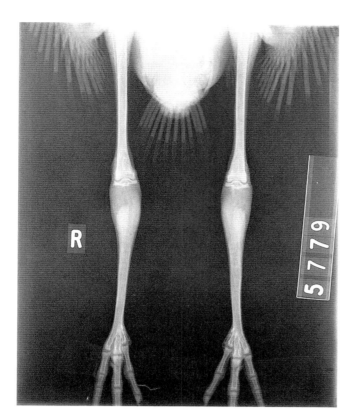

Fig. 7.3 Radiograph of demoiselle crane (*Anthropoides virgo*) chick with rickets. The growth plates are abnormally thick (proximally to distally), even for this very rapidly growing bird, and the line of mineralization of the growth plate is irregular.

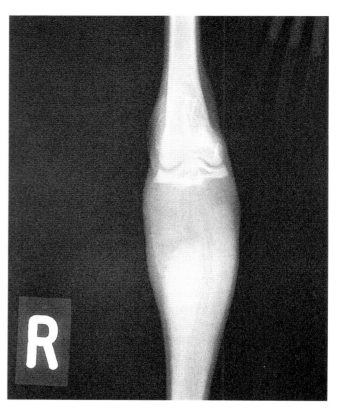

Fig. 7.4 Radiograph of the intertarsal joint of a demoiselle crane chick with rickets (higher magnification of Fig. 7.3). The growth plate is abnormally thick and mineralization of the plate is irregular.

- *Rickets*: a failure of mineralization of osteoid or of the maturing part of the cartilaginous growth plate in young, growing animals. Radiography reveals widening and distortion of the growth plates. Rickets can be caused by a variety of nutrient imbalances, although the term is often used to imply a specific nutrient (usually vitamin D_3) deficiency
- *Fibrous osteodystrophy*: a condition in which there is osteoclastic resorption of osteoid and replacement with highly cellular connective tissue in response to bone weakness. This may occur in response to osteoporosis (due to prolonged protein deficiency) or to osteomalacia (due to prolonged dietary calcium imbalance)
- *Nutritional secondary hyperparathyroidism*: hypocalcemia (typically due to dietary calcium deficiency) stimulates the release of parathyroid hormone and this, in turn, stimulates the mobilization of calcium from bone. This leads to osteomalacia in adults and rickets in young.

Etiology

In birds the most common metabolic bone diseases are those arising as a result of disturbances of mineralization,

and these are usually due to dietary imbalances. Reduced availability of calcium for deposition in bone is, in my experience, most commonly due to straightforward dietary calcium deficiency but can be related to a number of other factors. Calcium may be unavailable because of either dietary deficiency or reduced absorption. Reduced absorption may occur in vitamin D deficiency, if the diet contains excess fat or phytic acid or if the ratio of phosphorus to calcium is high. Vitamin D deficiency may be due to low dietary levels, malabsorption or failure of the processes of synthesis, and the latter may occur in liver or kidney disease or under conditions of inadequate exposure to ultraviolet light. Rickets can also be caused by dietary phosphorus inadequacy, as has been reported in rheas (*Rhea americana*) (Gröne *et al.*, 1995).

Species susceptible

All species of bird are susceptible. Metabolic bone disease has been reported in free-living birds (e.g. where acid rain has led to a reduction in available calcium in the environment) and when vultures select pieces of china or plastic instead of bone to supplement the diets of their chicks. However, considering how readily metabolic bone disease occurs in free-living birds reared in captivity, it is striking how rare it appears to be in the wild.

A key point that is rarely grasped in the literature is that, because of their very rapid growth rates, birds have higher calcium requirements during growth than other taxa. Altricial birds, those reared in nests by their parents, reach their adult size some five times sooner than is typical for mammals of the same adult size (Kirkwood and Webster, 1984). The calcium density of adult birds is very similar to that of mammals (all vertebrates contain about 2.5% calcium on a dry matter basis), so growing altricial birds typically have to deposit about five times more calcium each day than mammals of the same adult size. They therefore require a greater calcium to energy ratio in the diet than other taxa (Kirkwood, 1996) and, when dietary calcium concentration is too low, can develop severe metabolic bone disease in a few days.

The species most at risk of calcium deficiency are those that grow very rapidly (altricial species) and that are reared artificially (i.e. hand-reared) by uninformed or inexperienced persons. It is often seen in young carnivorous birds that have been fed diets that do not contain bone. It is known that some species of birds select calcium-rich foods for their young, and this ability may be widespread in birds. So long as such items are available in their aviaries, parent birds are less likely than humans to provide unbalanced diets. Parent-reared captive birds are therefore at less risk than those reared artificially.

Clinical signs

The clinical signs depend on species, age, duration of predisposing cause (e.g. dietary deficiencies) and other factors. A gradual weakening of the skeleton in an adult, or failure of skeletal mineralization during growth may become apparent suddenly if pathological fracture occurs. Birds with severe metabolic bone disease typically show lameness and reluctance to move but even very severe skeletal abnormalities are sometimes overlooked in nestling birds and a drop in appetite may be the reason why such cases are initially presented. Metabolic bone disease should be suspected in any growing bird that is failing to thrive. There can be distortion of the beak, curves in the line of the sternum and, if pathological fractures are present, gross distortions of the limbs may be apparent.

Post-mortem changes

At post-mortem pathological fractures may be apparent and long bones may be abnormally flexible (in young chicks in which mineralization have failed to proceed) or easily fractured. Distortions of the beak and/or sternum and of other parts of the skeleton may also be apparent. There may also be evidence of poor body condition.

Radiography

Radiography is very valuable in confirming the diagnosis and assessing the severity of the lesions. Considerable demineralization can occur before any changes can be detected on radiography. Thinning of the cortices and a more pronounced trabecular pattern may be apparent in relatively mild cases. Pathological fractures and subperiosteal new bone deposition may be seen.

Hematology/blood biochemistry

In metabolic bone disease alkaline phosphatase levels are likely to be elevated and, in the late stages, there may be hypocalcemia. Hematology and blood biochemistry are not particularly valuable in the diagnosis of metabolic bone disease but are very helpful in the process of determining the cause. From these results, it may be possible to rule out the possibility that other underlying diseases (e.g. of the liver or kidney, see above) may be playing a part in the etiology.

Diet evaluation

Detailed assessment of the daily food intake and the nutrient composition of the diet is an important component of the investigation into pinpointing the cause of the problem. Information should be sought from the owner about the diet. A full list of all the components of the diet is required with good estimates (or precise measures, if they can be obtained) of the quantity of each consumed by the bird each day. From this, using a nutrition database (e.g. Animal Nutritionist, N-Squared Computing, OR) or data tables on the nutrient composition of foods (e.g. Paul and Southgate, 1987), estimates of the daily intake of energy, calcium, phosphorus and other nutrients can be obtained. Dietary calcium deficiency is often easy to demonstrate in this way. Since the vitamin concentrations of foods are more variable and harder to predict, estimates of daily vitamin intakes obtained in this way must be interpreted with more caution.

Treatment

Relatively mild cases of metabolic bone disease caused by dietary imbalances or deficiencies and in which there is no other underlying disease respond well and rapidly if the diet is corrected and it may be possible to correct mild distortions of limb bones by splinting. If the condition is severe, with multiple pathological fractures, euthanasia is indicated.

Prevention

Provision of a diet with an appropriate balance of nutrients is the key to preventing all but the rarest forms of metabolic bone disease (i.e. except those due to underlying liver or kidney disease). However, this is more easily said than done. There are two difficulties. The first is that knowledge of the nutritional requirements of all but a few species is scant (see, for example, Scott, 1986;

Robbins, 1983); secondly, preparation of well-balanced diets for insectivores or fructivores, for example, can be a complex task. Having decided the components on which the diet should be based and roughly the proportions in which they should be offered (both of which should be based on knowledge of the feeding habits of the species in the wild), the nutrient composition of the diet should be either estimated using the method described above or, better still, analyzed. The dietary concentrations at least of calcium, phosphorus and vitamin D_3 can then be compared with appropriate recommendations.

Twisting and bending deformities of the long bones in growing birds

James Kirkwood

Description

Twisting and/or bending deformities of the tibiotarsus and tarsometatarsus (Figs 7.5–7.11) and/or of the wing bones, other than those attributable to metabolic bone disease (see above), can be common during growth of some species of birds reared in captivity (Kirkwood, 1993). These deformities can result in medial or lateral deviations or inward or outward rotations of the lower parts of the limb or limbs. The syndrome is variously known as 'spraddle leg', 'bow-leg syndrome' or 'leg weakness'. The etiology of comparable deformities of wing bones resulting in 'angel wing' or 'slipped wing', in which there is outward rotation of the manus, is probably similar. Some of these distortions of the leg bones can develop quite rapidly (hours to days) and, if severe,

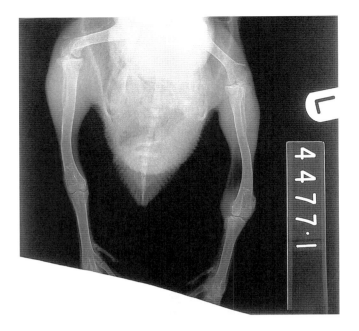

Fig. 7.6 Inward deviation of the distal part of the tibiotarsus in a mallard (*Anas platyrhynchos*). This may have been associated with excessive rates of weight gain during the early stages of growth.

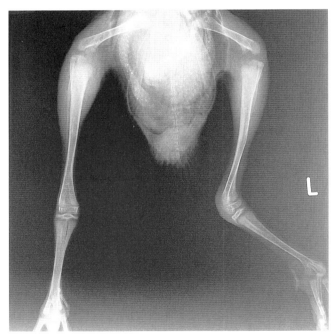

Fig. 7.7 Severe (approximately 90°) rotation of the left tibiotarsus of a Hawaiian goose (*Branta sandvicensis*) during growth.

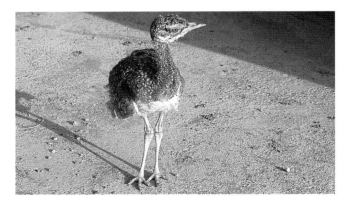

Fig. 7.5 Mild distortion of the left leg of a buff-crested bustard (*Eupodotis ruficrista*). This appears to be due to rotation of the tibiotarsus rather than outward bending of the tarsometatarsus.

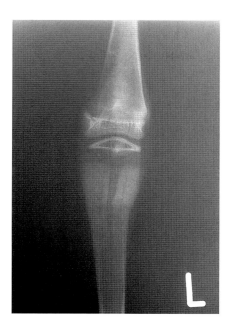

Fig. 7.8 Intertarsal joint of a growing rhea (*Rhea americana*). A lesion is visible in the left side of the recently mineralized part of the proximal tarsometatarsus. This could have been caused by trauma or possibly by a metabolic disturbance to the growth plate a few days earlier. It has caused a slight bend in the proximal tarsometatarsus.

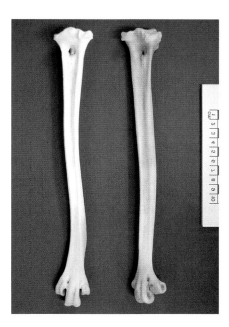

Fig. 7.9 The tarsometatarsus bones of a young rhea, showing twisting and bending deformities.

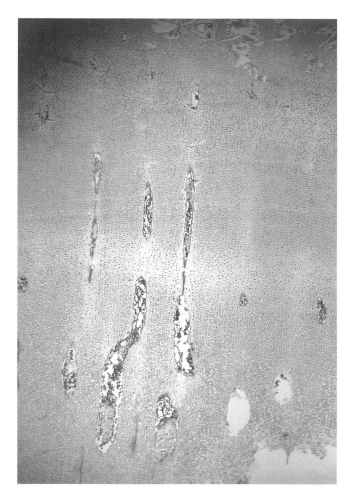

Fig. 7.10 Section through the proximal tarsometatarsus growth plate of a growing rhea. This illustrates the depth of the proliferation (flat cell) zone, into which blood vessels penetrate deeply from the metaphyseal (distal) side.

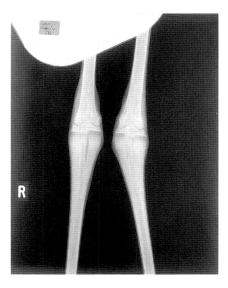

Fig. 7.11 Lateral bending deformity of the proximal tarsometarsus of a growing sarus crane (*Grus antigone*). The proximal end of the tarsometatarsus of this species grows rapidly and it seems likely, therefore, that this deformity was caused by a disturbance to the growth plate (trauma or metabolic), resulting in slowing of the lateral side of the plate a few days before this radiograph was taken.

seriously compromise locomotion and the ability to stand and can thus lead to life-threatening complications. Like metabolic bone disease, these deformities can be common in birds reared in captivity but appear to be very rare in free-living birds (although they have been reported, e.g. by Kreeger and Walser, 1984).

Etiology

Several factors appear to influence the incidence of these diseases. There seem to be some genetic factors, in that the deformities appear to be most common in large, long-legged, precocial species. They occur also, however, in small waterfowl and Galliformes and other species and have been reported at a very high incidence in some strains of domestic broiler fowl reared under some conditions. The incidence appears to be influenced by environmental factors that may facilitate rapid growth, including *ad libitum* access to energy- or protein-rich diets and lack of exercise. A variety of nutrient imbalances or deficiencies have been implicated in the etiology but these deformities appear, in some cases, to arise even when diets are apparently well balanced (Riddell, 1981).

Some, and possibly all, of these distortions arise through disturbance of the growth plate. The rate at which the tip of a growing bone advances is a function of the number of dividing cells in the cartilaginous growth plate, the frequency with which they divide and the size to which they grow prior to being mineralized. Long-legged birds are so because their leg bones grow rapidly, rather than for an extended period, compared with those with shorter legs, and growth rates in excess of 1 mm/d are not uncommon (Kirkwood *et al.*, 1989). Variation in bone growth rates between species is largely due to variation in numbers of dividing cells and thus in the thickness of the cartilaginous growth plate (Kember *et al.*, 1990); thus the price of rapid growth is the necessity for relatively thick (in the plane of growth) growth plates. These highly metabolically active structures are supplied with nutrients by blood vessels that protrude deeply into them from above and below (Wise and Jennings, 1973) and their function is easily disturbed by trauma and other insults. Any disturbance, such as local disruption of blood supply, thus results in a slowing of growth on one side of the plate and will rapidly cause a bend.

Clinical and post-mortem signs

These include rotation or deviation of the lower limbs. On radiography, apart from the distortion, the appearance of the bone and growth plates may be normal. Because of the rapid rate of growth, the growth plate lesion that led to the distortion is soon left 'downstream' of the advancing plate and is likely to be hidden as it becomes mineralized just hours after the problem occurred.

Treatment

If detected at an early stage, changes to management aimed at limiting intake of high-energy or high-protein foods and increasing activity level may halt the progress of limb bone distortions. Severe distortions are difficult to treat and the management of birds with severe distortions is difficult. Approaches to treatment, including derotational osteotomy, have been described by Stewart (1989), Jensen *et al.* (1992), Greenacre *et al.* (1994), Gilsleider (1992).

Prevention

The incidence of these distortions of the limb bones can be minimized by feeding appropriately balanced diets, avoiding *ad libitum* access to high-protein, high-energy diets, encouraging activity in outdoor runs with access to sunlight, and taking steps to minimize the risk of trauma (and sudden strains) to the limbs.

Slipped tendon, angel wing and rolled toes

James Kirkwood

Slipped tendon

Definition

Slipped tendon is the name given to the condition, in which the gastrocnemius tendon, instead of running over the caudal part of the intertarsal joint, becomes displaced laterally or medially. This precludes effective extension of the lower limb. Affected birds are severely lame and unable to walk normally. The condition is sometimes referred to as perosis.

Etiology

In many old textbooks of poultry nutrition, the cause of perosis is stated to be manganese deficiency. However, a variety of other nutrient deficiencies (including deficiencies of vitamins B_6 and B_{12}, biotin, choline and methionine) and other factors may also cause or predispose to the condition. It can occur as a sequel to medial or lateral distortions of the tarsometatarsus (of which the etiology is complex and multifactorial, see above) because, once the tibiotarsus and the tarsometatarsus become out of line, there are considerable sideways forces on the tendon, particularly when the joint is being extended.

Clinical and post-mortem signs

Affected birds are unable to extend the intertarsal joint effectively and cannot therefore walk or stand normally on the affected leg. On palpation, the tendon can be felt to be mobile and, when the intertarsal joint is flexed, tends to slip to the medial or lateral aspect of the joint. It is typically a disease of young, growing, precocial birds but can also occur as a result of trauma in adults of any species.

Treatment and prevention

Treatment is difficult and, although the etiology is not entirely clear, it is thought to be mainly related to dietary deficiencies; provision of a well balanced diet is thus the main approach to prevention. Over the years, several surgical techniques have been proposed to correct slipped tendons, mainly in Anseriformes. One particularly useful technique involves dissecting the displaced tendon from any adhesion and returning it to the trochlear groove. The tendon sheath is then sutured to the lateral periosteum and retinaculum using simple interrupted stitches with fine, absorbable material (Olsen, 1994). An innovative technique to repair slipped tendon in a gosling was recently described. The technique involved the placement of a surgical staple on each condyle of the distal tibiotarsus. The tendon was replaced on the trochlea between the two staples and was held in placed using a sterile cable tie woven over the tendon and through the staples (Brown, 2000). The skin was sutured using simple interrupted stitches. The staples and cable tie were removed 4 d later since the bird was unable to walk freely using the leg and it was found that the tendon was trapped with the cable tie and could not move freely along the trochlea. Despite this, the bird recovered uneventfully and continued growing into adulthood (Brown, 2000). A noninvasive procedure involving placing stitches on the skin to reduce the displaced tendon temporarily may also prove useful.

Angel wing

Definition

Angel wing or slipped wing can be defined as the lateral rotation of the distal wing in young growing birds. The condition seems to affect mainly some species of waterfowl (Kear, 1973; Olsen, 1994) and bustards (Sukhanova, 1992; Naldo et al., 1998).

Etiology

Different factors may contribute to the development of angel wing, including the added weight of the blood-filled quills during rapid growth of the primary feathers, which can appear as early as 2 d of age (Sukhanova, 1992), causing the wing tip to rotate outwards (Kear, 1973; Olsen 1994), excessive heat during the early growing period (White, 1985), high protein intake (Olsen, 1994), manganese deficiency (Olsen, 1994) and genetic factors (Wallach and Boever, 1983).

Treatment and prevention

Angel wing is usually corrected by taping the wing on itself (rather than around the body) in the normal anatomical position for 3–5 d.

Rolled toes

Definition

Rolled toe is the medial rotation of the phalanges of young growing birds. This condition is most often seen in bustards (Naldo et al., 1998) and ratites (Stewart, 1994).

Etiology

It has been suggested that rolled toes develop secondary to perosis (Gewalt and Gewalt, 1966). Riboflavin deficiency and embryo malpositioning are factors that may cause this condition (Anderson, 1983). In ostriches, the incidence of rolled toes appears to be related to genetic abnormalities, incubation problems and unsuitable substrates during the first week of life (Stewart, 1994).

Treatment and prevention

Rolled toes are commonly corrected by applying splints using tape. In larger species, the use of thermoplastic tape, rubber tubing or aluminum-padded splints is more indicated.

Inanition

James Kirkwood

Definition

Starvation is the condition of severe depletion of energy reserves resulting from total cessation of food intake. Chronic reduction of intake to a level below that required to meet energy demands is termed inanition. Unless reversed, both lead to death through exhaustion of energy reserves or secondary complications (metabolic or infectious). At death, all nonstructural lipid may have been utilized. Food supply sets an ultimate limit to population sizes and, since in free-living populations demand often exceeds supply, starvation is a common cause of death in animals of many species and a cause of mass mortality incidents.

In captive animals starvation is rare but inanition may result from misjudgment of requirements (especially of hatchlings) or through overzealous restriction of the food intake of birds kept for falconry to keep them 'keen' to return to the lure.

Etiology

Inanition may be due to: 1) environmental factors that cause a reduction in food intake (e.g. failure of food supply or climatic conditions that prevent foraging) or an increase in energy expenditure (e.g. cold weather); and 2) intrinsic factors that depress appetite or that compromise ability to find, prehend, ingest, digest or metabolize food. Complete cessation of food intake leads to rapid depletion of glycogen stores and switch to fat and protein catabolism. In starvation carbohydrate is derived from protein catabolism by gluconeogenesis. During fasting, weight loss is due to loss of fat, protein and water in such proportions that the energy density of tissue (weight) lost is typically about 2–3 kcal/g (Kirkwood, 1981; Robbins, 1983).

Clinical signs

In the later stages there is weakness and lethargy. Starving birds are palpably thin and may weigh as little as 66% of normal. There may be anemia, leukopenia, raised urea and creatinine, hypoproteinemia and perhaps hypocalcemia. (Fig 7.12)

Post-mortem findings

There may be weak or absent rigor mortis, absence of fat, muscle wasting and the absence of other significant pathology (although there may be evidence of opportunist infections). The digestive tract will often, but not always, be empty.

Treatment and prevention

Except in extreme cases, affected birds are likely to respond well when provided with an adequate supply of good-quality food. In extreme cases, parenteral fluids and nutrition are important in initial treatment. Prevention, in captive animals, obviously depends upon adequate food. Ideally, body condition (weight) should be monitored and, if food is not provided *ad libitum*, then monitoring must be close.

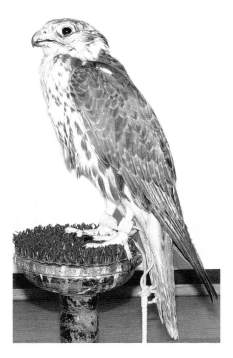

Fig. 7.12 The saker falcon (*Falco cherrug*) depicted on the photograph was presented with a history of reduced appetite of two weeks. The falcon was severely emaciated and dehydrated. On examination the falcon was found to be undergoing a severe candidiasis infection affecting the crop.

ACKNOWLEDGMENTS

Most of my work on avian bone growth was carried out at the Institute of Zoology, London. I am most grateful to the late Mr. Tony Fitzgerald and other staff of the Veterinary Science Department of the Institute of Zoology for taking the radiographs and to Mr. Terry Dennett for the photography.

REFERENCES

Anderson MP (1983) Bone disease in neonatal and juvenile birds. *Proceedings of the American Association of Zoo Veterinarians*, pp. 171–175.

Brown CS (2000) An innovative repair method for slipped tendon. *Proceedings of the Association of Avian Veterinarians*, Portland, pp. 127–131.

Fowler ME (1986) Metabolic bone disease. In: Fowler ME (ed.) *Zoo and Wild Animal Medicine*, 2nd edn, pp. 70–99. WB Saunders, Philadelphia.

Gewalt W, Gewalt I (1966) Über Haltung und Zucht der Grosstrappe (*Otis tarda*). *Zoologische Garten NF* **32**: 265–322.

Gilsleider E (1992) Surgical corrections of ratite musculoskeletal defects. *Proceedings of the American Association of Zoo Veterinarians*, Oakland, pp. 174–175.

Greenacre CB, Aron DL, Ritchie BW (1994) Dome osteotomy for successful correction of angular limb deformities. *Proceedings of the Association of Avian Veterinarians*, Reno.

Gröne A, Swayne DE, Nagode LA (1995) Hypophosphataemic rickets in rheas (*Rhea americana*). *Veterinary Pathology* **32**: 324–327.

Jensen JM, Harvey-Johnson J, Weiner ST (1992) *Husbandry and Medical Management of Ostriches, Emus and Rheas*. Wildlife and Exotic Animal Teleconsultants, College Station, TX.

Kear J (1973) Notes on the nutrition of young waterfowl, with special reference to slipped wing. In: Duplaix-Hall N (ed.) *International Zoo Yearbook* **13**, pp. 97–100, Zoological Society of London, London.

Kember NF, Kirkwood JK, Duignan PJ *et al.* (1990) Comparative cell kinetics of avian growth plates. *Research in Veterinary Science* **49**: 283–288.

Kirkwood JK (1981) Maintenance energy requirements and rate of weight loss during starvation in birds of prey. In: Cooper JE, Greenwood AG (eds) *Recent Advances in the Study of Raptor Diseases*, pp. 153–157. Chiron Publications, Keighley.

Kirkwood JK (1993) Bone diseases in captive and free-living wild birds. Presented at the Meeting of the British Ornithologists' Union, Symposium on Diseases and Parasites of Birds, Cambridge.

Kirkwood JK (1996) Nutrition of captive and free-living wild animals. In: Kelly N, Wills J (eds) *Manual of Companion Animal Nutrition*, pp. 235–243. British Small Animal Veterinary Association, Cheltenham.

Kirkwood JK, Duignan P, Kember NF *et al.* (1989) The growth of the tarsometatarsus bone in birds. *Journal of Zoology* 217: 403–416.

Kirkwood JK, Webster AJF (1984) Energy budget strategies for growth in mammals and birds. *Animal Production* 38: 147–155.

Kreeger TJ, Walser MM (1984) Carpometacarpal deformity in giant Canada geese (*Branta canadensis maxima*). *Journal of Wildlife Diseases* 20: 245–248.

Naldo JL, Bailey TA, Samour JH (1998) Musculoskeletal disorders in bustard pediatric medicine. *Journal of Avian Medicine and Surgery* 12: 82–90.

Olsen JH (1994) Anseriformes. In: Ritchie BW, Harrison GJ, Harrison LR (eds) *Avian Medicine: Principles and Application*, pp. 1237–1275. Wingers Publishing, Lake Worth, FL.

Paul AA, Southgate DAT (1987) *McCance and Widdowson's the Composition of Foods*, 4th edn. HMSO, London.

Riddell C (1981) Skeletal deformities in poultry. *Advances in Veterinary Science and Comparative Medicine* 25: 277–310.

Robbins CT (1983) *Wildlife Feeding and Nutrition*. Academic Press, New York.

Scott ML (1986) *Nutrition of Humans and Selected Animal Species*. John Wiley & Sons, New York.

Stewart J (1994) Ratites. In: Ritchie BW, Harrison GJ, Harrison LR (eds) *Avian Medicine: Principles and Application*, pp. 1284–1326. Wingers Publishing, Lake Worth, FL.

Stewart JS (1989) Husbandry, medical and surgical management of ratites, Part II. *Proceedings of the American Association of Zoo Veterinarians*, Greensboro, pp. 119–122.

Sukhanova OV (1992) Ontogenesis of great bustard chicks reared in captivity. *Bustard Studies* 5: 150–163.

Wallach JD, Boever WJ (1983) Gamebirds, waterfowl and ratites. In: *Diseases of Exotic Animals: Medical and Surgical Management*, pp. 831–888. WB Saunders, Philadelphia.

White DM (1985) A report on the captive breeding of Australian bustards at Serendip Wildlife Research Station. *Bustard Studies* 3: 195–211.

Wise DR, Jennings AR (1973) The development and morphology of the growth plates of two long bones of the turkey. *Research in Veterinary Science* 14: 161–166.

Behavioral osteodystrophy

Nigel H. Harcourt-Brown

There seems little doubt that the cause of osteodystrophy in captive bred birds, such as parrots, is mostly poor nutrition but other factors can play a part in causing bone deformity. There are few studies that review the incidence of juvenile osteodystrophy in a species of bird. In a group of 36 unrelated, hand-reared African gray parrots (*Psittacus erithacus*), whole body radiographs were made as part of their clinical examination. All the birds were fully grown and skeletally mature and were not thought by their owners to be suffering from any orthopedic problems. In this group, 44% were found to have radiographic signs of previous juvenile osteodystrophy that had occurred while growing, presumably during hand-rearing (Harcourt-Brown, 2003). While many of the long bones were variously affected, the tibiotarsus was deformed in all the affected birds. This bone appears to take the majority of the strain when the bird is walking or standing. Bony deformity caused by juvenile osteodystrophy has not been reported in adult, wild-caught, imported African gray parrots.

Rapidly growing bone is relatively weak, easily deformed and has a low resistance to physical stress and strain. The bone has to be strong enough to provide support as well as give purchase for normal muscle function. The growth rate of birds is related to their final bodyweight, metabolic rate and food intake. In wild birds there is a balance between the rate of growth and the length of time that the bird is dependent on its parents. There are many reasons why it is advantageous for a young bird to grow to independence quickly but the rate is balanced by the risk to the parents (Starck and Ricklefs, 1998). Altricial nestlings (such as parrots) are totally dependent on their parents for food and protection during growth and are confined to a nest; however, they grow rapidly. This rapid growth is made possible by allowing the bone to remain weak; deformity is prevented by confining the bird to a small nest space where its behavior prevents it from moving around excessively. Except when being fed, these babies lie in an intertwined, self supporting huddle (Fig. 7.13).

Carrier and Leon (1990) examined the bone growth pattern of the California gull (*Larus californicus*). Newly hatched gulls can run and swim starting within the first 2 d after hatching. However they do not fly until they are at least 42 d old. The strength of the long bones was assessed by breaking strain; this showed that the leg bones were of similar relative strength to the adult

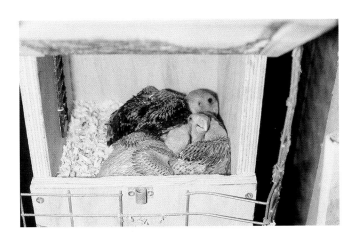

Fig. 7.13 In a nest of parrots (*Pionus fuscus*) the young birds lie in a self-supporting huddle. There are many advantages to this behavior; aiding normal bone growth is one.

birds' throughout the whole period of growth because of increased thickness; the wing bones were relatively less developed and weak throughout the whole growth period. When the birds reached maximum body mass and started to exercise their wings, the strength of the wing bones increased rapidly to match that of the adult bird. Based on several parameters, Carrier and Leon (1990) suggested that there was a trade-off between development and energy requirements: early development of the wing requires an investment of energy that could be used 'better' for other functions more critical to development.

In a typical parrot (e.g. dusky parrot, *Pionus fuscus*), Harcourt-Brown (2003) showed that in 'normal' circumstances parrots do not become ambulant until skeletal maturity is completed and until the majority of the feathers have stopped growing, become pneumatized and therefore weigh the least. In the nest these birds moved relatively very little, lying in an intertwined huddle that supported their relatively weak, growing skeleton (Fig. 7.13). At 50 d old, by which time their bones had stopped growing, they would climb to the nest entrance, retreating if scared. From day 51 they would flap their wings vigorously inside the nest. At 53 d old the parrots emerged from the nest. Using measurements made from radiographs, the bones in the legs appeared to be no thicker (therefore stronger) than the wings. During the course of this study a behavioral reflex was noted: growing birds removed from the nest and placed singly on a flat surface would stand up and walk about until restrained (Fig. 7.14). As soon as they were placed back with their siblings they rejoined the huddle and lay down. This behavioral reflex has great advantages in a large nest cavity. A baby bird that has been separated from its siblings will walk around until it bumps into

them and then resumes its place in the pile, which provides warmth, protection and skeletal support as well as an 'even chance' at feeding time. The huddling/walking reflex is shared by other groups of altricial birds. Zoologists have observed it in raptors (Newton, 1978) and small passerines, such as reed warblers (*Acrocephalus scirpaceus*) (A. Radford, personal communication).

Many parrots are now hand-reared and as a result of this reflex are often allowed and even encouraged to move around in this abnormal manner. It was postulated that this abnormal increase in activity and the lack of support from siblings might predispose these hand-reared birds to develop pathological bony deformity. As the birds stand and walk, great strain is placed on the tibiotarsus, causing this bone to deform first. If the birds are fed a diet that is deficient in calcium and vitamin D_3, poor mineralization of the skeleton will increase the incidence as well as the severity of these skeletal abnormalities.

It seems a sensible precaution when hand-rearing young birds of any species to attempt to mimic their behavior in the wild while under the care of their parents (Figs 7.15 and 7.16). Ideally birds that grow in nests should be provided with a nest of the same dimensions. In one instance, white-cheeked touracoes (*Turaco leucotis*) were being hand-reared on an apparently well balanced diet and were still being affected with bony deformity while growing. With no dietary change, this was prevented in the next clutch by keeping the birds in a touraco nest during the period of growth; they moved less and appeared to be better supported (J. Wayne, personal communication). Many long-legged birds, such as cranes (Gruidae) and flamingoes (Phoenicopteridae) are relatively overactive when they lack parental care and guidance (Fig. 7.17). This encourages rotational deformity of the long bones as well as bending deformities. Similar

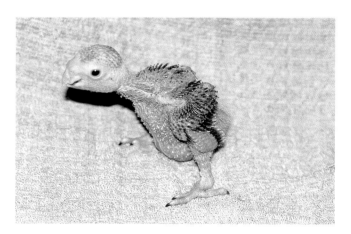

Fig. 7.14 A half grown parent-reared parrot (*Pionus senilis*) isolated from its siblings will, without encouragement, stand up and walk around. Its heavy visceral compartment makes it necessary for it to splay out its legs, placing abnormal strains on the tibiotarsus and femur; the potential for bending and rotational deformity is obvious.

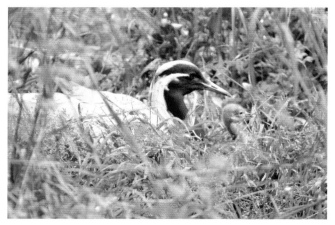

Fig. 7.15 Demoiselle cranes (*Anthropoides virgo*) spend time protecting and foraging on behalf of their offspring. The legs of this young bird grow very rapidly. The parents find food, which they take to the young bird. If they call it to eat the chicks arrives in a slow and deliberate manner; alarm calls elicit a crouching response. (Courtesy of S. Parkes).

often lined with absorbent paper such as kitchen roll; on top of plastic this can make a slippery surface. The birds are usually removed from their box for feeding, which again is a hygiene measure. They often have to be restrained manually while they are being fed, which can force the legs into abnormal positions. As the birds grow they try to get out of their boxes and will frequently use their wings to climb. They rest on their sternum and in small boxes they lie with their wings hanging over the side. When the birds are half to two-thirds grown they are often placed, as a group, in a large box that allows them to walk about. Young pet parrots are often sold to their new owners before their feathers are fully grown and while they are still being hand-fed. From an early age the young birds respond to feeding, and the feeder, enthusiastically. It is very common for half-grown baby birds to be allowed to run around following the feeding-spoon or syringe.

Hand rearing encourages abnormal physical behavior in growing parrots, and other birds, that will exacerbate the effects of a deficient diet and encourage the appearance of skeletal deformity. It is possible that in some birds overexercise is a major rather than a minor causative factor of their bone deformity.

Limiting the movement of birds during hand-rearing can be accomplished by mimicking natural nesting conditions as closely as possible: a limited nest area with high solid sides and a soft floor that molds to the shape of the body (e.g. wood shavings covered with kitchen roll); the presence of siblings, other similar sized parrots, or adequate padding to replace sibling support for single birds; subdued lighting between feeds; and considerable care taken when moving and feeding the young birds. Many breeders already do this with their birds.

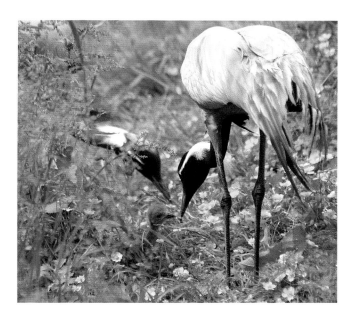

Fig. 7.16 When cranes are not foraging they sit in a protective manner and the baby sits with them, allowing the young bird to rest. It has been shown in lambs that the growth of bones takes place during the rest period (Noonan *et al.*, 2004); it is likely that the same occurs in birds, making rest for rapidly growing bones very important. (Courtesy of Mr. J. Chitty).

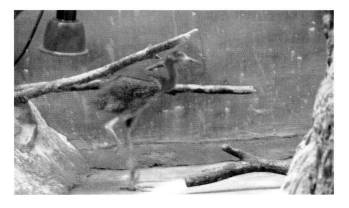

Fig. 7.17 The photograph shows a crane chick (*Grus japonensis*) being artificially reared. The bird is far more active than parent-reared chicks, spending more time walking and running unimpeded on a concrete surface. Alarm causes increased and panicky movements. (Courtesy of Mr. J. Chitty).

changes have been reported in poultry where *ad libitum* feeding and overactivity caused by excessive photoperiod (23 h light) while growing increase the incidence of bony abnormalities, including rotational deformity; this subject was reviewed by Whitehead (1992).

For hand-rearing, the age at which the young bird is removed from the parent's care varies but it is possible to hand-rear from hatching. Younger parrots are easier to train to hand feeding than older ones are. It is very difficult to keep the birds clean. To combat this problem the growing birds are kept in plastic boxes, which are of various sizes but usually relatively large. The box is

REFERENCES

Carrier D, Leon LR (1990) Skeletal growth and function in the California gull (*Larus californicus*). *Journal of the Zoological Society of London* **222**: 375–389.

Harcourt-Brown NH (2003) The incidence of juvenile osteodystrophy in hand-reared grey parrots (*Psittacus e. erithacus*). *Veterinary Record* **152**: 438–439.

Newton I (1978) Feeding and development of sparrowhawk *Accipiter nisus* nestlings. *Journal of the Zoological Society of London* **184**: 465–487.

Noonan KJ, Farnum CE, Leiferman EM *et al.* (2004) Growing pains: are they due to increased growth during recumbency as documented in a lamb model? *Journal of Pediatric Orthopaedics* **24**: 726–731.

Starck JM, Ricklefs RE (1998) *Avian Growth and Development*. Oxford University Press, New York.

Whitehead CC (1992) *Bone Biology and Skeletal Disorders in Poultry*. Carfax Publishing, Abingdon.

FURTHER READING

Classen HL, Riddell C (1989) Photoperiodic effects on performance and leg abnormalities in broiler chickens. *Poultry Science* **68**: 873–879.

Harcourt-Brown NH (2004) Development of the skeleton and feathers of dusky parrots (*Pionus fuscus*) in relation to their behaviour. *Veterinary Record* **154**: 42–48.

Huff WE (1980) Evaluation of tibial dyschondroplasia during aflatoxicosis and feed restriction in young broiler chickens. *Poultry Science* **59**: 991–995.

Kestin SC, Su G, Sorensen P (1999) Different commercial broiler crosses have different susceptibilities to leg weakness. *Poultry Science* **78**: 1085–1090.

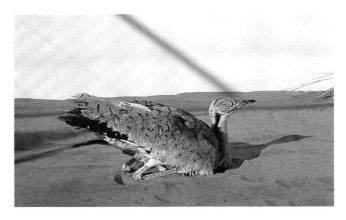

Fig. 7.18 Recumbent houbara bustard (*Chlamydotis undulata*) with capture-related paresis.

Capture paresia

Thomas A. Bailey

This section is concerned with capture paresia, which is an important cause of mortality of birds during capture and translocation episodes (Spraker *et al.*, 1987). Although a similar condition is a well recognized complication in the capture of wild ungulates (Harthoorn and Young, 1974; Harthoorn, 1976; Wallace *et al.*, 1987; Robinson *et al.*, 1988; Spraker, 1993), it has received less attention in birds.

It is known by a spectrum of names such as muscular dystrophy, capture disease, capture myopathy, degenerative polymyopathy, overstraining disease, white muscle disease, leg paralysis, muscle necrosis, idiopathic muscle necrosis, exertional rhabdomyolysis, stress myopathy, transit myopathy, diffuse muscular degeneration and white muscle stress syndrome (Spraker, 1993).

Definition

Paresis is defined by Blood and Studdert (1988) as 'slight or incomplete paralysis, and includes animals that can make purposeful attempts to rise without being able to do so, those that are able to rise with assistance, those that are able to rise and walk with major difficulty including frequent falling, and those able to stand and walk without assistance, but with slight errors'.

Species affected

Capture paresia and other similar degenerative myopathies have been described in the following species:

- Greater flamingoes (*Phoenicopterus ruber roseus*) and lesser flamingoes (*Phoeniconaias minor*) (Young, 1967)
- Secretary birds (*Sagittarius serpentarius*) (Heerden, 1977)
- Ostriches (*Struthio camelus*), emus (*Dromaius novaehollandiae*) and rheas (*Rhea americana*) (Heerden, 1977; Rae, 1992; Stewart, 1994; Tully *et al.*, 1996)
- Bar-tailed godwits (*Limosa lapponica*) (Minton, 1980)
- Sandhill cranes (*Grus canadensis*) (Windingstad *et al.*, 1983; Carpenter *et al.*, 1991)
- Whooping cranes (*Grus americana*) (Gainer, 1988)
- Canada geese (*Branta canadensis*) (Chalmers and Barrett, 1982)

- Free-living turkeys (*Meleagris gallopavo*) (Atkinson and Forrester, 1987; Spraker *et al.*, 1987; Jessup, 1993)
- East African crowned cranes (*Balearica regulorum gibbericeps*) (Brannian *et al.*, 1981)
- Houbara (*Chlamydotis undulata macqueenii*), kori (*Ardeotis kori*) and rufous-crested bustards (*Eupodotis ruficrista*, Fig. 7.18) (Bailey *et al.*, 1996a, 1996b).
- Domestic turkey (*Meleagris gallopavo*) (Cardona *et al.*, 1992).

Pathogenesis

The exact pathogenesis of capture paresia is not clear but it involves anaerobic metabolism during intense muscular activity (Harthoorn, 1976; Wallace *et al.*, 1987). Lactic acid produced in muscle causes local and systemic acidosis, resulting in the lesions and clinical signs of paresis (Harthoorn, 1976; Chalmers and Barrett, 1982). Low pH at the tissue level results in increased permeability of cell membranes and cell lysis, releasing intracellular enzymes including creatine kinase (CK), lactate dehydrogenase (LDH) and aspartate aminotransferase (AST) into the blood (Harthoorn, 1975; Chalmers and Barrett, 1982). Elevated concentrations of CK and AST in serum or plasma thus reflect damage to skeletal and cardiac muscle. Elevation of serum CK concentration appears to be the most sensitive and specific index of muscle damage in both mammals (Chalmers and Barrett, 1982) and birds (Franson, 1982; Lumeij, 1988a, 1988b, 1993; Cardona *et al.*, 1992). It should be noted that not all elevations in plasma CK activities are an indication of disease: for example, it is known that CK levels dramatically increase in healthy bustards that are handled (Bailey *et al.*, 1997).

Clinical signs and history

A number of factors are considered to predispose birds to capture paresia, including:

- Strenuous pursuit during capture operations
- Prolonged handling
- Translocation
- Poor transport conditions
- Possible vitamin E and selenium deficiencies
- Intercurrent disease
- Hot weather
- Cramping of the limbs.

The clinical signs of capture paresia include:

- Depression
- Limb paresis or paralysis
- Hock-sitting
- Lateral or sternal recumbency with reluctance to rise or move
- Death during or after capture, handling or translocation.

Acute death occurs in many cases and is thought to be caused by myocardial necrosis and trauma, while necrosis of the muscles of the thighs and flank causes limb paralysis (Young, 1967). The generally excitable disposition of ratites predisposes these animals to myopathy, especially in poorly managed facilities. Dietary factors are important when investigating outbreaks of myopathy. Myopathy in pelicans (*Pelicanus occidentalis*) has been reported following vitamin E deficiency caused by feeding rancid food (Shivaprasad *et al.*, 2002). Monensin toxicity has been linked to degenerative myopathy in ostriches (Baird *et al.*, 1997).

Differential diagnosis

Other causes of hind-limb paresis or paralysis must be considered and ruled out in the differential diagnosis of this condition. A full list of the possible causes of paresia and paralysis in birds is presented in Table 7.1.

Diagnosis

Diagnosis of capture paresia is based on consideration of the history, clinical signs and detection of elevated plasma levels of CK, AST and LDH.

Post-mortem changes

The following macroscopic findings have been observed in birds examined post-mortem that died from capture paresia (Young, 1967; Windingstad *et al.*, 1983; Spraker *et al.*, 1987; Carpenter *et al.*, 1991; Cardona *et al.*, 1992; Rae, 1992):

- Small to large white or pale foci and streaks on the myocardium, muscles of the hindlimbs and the pectoral muscles
- Ruptured muscles

TABLE 7.1 Differential diagnosis of the causes of paresia and paralysis in birds	
History	**Possible cause**
Traumatic	Vertebral fractures or luxations
	Multiple fractures
	Pelvic fractures
	Dislocations or sprains
Infectious	Neuritis (peripheral nerve)
	Encephalitis or encephalomyelitis
	Intervertebral abscess
	Septicemia with spinal infection
	Nephritis
	Viral infections including paramyxovirus group 3, reovirus, papovirus, Pacheco's virus
	Bacterial infection including *Chlamydia, Listeria, Yersinia, Salmonella, Streptococcus*
	Fungal infection, including aspergillosis, involving the central nervous system
Metabolic/nutritional	Suspected vitamin E/selenium deficiency
	Multiple fractures secondary to metabolic bone disease
Reproductive	Obturator paralysis from difficult delivery
	Egg binding
	Broken leg from calcium deficiency
	Ectopic egg
Neoplastic	Renal adenocarcinoma
	Fibrosarcoma
	Other neoplasia or space-occupying lesion
Poisons	Botulism
	Lead toxicosis
	Furazolidone and ionophore toxicity
Miscellaneous	Cloacal lithiasis

- Hemorrhages in the musculature of the thighs and flank
- Petechiae in the myocardium.

Histopathology is important in diagnosing this condition because macroscopically visible lesions may not always be detected on post-mortem examination (Gainer, 1988). Microscopically the main changes include necrosis of myocardial and skeletal muscle. Signs of renal failure may also be detected. The microscopic changes associated with this condition are fully described elsewhere (Young, 1967; Windingstad *et al.*, 1983; Spraker *et al.*, 1987; Carpenter *et al.*, 1991; Rae, 1992).

Treatment

The primary goal of treatment is the control of shock and hyperthermia (Fig. 7.19):

- Intravenous and oral sodium bicarbonate to correct acidosis
- Fluid therapy to restore blood pressure and volume
- Parenteral vitamin E and selenium and multiple vitamins
- Corticosteroids
- Cooling the bird if it is hyperthermic
- Possible cardiac and respiratory stimulants.

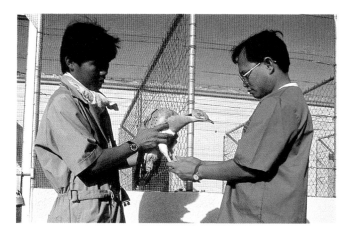

Fig. 7.19 Supportive therapy, including physiotherapy, is an important consideration in the management of birds with capture-related paresia.

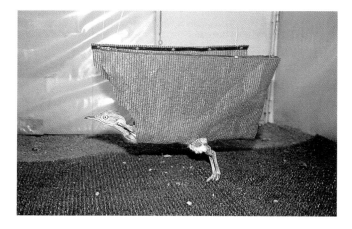

Fig. 7.20 Slings can be made to support birds with paresia.

Attempts have been made to support affected birds in slings (Fig. 7.20) and to provide physiotherapy in the form of massage and placing limbs in lukewarm water. Mild cases of paresia may recover, but the prognosis is poor for severe cases.

Prevention

Capture myopathy is difficult to treat and every effort should be made to prevent the problem. Recommendations for minimizing the problem include:

- Supplemental vitamin E and selenium prior to episodes of capture, handling and/or translocation (Mushi *et al.*, 1998)
- Capturing birds on days that have acceptable environmental conditions
- Keeping handling times and struggling to a minimum and avoiding hyperthermia

- Using proven capture techniques for the species to be caught
- Being aware that certain species, such as free-living turkeys, appear to be more susceptible to this condition than others (Spraker *et al.*, 1987)
- Transporting birds in well ventilated containers
- Conditioning and training groups of animals, which can reduce the mortality associated with older methods of capture that involve them in exertion.

REFERENCES

Atkinson CT, Forrester DJ (1987) Myopathy associated with megaloschizonts of *Haemoproteus meleagridis* in a wild turkey from Florida. *Journal of Wildlife Diseases* **23**: 495–498.

Bailey TA, Samour JH, Naldo J et al. (1996a) Causes of morbidity in bustards in the United Arab Emirates. *Avian Diseases* **40**: 121–129.

Bailey TA, Nicholls PK, Samour JH et al. (1996b) Post-mortem findings of bustards in the United Arab Emirates. *Avian Diseases* **40**: 296–305.

Bailey TA, Wernery U, Naldo J, Samour JH (1997) Concentrations of creatine kinase and lactate dehydrogenase in captive houbara bustards (*Chlamydotis undulata macqueenii*) following capture. *Comparative Haematology International* **7**: 113.

Baird GJ, Caldow GL, Peek IS, Grant DA (1997) Monensin toxicity in a flock of ostriches. *Veterinary Record* **140**: 624–626.

Blood DC, Studdert VP (1988) *Baillière's Comprehensive Veterinary Dictionary*. Baillière Tindall, London.

Brannian RE, Graham DL, Creswell J (1981) Restraint associated myopathy in East African crowned cranes. *Proceedings of the American Association of Zoo Veterinarians*, Seattle, pp. 21–23.

Cardona CJ, Bickford AA, Galey FD et al. (1992) A syndrome in commercial turkeys in California and Oregon characterized by rearlimb necrotizing myopathy. *Avian Diseases* **36**: 1092–1101.

Carpenter JW, Thomas NJ, Reeves S (1991) Capture myopathy in an endangered sandhill crane (*Grus canadensis pulla*). *Journal of Zoo and Wildlife Medicine* **22**: 488–493.

Chalmers GA, Barrett MW (1982) Capture myopathy. In: Hoff GL, Davis JW (eds) *Non-infectious Diseases of Wildlife*, pp. 84–89. Iowa State University Press, Ames, IA.

Franson JC (1982) Enzyme activities in plasma, liver, and kidney of black ducks and mallards. *Journal of Wildlife Diseases* **18**: 481–485.

Gainer RS (1988) Capture mortality of a young whooping crane (*Grus americanus*). *Proceedings of the American Association of Zoo Veterinarians and American Association of Wildlife Veterinarians*, Toronto, p. 57.

Harthoorn AM (1975) Operative factors in capture myopathy. *Proceedings of the World Veterinary Congress*, Thessalonika.

Harthoorn AM (1976) *The Chemical Capture of Animals*, pp. 103–106. Baillière Tindall, London.

Harthoorn AM, Young E (1974) A relationship between acid–base balance and the acute phase of capture myopathy (so-called over-straining disease) in zebra (*Equus burchelli*) and an apparent therapy. *Veterinary Record* **95**: 337–342.

Heerden JV (1977) Leg paralysis in birds. *Ostrich* **48**: 118–119.

Jessup DA (1993) Translocation of wildlife. In: Fowler ME (ed.) *Zoo and Wild Animal Medicine Current Therapy* 3, p. 496. WB Saunders, Philadelphia.

Lumeij JT (1988a) Enzyme activities in tissues and elimination half-lives of homologous muscle and liver enzymes in the racing pigeon (*Columba livia domestica*). *Avian Pathology* **17**: 851–864.

Lumeij JT (1988b) Changes in plasma chemistry after drug-induced liver disease or muscle necrosis in racing pigeons (*Columba livia domestica*). *Avian Pathology* **17**: 865–874.

Lumeij JT (1993) Avian plasma chemistry in health and disease. *Proceedings of the European Association of Avian Veterinarians*, Utrecht, pp. 558–566.

Minton CDT (1980) Occurrence of 'cramp' in a catch of bar-tailed godwits (*Limosa lapponica*). *Wader Study Group Bulletin* **28**: 15–16.

Mushi EZ, Isa JEW, Chabo RG, Binta MG (1998) Selenium-vitamin E responsive myopathy in farmed ostriches (*Struthio camelus*) in Botswana. *Avian Pathology* **27**: 326–328.

Rae M (1992) Degenerative myopathy in ratites. *Proceedings of the Association of Avian Veterinarians*, New Orleans, pp. 328–335.

Robinson WF, Wyburn RS, Grandage J (1988) The skeletal system. In: Robinson WF, Huxtable CRR (eds) *Clinicopathologic Principles for Veterinary Medicine*, pp. 383–384. Cambridge University Press, Cambridge.

Shivaprasad HL, Crespo R, Puschner B *et al.* (2002) Myopathy in brown pelicans (*Pelicanus occidentalis*) associated with rancid feed. *Veterinary Record* **150**: 307–311.

Spraker TR (1993) Stress and capture myopathy in artiodactylids. In: Fowler ME (ed.) *Zoo and Wild Animal Medicine Current Therapy 3*, pp. 481–489. WB Saunders, Philadelphia.

Spraker TR, Adrian WJ, Lance WR (1987) Capture myopathy in wild turkeys (*Meleagris gallopavo*) following trapping, handling and transportation in Colorado. *Journal of Wildlife Diseases* **23**: 447–453.

Stewart J (1994) Ratites. In: Ritchie BW, Harrison GJ, Harrison LR (eds) *Avian Medicine: Principles and Application*, pp. 1307–1308. Wingers Publishing, Lake Worth, FL.

Tully TN, Hodgin C, Morris M *et al.* (1996) Exertional myopathy in an emu (*Dromaius novaehollandiae*). *Journal of Avian Medicine and Surgery* **10**: 96–100.

Wallace RS, Bush M, Montali RJ (1987) Deaths from exertional myopathy at the National Zoological Park from 1975 to 1985. *Journal of Wildlife Diseases* **23**: 454–462.

Windingstad RM, Hurley SS, Sileo L (1983) Capture myopathy in a free-flying greater sandhill crane (*Grus canadensis tabida*) from Wisconsin. *Journal of Wildlife Diseases* **19**: 289–290.

Young E (1967) Leg paralysis in the greater flamingo and lesser flamingo. *International Zoo Yearbook* **7**: 226–227.

Toxicology

Jaime Samour

Toxicology is the area of medical sciences that studies the actions of chemical compounds on biological systems. These compounds are normally referred to as toxicants or toxic agents, poisons and toxins. The term toxin should be used only and exclusively to define a protein produced by a biological organism such as a higher plant, certain animals and pathogenic bacteria that is toxic to other living organisms. Toxicosis, poisoning and intoxication relate to the disease caused by the action of the chemical compound. Toxic agents may be exogenous or endogenous. Exogenous agents are those originating from outside the body. These include: 1) man-made or synthetic compounds, such as pesticides, and 2) naturally occurring or natural compounds, such as those found in toxic plants and fungi. Endogenous toxic agents are those originating from within the body and include mainly toxins produced by pathogenic bacteria or fungi.

Captive birds are particularly susceptible to various toxicoses because of their inquisitive nature. Very commonly pet birds are allowed to fly freely within the house and can easily have access to household goods such as detergents, pesticides, disinfectants, toxic plants and inhalant agents that could be harmful to them. In bird gardens, zoological collections, parks and farms, birds can be exposed to building materials, toxic plants or items thrown by members of the public that could also be detrimental to their health. Free-living birds very frequently come into contact with toxic agents such as pesticides, fertilizers and herbicides in farm and cultivated lands, lead from shotgun pellets or fishing weights in ponds, lakes and rivers and a myriad of potentially harmful compounds in industrial areas, construction sites and rubbish dumps.

Avian toxicology is a vast area and to include a full description of all agents potentially toxic to birds is beyond the scope of this book. This section deals with the most common toxicoses reported by clinicians in avian species. For further information on avian toxicology the reader is referred to Petrak, 1982; Cooper, 1985; Harrison, 1986; Osweiler, 1986; Rosskopf and Woerpel, 1986; Humphreys, 1988; LaBonde, 1991, 1996a; Lumeij *et al.*, 1993; Porter, 1993; Dumonceaux and Harrison, 1994; Bauck and LaBonde, 1997; Lang, 1997.

Ammonium chloride toxicosis in Falconiformes

Ammonium chloride (NH_4Cl) or ammonium muriate is an inorganic salt, commercially available as hygroscopic colorless crystals or as a white crystalline powder with a cool saline taste. The dose producing a 50% probability of death (LD_{50}) in the rat is 1650 mg/kg. Its application in both human and veterinary medicine is primarily for acidifying the urine and increasing the rate of urine flow but it is also widely used as a secretory expectorant and cilia augmentor. This is probably achieved by directly or indirectly increasing the beat frequencies of the cilia in the respiratory tract, but the exact mode of action or the mechanism involved is poorly understood (Brander *et al.*, 1991).

Following ingestion in domestic animals and humans, ammonium chloride is metabolized in the liver and converted into urea and hydrochloric acid, resulting in severe acidosis. Excretion takes place via the urinary pathway (Gilman *et al.*, 1985). Birds are uricotelic, excreting the end product of nitrogen metabolism as uric acid. This is synthesized in the liver and excreted by glomerular filtration but mainly by tubular secretion (King and McLelland, 1984). Thus in mammals, and presumably in birds, when a high dose of ammonium chloride is administered orally or in the presence of liver insufficiency, acute hyperammonemia is experienced. As a result, the levels of NH_3 are too high for the liver detoxifying capacity, acting subsequently as a cytotoxic agent, mainly in the brain. Sometimes, depending on the dose ingested and the digestive process, carbamates appear as toxic metabolites, acting as reversible inhibitors of cholinesterase (Forth *et al.*, 1983).

In the countries around the Persian Gulf, ammonium chloride is best known as *schnather*, an Arabic word widely used by falconers and by people trading in traditional Arab medicine, who normally sell it in the form of crystals.

During the initial phase of the hunting period (November), a considerable number of falconers in the Gulf routinely administer ammonium chloride to the falcons under their charge with the aim of improving their hunting ability. There are other falconers who will administer ammonium chloride to a particular bird that failed to kill or did not show interest in its prey during the first hunting trip. The method normally requires two handlers, one for casting the falcon and the second for forcing a small (10–25 mm diameter) crystal of ammonium chloride down into the crop of the immobilized bird. As an alternative, it is also a common practice to wrap several small crystals of ammonium chloride in a piece of cotton cloth, forming a small sac and tied at one end with a piece of thin string about 25 cm long. When the small sac is force-fed, the other end of the string is left protruding from the mouth so it can be used to retrieve the sac after a few minutes. The theory behind this procedure is that the chemical action of ammonium chloride will remove the 'fat deposits within the stomach', resulting in a hungrier bird and one therefore more interested in hunting.

Clinical signs

Two or three minutes after the administration of the ammonium chloride the falcon usually vomits violently, bringing up large quantities of a thick, green-yellow mucus (Fig. 7.21), sometime with whitish strands and the

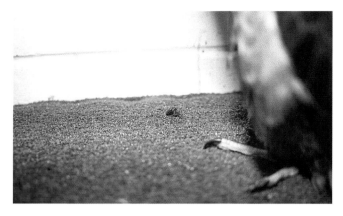

Fig. 7.22 The same bird as in Fig. 7.21. The bird has cast the 'bag' used to wrap the ammonium chloride crystals. Falcons very often die when large crystals are broken down into smaller fragments and the bird fails to vomit all the ammonium chloride ingested.

partially dissolved crystal. Nevertheless, falconers are very familiar with the toxic effects of this substance and know quite well, probably from previous painful experience, that if the bird is not able to vomit the ingested crystal within 5–10 min it will undoubtedly die. In this respect, I have witnessed the death of several individuals within 15 min following ingestion. Sometimes a large ingested crystal breaks down into smaller fragments within the crop (Fig. 7.22), resulting only in the partial vomition of the ammonium chloride crystal originally swallowed, an event that usually goes unnoticed by the falconer. In this case, the bird soon becomes lethargic and anorexic, loses weight rapidly and begins passing characteristic, dark metallic-green mutes. During the terminal phase, the bird is unable to stand on its block, remaining on the floor most of the time, and the breathing becomes dyspneic. This is followed by a short period, usually 4–8 h, characterized by fits and opisthotonos followed by death. The clinical signs develop over 3–7 d, depending on the total amount of ammonium chloride ingested, although there have been occasions in which the bird died up to 2 weeks later.

Pathological changes

Gross pathological changes observed at post-mortem examinations of affected birds included generalized congestion of the mucosa and the presence of dark, metallic-green mucus along the entire digestive tract. The liver was friable and of a uniform dark, metallic-green color. The kidneys showed mild perirenal edema and mild to severe cortical and medullary congestion. Histopathological findings were nonspecific. The livers showed moderate to severe congestion and golden-brown pigment (possibly hemosiderin) within Kupffer's cells and macrophages. Other lesions were variable.

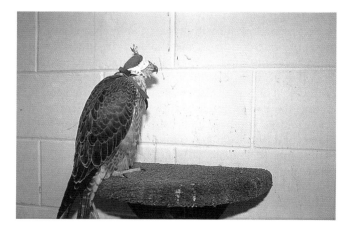

Fig. 7.21 Ammonium chloride toxicosis in a peregrine falcon (*Falco peregrinus*). Three minutes after force-feeding the toxic agent, the bird started vomiting. Note the wall smeared with green mucus.

In some birds these included perivascular cuffing by plasma cells and other mononuclears. Subcapsular, well scattered, small foci of early coagulative necrosis and vacuolation of the hepatocyte cytoplasm were also found. Sometimes the necrosis was associated with mononuclear cell infiltration. It is possible that some of these lesions were secondary to bumblefoot. The kidneys showed mild to severe tubular nephrosis. Many tubules were dilated and/or partially occluded with acidophilic or slightly basophilic amorphous material, probably due to urate nephrosis.

Physiology and pathological considerations

The biochemical action of ammonium chloride as an acidifier may be responsible for the stimulation of appetite at the central nervous system level. In domesticated animals, it is known that groups of neurons in the lateral hypothalamus promote hunger and that noradrenergic and cholinergic transmitter systems are also implicated in the stimulation of appetite (Klemm, 1984). Probably and perhaps more correctly, ammonium chloride may be responsible for a chronic chemical irritation of the hunger terminals in the upper digestive tract. In Falconiformes, the taste buds are located on the base of the tongue. There are 30–40 axons connecting each taste bud to the central nervous system through the glossopharyngeal nerve (King and McLelland, 1984). The autonomic terminals in the crop, esophagus and gizzard may also be stimulated by this chemical action, sending constant messages of hunger to the hypothalamus.

Falconers often report that, following administration of ammonium chloride, the falcon looks more alert during hunting and is hungry all the time. It is difficult to assess the validity of this statement but, despite its apparently favorable effect, ammonium chloride remains a highly toxic agent responsible for the death of a significant number of falcons.

ACKNOWLEDGMENT

I am grateful to the *Veterinary Record* for allowing me to reproduce part of Samour JH, Bailey TA, Keymer IF (1995) Use of ammonium chloride in falconry in the Middle East. *Veterinary Record* **137**: 269–270.

Lead toxicosis

Lead toxicosis or plumbism is the most common heavy metal toxicity in free-living and captive birds and is perhaps the most frequent form of intoxication in avian species worldwide. Birds can ingest lead deliberately, as in the case of waterfowl ingesting shotgun pellets as grit, or accidentally, as in the case of a captive bird of prey ingesting hidden shotgun pellets from a bird or

TABLE 7.2 Sources and clinical signs related to lead toxicosis

Source	Clinical signs
Lead-based paint, lead-free paint with leaded drying agents, fishing weights, shotgun pellets, batteries, linoleum, plaster, masonry putty, petrol fumes, lead-coated household and industrial items	General signs: Weakness, weight loss, lethargy, anorexia Hematological signs: basophilic stippling, red blood cell intracytoplasmic vacuolization Renal signs: Polyuria, hematuria, hemoglobinuria Gastrointestinal signs: diarrhea, dark feces, ileus of upper digestive tract, regurgitation Neurological signs: ataxia, head tremors, circling, head tilt, dropped wings, paresis, hyperesthesia, paralysis, blindness, convulsions

a mammal that has been shot. Lead is relatively insoluble but small amounts are absorbed throughout the gastrointestinal tract, causing a wide variety of clinical signs. The clinical signs may be encountered as acute or chronic forms and the severity of these usually depends on the amount of lead ingested. Bailey *et al.* (1995) recently reported lead toxicosis in a flock of houbara bustards (*Chlamydotis undulata*) after ingestion of lead-based paint flakes. For further information on lead toxicosis in other species of birds, refer to Redig *et al.*, 1980; MacDonald *et al.*, 1983; Harrison, 1986; Dement *et al.*, 1986; Mautino, 1990; Dumonceaux and Harrison, 1994; LaBonde, 1996b; and Bauck and LaBonde, 1997. Table 7.2 shows the most common sources of lead and toxic-related clinical signs in birds.

Diagnosis

Figs 7.23–7.35 illustrate signs, clinical and post-mortem, diagnosis and treatment in lead poisoning.

The diagnosis of lead toxicosis in birds is based on:

- Clinical history
- Radiology (presence of radiopaque foreign bodies in the crop and gastrointestinal tract)
- Blood chemistry (increased AST, LDH, CPK)
- Hematology (low hemoglobin (Hb) and red blood cell (RBC) count, intracytoplasmic vacuoles, basophilic stippling)
- Blood analysis (blood levels of 20 μg/dl are indicative of lead toxicity and levels of 50 μg/dl or more confirm the diagnosis)
- Tissue analysis (tissue wet levels of 3 and 6 ppm are indicative of lead toxicity and wet levels of 6 ppm or more confirm the diagnosis).

Traditionally, blood lead level in veterinary medicine has been estimated using graphite furnace atomic absorption spectrometry. However, a new electrochemical method

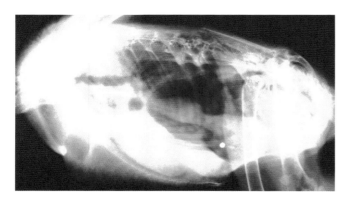

Fig. 7.23 Laterolateral radiograph of a saker falcon (*Falco cherrug*) showing a lead pellet from a shotgun within the ventriculus. In the Middle East, in common with other countries, falcons are commonly intoxicated with lead when fed on small birds shot with air rifles or shotguns and containing lead pellets or lead pellet fragments within their bodies.

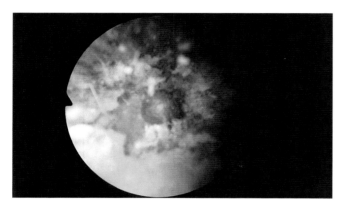

Fig. 7.24 Endoscopic view of the lead pellet within the ventriculus of the same falcon as in Fig. 7.23.

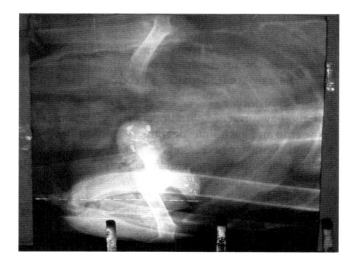

Fig. 7.25 Radiograph of a mute swan (*Cygnus olor*) affected with lead toxicosis. Swans and other waterfowl become intoxicated with lead after ingesting shotgun pellets and weights, commonly used by fishermen, from the bottom of shallow pools and lakes. (Courtesy of Mr. N. A. Forbes).

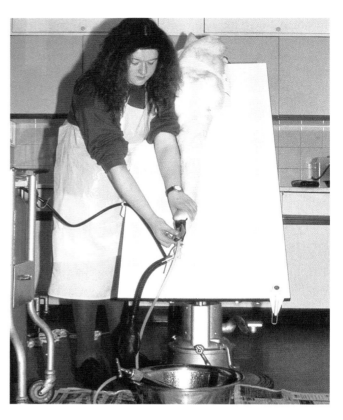

Fig. 7.26 The same bird as in Fig. 7.25. Flushing of the proventriculus and gizzard to remove lead shot and lead particles is an essential component of the primary treatment for lead toxicosis. (Courtesy of Mr. N. A. Forbes.)

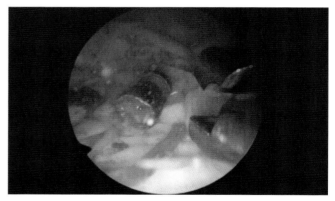

Fig. 7.27 A pellet from an air rifle within the ventriculus of a gyrfalcon (*Falco rusticolus*). Endoscopic-assisted pellet removal using either flexible or rigid endoscopes is sometimes necessary when stomach flushing fails to dislodge them from the ventriculus.

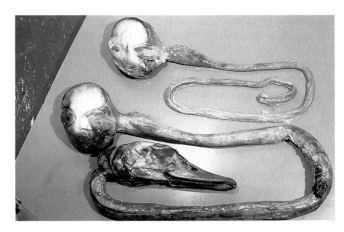

Fig. 7.28 Mute swan. **Top:** Unopened normal esophagus (note, no crop in this species), proventriculus and gizzard. **Bottom:** Distention of esophagus and proventriculus caused by impaction with vegetable matter caused by lead poisoning. (Courtesy of Mr. A. Hunt).

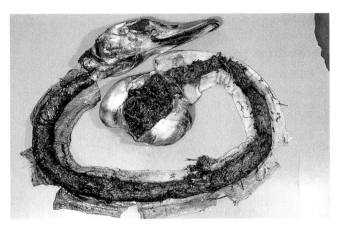

Fig. 7.29 Mute swan with esophagus, proventriculus and gizzard opened to show impaction with vegetable matter. Lead poisoning. (Courtesy of Mr. A. Hunt).

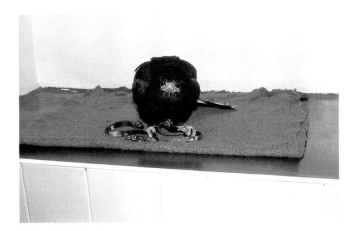

Fig. 7.30 Harris hawk (*Parabuteo unicinctus*) affected with lead toxicosis. Note the depressed, 'dog sitting' position as a result of general weakness and progressive paralysis of the legs. (Courtesy of Mr. N. A. Forbes).

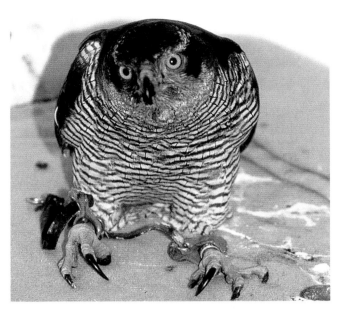

Fig. 7.31 A similar case of lead poisoning in a goshawk (*Accipiter gentilis*). (Courtesy of Mr. N. A. Forbes).

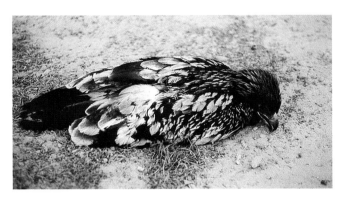

Fig. 7.32 Immature spotted eagle (*Aquila clanga*) affected with lead toxicosis. Nervous signs, such as ataxia, head tremors, blindness, dropped wings, paralysis and convulsions, are characteristic of advanced lead toxicosis. (Courtesy of Dr. U. Wernery).

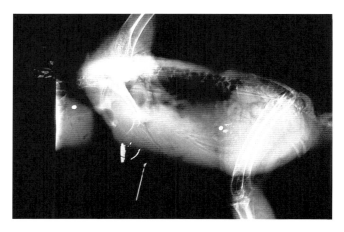

Fig. 7.33 X-ray of a peregrine falcon with lead pellets within the crop and proventriculus. (Courtesy of Mr. N. A. Forbes).

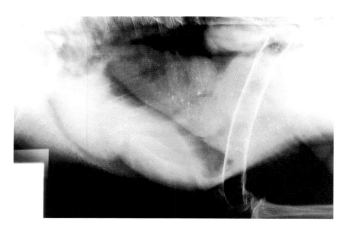

Fig. 7.34 Golden eagle (*Aquila chrysaetos*) affected with chronic lead poisoning. Note the dilated proventriculus. (Courtesy of Mr. N. A. Forbes).

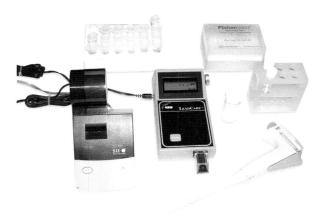

Fig. 7.35 The LeadCare System® is widely used in the diagnosis of lead toxicosis in birds. The system relies on electrochemistry and a sensor to detect lead levels in whole blood.

(LeadCare System®) has recently been introduced into the market for use with avian species (Samour and Naldo, 2002). This system relies on electrochemistry and a sensor to detect lead levels in whole blood (Fig. 7.30). Most of the lead is carried in the erythrocytes. When whole blood is mixed with the treatment reagent, the lead present in the erythrocytes is removed and made available for detection. When a test is run, the analyzer causes the lead to collect on the sensor. After a short period of time, the analyzer removes the lead, measures it and converts the results into a displayed blood lead level. The results are expressed in µg/dl. The upper measuring range of the analyzer is 65 µg/dl. Results above this value are expressed as 'high'.

Treatment

Primary treatment

- Removal of foreign bodies (crop or gastric lavage, endoscopy, surgical).

Chelative therapy

- Calcium disodium ethylene diamine tetra-acetate (CaNa$_2$ EDTA) 10–40 mg/kg IM twice daily. A recent publication reported the use of a 25% solution of Ca Na$_2$ EDTA in falcons at the dose rate of 100 mg/kg, undiluted IM b.i.d. for 5–25 consecutive days (Samour and Naldo, 2004) without observing any deleterious effect
- D-penicillamine (PA) 55 mg/kg PO twice daily × 10 d
- Dimercaprol (BAL) 2.5 mg/kg IM every 4 h for 2 d, followed by twice-daily administration until the clinical signs are resolved
- Dimercaptosuccinic acid (DMSA) 25–35 mg/kg PO twice daily/5 d/week × 3–5 weeks.

Support therapy

- IV or SC glucose/electrolyte fluids, corticosteroids, antibiotics, vitamin B$_{12}$, vitamin B$_1$, antifungal agents and magnesium sulfate.

Zinc toxicosis

Zinc toxicosis or 'new wire disease' is a relatively common toxic condition affecting mainly captive birds. Newly manufactured galvanized wire and newly manufactured galvanized watering and feeding containers are usually the main source of zinc toxicosis in captive birds. Some galvanized coatings may contain up to 99.9% zinc, while others may have 98% zinc and 1% lead (Howard, 1992). Some coins also have a high percentage of zinc. A mallard duck (*Anas platyrhynchos*) was brought to a clinic for clinical examination. The bird was weak,

TABLE 7.3 Sources and clinical signs related to zinc toxicosis

Source	Clinical signs
Galvanized wire and mesh, galvanized feeding and watering containers, some coins	Lethargy, weight loss, anemia, regurgitation, polydipsia, polyuria, hyperglycemia, ataxia, convulsions

lethargic and unable to walk. An X-ray showed a large, irregularly shaped foreign body in the gastric area. Surgery was performed and a stack of 12 worn out British 2p coins were retrieved from its gizzard. Tissues were not analyzed but a presumptive diagnosis of zinc toxicosis was made (J. Samour, unpublished observation). Zinc toxicosis has been recorded in a black bustard (*Eupodotis afra*) (Lloyd, 1992) and in a hyacinth macaw (*Anodrhynchus hyacinthus*) (Romagnano *et al.*, 1995). More recently, zinc toxicosis was diagnosed in a flock of orange-bellied parrots (*Neophema chrysogaster*) housed in a newly built aviary. The parrots did not show any sign of disease prior to death. Most birds were found dead with no obvious histological lesions. Affected birds had a mean zinc level of 154.3 μg/g in the kidneys, 289.8 μg/g in the liver and 723.6 μg/g in the pancreas (Holz *et al.*, 2000). A recent report gave a detailed description of the diagnosis and treatment of zinc toxicosis in a wattled crane (*Bugeranus carunculatus*) from a zoological collection (Barrows *et al.*, 2005). The clinical signs of zinc toxicosis are very similar to those described for lead. For additional information on zinc toxicosis in other species of birds the reader is referred to Harrison, 1986; Howard, 1992; Dumonceaux and Harrison, 1994; LaBonde, 1996a; Bauck and LaBonde, 1997; and Van Sant, 1997. Table 7.3 presents the most common sources of zinc and toxicity-related signs.

Diagnosis

Zinc toxicosis is usually diagnosed by:

- Clinical history
- Radiology
- Blood analysis (zinc levels of 200 μg/dl are suggestive of zinc toxicosis)
- Tissue analysis (pancreatic tissue zinc levels greater than 1000 μg/g are suggestive of zinc toxicosis).

Treatment

Treatment of zinc toxicosis is very similar to the treatment described for lead toxicosis.

Primary treatment

- Removal of foreign bodies (crop or gastric lavage, endoscopy, surgical).

Chelative therapy

- Calcium disodium ethylene diamine tetraacetate (Ca EDTA) 10–40 mg/kg IM twice daily
- D-penicillamine (PA) 55 mg/kg PO twice daily × 10 d
- Dimercaprol (BAL) 2.5 mg/kg IM every 4 h × 2 d, followed by twice-daily administration until the clinical signs are resolved.

Note: Ca EDTA or PA are useful chelative agents, but BAL is perhaps the most indicated agent in the case of zinc toxicosis.

Support therapy

As described for lead toxicosis.

Copper toxicosis

There are scant reports in the literature concerning copper toxicosis in avian species. This may be due to the fact that copper is less widely used around birds or bird facilities than lead or zinc. Frank and Borg (1979) reported a liver copper level greater than 3000 mg/kg and a kidney copper level greater than 50 mg/kg in a case involving a mute swan (*Cygnus olor*) displaying typical clinical signs associated with copper toxicosis. I witnessed a case of copper toxicosis in a brown kiwi (*Apteryx australis*) in a zoological collection after the ingestion of three segments, 3–5 cm long, of electrical copper wire left in the enclosure by electricians on routine maintenance work. The liver copper level in the kiwi was nearly 3500 mg/kg (J. Samour, unpublished observation). For more information concerning copper toxicosis in other species of birds the reader is referred to Dumonceaux and Harrison, 1994. The potential sources of copper and related clinical signs of copper toxicosis are listed in Table 7.4.

Diagnosis

Copper toxicosis can be diagnosed by:

- Clinical history
- Radiology
- Tissue analysis.

TABLE 7.4 Sources and clinical signs related to copper toxicosis

Source	Clinical signs
Electrical wire, some coins, excessive copper dietary supplementation, anti-algae agents (copper sulfate)	Anemia, weakness, weight loss, lethargy. Post-mortem finding: metal-black liver appearance

Treatment

Chelative therapy

- D-penicillamine (PA) 52 mg/kg/d PO × 6 d has been recommended for mammals.

Support therapy

As described for lead toxicosis.

Botulism

Botulism (Figs 7.36–7.37) is a toxic neuroparalytic disease produced by the ingestion of toxins of *Clostridium botulinum*. There are at least seven types of toxin produced by the different strains of *C. botulinum*. Type C is responsible for most of the toxicosis reported in birds worldwide. Types A and E, which are more relevant to human botulism, have also been implicated in toxicity outbreaks in birds. *C. botulinum* is an anaerobic, spore-forming, motile and Gram-positive bacillus commonly found associated with putrefying vegetable matter in marshes and wetlands and decomposing animal carcasses. The bacillus can also be found in badly stored and decomposing grain, silage and hay. Outbreaks of botulism have been widely documented in waterfowl, but seagulls, terns and other aquatic species can be affected. Botulism has also been documented in captive ostriches (Shakespeare, 1995). In the Middle East, this disease has been observed in feral domestic pigeons (*Columba livia*) and collared doves (*Streptopelia decaocto*) after eating proprietary pellets that had been badly stored in a silo (J. Samour, unpublished observation). This toxic condition is more frequently reported during the hottest months of the year because of the increased alkalinity of stagnant water and the anaerobic conditions created on the substrate of ponds and marshes. The toxins of *C. botulinum* affect the releasing mechanism of acetylcholine at the terminal sections of the peripheric nerves, causing an acute, flaccid and descending paralysis. Other clinical signs include dyspnea, hypersalivation, nasal and ocular discharge and diarrhea. For more information on botulism in avian species, refer to Bennett, 1994; LaBonde, 1996a; and Gerlach, 1997. (Figs 7.38–7.39)

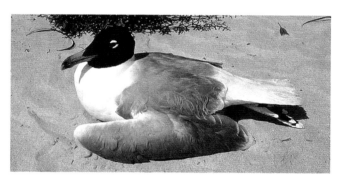

Fig. 7.36 A great black-headed gull (*Larus ichthyaetus*) affected with *Clostridium botulinum* toxicosis. Note the typical clinical sign of wing paralysis manifested through the 'dropped wing' appearance. Gulls have scavengers' feeding habits and are very often affected with *C. botulinum* toxicosis when feeding from rubbish dumps near human habitation. (Courtesy of Dr. U. Wernery).

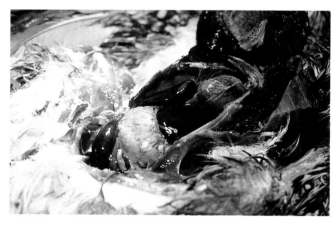

Fig. 7.38 Post-mortem examination of a gyrfalcon (*Falco rusticolus*). The falcon died of enterotoxemia caused by *Clostridium perfringens*. Note the highly congested intestine. (Courtesy of Dr. U. Wernery and Dr. J. Kinne).

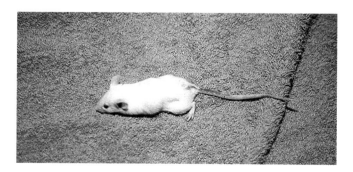

Fig. 7.37 Typical wasp-waist appearance of a white mouse after intraperitoneal inoculation with *Clostridium botulinum* toxin. (Courtesy of Dr. U. Wernery).

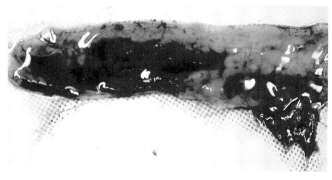

Fig. 7.39 Intestinal mucosa of the gyrfalcon in Fig. 7.38. Note the extensive hemorrhagic changes due to severe enteritis. (Courtesy of Dr. U. Wernery and Dr. J. Kinne).

Diagnosis

- Clinical history
- Culture
- Tissue toxin analysis (submit frozen liver and kidneys)
- Water and feed toxin analysis (submit frozen)
- Mouse inoculation neutralization assay.

Treatment

Primary therapy

- Antitoxin administration (0.05–1 ml/d).

Support therapy

- Drenches, cathartics and laxatives
- Tube feeding
- IV or SC glucose/electrolyte fluids, antibiotics and vitamins B_{12} and B_1.

Mycotoxicosis

Mycotoxicosis is a general term used to describe a series of toxic conditions caused by the ingestion of feed contaminated with the toxins of different saprophytic and phytopathogenic fungi and molds. These toxins are normally referred to as mycotoxins. Mycotoxins are secondary metabolites, which are not produced for the benefit of the fungus or mold.

Fungi and molds commonly grow on basic feed ingredients and pelletized commercial feed if these are stored for a long period of time and under suboptimal temperature and relative humidity conditions. Some fungi even grow on the crop itself when the environmental conditions are suitable. Dumonceaux and Harrison (1994) provided a more detailed account of mycotoxicosis in birds. An account of the effect of mycotoxins (aflatoxin B_1 and vomitoxin) in young ostrich chicks was described by Scheideler and Kunze (1997). As outlined by Pier (1990), aflatoxin is toxic to ducklings in an oral LD_{50} dose of 0.36 mg/kg, and to chicks in an oral LD_{50} dose of 6.5 mg/kg. The most important mycotoxins relevant to birds produced by fungi or molds are listed in Table 7.5.

Diagnosis

- Clinical history
- Post-mortem changes
- Histopathological analysis
- Toxin quantitative analysis in food and gastrointestinal contents.

TABLE 7.5 Relevant mycotoxins in avian medicine produced by fungus or mold

Mycotoxin	Fungus or mold	Clinical and pathological signs
Aflatoxin B_1	Aspergillus flavus, A. parasiticus	Anorexia, lethargy, CNS signs, sudden death, hepatitis, splenitis, pancreatitis
Ochratoxin A	Aspergillus ochraceus, Penicillium citrinum, P. viridicatum	CNS signs, hepatotoxic and nephrotoxic signs, immune system and bone marrow suppression
Vomitoxin (deoxynivalenol)	Fusarium roseum, Gibberella zeae	Vomiting, regurgitation, diarrhea
Trichothecenes, satratoxins, T_2 toxin, diacetoxyscirpenol	Stachybotrye atra, Fusarium roseum, F. scirpi, F. tricinctum, F. equiseti, F. culmorum	Necrotic ulcerative lesions of the upper digestive tract, flaccid neck and wing paralysis, contact dermatitis, distal necrosis

Treatment

Attempting treatment of clinical cases affected with aflatoxicosis is usually unrewarded. However, with other mycotoxicosis, if not chronic or severe, the cases usually resolve when the source of toxicity is withdrawn, with the aid of support therapy.

Pharmacological compounds toxicosis

There are numerous pharmacological compounds that are potentially toxic to birds. In most cases, the toxic effect of a particular compound is related to the administration of a dose higher than that recommended. Conversely, the toxicity may be due to the administration of a particular compound for a period of time longer than normally recommended (Harrison, 1986; Dumonceaux and Harrison, 1994; LaBonde, 1996a; Bauck and LaBonde, 1997). A recent study reported suspected fenbendazole toxicosis in two vulture species and Marabou storks. A group of ten African white-backed vultures (*Gyps africanus*), three lappet-faced vultures (*Torgos tracheliotus*) and six Marabou storks (*Leptoptilos crumeniferus*) were routinely treated for gastrointestinal parasites using 47–60 mg/kg for three consecutive days. Six white-backed and one lappet-faced vultures and one Marabou stork died after a short period of depression and anorexia. Hematology analyses revealed profound leukopenia in all cases. On histology examination, severe necrotizing enteritis, bacterial hepatitis and evidence of septicemia was found (Bonar *et al.*, 2003).

The past 10 years have seen a sharp decline in the population of at least three vulture species in the Indian

TABLE 7.6 Potential toxic effects of common pharmacological compounds in birds

Pharmacological compound	Clinical and pathological signs
ANTIBIOTICS	
Cefalosporins	Nephrotoxic, hepatotoxic
Chloramphenicol	Nephrotoxic
Gentamicin	Nephrotoxic
Doxycycline	Tissue necrosis, cartilage abnormalities in growing birds
Ticarcillin	In combination with tobramycin may be hepatotoxic
Oxytetracyclines	Tissue necrosis, inflammation, nephrotoxic, prolonged use may depress gut flora
Trimethoprim–sulfa drug combinations, furazolidone	Regurgitation, general depression, gastrointestinal tract stasis
Tylosin	Convulsions
ANTIFUNGAL	
Amphotericin B	Nephrotoxic, hepatotoxic, vomiting, convulsions
Flucytosine	Anemia, bone marrow depression, leukopenia
ANTHELMINTICS/ANTIPARASITICS	
Fenbendazole	CNS signs
Ivermectin	Lethargy, depression and death in some small psittacines when administered IM
Levamisole	Regurgitation, ataxia, dyspnea, hepatotoxic
Praziquantel	General depression, death
ANTIPROTOZOAL	
Dimetridazole	CNS signs, hepatotoxic
VITAMINS	
A	Osteodystrophy, parathyroid hyperplasia, dermatitis
D_3	Mineralization of organs, nephrosis, increase serum calcium level
ANTICOCCIDIAL/ANTIPROTOZOAL	
Monensin	Ataxia, dyspnea, degenerative myopathy, death (Baird *et al.*, 1997)

subcontinent. The species involved include the long-billed vulture (*Gyps indicus*), slender-billed vulture (*Gyps tenuirostris*) and Oriental white-backed vulture (*Gyps bengalensis*) (Prakash 1999; Gilbert *et al.*, 2002). This crisis prompted an international response to investigate the cause of the decline. Extensive health screening failed to detect a common cause for the extensive mortality. Post-mortem examination, however, found severe visceral gout in over 85% of the carcasses examined. Extensive toxicological investigation for heavy metals, pesticides and herbicides did not reveal any significant finding. On further toxicological examination, the nonsteroidal anti-inflammatory drug diclofenac, in residues of 0.051–0.643 µg per gram of kidney, was detected in 25 out of 25 vultures that had visceral gout (Risebrough, 2004; Oaks *et al.*, 2004; Green *et al.*, 2004). The control group, consisting of vultures that had died of other causes, proved negative for the presence of diclofenac. In 2005 the government of India announced the phasing out of diclofenac for veterinary use within 6 months (Anonymous, 2006).

Table 7.6 shows the clinical and pathological signs associated with the use of certain pharmacological compounds in birds.

Pesticide toxicosis

Pesticide is a broad term that encompasses groups of chemicals commonly used to eradicate unwanted and destructive animals and plants. These different chemical compounds can be classified under three main groups: insecticides, rodenticides and herbicides.

Most cases of pesticide toxicosis in birds occur by negligence or by accident. Very often the instructions of manufacturers are not properly followed and the pesticide is applied directly to birds or in the surrounding of aviaries. In this respect, I have witnessed several cases in which bird owners trying to treat their birds for flea or lice infestation had sprayed the birds directly with products commonly used for flies and cockroaches. Conversely, pesticides are commonly applied or placed in areas where birds have direct access to and ingest them, either in their pure form or through contaminated food or water.

The clinical signs vary significantly depending on the compound and degree of toxicosis. The most commonly encountered clinical signs include gastrointestinal disorders, such as anorexia, regurgitation, vomiting and diarrhea, central nervous system signs, convulsions, dyspnea, cyanosis and death. For more detailed accounts of pesticide toxicosis in birds, the reader is referred to Harrison, 1986; Lumeij *et al.*, 1993; Porter, 1993; Dumonceaux and Harrison, 1994; LaBonde, 1996a; and Bauck and LaBonde, 1997. Tables 7.7–7.9 illustrate the most common pesticides that are potentially toxic to birds.

The diagnosis is usually based on clinical history and forensic examination for a particular toxic compound. The treatment of severe cases of pesticide toxicosis is

TABLE 7.7 Common insecticides potentially toxic to birds

Toxic compound	Source/action
Chlorinated hydrocarbons	Currently used around live animals: lindane, methoxychlor, toxaphene. Toxic for use around live animals: aldrin, dieldrin, benzene hexachloride, chlordane, endrin
Organophosphates	Dichlorvos, malathion, parathion, diazinon, fenthion, trichlorfon, coumaphos
Carbamates	Carbaryl, carbofuran, methomyl, propoxur
Compounds of plant origin	Pyrethrins: pyrethrum is a widely used insecticide extracted from the flowers of *Chrysanthemum cinerariaefolium* Pyrethroids: These are synthetic preparations made from pure pyrethrins. These include allethrin, cypermethrin, decamethrin, fenvalerate, fluvalinate, permethrin, tetramethrin

TABLE 7.8 Common rodenticides potentially toxic to birds

Toxic compound	Source/action
Anticoagulant rodenticides	Warfarin, brodifacoum, coumafuryl
Pyraminyl	Vacor
Zinc phosphide	Used widely since affected rodents commonly die in the open
Crimidine	Castrix

TABLE 7.9 Common herbicides potentially toxic to birds

Toxic compound	Source/action
Plant hormone herbicides	2–4-dichlorophenoxyacetic acid, 2,4,5-trichlorophenoxyacetic acid, 2-methyl-4 chlorophenoxyacetic acid, 2,2-dichloropropionic acid
Triazine compounds	Atrazine, cyanazine, prometryn, propazine, metribuzin, simazine
Thiocarbamate compounds	Barban, chlorpropham, diallate, pebulate, triallate, vernolate
Phenylurea compounds	Diuron, fenuron, linuron, monolinuron, norea
Pentachlorophenol	Also used as fungicide, insecticide, wood preservative and molluscicide

usually unrewarded, but in some cases health can be restored to normal by withdrawing the toxic source and by additional support therapy.

Toxic plants

There is widespread controversy in the literature as to which species of plants and which part of the plant offer a definite risk of toxicity to birds. There also appears to be discrepancy as to which bird species are susceptible to toxicosis after the ingestion of certain plants.

Recently, a large number of greater flamingos (> 579) (*Phoenicopterus rubber*) died during the summer of 2001 in Doñana National park. Other species of waterfowl also perished in the same outbreak. The suspected

cause was the sudden presence of a dense water bloom of cyanobacteria but mainly *Microcystis aeruginosa* and *Anabaena flos-aquae* (Alonso-Andicoberry *et al.* 2002)

Other toxic compounds

There is a wide range of household and industrial products that are potentially toxic to birds (Fig. 7.40). Sporadic reports appear in the literature with definite accounts of toxicosis due to a particular compound (Dumonceaux and Harrison, 1994; LaBonde, 1996a; Lang, 1997). Table 7.10 illustrates some of the most common toxicoses related to various miscellaneous compounds.

Most of the plant species listed as toxic to birds have been widely documented as toxic to mammals, especially herbivores, or to humans. However, there are only a handful of clinical cases in which toxicosis due to toxic plants has been diagnosed (Harrison, 1986; Dumonceaux and Harrison, 1994; LaBonde, 1996a; Bauck and LaBonde, 1997). Table 7.11 lists the plant species mentioned in the literature as potentially toxic to birds.

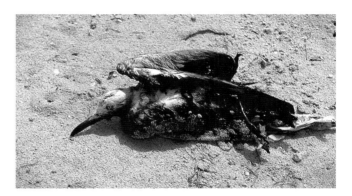

Fig. 7.40 An immature tern partially covered with crude oil. Oil spills are very common around coastal areas of the world and every year are responsible for the death of hundreds of seashore birds. Death usually occurs as a result of the feathers becoming coated with oil and birds are unable to move freely and to feed. Death may also occur due to hypothermia and by direct ingestion of oil.

TABLE 7.10 Miscellaneous compounds potentially toxic to birds

Toxic compound	Source
Ethylene glycol	Antifreeze compounds
Chocolate	Commercially available
Nicotine	Tobacco products, tobacco smoke
Ammonia, chlorine, sodium hydroxide	Disinfectants, cleaners
Selenium sulfide	Dog shampoo
Arsenic	Contaminated mineral block
Carbon monoxide	Automobile engine, combustion oven and domestic oven/cooker fumes
Mercury	Mirror linings
Sodium chloride	Household salt, rock salt
Silicone	Peat moss
Nitrates	Fertilizers
Polytetrafluoroethylene gas	Overheated Teflon-lined cooking pans, ironing board covers, some heating elements, some lampshades
Petroleum	Crude petroleum or its derivatives

TABLE 7.11 Plants potentially toxic to birds

Scientific name	Common name	Scientific name	Common name
Amarylidaceae	Amaryllis	Convallaria majalis	Lily of the valley
Rhododendron occidentale	Azalea	Lobelia spp.	Lobelia
Persea americana	Avocado	Astragalus and Oxtropis spp.	Locoweed
Poinciana gilliesii	Bird of paradise	Kalanchoe spp.	Maternity plant
Acepodium podograria	Bishop's weed	Cannabis sativa	Marijuana
Robinia pseudoacacia	Black locust	Phoradendron villosum	Mistletoe
Microcystis aeruginosa	Blue-green algae	Asclepias spp.	Milkweed
Buxus sempervirens	Boxwood	Prunus caroliniana	Mock orange
Arctium minus	Burdock	Aconitum spp.	Monkshood
Ranunculaceae	Buttercup	Ipomoea spp.	Morning glory
Caladium spp.	Caladium	Kalmia latifolia	Mountain laurel
Trichodesma incanum	Camel bush	Narcissus spp.	Narcissus
Ricinus communis	Castor bean	Solanum spp.	Nightshade
Prunus spp.	Cherry	Quercus spp.	Oak
Montana rubens	Clematis	Nerium oleander	Oleander
Sesbania vesicaria	Coffee bean	Petroselinum sativum	Parsley
Caltha polustris	Cowslip	Philodendron scandens	Philodendron
Datura spp.	Datura	Euphorbia pulcherrima	Poinsettia
Daphne spp.	Daphne	Phytolacca americana	Pokeweed
Dieffenbachia spp.	Dieffenbachia	Conium maculatum	Poison hemlock
Hedera helix	English ivy	Solanum tuberosum	Potato (shoots)
Alocasia and Colocasia spp.	Elephant's ear	Arbus precatoius	Precatory bean
Claviceps purpurea	Ergot	Ligustrum vulgare	Privet
Digitalis purpurea	Foxglove	Rhododendron simsii	Rhododendron
Conium maculatum	Hemlock	Rheum rhaponticum	Rhubarb
Hyacinthus orientalis	Hyacinth	Abrus precatorius	Rosary pea
Hydrangea spp.	Hydrangea	Symplocarpus foetidus	Skunk cabbage
Iris spp.	Iris	Ornithogalum umbellatum	Snowdrop
Arisaema spp.	Jack-in-the-pulpit	Nicotiana spp.	Tobacco
Solanum pseudocapsicum	Jerusalem cherry	Parthenocissus spp.	Virginia creeper
Datura stramonium	Jimsonweed	Wisteria spp.	Wisteria
Juniperus virginiana	Juniper	Taxus media	Yew
Delphinium spp.	Larkspur		

Source: adapted from Harrison 1986 and LaBonde 1996a.

Figure 7.36 illustrates an unusual case of toxicosis in a saker falcon (*Falco cherrug*) bitten on the hind talon by a sand snake (*Psammophis schokari*). Snake bite is commonly reported in domestic mammals but, to my knowledge, has never been documented in a bird.

Recently, an interesting incident of suspected chocolate toxicity was reported in an adult, male African gray parrot (*Psittacus erithacus*). The parrot was taken to a veterinarian approximately 12 h after ingesting a large chocolate doughnut. The bird died 24 h after presentation. The gross post-mortem changes observed and subsequent histopathology findings in the parrot were consistent with changes observed in canines after ingesting a lethal dose of theobromine, the methylxanthine found in chocolate (Cole and Murray, 2005). (Fig. 7.41)

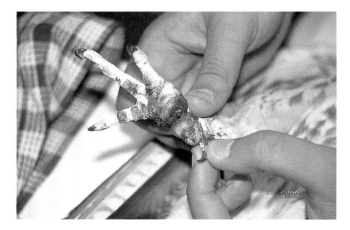

Fig. 7.41 An unusual case of a saker falcon bitten on the back talon by a sand snake (*Psammophis schokari*), a mildly poisonous snake inhabiting areas of sparse vegetation in the Middle East. The falcon was bitten during a training exercise when it unknowingly landed close to the spot where the snake was hiding. The falcon was taken for veterinary attention 12 h after the incident but it was too late and the bird died immediately after admission.

REFERENCES

Alonso-Andicoberry C, García-Villada L, Lopez-Rodas V, Costas E (2002) Catastrophic mortality of flamingos in a Spanish national park caused by cyanobacteria. The Veterinary Record 151: 706–707.

Anonymous (2006) Action plan for vulture conservation in India. Ministry of Environment and Forests, New Delhi, India, pp. 1–18.

Bailey TA, Samour JH, Naldo J, Howlett JC (1995) Lead toxicosis in captive houbara bustards (Chlamydotis undulata macqueenii). Veterinary Record 137: 193–194.

Baird GJ, Caldow GL, Peek IS, Grant DA (1997) Monensin toxicity in a flock of ostriches. Veterinary Record 140: 624–626.

Barrows M, Hartley M, Pittman JM (2005) Zinc toxicosis in a wattled crane (Bugeranus carunculatus). Proceedings of the European Association of Avian Veterinarians, Arles, pp. 491–494.

Bauck L, LaBonde J (1997) Toxic diseases. In: Altman RB, Clubb SL, Dorrestein GM, Quesenberry K (eds) Avian Medicine and Surgery, pp. 604–613. WB Saunders, Philadelphia.

Bennett RA (1994) Neurology. In: Ritchie BW, Harrison GJ, Harrison LR (eds) Avian Medicine: Principles and Application, pp. 738–747. Wingers Publishing, Lake Worth, FL.

Bonar CJ, Lewandowski AH, Schaul J (2003) Suspected fenbendazole toxicosis in 2 vulture species (Gyps africanus, Torgos tracheliotus) and marabou storks (Leptoptilos cremeniferus). Journal of Avian Medicine and Surgery 17: 16–19.

Brander GC, Pugh DM, Bywater RJ, Jenkins WL (1991) Drugs used in the modification of cell, tissue, organ and system function. In: Daykin PW (ed.) Veterinary Applied Pharmacology and Therapeutics, 5th edn, p. 194. Baillière Tindall, London.

Cole G, Murray M (2005) Suspected chocolate toxicity in an African gray parrot (Psittacus erithacus). Proceedings of the Association of Avian Veterinarians, Monterey, pp. 339–340.

Cooper JE (1985) Veterinary Aspects of Captive Birds of Prey, 2nd edn. Standfast Press, Saul, Gloucestershire.

Dement SH, Chisolm JJ, Barber JC, Strandberg JD (1986) Lead exposure in an 'urban' peregrine falcon and its avian prey. Journal of Wildlife Diseases 22: 238–244.

Dumonceaux G, Harrison G (1994) Toxins. In: Ritchie BW, Harrison GJ, Harrison LR (eds) Avian Medicine: Principles and Application, pp. 1030–1052. Wingers Publishing, Lake Worth, FL.

Forth W, Heuschler D, Rummel W (1983) Infusionstherapie. Allgemeine und Spezielle Pharmakologie und Toxicologie, 4th edn, p. 283. Bibliographisches Institut, Mannheim.

Frank A, Borg K (1979) Heavy metals in tissue of the mute swan (Cygnus olor). Acta Veterinaria Scandinavica 20: 447–465.

Gerlach H (1997) Anatiformes. In: Altman RB, Clubb SL, Dorrestein GM, Quesenberry K (eds) Avian Medicine and Surgery, pp. 960–972. WB Saunders, Philadelphia.

Gilbert M, Virani MZ, Watson RT et al. (2002) Breeding and mortality of Oriental white-backed vulture Gyps bengalensis in Punjab Province, Pakistan. Bird Conserv Int 12: 311–326.

Gilman GA, Goodman LS, Rall TW, Murad F (1985) Ammonium and acid-forming salts. In: Hardman JG, Limbird LE (eds) Goodman and Gilman's Pharmacological Basis of Therapeutics, 7th edn, p. 865. Macmillan, New York.

Green RE, Newton I, Shultz S et al. (2004) Diclofenac poisoning as a cause of vulture population decline across the Indian subcontinent. Journal of Applied Ecology 41: 793–800.

Harrison GJ (1986) Toxicology. In: Harrison GJ, Harrison LR (eds) Clinical Avian Medicine and Surgery, pp. 491–499. WB Saunders, Philadelphia.

Holz P, Phelan J, Slocombe R et al. (2000) Suspected zinc toxicosis as a cause of sudden death in orange-bellied parrots (Neophema chrysogaster). Journal of Avian Medicine and Surgery 14: 37–41.

Howard BR (1992) Health risks of housing small psittacines in galvanized wire mesh cages. Journal of the American Veterinary Medical Association 200: 1667–1674.

Humphreys DJ (1988) Veterinary Toxicology, 3rd edn. Baillière Tindall, London.

King AS, McLelland J (1984) Special sense organs. In: King AS, McLelland J (eds) Birds: Their Structure and Function, p. 284. Baillière Tindall, London.

Klemm WR (1984) Behavioral physiology. In: Swenson M (ed.) Duke's Physiology of Domestic Animals, 10th edn, p. 687. Cornell University Press, Ithaca, NY.

LaBonde J (1991) Avian toxicology. Veterinary Clinics of North America – Small Animal Practice 21: 1329–1342.

LaBonde J (1996a) Toxic disorders. In: Rosskopf WJ Jr, Woerpel RW (eds) Diseases of Cage and Aviary Birds, 3rd edn, pp. 511–522. Williams & Wilkins, Baltimore.

LaBonde J (1996b) Medicine and surgery of Anseriformes. In: Rosskopf WJ Jr, Woerpel RW (eds) Diseases of Cage and Aviary Birds, 3rd edn, pp. 956–1001. Williams & Wilkins, Baltimore.

Lang T (1997) Selected toxins in birds. Proceedings of the Association of Avian Veterinarians, Reno, pp. 287–292.

Lloyd M (1992) Heavy metal ingestion: medical management and gastroscopy foreign body removal. Journal of the Association of Avian Veterinarians 6: 25.

Lumeij JT, Westerhof I, Smit T, Spierenburg TJ (1993) Diagnosis and treatment of poisoning in raptors from the Netherlands: clinical case reports and review of 2,750 post-mortem cases 1975–1988. In: Redig PT, Cooper JE, Remple JD et al. (eds) Raptor Biomedicine, pp. 233–238. University of Minnesota Press, Minneapolis.

MacDonald JW, Randall CJ, Ross HM, Moon GM, Ruthven AD (1983) Lead poisoning in captive birds of prey. Veterinary Record 113: 65–66.

Mautino M (1990) Avian lead intoxication. Proceedings of the Association of Avian Veterinarians, Phoenix, pp. 245–247.

Oaks JL, Gilbert M, Virani MZ et al. (2004) Diclofenac residues as the cause of vulture population decline in Pakistan. Nature 427: 630–633.

Osweiler GD (1986) Household and commercial products. In: Kirk RW (ed.) Current Veterinary Therapy IX, pp. 193–195. WB Saunders, Philadelphia.

Petrak ML (1982) Diseases of Cage and Aviary Birds. Lea & Febiger, Philadelphia.

Pier AC (1990) Mycotoxins and mycotoxicoses. In: Biberstein EL, Zee C (eds) Review of Veterinary Microbiology, p. 348. Blackwell Science, Oxford.

Porter SL (1993) Pesticide poisoning in birds of prey. In: Redig PT, Cooper JE, Remple JD et al. (eds) Raptor Biomedicine, pp. 239–245. University of Minnesota Press, Minneapolis.

Prakash V (1999) Status of vultures in Keoladeo National Park, Bharatpur, Rajasthan, with special reference to population crash in Gyps species. Journal of the Bombay Natural History Society 96: 365–378.

Redig PT, Stowe CM, Barnes DM, Arent TD (1980) Lead toxicosis in raptors. Journal of the American Veterinary Medical Association 177: 941–943.

Risebrough R (2004) Fatal medicine for vultures. Nature 427: 596–597.

Romagnano A, Grindem CB, Degernes L, Mautino M (1995) Treatment of a hyacinth macaw with zinc toxicosis. Journal of Avian Medicine and Surgery 9: 185–189.

Rosskopf WJ Jr, Woerpel RW (1986) Heavy metal intoxication in caged birds: Parts I and II. In: Exotic Animal Medicine Practice, The Compendium Collection. Veterinary Learning Systems, Trenton, NJ.

Samour JH, Naldo J (2002) Diagnosis and therapeutic management of lead toxicosis in falcons in Saudi Arabia. Journal of the Association of Avian Veterinarians 16: 16–20.

Samour JH, Naldo J (2004) The use of Ca Na$_2$ EDTA in the treatment of lead toxicosis in falcons. Proceedings of the Association of Avian Veterinarians, New Orleans, pp. 125–129.

Scheideler SE, Kunze K (1997) A summary of mycotoxin (Aflatoxin B1 or vomitoxin) challenge in young ostrich chicks. Proceedings of the Association of Avian Veterinarians, Reno, pp. 167–168.

Shakespeare AS (1995) Compendium on Continuing Education for the Practicing Veterinarian: 1440.

Van Sant F (1997): Zinc and clinical disease in parrots. Proceedings of the Association of Avian Veterinarians, Reno, pp. 387–391.

Disorders of the digestive system

Ian F. Keymer, Jaime Samour

This is an abbreviated review of diseases of the digestive system of birds. The diseases listed and discussed apply mainly to psittacines unless otherwise stated. The object of this section is to aid the differential diagnosis of disorders of the digestive system. The review deals primarily with the pathological aspects of the subject; no attempt has been made to cover this vast subject in detail. The better known disorders are merely listed, and discussion is mostly confined to those thought to be of special interest, previously unpublished work and poorly documented data on which there is limited information. For more detailed information the reader should consult other chapters in this book, and textbooks by Arnall and Keymer (1975), Burr (1982), Petrak (1982), Griner (1983), Gabrisch and Zwart (1984), Cooper (1985), Fowler (1986), Ritchie *et al.* (1994), Beynon *et al.* (1996a, 1996b), Randall and Reece (1996), Ritchie (1996), Rosskopf and Woerpel (1996) and Altman *et al.* (1997).

Although a great deal is known about disorders of the digestive system, there are still many gaps in our knowledge. The diseases are listed according to the main anatomical structures that are affected: the beak; buccal and oral cavity, including pharynx (oropharynx) and tongue; crop or ingluvies; proventriculus; gizzard or ventriculus; intestine (duodenum, small and large intestine, including cecum); pancreas; cloaca; and liver. Ceca are rudimentary in many species and are not present in most psittacines, including the budgerigar (*Melopsittacus undulatus*), in spite of the report of *Heterakis gallinae* in the ceca of budgerigars by Shanthikumar (1987).

It is worth noting that, although there appears to be a higher incidence of neoplasia in budgerigars than in any other species of vertebrate, neoplasms of the digestive system are relatively rare in most species. For more detailed information, especially regarding Psittaciformes, see Latimer, 1994.

Beak

Some beak abnormalities are presented in Box 7.1 and in Figures 7.42–7.52.

When the beak is examined for abnormalities, it is important to be aware of the normal appearance, because this often differs in shape and coloration according to the species (see Arnall and Keymer, 1975, for illustrations). A healthy beak should be smooth, with a sheen, and be symmetrically colored and shaped. The coloration and sharpness or bluntness of the beak is often specific to the species. In some species of Psittaciformes, for example, a light coloration may indicate that the bird is young, because the beak becomes darker as the bird matures. In some other species the reverse applies, with the young of the species having a darker beak.

There are many types of beak abnormality, the causes of which in many cases are conjectural rather than proven (as stated in Box 7.1). For example, various types of deformity and poor beak quality have been attributed to malnutrition such as deficiencies of vitamins

Box 7.1. Abnormalities of the beak
Poor quality: Dry, flaky surface and overgrown; malnutrition, liver disease, senility, cnemidocoptic mange, PBFD (see below)

Psittacine beak and feather disease (PBFD): Circovirus infection. Color change and progressive growth. Elongation of beak with the development of fault lines associated with feather loss

Transverse grooving: Chronic respiratory disease, PBFD

Splitting: Sequel to trimming or trauma, malnutrition

'Rubber beak': Nutritional secondary hyperparathyroidism in all species

'Scissors beak': Uncertain etiology but believed to be caused by feeding neonates placing the syringe always on the same side of the oropharynx

Malocclusion and crookedness: Causes include insufficient wear and tear, malnutrition, metabolic bone disease, trauma. Mange (*Cnemidocoptes pilae* infestation) in smaller Psittaciformes

Upper beak elongation: Causes include insufficient wear and tear, with neglect

Lower beak elongation: Obsessive biting of cage wire in Psittaciformes considered to be one cause

Hyperkeratosis: Changes due to senility and possible chronic hypovitaminosis A

Neoplasia causing deformities: In Psittaciformes – carcinoma, fibrosarcoma, adenocarcinoma, keratoma, osteosarcoma

Beak deformities of nestlings and juveniles: Hereditary and/or congenital. In Psittaciformes sometimes associated with feeding sticky, wet food when hand rearing

Beak deformity of unknown etiology

Other deformities: Trauma (e.g. sequel to trimming); burning from biting electric wiring or cooking utensils, especially Psittaciformes; localized bacterial infections with osteomyelitis; beak necrosis caused by zygomycosis (*Zygomycetes* infection); cnemidocoptic mange, etc.

A and D, pantothenic acid, biotin and folic acid, but supporting experimental evidence is lacking. Of all these deficiencies in Psittaciformes, hypovitaminosis A is the most convincing, especially when there is evidence of hyperkeratosis.

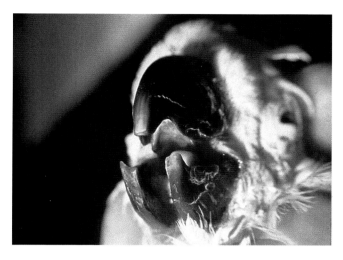

Fig. 7.42 Sulfur-crested cockatoo (*Cacatua galerita*) with longitudinal split and separation of the lower mandible. Malnutrition and subsequent trauma are possible causes. Note also flaky uneven surface of the horny sheaths of the mandibles, i.e. the maxillary rhamphotheca (upper) and the mandibular rhamphotheca (lower). (Courtesy of Mr. T. Dennett, Zoological Society of London).

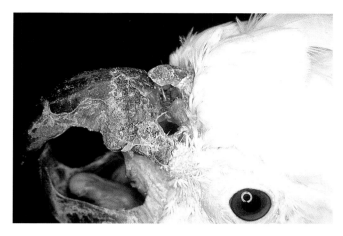

Fig. 7.43 Sulfur-crested cockatoo showing osteomyelitis originating at the base of the upper mandible and involving the external nares. This has interfered with the growth of the beak and may have caused the flakiness of the surface of the rhamphotheca. (Courtesy of Mr. A. D. Malley).

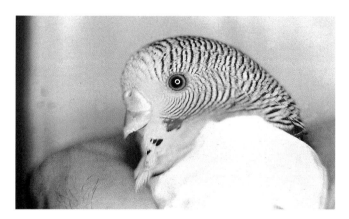

Fig. 7.44 Immature budgerigar (*Melopsittacus undulatus*) showing malocclusion, possibly hereditary or congenital in origin. (Courtesy of Mr. A. D. Malley).

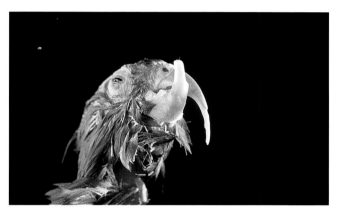

Fig. 7.45 Senegal parrot (*Poicephalus senegalus*) showing so-called 'scissors beak'. The upper mandible is deviated to the bird's left and the lower to the right. Sometimes this occurs when the bird is young and is fed sticky, wet food during hand rearing. (Courtesy of Mr. T. Dennett, Zoological Society of London).

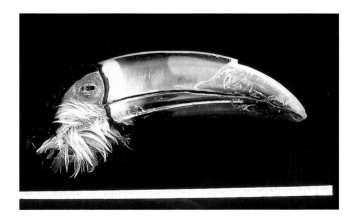

Fig. 7.46 Aged toucan (*Ramphastos* sp.) showing flakiness of the beak as frequently seen associated with senility. (Courtesy of Mr. T. Dennett, Zoological Society of London).

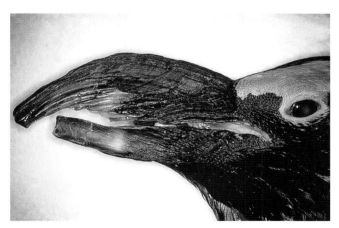

Fig. 7.47 An aged jackass or black-footed penguin (*Spheniscus demersus*) showing hyperkeratosis of both mandibles. Chronic hypovitaminosis A is a possible contributory factor. (Courtesy of Mr. T. Dennett, Zoological Society of London).

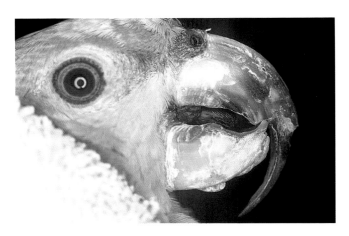

Fig. 7.48 Orange-winged amazon parrot (*Amazona amazonica*) showing deformity and overgrowth of the maxillary rhamphotheca of unknown etiology. The flakiness, elongation of rhamphotheca and fault lines showing on both mandibles (especially near the base of the beak) resemble psittacine beak and feather disease (PBFD) but this disease is less common in *Amazona* spp. than in some other psittacines such as *Cacatua* spp. (Courtesy of Mr. A. D. Malley).

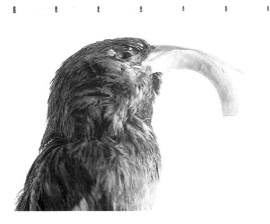

Fig. 7.49 Melanistic house sparrow (*Passer domesticus*) showing marked overgrowth of the beak. The upper mandible is grossly elongated and the lower is thickened, curved ventrally and overgrown. Cause unknown. The plumage shows almost complete melanism. (Courtesy of Mr. T. Dennett, Zoological Society of London).

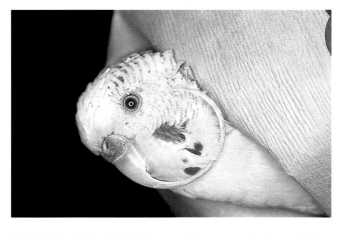

Fig. 7.50 Budgerigar displaying a grossly overgrown beak caused by neglect. (Courtesy of Mr. A. D. Malley).

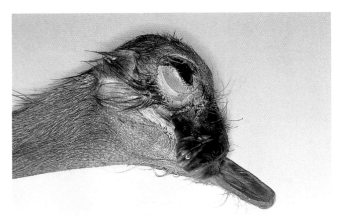

Fig. 7.51 Lateral view of the head of a 4-month-old ostrich (*Struthio camelus*) chick showing a grossly deformed upper beak associated with incorrect temperature settings during artificial incubation. The ostrich was destroyed on humane grounds. (Courtesy of Dr. J. Samour).

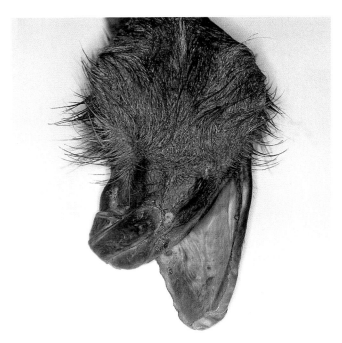

Fig. 7.52 The same ostrich chick as in Fig. 7.51. Dorsal view. (Courtesy of Dr. J. Samour).

Psittacine species appeared to be prone to two common beak deviation presentations during the growth period: the so-called 'scissors beak', where the upper beak grows towards the side of the lower beak (Speer, 2003a); and prognathism, where the lower beak is longer than the upper beak (Clipsham, 1989, 1992; Speer, 1995, 2003b). Different techniques and materials to correct these abnormalities have been proposed by Clipsham (1992) and Martin and Ritchie (1994) and more recently by Tully *et al.* (2005).

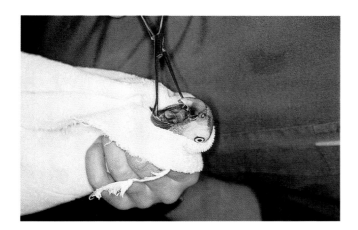

Fig. 7.53 African gray parrot (*Psittacus erithacus*) affected with a sublingual keratoma probably caused by hypovitaminosis A. (Courtesy of Mr. A. D. Malley).

Buccal cavity and pharynx (oropharynx), tongue and salivary glands

Hypovitaminosis A

Hypovitaminosis A (Fig. 7.53) produces metaplasia of salivary and lachrymal gland epithelium and is a common problem in the larger seed-eating Psittaciformes kept on a restricted seed diet. There is evidence that some species, such as the eclectus parrot (*Eclectus roratus*), have a particularly high requirement for this vitamin. Fungal and bacterial infections are usually a sequel to this form of malnutrition. Histologically the lesions are characterized by squamous metaplasia of the epithelium of the salivary gland ducts, which in chronic cases causes occlusion due to formation of the homogenous masses of keratin and necrotic, cellular debris.

Necrosis of mucous membrane

This is associated with *Escherichia coli*, *Pseudomonas* spp., *Mycobacterium avium* and other bacterial infections. These infections can be a sequel to trauma. Trichomonosis (*Trichomonas gallinae* infection) may be a cause, especially in pigeons (Columbidae) and birds of prey (Falconiformes). Can be a sequel to vitamin A deficiency. *Pseudomonas aeruginosa* stomatitis has been recently described in captive saker falcons (*Falco cherrug*) as a sequel to *Trichomonas* infection (Samour, 2000a).

Pox

The virus causes diphtheritic membranes and ulceration on the mucosa. It occurs mainly in Falconiformes,

Galliformes, Columbiformes, Psittaciformes and Passeriformes. It affects birds in other orders less frequently.

The diphtheroid or so-called 'wet pox' which affects the buccal cavity sometimes extends down the pharynx and affects the larynx and even the proximal trachea. This viral infection can also produce a septicemia, especially in small passerines (e.g. the canary (*Serinus canaria*)). It may or may not be associated with the cutaneous form. In psittacines the disease is most common in larger, recently imported birds. In the early stage of 'wet pox' fibrinous exudate lines the buccal mucosa and later becomes grayish-brown and caseous. Focal areas rapidly become confluent so that in advanced cases the entire mucosa is affected. If these caseous lesions are scraped away a bleeding surface with destruction of the epithelium is revealed.

Anatid herpesvirus (duck virus enteritis or duck plague) (Fig. 7.55)

This may cause diphtheritic membranes and ulceration of buccal mucosa, and of mucosa elsewhere in the gastrointestinal tract (see Esophagitis below).

Candidiasis (*Candida albicans* infection)

This occurs secondary to malnutrition (e.g. hypovitaminosis A), prolonged antibiotic therapy or feeding sticky, sloppy food when hand-rearing neonates. It occurs in many species of bird, sometimes associated with *Aspergillus* spp. The diagnosis and a novel treatment of candidiasis in falcons (Falconiformes) in Saudi Arabia was recently described (Samour and Naldo, 2002a).

Mucormycosis of tongue (*Absidia corymbifera* infection)

Sometimes referred to as zygomycosis or phycomycosis, this is secondary to malnutrition and prolonged antibiotic therapy.

Capillaria spp., especially *C. contorta*, infestation

This is rare in psittacines and is more frequently seen in Galliformes and Falconiformes.

Trauma

This may result from a foreign body lodged under the tongue (Fig. 7.54) or in the throat, or by burns.

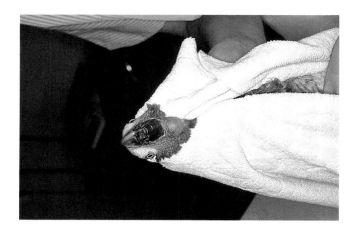

Fig. 7.54 African gray parrot with an abscess of the tongue. Note the rounded swelling at its base on the bird's left side. The anterior part of the tongue is normal. Cause may have been puncture of the tongue by a sharp foreign body. (Courtesy of Mr. A. D. Malley).

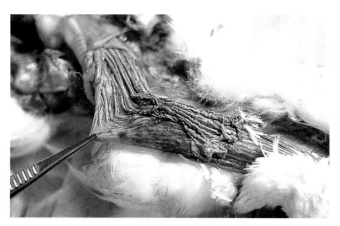

Fig. 7.55 Severe esophagitis due to anatid herpesvirus infection in a mute swan (*Cygnus olor*). Note the reddened, hemorrhagic lesions and the more advanced, brownish-colored, confluent necrotic lesions affecting the longitudinal folds of the esophagus. The virus also causes vascular damage to other areas of the gastrointestinal tract. The esophageal–proventricular junction may appear as a hemorrhagic ring. Free blood is often found in the small intestine of several species of waterfowl. At a later stage, whitish necrotic plaques form on the intestinal mucosa. Cecal lesions also occur and cloacal hemorrhages and/or necrosis are common. Lesions found in swans and geese (*Anser* spp.) differ somewhat from those in ducks (Keymer and Gough, 1986). (Crown copyright).

Hemorrhage

Hemorrhage may be caused by trauma, bacterial infections or a deficiency of vitamin A or K, or of calcium.

Neoplasia

In Psittaciformes this may be fibrosarcoma or squamous cell carcinoma.

The tongues of seed-eating psittacines are short, blunt, smooth and muscular, but those of fruit eaters (e.g. lories (Loridae)), have papillae at the tip that must not be mistaken for lesions.

Halitosis

Halitosis is sometimes clinical evidence of mouth (Fig. 7.54), crop or proventricular lesions, other digestive disorders (see later) and also upper respiratory diseases, especially when this is of bacterial and/or fungal etiology.

Esophagus and crop

Esophagitis, ingluvitis and necrosis

These are caused by mixed bacterial and/or fungal infections, herpesvirus infection in pigeons and duck virus enteritis or anatid herpesvirus infection of waterfowl (Fig. 7.55).

The esophageal and crop necrosis syndrome in budgerigars (*Melopsittacus undulatus*) first reported by Keymer (1958a), which was associated with a mixed bacterial flora, is illustrated by Arnall and Keymer (1975). It is characterized by raised, parallel, yellowish ridges of necrotic material on the mucosa. In severe cases the lesions

may extend from the cervical to the thoracic esophagus and involve most of the crop. It seems likely, in some cases at least, that these lesions are a sequel to trichomonosis. Affected birds usually vomit and have diarrhea. Trichomonosis is an especially important disease of the upper digestive and respiratory tracts in Columbiformes and Falconiformes (Samour and Cooper, 1995; Samour, 2000b; Samour and Naldo, 2003, 2005), in which it is known as 'frounce'. Ingluvial stasis occurs mainly in hand-fed neonates and old, debilitated birds. In avian polyomavirus (APV) of psittacines, including budgerigar fledgling diseases (BFDs), a vesicular degeneration of the epithelium occurs with inclusion body formation. In a recent report comprising 1994–2004 sclerosing ingluvitis was described in 12 avian species including three cockatiels (*Nymphicus hollandicus*), two macaws (*Ara* spp.), two Amazon parrots (*Amazona* spp.), one umbrella cockatoo (*Cacatua alba*), one African gray parrot (*Psittacus erithacus*), one nanday conure (*Nandayus nenday*), one elegant crested tinamou (*Eudromia elegans*) and one domestic fowl (*Gallus gallus* var. *domestica*). The diagnosis was made by histopathology and was characterized by thickening or increase in the density of the serosal tunic of the ingluvies due to fibrosis and neovascularization and, on occasion, edema (Garner, 2005).

Esophageal and/or ingluvial impaction

This is caused by nibbling and ingestion of cloth cage covering in psittacines; extreme debility and malnutrition; and lead poisoning, especially in Anseriformes. Can be a sequel to ingluvial stasis (see below) and cause autointoxication.

Capillaria contorta and other *Capillaria* spp. infestation of the esophagus and/or crop

Rare in psittacines, mainly seen in Falconiformes (Cooper, 1969) and Galliformes.

Esophageal and/or ingluvial candidiasis

See buccal cavity above.

Esophageal and/or ingluvial trichomonosis

See abscessation of buccal cavity above.

Ingluvial calculi (Fig. 7.56)

One example in a budgerigar (*Melopsittacus undulatus*) was of mixed composition (Arnall and Keymer, 1975). Urate calculi may represent ingested urates from the excreta. All types are rare.

Ingluvial stasis (Fig. 7.57)

Associated with bacterial and/or fungal infections, APV including BFD, unsuitable diet and foreign bodies.

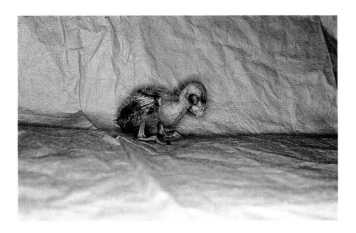

Fig. 7.57 Nestling cockatiel (*Nymphicus hollandicus*) showing gross impaction of the crop. (Courtesy of Mr. A. D. Malley).

Ingluvial inflation

This may be caused by formation of gas due to stasis and bacterial infection.

'Sour crop syndrome'

This is ingluvitis and ulceration of mucosa due to poor quality stale food, or localized bacterial/fungal infections. Also associated with candidiasis Figs 7.58 and 7.59) and trichomonosis. Sequel to stasis.

Pendulous crop

Distension is a sequel to ingluvial stasis and/or inflation. Often associated with Gram-negative bacteria. May get hypertrophy of ingluvial mucosa and flaccidity with slow emptying of crop.

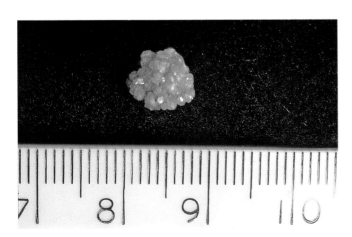

Fig. 7.56 Ingluvial calculus from a budgerigar that contained potassium, phosphates and oxalates and had a strongly cystine-positive reaction. (Courtesy of Mr. G. Dibley).

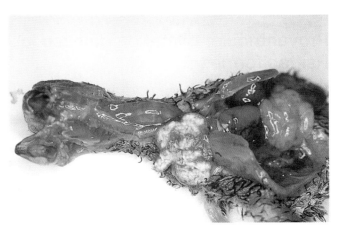

Fig. 7.58 Crop candidiasis in a nestling lorikeet (Family Loriidae). Note the creamy white, necrotic, epithelial material involving the crop mucosa. Less extensive lesions are also present in the buccal cavity. (Courtesy of Mr. A. D. Malley).

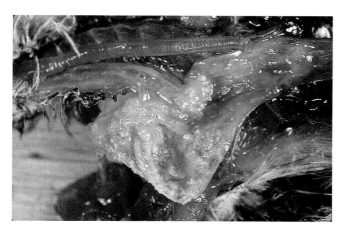

Fig. 7.59 Ingluvial candidiasis in a gray partridge (*Perdix perdix*). The crop epithelium shows extensive necrosis and marked sloughing of yellowish-white, necrotic material.

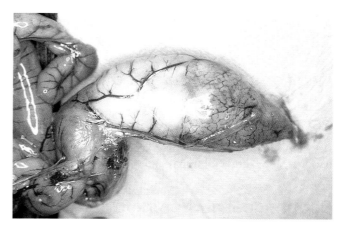

Fig. 7.60 Proventriculus of amazon parrot (*Amazona* sp.) showing dilatation and impaction due to proventricular dilatation disease. A similar appearance can occur in lead poisoning and debilitated birds. (Courtesy of Mr. A. D. Malley).

Regurgitation of crop contents

Courtship display in some healthy psittacine birds (e.g. budgerigars). Represents vomiting in sick birds (multifactorial cause).

Neoplasia

In Psittaciformes this includes leiomyosarcoma and squamous cell carcinoma.

Proventriculus

The proventriculus is the glandular stomach. Regurgitation of the gastric juices may be responsible for some cases of sour crop (see above). In comparison with esophagus and crop, the proventriculus only infrequently shows lesions.

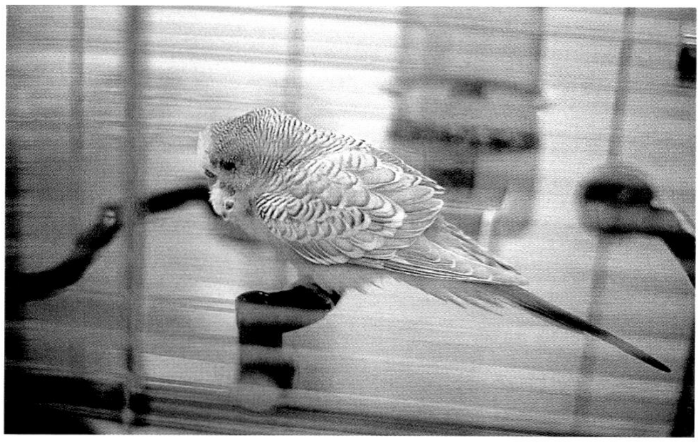

Proventricular dilatation disease in Psittaciformes

Also known as psittacine proventricular dilatation syndrome (PPDS), macaw wasting disease (MWD), neuropathic gastric dilatation, mesenteric ganglio-neuritis and encephalomyelitis, neuropathic gastric dilatation and infiltrative splanchnic neuropathy, this is probably caused by a viral infection.

Proventricular dilatation disease (PDD) is the most important disease of the proventriculus in Psittaciformes (Figs 7.60–7.62). Typical cases show multifocal, lymphocytic leiomyositis, sometimes with lymphocytic infiltration of nerve ganglia. Clinical signs include weight loss, intermittent regurgitation, diarrhea and the presence of undigested seed in the excreta. Neurological signs are

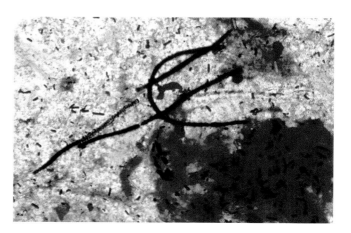

Fig. 7.61 Budgerigar affected with avian gastric yeast. Note fluffed up, depressed appearance with wings held slightly away from the body. (Courtesy of Mr. A. D. Malley)

Fig. 7.62 Avian gastric yeast (*Macrorhabdus ornithogaster*) from the proventriculus of a budgerigar. Gram stain, ×100. (Courtesy of Mr. A. D. Malley).

a sequel, with incoordination and lameness. This disease is characterized histologically by lymphoplasmacytic cell infiltration of the splanchnic nerves of the gastrointestinal tract (Lumeij, 1994; Boutette and Taylor, 2004). Clark (1984) suggested that malnutrition may be an important cause of the proventricular dilatation. He believes that the impaction that occurs in this disease may be associated with rapid swelling of dry seed upon contact with the proventricular secretions. The pressure and ischemia that result may be sufficient to interfere with peristalsis. As few seeds succeed in passing through to the gizzard, the bird continues to eat to satisfy its hunger, leading to further distension of the organ. However, more recent research (Gough and Drury 1996; Gough *et al.*, 1996; Gregory *et al.*, 1997) indicates that an enveloped virus approximately 80 nm in diameter may be the cause of the disease. The possibility that malnutrition may be a predisposing factor cannot be excluded.

Although this disease appears to affect mainly psittacine birds, an interesting case of PDD was recently reported in a peregrine falcon (*Falco peregrinus*) (Shivaprasad *et al.*, 2005). This appears to be the first report of this disease in birds of prey.

Proventricular and gizzard impaction (Figs 7.63 and 7.64)

In addition to causing impaction in Psittaciformes, PDD has also been suspected in individual species of non-psittacines (i.e. Ciconiiformes, Anseriformes, Piciformes and Passeriformes). Impactions can also be associated with lead poisoning, malnutrition, bacterial and/or fungal infections and occasionally parasitism.

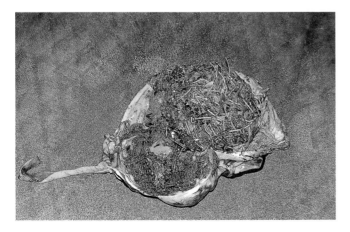

Fig. 7.63 Proventricular and gizzard impaction in a 3-month-old ostrich chick caused by repeated ingestion of coarse and fibrous vegetable matter. (Courtesy of Dr. U. Wernery).

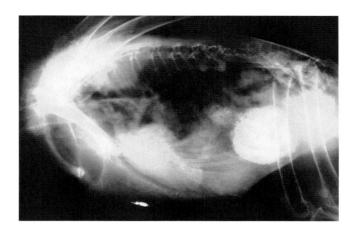

Fig. 7.64 Laterolateral radiograph of a saker falcon (*Falco cherrug*) showing severe impaction of the ventriculus with fine desert sand. In the Middle East, falcons are commonly fed on their blocks. However, it is common for falcons to take the food to the floor and ingest fine sand adhered to the food leading to impaction. (Courtesy of Dr. J. Samour).

Candidiasis (*Candida albicans* infection)

Candidiasis is uncommon in psittacines and is usually an extension of the infection from the crop and the thoracic esophagus.

Stomach (Proventriculus) worm infestation (Fig. 7.65)

This occurs mainly in the following: Struthioniformes (ostriches), *Libostrongylus* (= *Ornithostrongylus*) *douglassi*; Pelecaniformes and Charadriiformes, *Contracaecum* spp.; Anseriformes, *Echinuria* spp.; Columbiformes, *Tetrameres fissipina* and *Dispharynx nasuta*; and Psittaciformes, *Synhimantus (Dispharynx) nasuta* (several synonyms; also known as *Spirura incerta, Habronema incertum* and *Cyrnea incerta*).

Stomach worms are confined almost entirely to recently imported, free-living birds. Considerable confusion exists regarding the nomenclature of these nematodes in psittacines. Helminthological taxonomists, especially in the past, have changed not only the species names but also the genera of these worms. Veterinarians are also often guilty of causing confusion by not having the parasites accurately identified by helminthologists. According to Linda Gibbons, International Institute of Parasitology, St Albans, UK (personal communication, 1991), the genus *Spiroptera* is now obsolete and worms in that genus have now been allocated to either *Acuaria* or *Spirura*. This means that *Spiroptera incerta* referred to by Keymer (1982) and by Shanthikumar (1987), is now *Spirura incerta*. The genus *Dispharynx* has been relegated to a subgenus of the genus *Synhimantus* and should therefore be shown in parentheses following the genus name. According to

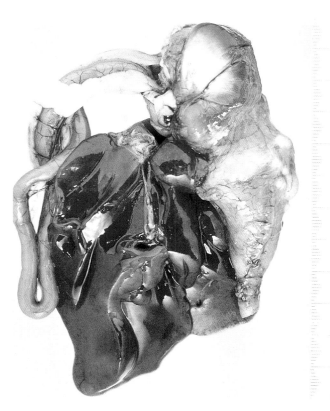

Fig. 7.65 Mallard duck (*Anas platyrhynchos*). Distension and partial impaction of proventriculus (stomach) caused by infestation with the nematode *Echinuria* (Syn. *Acuaria*) sp. (Courtesy of Mr. T. Dennett, Zoological Society of London).

Shanthikumar, *Synhimantus (Dispharynx) nasuta* occurs in budgerigars and other psittacines. However, as all stomach worms require an intermediate, invertebrate host they will only be found in free-living and recently captured birds or in those kept in outdoor aviaries with soil and growing plants.

Atony

In Psittaciformes it is often associated with stasis of the crop leading to autointoxication. It is a typical finding in lead poisoning (see Esophagus and crop, above).

Hypertrophy of unknown etiology

This occurs in macaws (*Ara* spp.) and cockatoos (*Cacatua* spp.).

Proventriculitis

This is associated with avian gastric yeast (*Macrorhabdus ornithogaster*) especially in Psittaciformes and less frequently in Passeriformes and birds in other orders. The cause was originally attributed to Megabacteria. Viruses (e.g. adenovirus), may be involved. Contributory factors may be dietary deficiencies, especially hypovitaminosis A.

Foreign bodies

Seen especially in Struthioniformes and Rheiformes, but also in others such as Anseriformes, Galliformes, Psittaciformes and Passeriformes.

Neoplasia

In Psittaciformes: adenocarcinoma.

Gizzard or ventriculus

Gizzard lesions are relatively uncommon.

Proventricular dilatation disease

See Proventriculus, above.

Erosion of koilin lining

Possible nutritional causes and foreign bodies. Excessive ingestion of very sharp, fine sand in Psittaciformes. Erosion of the koilin layer, especially at the proventricular junction, may be caused by hypovitaminosis A or by eating highly polyunsaturated fatty acids, such as those present in cod liver oil, when these are not protected by an adequate dietary level of vitamin E.

Stomach worm infestation

See also Proventriculus, above. *Amidostomum anseris* infestation occurs in goslings (Anseriformes) (Fig. 7.66). The nematode *Porrocaecum ensicaudatum* has been reported by Burr (1982) as occurring in the gizzard of

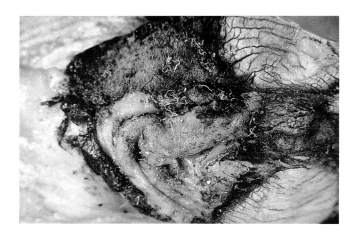

Fig. 7.66 Gizzard worm (*Amidostomum anseris*) in a goose (*Anser* sp.). The whitish, thread-like nematodes are clearly visible and have caused considerable damage to the bile- and blood-stained, blackish koilin layer of the ventriculus. (Crown copyright).

Psittaciformes. However, this may be an example of incorrect identification, because the parasite is normally found in the small intestine of passerine birds (Keymer, 1982).

Muscular atrophy

Possible vitamin E and selenium deficiency.

Mycotic malfunction syndrome

Fungi species penetrating wall of gizzard.

Traumatic ventriculitis

Perforation and/or erosions and ulcerations (see also Proventriculus, above) of the koilin layer ('horny lining'), caused by foreign bodies such as pieces of cage wire. Sometimes, because of the muscular action of the gizzard, sharp objects penetrate and perforate the wall and cause peritonitis.

Hemosporidiosis

In Psittaciformes, megaloschizonts occur in the gizzard musculature. The precise identification is uncertain and they are variously attributed to *Leucocytozoon*, *Akiba* or *Haemoproteus* spp.

Neoplasia

In Psittaciformes, neoplasia confined to the gizzard is uncommon: e.g. a mucus-secreting adenocarcinoma in the gizzard of a purple capped lory (*Domicella domicella*) recorded by Appleby and Keymer (1971) and an adenoma in a vernal hanging parrot (*Loriculus vernalis*) by Griner (1983). (Figs 7.67–7.73)

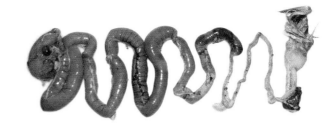

Fig. 7.68 Severe impaction of the intestinal tract in a peregrine falcon (*Falco peregrinus*). The impaction was caused by the formation of a solid fecal pellet formed by sand, feather particles and dried feces. The falcon was severely dehydrated.

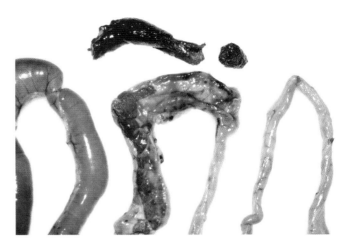

Fig. 7.69 Dissection of the impacted intestinal tract of the same falcon as in Fig. 7.68 showing the pellet responsible for the impaction and a cross-section of the pellet.

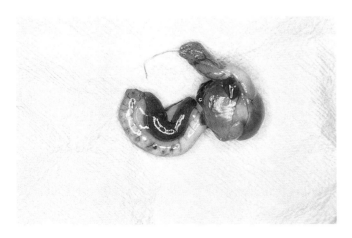

Fig. 7.67 Splendid parakeet (*Neophema splendida*) showing impaction of the proximal loop of the duodenum and intense congestion of the distal loop associated with pseudomoniasis. (Courtesy of Mr. A. D. Malley).

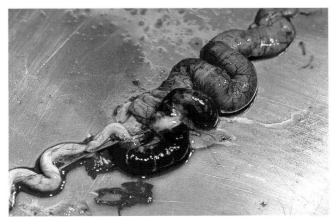

Fig. 7.70 Intussusception or invagination of a segment of the large intestine in a 6-month-old ostrich. Note the highly congested and almost necrotic intestinal loop. (Courtesy of Dr. U. Wernery).

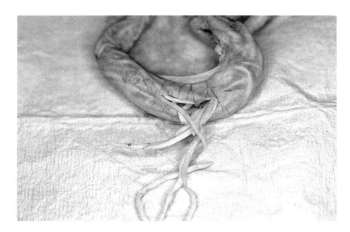

Fig. 7.71 Splendid parakeet. The small intestine is impacted with numerous roundworms (*Ascaridia* spp.). (Courtesy of Mr. A. D. Malley).

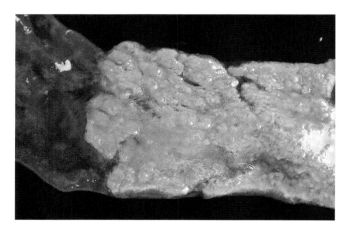

Fig. 7.72 Toucan (*Ramphastos* spp.). Severe diphtheritic enteritis of the small intestine caused by a heavy infestation of threadworm (*Capillaria* spp.). Note the yellowish-white necrotic diphtheritic membrane covering most of the mucosa, the exposed adjacent part of which shows intense reddening and congestion of the epithelial surface. (Courtesy of Mr. T. Dennett, Zoological Society of London).

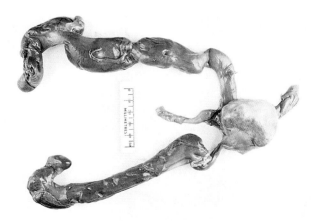

Fig. 7.73 Tuberculosis (*Mycobacterium avium* infection) showing a large, rounded and sessile caseous necrotic lesion involving the ileocecal junction of a peafowl (*Pavo cristatus*). Note the presence of well developed ceca. (Courtesy of Mr. T. Dennett, Zoological Society of London).

Intestine, including ceca

Figures 7.67–7.78 give some examples of intestinal disorders.

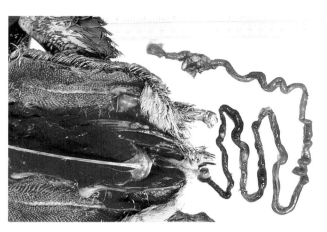

Fig. 7.74 Intestinal tuberculosis (*Mycobacterium avium* infection) showing widely scattered, multiple, necrotic nodules involving the gut of a guillemot (*Uria aalge*). Both the mucosa and wall of the intestine were affected. Note absence of ceca. The alimentary tract, anterior to the duodenum, has been removed. (Courtesy of Mr. T. Dennett, Zoological Society of London).

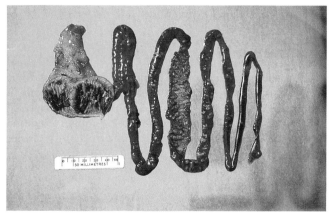

Fig. 7.75 Salmonellosis (*Salmonella typhimurium* infection) involving the intestinal tract of a macaw (*Ara* sp.). The mucosa of the proventriculus is slightly reddened but the duodenum and pancreas, and the remainder of the intestinal tract, are purplish-black in color. The intestinal epithelium was found to be markedly congested and multiple, mainly discrete, necrotic nodules were found throughout the intestinal tract. Many of these are visible through the intestinal wall, as well as on the mucosal surface where the gut has been opened. The gizzard is empty and shows greenish bile staining of the koilin layer. Note the absence of ceca. (Courtesy of Mr. T. Dennett, Zoological Society of London).

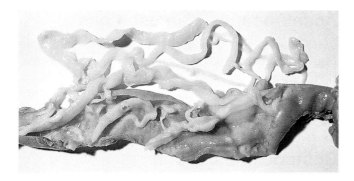

Fig. 7.76 Great crested grebe (*Podiceps cristatus*). Portion of small intestine opened to reveal a heavy infestation of cestodes (species not identified). This bird was in good condition and was killed accidentally. There was no evidence that the tapeworms were playing a pathogenic role.

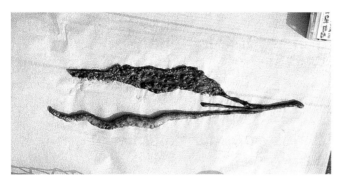

Fig. 7.77 Nodular typhlitis (*Heterakis isolonche* infestation) in a brown-eared pheasant (*Crossoptilon mantchuricum*). Both ceca are severely affected by the formation of nodules in the cecal wall, which are visible exteriorly. These nodules contain the parasite imbedded in proliferative connective tissue. (Crown copyright).

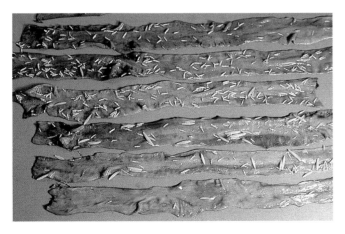

Fig. 7.78 Mute swan. The small intestine has been opened to reveal a heavy infestation of Acanthocephalid or thorny-headed worm (species not identified). These worms require an aquatic, invertebrate intermediate host and can be pathogenic. (Courtesy of Mr. A. Hunt).

Bacterial infections

Salmonellosis (*Salmonella* spp., especially *S. typhimurium* infection) (Fig. 7.75); *Escherichia coli* infection; pasteurellosis (*Pasteurella* spp. infection); yersiniosis (*Yersinia pseudotuberculosis* and rarely *Y. enterocolitica* infections); tuberculosis (*Mycobacterium avium* in all avian orders (Figs 7.73–7.74) and *M. tuberculosis* and *M. bovis* infections in Psittaciformes); pseudomoniasis (*Pseudomonas aeruginosa* infection, Fig. 7.74); aeromoniasis (*Aeromonas hydrophila* infection); necrotic enteritis associated with *Clostridium* spp. in rainbow lorikeets (*Trichoglossus haematodus*) (see below); and chlamydiosis or psittacosis (*Chlamydophila psittaci* infection). The role of other organisms in enteric infections of the Psittaciformes (e.g. *Campylobacter jejuni* and *Serratia* and *Citrobacter* spp.) is unclear. Almost all these bacteria, with the exception of *M. tuberculosis* and *M. bovis*, infect most other avian species. Clostridial enteritis caused by *Clostridium perfringens* is well known in Galliformes but *C. colinum* is the cause in quail (*Colinus virginianus* and *Coturnix coturnix*). *C. perfringens* infection has also been recorded in Sphenisciformes, Columbiformes and Passeriformes. Typhlitis caused by *Treponema* spp. also occurs occasionally in other species (e.g. Galliformes and Anseriformes). In order to assess the pathogenicity of bacteria, much more study is needed on normal flora of the gut of birds.

Viral infections

In Psittaciformes, these include paramyxovirus (PMV) group 1 (Newcastle disease), group 5 (Kunitachi virus of budgerigars) and possibly groups 2 and 3; and Pacheco's disease (herpesvirus) causing hemorrhagic diarrhea and suspected viral (enterovirus-like) enteritis in cockatoos (*Cacatua* spp.). Anatid herpesvirus enteritis with cloacitis occurs in Anseriformes; adenovirus in psittacines and pigeons; rotavirus enteritis in pheasants (*Phasianus colchicus*); and possibly reoviruses in some species.

Although the pathogenicity of most species of bacteria as a cause of enteritis is well known, the same cannot be said for viruses, especially coronaviruses, reoviruses and rotaviruses. An example of viral enteritis in free-living cockatoos, thought to be caused by an enterovirus-like agent, has been reported by McOrist (1991). It was encountered in galahs (*Eolophus roseicapilla*) and in sulfur-crested cockatoos (*C. galerita*). Clinical signs were diarrhea and weight loss. At necropsy the duodenum was found to be distended with yellow liquid. Histological examination revealed proliferation of crypts and villus stunting. Small intracytoplasmic inclusion bodies of an enterovirus were found in the enterocytes on electron microscopy. Circovirus-like particles have been found (associated with 'watery' droppings) in the cloacal bursae of young pigeons (*Columba livia*), but their etiological role has not been established (Gough and Drury, 1996).

Avian virology is a rapidly expanding field of study. For further information regarding viral infections of the digestive system, the reader should consult the relevant textbooks mentioned in the introductory paragraphs. More research is needed concerning the pathogenicity of avian viruses, especially in psittacines and other non-gallinaceous birds.

Fungal infection

Candida albicans infection.

Protozoal infection

Giardiasis (*Giardia* spp. infection) occurs especially in Psittaciformes nestlings but also in Anseriformes and Galliformes; hexamitiasis (*Hexamita* spp. infection) occurs in Galliformes, Columbiformes and more rarely Psittaciformes, including budgerigars; so-called protozoan dysentery associated with *Hexamita, Trichomonas* and *Blastocystis* spp. occurs in game birds (Galliformes); and coccidiosis (*Eimeria* and *Isospora* spp. infections) occurs mostly in Galliformes but also in several other orders (e.g. Anseriformes, Columbiformes and Psittaciformes). Microsporidiosis is occasionally recorded in Psittaciformes. *Histomonas meleagridis* causes typhlitis and hepatitis in some gallinaceous birds (see Liver, below). Cochlosomiasis (*Cochlosoma* spp.) in Passeriformes.

Giardiasis is stated by Fudge (1991) to be very common in cockatiels in North America. Coccidiosis in Psittaciformes is a frequent, but incorrect, diagnosis made by laymen, probably because it is common in poultry and game birds. The first confirmed record of the infection in Psittaciformes appears to be that made by Keymer (1958b), who identified an *Eimeria* sp. in a budgerigar. The parasite was found 2 years later by Farr (1960) in Mexico and named *Eimeria dunsingi*. Since then, coccidiosis has been recorded in other psittacines but it remains an uncommon disease. However, it is likely that many birds have subclinical infections over a long period of time, as suggested by Hooimeijer and Fortune (1991), who found an *Eimeria* sp. in a blue-fronted Amazon parrot (*Amazona aestiva*) that had been totally isolated for over 2 years.

Nematode infestation

This includes *Ascaridia* spp., especially *Ascaridia hermaphrodita*, in the small intestine of Psittaciformes (Fig. 7.71); *Capillaria* spp. infestations of small intestine in Psittaciformes and some other orders (Fig. 7.72); *Ascaridia columbae, Capillaria columbae* and *C. longicollis* in pigeons; *Heterakis gallinae* infestation of ceca in several species of Galliformes and *H. isolonche* in peafowl (*Pavo* spp.) and some species of pheasant (Phasianinae). (Fig. 7.77) Numerous other nematodes occur in all avian species.

Acanthocephalid infestations

Mediorhynchus grande in a varied lorikeet (*Trichoglossus: Psitteuteles versicolor*) was reported by Shanthikumar (1987). Acanthocephalids are very rare in psittacines. Waterfowl are common hosts but (Fig. 7.78) these worms also infest many species of the Passeriformes and birds of prey (Falconiformes).

Cestode infestations

Several species occur in Psittaciformes but *Raillietina* spp. are probably the most common. Cestodes sometimes cause impactions of the gut, being especially prevalent in African gray parrots (*Psittacus erithacus*) and cockatoos (*Cacatua* spp.). A considerable number of species occur in a wide variety of birds, the genera *Dilepis* and *Choanotaenia* being particularly common in Passeriformes, *Raillietina* in Galliformes and Columbiformes, and *Hymenolepis* in Anseriformes.

Trematode infestations

These are rarely encountered in Psittaciformes, the incidence of infestation being highest in Anseriformes and other aquatic species.

Villous atrophy/malabsorption syndrome

Chronic, often fatal disease, associated with weight loss in budgerigars. Villous atrophy leading to a malabsorption syndrome has been described in budgerigars by Baker (1985). The only gross post-mortem finding was a dilatation of the proximal two-thirds of the intestine. The intestinal contents may be normal or slightly mucoid. However, histological examinations initially reveal a massive inflammatory reaction, which fills and grossly distends the lamina propria of the villi. The inflammatory cells are predominantly lymphocytes, with a smaller number of plasma cells. This inflammatory reaction persists and the villi become shortened and tend to fuse. The crypts increase both in size and in the number of cells lining them. It is thought that this state can persist for months. In long-standing cases apparently normal mucosal cells become replaced by goblet cells. Eventually the disease can lead to death. The cause of the disease is unknown. However, it is reported to resemble immunoproliferative disease of the small intestine of Basenji dogs and therefore an immune reaction may play a role.

Volvulus

Uncommon, but reported in Struthioniformes (Wade, 1992).

Nonspecific enteropathies

These cause enteritis and diarrhea. 'Enteritis' is probably the most common disease referred to in books on cage and aviary birds written by bird fanciers and other non-veterinarians. In fact, proven enteritis as a specific entity is not as common as is generally believed. This is because, at post-mortem examination, the intestinal tract is often too autolyzed for enteritis to be confirmed histopathologically and diarrhea is not necessarily indicative of enteritis, as is frequently assumed by non-veterinarians. In some species of bird the normal appearance of feces is sometimes mistaken for diarrhea. It is essential, therefore, for the clinician to be aware of the appearance of the normal excreta for the species being examined (e.g. frugivorous species have fluid droppings). In addition to enteritis, diarrhea can be associated with liver disease. Visceral gout and renal disorders also often cause excessive excretion of urates, and this can be mistaken for diarrhea. Pressure on the gut from abdominal neoplasms, especially in budgerigars, can produce signs of diarrhea. Although true enteritis can be associated with dietary disorders, it is usually due to septicemias caused by bacterial and viral infections. It also occurs in protozoal infections of the gut (see above) and is sometimes caused by helminths, especially *Capillaria* spp. In psittacines *Ascaridia* spp. are more likely to cause intestinal impaction than enteritis. This is because the worms usually occur in the duodenum and upper jejunum, where in psittacines the lumen of the gut is wider than it is more caudally.

McOrist (1991) has recorded a necrotic enteritis in free-living rainbow lorikeets in Australia. Bacteria of the *Clostridium perfringens* complex were thought to be the cause. At necropsy, the disease was characterized by acute dilatation and inflammation of the small intestine. Histological examination revealed 'acute mucosal necrosis and inflammation, with rows of clostridial bacteria attached to the luminal surface of villus enterocytes'. Although clostridial enteritis is well known in some gallinaceous species, it appears to be rare in psittacines. Indeed, most of the bacterial infections listed above are well known in other species of birds. However, aeromoniasis is an exception, being better known as a disease of amphibians and fish. It has been described in cockatiels (*Nymphicus hollandicus*) by Panigrahy *et al.* (1981).

One common type of enteropathy is that seen in recently imported small Psittaciformes and Passeriformes (G. Jackson and I. F. Keymer, unpublished data). It appears to be linked to stress and probably hypoglycemia. Birds die in reasonably good bodily condition with a contracted and usually empty gizzard. The small intestine contains black mucoid material and digested or partially digested blood. This syndrome appears to follow starvation as the result of receiving no food for several hours or following a change of diet that is unfamiliar and unacceptable to the bird. The intestinal mucosa is frequently hemorrhagic in appearance. On bacteriological examination, non-hemolytic *Escherichia coli* can usually be isolated in pure culture.

Intestinal perforation frequently leads to peritonitis. Causes include foreign bodies of many kinds; heavy infestations of *Ascaridia* spp. (especially in Australian parakeets), other nematodes and cestodes.

Impaction of the colorectum

Usually secondary to impactions of the oviduct, including 'egg binding' and renal neoplasia.

Enterolithiasis

A rare condition that has been observed by Kollias *et al.* (1984). An umbrella cockatoo (*Cacatua alba*) was found to have an enterolith weighing 11.5 g in the lumen of the duodenal flexure. It was subcrystalline in texture and contained a high proportion of oxalates.

Rectal prolapse

Caused by straining, resulting also in prolapse of the cloaca (see below). Secondary to intestinal disorders and others.

Neoplasia

In Psittaciformes: adenocarcinoma, leiomyosarcoma.

Pancreas

The pancreas is enclosed by the duodenal loop and has both endocrine and exocrine functions. For endocrine malfunction of the pancreas the reader should refer to the section on Endocrine disorders. Diseases of the pancreas in Psittaciformes are relatively rare but are becoming recognized more frequently with the increasing use of blood chemistry in clinical diagnosis.

Pancreatitis

Inclusion body pancreatitis (IBP) appears to have been first described by Wallner-Pendleton *et al.* (1983) in love birds (*Agapornis* sp.). It is believed to be caused by an adenovirus. Adenoviruses also cause pancreatitis in some species of Galliformes. Other viruses causing pancreatitis are paramyxovirus 1 in domestic pigeons; paramyxovirus 3 in Psittaciformes (*Neophema* spp., see Atrophy below); avian influenza viruses in some Galliformes; Herpesvirus in Psittaciformes; and anatid Herpesvirus in Anseriformes. Pancreatitis often causes polyuria.

Acute pancreatic necrosis

Unknown cause. An acute pancreatic necrosis has been described by Pass *et al.* (1986) in galahs or roseate cockatoos. The lesions are stated to differ considerably from those of IBP and involve massive necrosis of both the endocrine and exocrine tissues. Affected birds are very fat and the pancreas becomes swollen and edematous. Calcium salts are found in the necrotic tissue. Lesions were also present in the abdominal fat, liver and spleen. The precise cause was not ascertained, although the lesions were believed to be due to the release of pancreatic proteolytic enzymes into tissues and the circulation.

Diabetes mellitus

This was infrequently diagnosed until relatively recently (see Endocrine Disorders, below).

Atrophy

Pancreatic atrophy appears to have been first recognized by Beach (1962) in a budgerigar. The signs shown by the bird suggested exocrine rather than endocrine dysfunction. In the early 1980s in England, Keymer (unpublished data) found pathological lesions associated with atrophy of the organ in splendid parakeets (*Neophema splendida*). The lesions were very extensive. In three birds a severe pancreatitis was present, which appeared to be primary and may have resulted in the eventual atrophy. There was severe mononuclear cell and some fibroblast infiltration of the interstitial tissues. The infiltrating cells were mainly lymphocytes and plasma cells. Very few granulocytes were present. Acinar cells showed some loss of zymogen granules. Attempts to isolate a virus using embryonating domestic fowls' eggs and tissue culture were unsuccessful. Simpson (1993) recorded similar findings in *Neophema* spp. and strongly suspected the cause of the pancreatitis to be PMV-3 infection as found by workers in Belgium and the Netherlands. Since the record by Beach (1962), pancreatic atrophy has also been described by Hasholt (1972) and Quesenberry and Liu (1986). The lesions described by the latter workers are not unlike the infectious stunting syndrome of broiler chickens, according to C. J. Randall (personal communication, 1986). Obviously, more investigations are needed in order to ascertain the precise causes of pancreatic disease in psittacines. Recently, a case of pancreatic atrophy in a peregrine falcon (*Falco peregrinus*) was described. The falcon was presented with a history of progressive weight loss despite a normal food intake. The bird was admitted for treatment but continued losing weight despite the provision of two meals a days. Blood chemistry revealed a serum amylase of 2508 U/l (normal range 350–1050 U/l). By day 10, the falcon started showing signs of coprophagia, eating any fecal pellet as soon as it was passed. The falcon died immediately after, without having any specific treatment instituted (Samour and Naldo, 2002b).

Neoplasia

In Psittaciformes: embryonal nephroma, adenoma, islet cell carcinoma. Adenocarcinoma also in Columbiformes and Anseriformes.

Cloaca

Cloacitis

Frequently a sequel to chronic oviductitis, enteritis, digestive and/or renal disorders, and seldom primary. It may lead to so-called 'pasting of the vent' or 'vent gleet'. The feathers become matted with excreta around the cloaca. In budgerigars this is known as 'wet vent' and has a multifactorial etiology (Baker, 1987).

'Vent gleet' (cloacitis)

Associated with intestinal infections of bacteria, protozoa and other intestinal disorders. Synonymous with other lay terms: 'wet vent' and 'pasting of the vent'.

Prolapse

Caused by straining (Figs 7.79 and 7.80). Associated with chronic intestinal impactions, infections and irritations; foreign bodies in the alimentary tract, oviductitis; egg binding, pressure of intra-abdominal tumors; cloacal papilloma; and occasionally urate calculi (cloacaliths).

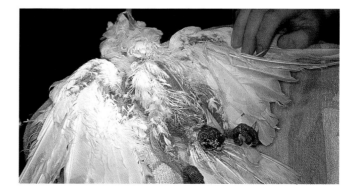

Fig. 7.79 Cockatoo (*Cacatua* sp.), showing prolapse of the cloaca. The mucosa is reddened, indicating intense congestion. Excreta covers the cloacal orifice. (Courtesy of Mr. A. D. Malley).

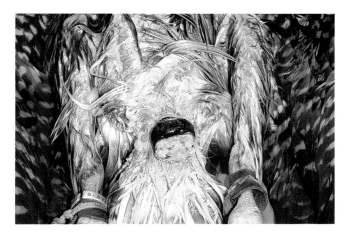

Fig. 7.80 Cloacal prolapse in a peregrine falcon. Note the severe 'burning' of the mucosal membrane due to the long-term contact with feces and urates. (Courtesy of Dr. J. Samour).

Liver

Gross lesions in the liver are seldom diagnostic. Hepatomegaly occurs in numerous infectious diseases, especially in *Chlamydophila psittaci* infection. However, histopathological examination can be more revealing, especially if special stains are used. Without the use of endoscopy, most liver disorders are difficult to diagnose in the live bird unless the enlarged liver causes distension of the abdomen or biochemical tests produce significant results. Figures 7.82–7.86 illustrate a variety of liver disorders.

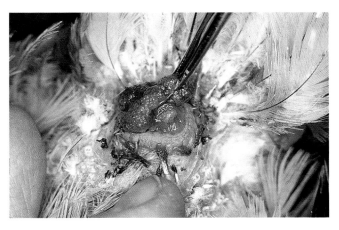

Fig. 7.81 Cloacal papilloma affecting an amazon parrot (*Amazona* sp.). Note the lobulated appearance with multiple small, raised, rounded areas visible beneath the surface of the lobules producing a cauliflower-like appearance. (Courtesy of Mr. A. D. Malley.)

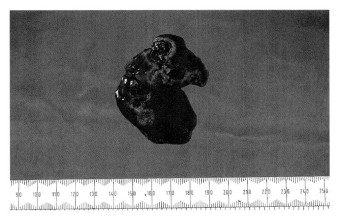

Fig. 7.82 Histomoniasis (*Histomonas meleagridis* infection) affecting the liver of a gray jungle fowl (*Gallus sonneratii*). Note the large, discrete and partly confluent, pale-yellowish, rounded areas of necrosis with dark centers. The lesions are similar to hepatic trichomonosis in Columbidae (see Fig. 7.84). (Courtesy of Mr. T. Dennett, Zoological Society of London).

Neoplasia

In Psittaciformes: cloacal papilloma (common; Fig. 7.81), adenocarcinoma, adenomatous polyp, undifferentiated sarcoma.

Papillomata are especially prevalent in conures (i.e. many species of the subfamily Psittacinae of the family Psittacidae), macaws (mainly *Ara* spp.), cockatoos (*Cacatua* spp.) and Amazon (*Amazona* spp.) parrots. Papillomata appear macroscopically as protruding swellings. In Psittaciformes they contain mucin-producing cells, in contrast to lesions induced by papillomaviruses in mammals that are formed by squamous cells. Sunberg *et al.* (1986) believed that papillomata in psittacines 'may not be caused by an infective agent' but by irritation of the cloacal mucosa. This results in hypertrophy and hyperplasia of the lining epithelium and may initiate the formation of papilloma.

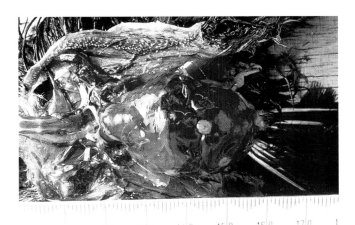

Fig. 7.83 Hepatic carcinoma. Black tanager (*Buthraupis melanochlamys*). Note the considerable enlargement and lobulated appearance of the liver and the presence of two rounded, slightly raised, whitish, cyst-like structures. Gelatinous material covers the anterior part of the liver distal to the heart. (Courtesy of Mr. T. Dennett, Zoological Society of London).

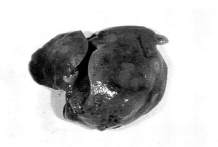

Fig. 7.84 Liver from a pigeon (*Columba livia*) showing lesions due to trichomonosis (*Trichomonas gallinae* infection). Lesions of this disease occur typically in the upper digestive tract and less frequently in the liver. The organ shows multiple, rounded areas of necrosis. The lesions are discrete or partly confluent. They usually have dark centers with a pale periphery, as can be seen in the smaller focal lesions. On gross appearance these lesions are similar to histomoniasis (*Histomonas meleagridis* infection), which appears to be confined to gallinaceous species. The overall dark coloration of the organ is due to autolysis.

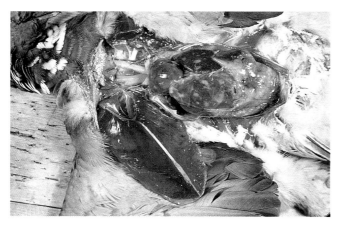

Fig. 7.85 Tuberculosis (*Mycobacterium* sp. infection) in a wood pigeon (*Columba palumbus*). The bird shows atrophy of the pectoral muscles and multiple yellowish-white, necrotic foci of varying sizes (mostly rounded in shape) throughout the liver. A sheet of fibrinous material covers the right lobe and the coils of the intestinal tract.

Bacterial infections

All the bacteria listed as intestinal pathogens are known to be capable of causing hepatitis in most species of bird, although infections with *Mycobacterium bovis* and *M. tuberculosis* appear to be confined to Psittaciformes. *M. avium* appears to infect birds in all orders. Other bacteria capable of causing hepatitis include *Pseudomonas pseudomallei,* causing melioidosis in Psittaciformes and a wide range of bacteria in other avian orders, including infections by *Erysipelothrix rhusiopathiae* (erysipelas); *Staphylococcus* spp., especially *S. aureus; Streptococcus* spp., including *S. bovis* in pigeons; and *Clostridium perfringens,* especially in Galliformes. Much more research needs to be done concerning the host range of *Campylobacter jejuni* infections. Hepatitis has been reported by Lawrence (1988) to occur with *C. jejuni* infection. However, little appears to be known about this infection in birds and more research is needed.

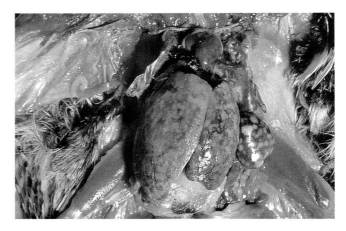

Fig. 7.86 Tuberculosis (*Mycobacterium* sp. infection) in a pheasant (*Phasianus colchicus*). The liver shows extensive areas of necrosis. The lesions in the spleen are more discrete and less confluent than in the liver. The lardaceous, rather swollen appearance of the liver (especially the right lobe) is due to amyloidosis.

Viral infections

In Psittaciformes these include: Pacheco's disease, caused by a herpesvirus; avian polyomavirus (APV including BFD); acute PBFD (circovirus infection); adenovirus inclusion body hepatitis (IBH); reovirus-associated hepatitis (A. A. Cunningham, personal communication, 1991); and suspected adenovirus and CELO virus infections. Vereecken *et al.* (1988) have reviewed adenovirus infection in pigeons. Falconiformes: IBH (herpesvirus infection) and possibly adenovirus. Columbiformes, Strigiformes and a few other orders: Herpesvirus. Anseriformes: goose virus hepatitis (parvovirus infection); and Galliformes: Marek's disease (herpesvirus infection), also suspected in a few other orders. Wheler (1993) has reviewed herpesvirus disease causing hepatosplenitis in a wide range of birds of several orders. Passeriformes: canary circovirus infection causing enlarged gallbladder and abdominal distension; and cytomegalovirus infection of Australian finches.

An inclusion body hepatitis has been described by Ramis *et al.* (1991) in a group of eclectus parrots. They provided evidence that this may have been the first report of an outbreak of avian adenovirus IBH in psittacines.

Fungal infections

Aspergillosis (usually *Aspergillus fumigatus* infection); aflatoxicosis or mycotoxicosis associated with eating moldy food contaminated with *Aspergillus flavus, Fusarium tricinctum*, etc. Lesions are characterized by bile duct hyperplasia and sometimes cirrhosis. Cryptococcosis (*Cryptococcus neoformans* infection) in kiwis (*Apteryx australis*) (Randall and Reece, 1996).

Trematodiasis

Liver and bile duct infestations with *Platynosomum* spp. in cockatoos (*Cacatua* spp.); 'Schistosomiasis' in the budgerigar. Very rare infestations.

Histomoniasis

Histomonas meleagridis infection: used to be a well-known cause of 'blackhead' in free-range domestic turkeys (*Meleagris gallopavo*). It is carried by the cecal worm *Heterakis gallinarum* and is occasionally encountered in jungle fowl (*Gallus* spp.) and peafowl, in which it also causes typhlitis (Fig. 7.82).

Trichomonosis

Trichomonas gallinae infection: sometimes causes focal necrosis of liver in pigeons (Fig. 7.84).

Lipidosis, fatty infiltration or degeneration

Common in budgerigars and cockatiels. Reported in many species in many orders. Multifactorial etiology but usually dietetic. Fatty liver–kidney syndrome (FLKS) of unknown etiology has been described in merlins (*Falco columbarius*) and reviewed in other species by Forbes and Cooper (1993). It is a well-known metabolic disorder of domestic fowl chicks, in which species a contributory cause may be biotin deficiency. The yellowish liver and musculature often seen in gouldian finches (*Choebia gouldiae*) resembles jaundice but this may not be correct, because using the Rimington test the results indicated that the yellow coloration is probably due to carotene (I. F. Keymer, unpublished data).

Hemochromatosis or iron storage disease

This is defined as excess iron in the liver accompanied by altered tissue storage morphology or function (Lowenstine and Petrak, 1980). It is especially common and severe in captive mynah birds (*Acridotheres* spp.). Other species are sometimes affected, including toucans and psittacines. Hemosiderosis is the deposition of hemosiderin in hepatocyte cytoplasm and Kupffer's cells, producing no evidence of pathogenicity. It occurs in many species of birds. Reduction of hepatocellular hemosiderin content in toco toucans (*Ramphastos toco*) with iron storage disease has been successfully achieved through chelation therapy (Cornelissen *et al.*, 1995) or dietary modification (Drews *et al.*, 2004).

Visceral gout

Whitish urate deposits on the hepatic capsule (Figs 7.87 and 7.88). A similar appearance may occur following injection of pentobarbital sodium.

Amyloidosis

Seen in some chronic infections (e.g. aspergillosis, tuberculosis, bumblefoot), especially in Anseriformes, Galliformes and Falconiformes (Figs 7.89 and 7.90). In Anseriformes also associated with stress.

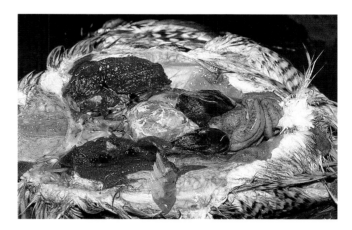

Fig. 7.87 Visceral gout in a hybrid gyr/saker falcon. Gout is a metabolic disorder caused primarily by kidney malfunction usually associated with urinary tract disease, prolonged dehydration, exogenous stressors and nutritional disorders, such as excessive intake of protein and calcium and vitamin–mineral deficiencies. In Falconiformes, this disorder has recently been associated with *Clostridium perfringens* infection. Note the whitish uric acid crystals deposited on the pericardium. (Courtesy of Dr. U. Wernery).

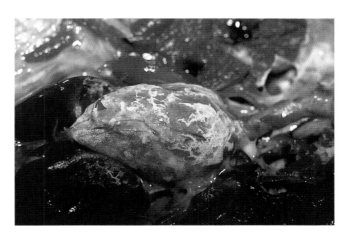

Fig. 7.88 Close-up view of the same specimen as in Fig. 7.87. (Courtesy of Dr. U. Wernery).

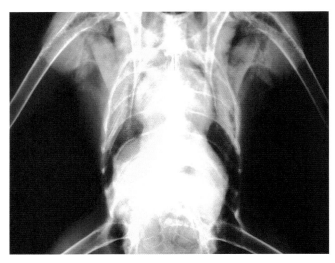

Fig. 7.89 Ventrodorsal radiograph of a gyrfalcon (*Falco rusticolus*) showing severe hepatitis. Histopathology from a biopsy obtained using key-hole celiotomy confirmed the diagnosis of absolute amyloidosis.

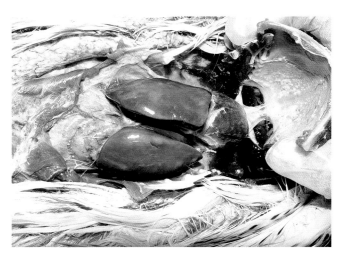

Fig. 7.90 Post-mortem examination of the falcon depicted in Figure 7.89. The liver was severely enlarged, hard to the touch and dark green in color. The condition was probably associated with severe bilateral chronic bumblefoot.

Toxic hepatitis

Various causes, including ingestion of heavy metals, chemical and plant poisons (e.g. aflatoxicosis).

Following ingestion of ammonium chloride in Falconiformes, Samour *et al.* (1995) found the liver of birds to be a uniform, dark green color and some showed early coagulative necrosis.

An unusual and interesting case of toxic hepatitis encountered by Keymer (unpublished data) was associated with the feeding of kidney beans. These beans of the genus *Phaseolus* contain the cyanogenetic glycoside phaseolunatin (Clarke and Clarke, 1975). Before they are used for feeding they must be soaked and boiled for at least 10 min. Many aviculturists use soaked seeds of leguminous plants (pulses) for hand-

rearing psittacine nestlings, so this type of toxicity may have been overlooked.

Diabetes mellitus

Fatty change may occur in the liver.

Pancreatic disease

See above.

Neoplasia

The following have been reported in Psittaciformes: undifferentiated carcinoma; fibrosarcoma; hemangioendothelioma; cholangiocarcinoma, cholangioma, 'biliary adenoma' and 'adenocarcinoma of intrahepatic bile ducts'; hepatocellular carcinoma; lymphoid leukosis-like syndrome (suspected oncornavirus type C), lymphosarcoma, 'malignant lymphoma', 'myeloblastic leukemia' and especially myeloblastosis in budgerigars.

In Passeriformes: lymphosarcoma, hepatocellular adenoma, carcinoma and 'avian leukosis'. The liver is a common site for neoplasia in all avian orders.

Cholangiocarcinomas are the most common avian hepatic tumor (Renner *et al.*, 2001). These authors reviewed the literature.

REFERENCES

Altman RB, Clubb SL, Dorrestein GM, Quesenberry K (eds) (1997) *Avian Medicine and Surgery*. WB Saunders, Philadelphia.

Appleby EC, Keymer IF (1971) More tumours in captive wild mammals and birds. A second brief report. In: *Sonderdruck aus Verhandlungsbericht des XIII Internationalen Symposiums über die Erkrankungen der Zootiere*, Helsinki. Academie-Verlag, Berlin.

Arnall L, Keymer IF (1975) *Bird Diseases: An Introduction to the Study of Birds in Health and Disease*. TFH Publications, Neptune City, NJ.

Baker JR (1985) Clinical and pathological aspects of 'going light' in exhibition budgerigars (*Melopsittacus undulatus*). *Veterinary Record* **116**: 406–408.

Baker JR (1987) A survey of the causes of 'wet vent' in budgerigars. *Veterinary Record* **121**: 448–449.

Beach JE (1962) Diseases of budgerigars and other cage birds. A survey of post-mortem findings. *Veterinary Record* **74**: 10–14, 63–68, 134–140.

Beynon PH, Forbes NA, Harcourt-Brown NH (eds) (1996a) *Manual of Raptors, Pigeons and Waterfowl*. British Small Animal Veterinary Association, Cheltenham.

Beynon PH, Forbes NA, Lawton MPC (1996b) *Manual of Psittacine Birds*. British Small Animal Veterinary Association, Cheltenham.

Boutette JB, Taylor M (2004) Proventricular dilatation disease: a review of research, literature, species differences, diagnostics, prognosis, and treatment. *Proceedings of the Association of Avian Veterinarians*, New Orleans, pp. 175–181.

Burr EW (1982) *Diseases of Parrots*. TFH Publications, Neptune City, NJ.

Clark FD (1984) Proventricular dilatation syndrome in large psittacine birds. *Avian Diseases* **28**: 813–815.

Clarke EGC, Clarke ML (1975) *Veterinary Toxicology*, p. 331. Baillière Tindall, London.

Clipsham R (1989) Surgical beak restoration and correction. *Proceedings of the Association of Avian Veterinarians*, Seattle, pp. 164–176.

Clipsham R (1992) Non-infectious disease of pediatric psittacines. *Seminars in Avian and Exotic Pet Medicine* **1**: 22–33.

Cooper JE (1969) Oesophageal capillariasis in captive falcons. *Veterinary Record* **84**: 634–636.

Cooper JE (1985) *Veterinary Aspects of Captive Birds of Prey*, 2nd edn. Standfast Press, Saul, Gloucestershire.

Cornelissen H, Ducatelle R, Roels S (1995) Successful treatment of a channel billed toucan (*Ramphastos vitellinus*) with iron storage disease by chelation therapy: sequential monitoring of the iron content of the liver during the treatment period by quantitative chemical and image analyses. *Journal of Avian Medicine and Surgery* **9**: 131–137.

Drews AV, Redrobe SP, Patterson-Kane JC (2004) Successful reduction of hepatocellular hemosiderin content by dietary modification in toco toucans (*Ramphastos toco*) with iron storage disease. *Journal of Avian Medicine and Surgery* **18**: 101–105.

Farr MM (1960) *Eimeria dunsingi* n. sp. (Protozoa, Eimeriidae) from the intestine of a parakeet, *Melopsittacus undulatus* (Shaw). *Libro homenaje al Dr Eduardo Cabberol y lal. Jubileo 1930–1960*, pp. 31–35. Instituto Politecnico Nacional, Mexico.

Forbes NA, Cooper JE (1993) Fatty liver–kidney syndrome of merlins. In: Redig PT, Cooper JE, Remple JD et al. (eds) *Raptor Biomedicine*, p. 288. University of Minnesota Press, Minneapolis.

Fowler ME (1986) *Zoo and Wild Animal Medicine*, 2nd edn. WB Saunders, Philadelphia.

Fudge AM (1991) Common medical conditions seen in the cockatiel, *Nymphicus hollandicus*. *Proceedings of the European Association of Avian Veterinarians*, Vienna, pp. 251–356.

Gabrisch K, Zwart P (1984) *Krankheiten der Heimtiere*. Schlutersche, Verlagsanstalt Bund Druckerei, Hannover.

Garner MM (2005) Sclerosing ingluvitis. *Proceedings of the Association of Avian Veterinarians*, Monterey, pp. 253–257.

Gough RE, Drury SE (1996) Circovirus-like particles in the bursae of young racing pigeons. *Veterinary Record* **138**: 167.

Gough RE, Drury SE, Harcourt-Brown NH, Higgins RJ (1996) Virus-like particles associated with macaw wasting disease. *Veterinary Record* **139**: 24.

Gregory CR, Ritchie BW, Latimer KS et al. (1997) Proventricular dilatation disease: a viral epornitic. *Proceedings of the Association of Avian Veterinarians*, Reno, pp. 43–52.

Griner LA (1983) *Pathology of Zoo Animals*. Zoological Society of San Diego, San Diego, CA.

Hasholt J (1972) Atrophy of the pancreas in budgerigars. *Nordisk Veterinaer-Medicin* **24**: 458–461.

Hooimeijer J, Fortune DG (1991) A case of coccidiosis in Psittaciformes. *Proceedings of the European Association of Avian Veterinarians*, Vienna, pp. 310–312.

Keymer IF (1958a) The diagnosis and treatment of common psittacine disease. *Modern Veterinary Practice* **39**: 21–26.

Keymer IF (1958b) Some ailments of cage and aviary birds. *Congress of the British Small Animal Veterinary Association*.

Keymer IF (1982) Parasitic diseases. In: Petrak ML (ed.) *Diseases of Cage and Aviary Birds*. Lea & Febiger, Philadelphia.

Keymer IF, Gough RE (1986) Duck virus enteritis (Anatid herpesvirus infection) in mute swans (*Cygnus olor*). *Avian Pathology* **15**: 161–170.

Kollias GV, Wehrmann S, Stetzer ER (1984) Enterolithiasis in an umbrella cockatoo. *Journal of the American Veterinary Medical Association* **185**: 1407–1408.

Latimer KL (1994) Oncology, digestive system. In: Ritchie BW, Harrison GJ, Harrison LR (eds) *Avian Medicine: Principles and Application*, pp. 655–659. Wingers Publishing, Lake Worth, FL.

Lawrence K (1988) The gastro-intestinal tract. In: *Manual of Parrots, Budgerigars, and other Psittacine Birds*, p. 76. British Small Animal Veterinary Association, Cheltenham.

Lowenstine LJ, Petrak ML (1980) Iron pigment in the livers of birds. In: Montali RJ, Migaki G (eds) *Comparative Pathology of Zoo Animals. The Symposia of the National Zoological Park, Smithsonian Institution*, pp. 127–135.

Lumeij JT (1994) Gastroenterology. In: Ritchie BW, Harrison J, Harrison LR (eds) *Avian Medicine: Principles and Application*, pp. 482–521. Wingers Publishing, Lake Worth, FL.

McOrist S (1991) Diseases of free-living Australian birds. *Proceedings of the Association of Avian Veterinarians*, Vienna, pp. 348–350.

Martin H, Ritchie BW (1994) Orthopedic surgical techniques. In: Ritchie BW, Harrison J, Harrison LR (eds) *Avian Medicine: Principles and Application*, pp. 1165–1169. Wingers Publishing, Lake Worth, FL.

Panigrahy B, Mathewson JJ, Hall CF, Grumbles LC (1981) Unusual disease conditions in pet and aviary birds. *Journal of the Veterinary Medical Association* **178**: 394–395.

Pass DA, Wylie SL, Forshaw D (1986) Acute pancreatic necrosis of galahs (*Cacatua roseicapilla*). *Australian Veterinary Journal* **63**: 340–341.

Petrak ML (1982) *Diseases of Cage and Aviary Birds*. Lea & Febiger, Philadelphia.

Quesenberry KE, Liu K (1986) Pancreatic atrophy in a blue and gold macaw. *Journal of the American Veterinary Medical Association* **189**: 1107–1108.

Ramis AJ, Domingo M, Ensenat C, Ferrer L (1991) Inclusion body hepatitis (IBH) in a group of *Eclectus roratus*. *Proceedings of the European Association of Avian Veterinarians*, Vienna, pp. 444–446.

Randall CJ, Reece R (1996) *Colour Atlas of Avian Histopathology*. Mosby-Wolfe, London.

Renner MS, Zaias J, Bossart GD (2001) Cholangiocarcinoma with metastasis in a captive Adelie penguin (*Pygoscelis adeliae*). *Journal of Zoo and Wildlife Medicine* **32**(3): 384–386.

Ritchie BW (1996) *Avian Viruses, Function and Control*. Wingers Publishing, Lake Worth, FL.

Ritchie BW, Harrison GJ, Harrison LR (eds) (1994) *Avian Medicine: Principles and Application*. Wingers Publishing, Lake Worth, FL.

Rosskopf WJ Jr., Woerpel RW (eds) (1996) *Diseases of Cage and Aviary Birds*, 3rd edn. Williams & Wilkins, Baltimore.

Samour JH (2000a) *Pseudomonas aeruginosa* stomatitis as a sequel to trichomoniasis in captive saker falcons (*Falco cherrug*). *Journal of Avian Medicine and Surgery* **14**: 113–117.

Samour JH (2000b) Supraorbital trichomoniasis infection in two saker falcons (*Falco cherrug*). *Veterinary Record* **146**: 139–140.

Samour JH, Naldo JL (2002a) Diagnosis and therapeutic management of candidiasis in falcons in Saudi Arabia. *Journal of Avian Medicine and Surgery* **16**: 129–132.

Samour JH, Naldo JL (2002b) Pancreatic atrophy in a peregrine falcon (*Falco peregrinus*). *Veterinary Record* **151**: 124–125.

Samour JH, Bailey TA, Keymer IF (1995) Use of ammonium chloride in falconry in the Middle East. *Veterinary Record* **137**: 269–270.

Samour JH, Cooper JE (1995) Trichomoniasis in birds of prey (Order Falconiformes) in Bahrain. *Veterinary Record* **136**: 358–362.

Samour JH, Naldo JL (2003) Diagnosis and therapeutic management of trichomoniasis in falcons in Saudi Arabia. *Journal of Avian Medicine and Surgery* **17**: 136–143.

Samour JH, Naldo JL (2005) Intra-auricular trichomoniasis in a saker falcon (*Falco cherrug*) in Saudi Arabia. *Veterinary Record* **156**: 384–386.

Shanthikumar SR (1987) Helminthology. In: Burr EW (ed.) *Companion Bird Medicine*, pp. 135–146. Iowa State University Press, Ames, IA.

Shivaprasad HL, Gilbert M, Watson RT et al. (2005) Decline of vultures on the Indian Subcontinent: the causes and its ramifications. *Proceedings of the Association of Avian Veterinarians*, Monterey, CA, pp. 109–112.

Simpson VR (1993) Suspected paramyxovirus 3 infection associated with pancreatitis and nervous signs in *Neophema* parakeets. *Veterinary Record* **132**: 554–555.

Speer BL (1995) Non-infectious diseases. In: Abramson J, Speer BL, Thomsen JB (eds) *The Large Macaws*, pp. 323–324. Raintree, Fort Bragg, CA.

Speer BL (2003a) Trans-sinus pinning technique to address scissors beak deformities in psittacines. *Proceedings of the European Association of Avian Veterinarians*, Tenerife, pp. 347–352.

Speer BL (2003b) Trans-sinus pinning technique for the correction of chronic mandibular prognathism in psittacines. *Proceedings of the European Association of Avian Veterinarians*, Tenerife, p. 3.

Sunberg JP, Junge RE, O'Banion MK et al. (1986) Cloacal papillomas in psittacines. *American Journal of Veterinary Research* **47**: 928–932.

Tully TN, Stevens AG, Diaz-Figaroa O et al. (2005) Use of a dental composite to correct beak deviation in psittacine species. *Proceedings of the European Association of Avian Veterinarians*, Arles, pp. 203–206.

Vereecken M, De Herdt P, Ducatelle R (1998) Adenovirus infections in pigeons: a review. *Avian Pathology* **27**: 333–338.

Wade JR (1992) Ratite pediatric medicine and surgery. *Proceedings of the Association of Avian Veterinarians*, New Orleans, pp. 1–12.

Wallner-Pendleton E, Helfer DH, Schimitz JA, Lowenstein L (1983) An inclusion-body pancreatitis in *Agapornis*. *Thirty-Second Western Poultry Conference*, California.

Wheler CL (1993) Herpesvirus disease in raptors. A review of the literature. In: Redig PJ, Cooper JE, Remple JD *et al.* (eds) *Raptor Biomedicine*, pp. 103–107. University of Minnesota Press, Minneapolis.

FURTHER READING

Beynon PH, Forbes NA, Lawton MPC (1996) *Manual of Psittacine Birds*. British Small Animal Veterinary Association, Cheltenham.

Cooper JE (1985) *Veterinary Aspects of Captive Birds of Prey*, 2nd edn, p. 256. The Standfast Press, Saul, Gloucestershire.

Cousquer G, Parsons D (2007) Veterinary care of the racing pigeon. *In Practice* **29**: 344–355.

McFerran JB, McNulty MS (1993) *Virus Infections of Birds*. Elsevier Science Publishers, Amsterdam.

Tudor DC (1991) *Pigeon Health and Disease*. Iowa State University Press, Ames, IA.

Endocrine disorders

Ian F. Keymer, Jaime Samour

Recent years have seen great advances in our knowledge of the anatomy, physiology and pathology of the endocrine system of birds. Although most of the published information comes from studies in the domestic fowl, there are occasional reports in the literature concerning mainly domestic pigeons (*Columba livia*), toucans (*Ramphastos* spp.), budgerigars (*Melopsittacus undulatus*) and other psittacines.

The endocrine system in birds includes the thyroid, parathyroid, adrenal and ultimobranchial glands, hypophysis, pancreas and gonads. The thymus is no longer considered to be an endocrine organ but forms part of the lymphatic system (King and McLelland, 1984). Although the pineal gland is an endocrine organ responsible for the regulation of the diurnal cycle, temperature and circadian locomotor activity (Ellis, 1976), there appears to be little recorded data on malfunction. However, there are at least two records of neoplasms in this organ, a pineoblastoma in a cockatiel (Wilson *et al.*, 1988) and a pinealoma in a dove (Reece, 1992).

The hormones secreted by the endocrine or ductless glands are released directly into the bloodstream and therefore reach all parts of the body. In this way they are able to stimulate or inhibit the functions of a wide range of other organs. Even small concentrations of a hormone can have a profound effect on body processes and therefore influence or cause pathological changes in tissues far removed from its source. This fact must be remembered when attempting clinical diagnosis of endocrine disorders and when hormones are used in the prevention or treatment of certain diseases.

There are several outstanding contributions, from both sides of the Atlantic, dealing with the anatomy, physiology and pathology of the endocrine system in birds. The reader is referred to Kronberger, 1973; Arnall and Keymer, 1975; Ebert, 1978; Epple and Stetson, 1980; Shöne and Arnold, 1980; Petrak and Gilmore, 1982; Gabrisch and Zwart, 1984; King and McLelland, 1984; Follett and Goldsmith, 1985; Leach, 1992; Joyner, 1994; Latimer, 1994; Lothrop, 1996; Lumeij, 1994; and Oglesbee *et al.*, 1997). A recent publication reviewed the neoplasms affecting birds of prey. Some of these neoplasms involved glands of the endocrine system (Forbes *et al.*, 2000).

Thyroid glands

Unlike mammals, birds have two thyroid glands, not one. They are situated at the base of the neck on either side of the trachea near the syrinx and jugular veins (Fig. 9.14). They are pinkish red or yellowish in color. Their size varies according to the species and in addition depends upon age and seasonal changes. The thyroids influence the growth rate of the young and govern the metabolic rate of all age groups. They increase in size when demands are greatest, for example during cold weather and egg laying. The normal thyroids weights are in the region of 0.02% of the total bodyweight. In a budgerigar weighing 35 g, each weighs approximately 3 mg and measures about 2 mm in length and 1 mm in width (Blackmore and Cooper, 1982). The left thyroid is usually slightly larger than the right. The normal thyroids of small passerine birds such as the canary (*Serinus canaria*) are rounded and pinhead in size. The size of the thyroid glands is also influenced by a number of factors, including sex, age, diet, environmental factors and secretory activity (King and McLelland, 1984). Disorders of the thyroids are listed in Table 7.12.

In response to thyroid stimulating hormone (TSH) released by the pituitary gland, the thyroids secrete 3,5,3′-triiodo L-thyronine (T_3) and 3,5,3′,5, tetraiodo L-thyronine (thyroxine, T_4). These hormones can be produced only when there is sufficient iodine and tyrosine available to the body. The secretion of TSH, T_3 and T_4 is influenced by the season, photoperiod, gonadal cycle and state of molting (Zenoble *et al.*, 1985). In contrast to that in mammals, the avian thyroid produces more T_4 than T_3 (Astier, 1980). For a useful and comprehensive review of the anatomy, physiology and physiopathology of the avian thyroid gland the reader is referred to the work by Merryman and Buckles (1998a, 1998b).

A recent pathological survey found thyroid hyperplasia in 30 birds (0.024%) from a total of 12 500 cases examined (Schmidt and Reavill, 2002). This condition was most common in the blue and gold macaw (0.012%). However,

TABLE 7.12 Disorders of the thyroid gland

Disorder	Species
GOITER	
Hypothyroidism (thyroid hyperplasia and dysplasia). Dietary iodine deficiency	Budgerigars, cockatiels, canaries, pigeons;[1-3] white backed vulture, southern caracara[4]
Hyperthyroidism (thyrotoxicosis). Excess dietary iodine or iodine supplementation	Not reported in non-domesticated species
NEOPLASIA	
Carcinoma	Budgerigar,[5] dwarf sulfur-crested cockatoo, European pochard[6]
Adenocarcinoma	Budgerigar, house sparrow,[7] Andean goose, laysan teal,[4] bald eagle[8]
Cystadenocarcinoma	Saker falcon[9]
Follicular cystadenoma	Caracara[10]
Cystic fibroadenoma	Black chested buzzard[11]
Adenoma	Budgerigar,[2,5,6] jackdaw,[6] canary[6]
Neoplasia (unspecified)	Budgerigar, cockatiel,[14] scarlet macaw[13]
OTHER DISORDERS	
Thyroiditis associated with septicemia	Budgerigar, various species,[2,14] red-vented cockatoo[15]
Amyloidosis	Various species[13]
Cyst formation	Budgerigar,[2] mandarin duck, Elliot's pheasant, Eleonora's falcon[12]
Atrophy and hypertrophy	Guillemots[16]
Hemiagenesis	Japanese quail[17]

[1] Blackmore, 1965. [2] Blackmore and Cooper, 1982. [3] Sasipreeyajan and Newman, 1988. [4] Griner, 1983. [5] Beach, 1962. [6] Wadsworth et al., 1985. [7] Petrak and Gilmore, 1982. [8] Bates et al., 1999. [9] Samour et al., 2001. [10] Forbes et al., 2000. [11] Hammmerton, 1943. [12] Wadsworth and Jones, 1979. [13] Schlumberger, 1955. [14] Von Zipper and Tamasohke, 1972. [15] Richkind et al., 1982. [16] Jefferies and Parslow, 1976. [17] Wight, 1986.

this number was considered unrepresentative, since the highest number of submissions (10.09%) was from macaws. The cause of thyroid hyperplasia was not established in this study.

Parathyroid glands

These are two very small yellow organs situated close to the posterior pole of each thyroid. They play an important role in calcium metabolism. The parathyroids secrete parathyroid hormone (PTH) in response to a decrease in the concentration of plasma calcium. PTH increases the plasma calcium concentration by increasing tubular reabsorption of calcium, by increasing bone resorption and calcium absorption from the gastrointestinal system. PTH is also involved in the synthesis of 1,25-dehydroxyvitamin D_3 and increasing the excretion of phosphorus through the renal system. Disorders of the parathyroids are given in Table 7.13.

When egg laying commences, there is a dramatic increase in the demand of calcium for eggshell production. In the domestic fowl, the shell gland in the oviduct secretes about 5 g of calcium carbonate in 20 h. This necessitates the withdrawal of 2 g of calcium ions from the blood each day at a rate of 100 mg/h. The calcium is resorbed from the bones. This procedure, however, cannot carry on indefinitely because the bones would soften and

TABLE 7.13 Disorders of the parathyroid glands

Disorder	Species
Nutritional secondary hyperparathyroidism. Dietary insufficiency of calcium, excess phosphorus, combination of both leading to hypocalcemia	Psittacines,[1] birds of prey[2]

[1] Altman, 1982. [2] Cooper, 1985.

fracture. Extra calcium therefore has to be absorbed from the food. Because the turnover of calcium is high, birds have developed a special type of medullary bone in the marrow of the long bones. At times when requirements for egg shell calcium are low, calcium ions in the blood are transferred to the medullary bone. When the calcium is required, PTH mobilizes this calcium, thus avoiding its withdrawal from the structural bones.

PTH also plays a role in the contraction of muscles, in blood clotting and in the secretion of phosphates by the tubules of the kidneys. It is believed that the parathyroid is not under the control of any other endocrine organ, but is stimulated by the level of calcium in the blood. The level of minerals in the blood of healthy birds is very constant, but in certain diseases it may fall markedly and result in softening of the bones (Epple and Stetson, 1980).

Adrenal glands

These are paired structures situated near the anterior pole of each kidney but in a few species, for example rheas (Rheidae), bald eagles (*Haliaëtus leucocephalus*) and others, the glands are fused into a single organ. The adrenals vary considerably in shape and size in different species and are directly related to bodyweight. They are just visible to the naked eye in the smaller passerines as pink or creamy-gray specks. In some species they have a yellowish tinge. Each gland is composed of two main sections as in mammals, but in birds the tissues are not demarcated into an outer cortex and inner medulla, the two types being mixed. Disorders of the adrenals are listed in Table 7.14.

The medullary or chromaffin tissue is composed of two types of cell. One type releases epinephrine while the second type releases norepinephrine. Epinephrine is involved in the process of glycogenolysis while norepinephrine is involved in gluconeogenesis. The cortical tissue is responsible for the secretion of corticosterone, aldosterone and 18-hydroxycorticosterone. The adrenal glands in birds secrete more corticosterone than aldosterone. In contrast to that in mammals, corticosterone in birds has both glucocorticoid and mineralocorticoid activities. The level of corticosterone in the blood plasma is increased under certain stressful conditions such as excessive cold, deprivation of water, surgical procedures, excessive handling or administration of certain drugs. Corticosterone plays an important role in carbohydrate,

fat and electrolyte metabolism. In addition, in marine birds this hormone appears to increase the secretion of sodium chloride by the nasal glands. When the intake of salt is excessive, the level of this hormone in the blood is dramatically increased. Aldosterone has the opposite effect in salt metabolism, because it acts on the kidney tubules and increases sodium reabsorption from the filtrate passing through the glomeruli in the renal cortex. Corticosterone levels in blood also increase during oviposition and follow a diurnal rhythm. The adrenal cortex is influenced by adrenocorticotropic hormone (ACTH) secreted by the anterior lobe of the pituitary gland (Epple and Stetson, 1980).

Ultimobranchial glands

These are small, pink, lentil-shaped glands situated at the entrance of the thoracic inlet, craniolaterally to the origin of the carotid arteries. They are about 2–3 mm in size in the adult domestic fowl. The ultimobranchial glands are integrated by the C cells, parathyroid nodules, vesicles and lymphoid tissue (King and McLelland, 1984).

The most important function of these glands is the secretion of calcitonin by the C cells. The exact role of calcitonin in birds is not fully understood but it appears to prevent excessive bone resorption by PTH (Baimbridge and Taylor, 1981).

Hypophysis

The hypophysis or pituitary is a small gland linked to the ventral aspect of the diencephalic brainstem (Table 7.15). This gland is integrated by the anterior lobe or adenohypophysis derived from the embryonic stomodeum and the posterior lobe or neurohypophysis derived from the diencephalon. The adenohypophysis is divided into the pars tuberalis and the pars distalis. Unlike mammals, the pars intermedia is not a separate entity, the equivalent cells of this being integrated within the pars distalis. The neurohypophysis is in direct communication with the brain and it is composed of the median eminence, the infundibulum and the neural lobe (King and McLelland, 1984).

TABLE 7.14 Disorders of the adrenal glands

Disorder	Species
Chronic recurrent disorders, associated in psittacines with such diseases as inclusion body hepatitis (IBH)	Psittacines, especially cockatoos and African gray parrots
Chronic disorders associated with long-standing infections such as aspergillosis, and tuberculosis, or permanent damage caused by a variety of factors	
NEOPLASIA	
Adenomas, cortical hyperplasia	Budgerigar,[1,2] white crowned parrot[3]
Carcinoma (unspecified, adrenal cortical cells)	Little owl,[2] pigeon[4]
Neoplasia of adrenal and ovary with metastases	Nicobar pigeon[3]
Adrenal cortical carcinoma	Long-crested eagle[5]
Adrenal adenocarcinoma	Scarlet macaw[6]
Adrenal carcinoma	Budgerigar[7]

[1] Beach, 1962. [2] Blackmore and Cooper, 1982. [3] Griner, 1983. [4] Gratzl and Köhler, 1968. [5] Halliwell and Graham, 1978. [6] Cornelissen and Verhofstad, 1999. [7] Latimer and Greenacre, 1995.

TABLE 7.15 Disorders of the hypophysis gland

Disorder	Species
Neoplasia and hyperplasia	Budgerigar,[1–6] cockatiel[7,8]
Adenoma	Yellow-naped Amazon parrot[9]

[1] Schlumberger, 1954. [2] Schlumberger, 1957. [3] Beach, 1962. [4] Blackmore and Cooper, 1982. [5] Petrak and Gilmore, 1982. [6] Bauck, 1987. [7] Curtis-Velasco, 1992. [8] Wheler, 1992. [9] Romagnano et al., 1995.

The adenohypophysis produces seven hormones, which are mostly named after the ductless glands that each controls. Adrenocorticotropic hormone (ACTH) maintains adrenal gland activity and controls the production of adrenal corticosteroids. Thyroid-stimulating hormone (TSH), as its name implies, controls the activity of the thyroid gland and the secretion of thyroid hormones. Follicle-stimulating hormone (FSH) stimulates the gonads in both sexes, as does luteinizing hormone (LH). Prolactin, or lactogenic hormone, suppresses FSH and appears to regulate the deposition of fat in birds prior to migration. It also causes broodiness and, in those species that have them, stimulates the production of brood patches. In pigeons this hormone also stimulates the production of 'crop milk'. The somatotropic hormones (STH) or growth hormones (GH) appear to regulate growth in immature birds. Finally, the function of the so-called melanocyte-stimulating hormone (MSH) is not clearly understood.

The neurohypophysis receives and stores two hormones, the arginine vasotocin and mesotocin. These are produced by the hypothalamic nuclei and transported by the hypothalamo-hypophyseal tract. Vasotocin is an antidiuretic hormone that differs slightly from the mammalian counterpart by one amino acid residue. Its main action in birds is to inhibit fluid loss from the kidneys by decreasing glomerular filtration. The other known actions of vasotocin include the control of water reabsorption and the stimulation of peristaltic movements of the oviduct during oviposition (Epple and Stetson, 1980).

Pancreas

The pancreas is situated at the first duodenal loop and is integrated in the majority of birds by the dorsal, ventral and splenic lobes. This organ has both endocrine and exocrine functions but only the islets of Langerhans, which contain endocrine cells, are dealt with in this section.

In birds, in contrast to mammals, there are three types of islet and not one. The dark islets contain alpha (α) and delta (δ) cells and the lighter islets contain beta (β) and δ cells. Mixed islets contain all three cell types. One type of α cell in the dark islets produces glucagon, a hormone that in birds plays a more important role than insulin in carbohydrate metabolism, by raising the plasma glucose. It also plays an important role in fat metabolism. The β cells produce the well known hormone insulin, but the levels of this hormone in the avian pancreas are considerably lower than in mammals. Insulin also plays a minor role in carbohydrate metabolism but its main role is as an anabolic hormone. The function of insulin in mammals is to take sugars out of the circulating blood and store them

in the liver in the form of glycogen, or to distribute them to the skeletal muscles and other organs, where they are temporarily stored for emergencies. When insulin is absent, as in diabetes, this leads to high levels of glucose in the blood. In birds, however, the role of insulin is much less clear. On occasions it seems that its role is reversed, so that the polypeptide hormone glucagon functions similarly to insulin in mammals. In some species of birds at least, however, it seems possible that insulin may help to prevent hyperglycemia. The δ cells secrete somatostatin, a hormone with a possible role in regulating the secretion of insulin and glucagon (Epple and Stetson, 1980).

For a comprehensive review of different disorders affecting the pancreas the reader is referred to the work of Lothrop (1996) and Speer (2001).

Until relatively recently, diabetes mellitus was considered to be quite rare and not to be expected in birds. Altman and Kirmayer (1976) reviewed the literature on the subject, since when there have been a few more reports (Table 7.16). As birds normally have a high fasting blood glucose level and insulin appears to play a relatively minor role in controlling carbohydrate metabolism, the definition of the disease in birds compared with that in mammals needs some modification. A definition modified from that of Stogdale (1986) is suggested as follows: 'A metabolic disorder in which the ability to oxidize carbohydrates is more or less completely lost, usually due to faulty pancreatic activity, especially of the islets of Langerhans, and to consequent disturbance of the normal insulin and glucagon

TABLE 7.16 Disorders of the pancreas

Disorder	Species
Diabetes mellitus	Budgerigar,[1,2] cockatiel,[1] racing pigeon,[3] canary, toco toucan,[4] Amazon parrots, macaws, cockatoos,[5] red-tailed hawk,[6] African gray parrot,[7] yellow-collared macaw, black-capped lory, yellow-naped amazon, parakeets[8]
Neoplasia (unspecified)	Budgerigar[9,10]
Islet cell tumor	Parakeet[10]
Adenocarcinoma	Peaceful dove[11]
Pancreatic atrophy	Budgerigar,[12,13] blue and gold macaw,[14] peregrine falcon[15]
Acute pancreatic necrosis	Galah cockatoo[16]
Exocrine pancreatic insufficiency	Yellow-naped amazon,[17] racing pigeon[18]
Pancreatic adenocarcinoma	Yellow-naped Amazon[17]
Pancreatic hypoplasia	Eclectus parrot[19]

[1] Altman and Kirmayer, 1976. [2] Appleby, 1984. [3] Murphy, 1992. [4] Douglass, 1981. [5] Woerpel and Rosskopf, 1984. [6] Waller-Pendleton et al., 1993. [7] Candeletta et al., 1993. [8] Lothrop, 1996. [9] Schlumberger, 1957. [10] Ryan et al., 1982. [11] Griner, 1983. [12] Beach, 1962. [13] Hasholt, 1972. [14] Quesenberry and Liu, 1986. [15] Samour and Naldo, 2002. [16] Pass et al., 1986. [17] Ritchey, 1997. [18] Amman et al, 2005. [19] Ritzman, 2000.

mechanism'. Appleby (1984) observed enlargement and pale-brown discoloration of the liver. Both he and Altman and Kirmayer (1976) found hepatic necrosis and evidence of lipidosis. The latter workers also recorded hepatic fibrosis and in their four cases in budgerigars could detect no pancreatic lesions, unlike Appleby (1984), who found evidence of degenerative changes in the islets. In a recent report, an adult male chestnut-fronted macaw (*Ara severa*) and an adult female military macaw (*Ara militaris*) were diagnosed with diabetes mellitus after extensive clinical diagnostic laboratory investigation. In addition, hemosiderosis in hepatic macrophages and hepatocytes was diagnosed through biopsies in the two birds. The authors highlighted the need to carry out further clinical investigations to ascertain a possible relationship between diabetes mellitus and hemosiderosis in large psittacines (Gancz *et al.*, 2005).

Ovary

In most bird species only the left ovary is functional. One exception is the brown kiwi (*Apterix australis*), in which it has been established that both ovaries are fully functional. Although there have been many reports of fully developed left and right ovary in Falconiformes, it seems very unlikely that both ovaries could be fully functional (King and McLelland, 1984). Ovarian disorders are set out in Table 7.17.

TABLE 7.17 Disorders of the ovary	
Disorder	**Species**
Neoplasia[1]	Budgerigar,[2–8] various psittacine and passerine species[2,5,9], barred shouldered dove[3]
Granulosa cell tumor	Budgerigar,[2,4,5,8,10,11] sulfur crested cockatoo,[10] Chinese painted quail,[11] red-legged honeycreeper,[11] pigeon,[12] military macaw[13]
Adenocarcinoma	Australian thicknee[14]
Diffuse papillary adenocarcinoma	Crimson rosella[11]
Adenoma	Pet birds[15] (unspecified)
Polyostotic hyperostosis	Budgerigars[5,16–18]
Sex reversal and other reproductive disorders of endocrine origin	Various species, poultry[17,19]
Ovarian cysts of possible endocrine origin	Canaries, budgerigars, pheasants and cockatiels[20]

[1] Mrzel *et al.*, 1979. [2] Petrak and Gilmore, 1982. [3] Keymer, 1980. [4] Frost C, 1961. [5] Beach, 1962. [6] Campbell, 1986. [7] Effron *et al.*, 1977. [8] Reece, 1992. [9] Neumann and Kummerfeld, 1983. [10] Ratcliffe, 1933. [11] Griner, 1983. [12] Chalmers, 1986. [13] Stoica *et al.*, 1989. [14] Appleby and Keymer, 1971. [15] Schmidt, 1997. [16] Schlumberger, 1959. [17] Arnall and Keymer, 1975. [18] Stauber E *et al.*, 1990. [19] Blount, 1947. [20] Speer, 1997. [21] Campbell and Stuart, 1984.

The ovary produces three hormones: estrogen, progesterone and an androgen. Both the ovary and the testes are influenced by the same pituitary hormones. The FSH stimulates the development of the ovarian follicles and secretion of estrogens by the ovary. Estrogens are steroid hormones involved in the development of the secondary female sex characteristics, such as change in beak color in some species; development of the incubation or brood patch by interaction with prolactin; development and maintenance of the female type of plumage and development of the oviduct by interaction with the steroid progesterone, although very little appears to be known about its functions. In addition estrogens are partly responsible for nest building behavior and the mobilization of calcium in the body for the production of eggshells. The latter is carried out in conjunction with hormone production by the parathyroid glands. Estrogens also stimulate the widening of the pelvic outlet to enable the eggs to be passed prior to egg-laying. The ovary, like the testes, decreases in size in winter, when the hours of daylight are short, and then enlarges again when the lengthening days of spring stimulate the hypothalamus and pituitary gland. Apparently very little is known about the action of the androgens produced by the ovary. LH secreted by the pituitary causes actual ovulation or shedding of the ova. As the ova enlarge, they form grape-like clusters, rupture from their follicles and drop into the funnel-shaped opening or infundibulum of the oviduct (Epple and Stetson, 1980).

In many species of birds the ovary is pale to dark yellow, related to lipid deposits. However, some species have a 'melanistic' ovary due to the presence of melanocytes. In these species the immature ovary tends to vary from black through dark green and gray to pale green in color. As the ovary develops and increases in size during the breeding season, the color also changes.

Testes

The testes are paired, cylinder-shaped gonads located, in most species, at the base of the anterior lobe of each kidney. As a general rule, in immature birds, the left testis tends to be larger than the right. Conversely, as birds mature, the right gonad becomes larger and heavier than the left. The morphometrics of the testis increase considerably during the breeding season. The color of the testes in many species is yellow, as a result of lipid deposits, while in other species, the color varies from pale-green through gray and dark-green to black, because of the presence of melanocytes. The color of the testes in these species changes according to sexual activity and size of the gonad. Disorders of the testes are listed in Table 7.18.

TABLE 7.18 Disorders of the testes

Disorders	Species
NEOPLASIA	
Seminoma	Budgerigar[1-8]
Sertoli cell tumor	Budgerigars,[1-3,9-11] Japanese quail[12]
Interstitial cell tumor	Budgerigar[1,3]
Leiomyosarcoma	Budgerigar[1]
Hemangioma	Budgerigar[1]

[1] Petrak and Gilmore, 1982. [2] Arnall, 1958. [3] Beach, 1962. [4] Rewell, 1948. [5] Lombard and Witte, 1959. [6] Blackmore, 1965. [7] Griner, 1983. [8] Turk et al., 1981. [9] Frost, 1961. [10] Effron et al., 1977. [11] Reece, 1992. [12] Gorham and Ottinger, 1986.

The testes produce testosterone in a small group of glandular cells situated between the sperm-producing tubules. It passes directly into the bloodstream and reaches all parts of the body. Testosterone generates and maintains the secondary sexual characteristics, such as the typical male head and body shape of a particular species, its posture, voice, sexual behavior, plumage and color. It is also responsible for the increase in size of the fleshy wattles and cere of some species (King and McLelland, 1984).

The sperm and testosterone output depends upon the pituitary hormones FSH and LH. FSH stimulates the growth of the testes and development of sperm and LH stimulates the interstitial glandular cells between the seminiferous tubules to produce testosterone (Epple and Stetson, 1980).

REFERENCES

Altman RB (1982) Disorders of the skeletal system. In: Petrak ML (ed.) Diseases of Cage and Aviary Birds, 2nd edn, pp. 383–384. Lea & Febiger, Philadelphia.

Altman RB, Kirmayer AH (1976) Diabetes mellitus in the avian species. Journal of the American Animal Hospital Association 12: 531–537.

Amman O, Visschers MJM, Dorrestein GM et al. (2005) Exocrine pancreatic insufficiency in a racing pigeon (Columba livia domestica). Proceedings of the European Association of Avian Veterinarians, Arles, pp. 179–183.

Appleby RC (1984) Diabetes mellitus in a budgerigar. Veterinary Record 115: 652–653.

Appleby EC, Keymer IF (1971) More tumours in captive wild mammals and birds. A second brief report. In: Sonderdruck aus Verhandlungsbericht des XIII Internationalen Symposiums über die Erkrankungen der Zootiere, Helsinki. Academie-Verlag, Berlin.

Arnall L (1958) Experiences with cage-birds. Veterinary Record 70: 120–128.

Arnall L, Keymer IF (1975) The endocrine system. In: Arnall L, Keymer IF (eds) Bird Diseases: An Introduction to the Study of Birds in Health and Disease, pp. 293–304. TFH Publications, Neptune City, NJ.

Astier H (1980) Thyroid gland in birds. In: Epple A, Stetson MH (eds) Avian Endocrinology, pp. 167–189. Academic Press, New York.

Baimbridge KG, Taylor TG (1981) The role of calcitonin in controlling hypercalcemia in the domestic fowl (Gallus domesticus). Comparative Biochemistry and Physiology 68: 647–651.

Bates G, Tucker RL, Ford S, Mattix ME (1999) Thyroid adenocarcinoma in a bald eagle (Haliaeetus leucocephalus). Journal of Zoo and Wildlife Medicine 30: 439–442.

Bauck LA (1987) Pituitary neoplastic disease in 9 budgerigars. Proceedings of the Association of Avian Veterinarians, Hawaii, pp. 87–90.

Beach JE (1962) Diseases of budgerigars and other cage birds. A survey of post-mortem findings. Veterinary Record 74: 10–14, 63–68, 134–140.

Blackmore DK (1965) The pathology and incidence of thyroid dysplasia in budgerigars (Melopsittacus undulatus). Veterinary Record 75: 1068–1072.

Blackmore DK, Cooper JE (1982) Diseases of the endocrine system. In: Petrak ML (ed.) Diseases of Cage and Aviary Birds, 2nd edn, pp. 478–490. Lea & Febiger, Philadelphia.

Blount WP (1947) Diseases of Poultry. Baillière Tindall & Cox, London.

Campbell TW (1986) Neoplasia. In: Harrison GJ, Harrison LR (eds) Clinical Avian Medicine and Surgery, pp. 500–508. WB Saunders, Philadelphia.

Campbell TW, Stuart LD (1984) Ovarian neoplasia in the budgerigar (Melopsittacus undulatus). Veterinary Medicine Small Animal Clinician 79: 215–218.

Candeletta SC, Homer BL, Garner MM et al. (1993) Diabetes mellitus associated with chronic lymphocytic pancreatitis in an African gray parrot (Psittacus erithacus erithacus). Journal of the Association of Avian Veterinarians 7: 39–43.

Chalmers GA (1986) Neoplasms in two racing pigeons. Avian Diseases 30: 241–244.

Cooper JE (1985) Veterinary Aspects of Captive Birds of Prey, 2nd edn with 1985 supplement. Standfast Press, Saul, Gloucestershire.

Cornelissen H, Verhofstad A (1999) Adrenal neoplasia in a scarlet macaw (Ara macao) with clinical signs of hyperadrenocorticism. Journal of Avian Medicine and Surgery 13: 92–97.

Curtis-Velasco M (1992) Pituitary adenoma in a cockatiel (Nymphicus hollandicus). Journal of the Association of Avian Veterinarians 6: 21–22.

Douglass EM (1981) Diabetes mellitus in a toucan. Modern Veterinary Practice 62: 293–295.

Ebert U (1978) Vogelkrankheiten, 2nd edn. Verlag Schaper, Hannover.

Effron M, Griner L, Benirschke K (1977) Nature and rate of neoplasia found in captive wild mammals, birds, and reptiles at necropsy. Journal of Natural Cancer Institute 59: 185–198.

Ellis LC (1976) Endocrine role of the pineal gland. American Zoologist 16: 100–101.

Epple A, Stetson MH (1980) Avian Endocrinology, pp. 167–189. Academic Press, New York.

Follett BK, Goldsmith AR (1985) In: Campbell B, Lack E (eds) A Dictionary of Birds, pp. 180–184. T & AD Poyser, Carlton, Staffordshire.

Forbes NA, Cooper JE, Higgins RJ (2000) Neoplasms of birds of prey. In: Lumeij JT, Remple JD, Redig PT et al. (eds) Raptor Biomedicine III, pp. 127–146. Zoological Education Network, Lake Worth, FL.

Frost C (1961) Experiences with pet budgerigars. Veterinary Record 73: 621–626.

Gabrisch K, Zwart P (1984) Krankheiten der Heimtiere. Schlütersche, Hannover.

Gancz AY, Wellehan JFX, Boutette J et al. (2005) Diabetes mellitus in large psittacines: a possible relationship with excessive iron storage. Proceedings of the Association of Avian Veterinarians, Monterey, CA, pp. 267–269.

Gorham SL, Ottinger MA (1986) Sertoli cell tumors in Japanese quail. Avian Disease 30: 337–339.

Gratzl E, Köhler H (1968) Spezielle Pathologie und Therapie der Geflügelkrankheiten. Ferdinand Enke, Stuttgart.

Griner LA (1983) Pathology of Zoo Animals, p. 213. Zoological Society of San Diego, San Diego, CA.

Halliwell WH, Graham DL (1978) Neoplasms in birds of prey. In: Fowler ME (ed.) Zoo and Wild Animal Medicine, p. 286. WB Saunders, Philadelphia.

Hammerton AE (1943) Proceedings of the Zoological Society of London, 112: 149.

Hasholt J (1972) Atrophy of the pancreas in budgerigar. Nordisk Veterinærmedicin 24: 458–461.

Jefferies DJ, Parslow JLF (1976) Thyroid changes in PCB-dosed guillemots and their indications of one of the mechanisms of action of these materials. Environmental Pollution 10: 293–311.

Joyner KL (1994) Theriogenology. In: Ritchie BW, Harrison GJ, Harrison LR (eds) Avian Medicine: Principles and Application, pp. 748–804. Wingers Publishing, Lake Worth, FL.

Keymer IF (1980) Disorders of the avian female reproductive system. *Avian Pathology* **9**: 405–419.

King AS, McLelland J (1984) *Birds: Their Structure and Function*, pp. 200–213. Baillière Tindall, London.

Kronberger (1973) *Haltung von Vögeln. Krankheiten der Vogel*. VEB Gustav Fischer, Jena.

Latimer KS (1994) Oncology. In: Ritchie BW, Harrison GJ, Harrison LR (eds) *Avian Medicine: Principles and Application*, pp. 640–672. Wingers Publishing, Lake Worth, FL.

Latimer KS, Greenacre CB (1995) Adrenal carcinoma in a budgerigar (*Melopsittacus undulatus*). *Journal of Avian Medicine and Surgery* **9**: 141–143.

Leach MW (1992) A survey of neoplasia in pet birds. In: Schmidt RE, Fudge AM (eds) *Neoplasia. Seminars in Avian and Exotic Pet Medicine* **1**(2): 52–64.

Lombard LS, Witte EJ (1959) Frequency and types of tumors in mammals and birds of the Philadelphia Zoological Gardens. *Cancer Research* **19**: 127–141.

Lothrop CD Jr (1996) Diseases of the endocrine system. In: Rosskopf WJ Jr, Woerpel RW (eds) *Diseases of Cage and Aviary Birds*, 3rd edn, pp. 368–379. Williams & Wilkins, Baltimore.

Lumeij JT (1994) Endocrinology. In: Ritchie BW, Harrison GJ, Harrison LR (eds) *Avian Medicine: Principles and Application*, pp. 582–606. Winger, Publishing, Lake Worth, FL.

Merryman JI, Buckles EL (1998a) The avian thyroid gland. Part one: a review of the anatomy and physiology. *Journal of Avian Medicine and Surgery* **12**: 234–237.

Merryman JI, Buckles EL (1998b) The avian thyroid gland. Part two: a review of the function and pathophysiology. *Journal of Avian Medicine and Surgery* **12**: 238–242.

MrzeL L, Pogacnik M, Josipovic D (1979) Frequency and characteristics of tumors in cage birds. *Veterinarski Glansnik* **33**: 989–993.

Murphy J (1992) Diabetes in toucans. *Proceedings of the Association of Avian Veterinarians*, pp. 165–170.

Neumann U, Kummerfeld N (1983) Neoplasms in budgerigar (*Melopsittacus undulatus*): clinical, pathomorphological and serological findings with special consideration of kidney tumors. *Avian Pathology* **12**: 353.

Oglesbee BL, Orosz S, Dorrestein GM (1997) The endocrine system. In: Altman RB, Clubb SL, Dorrestein GM, Quesenberry K (eds) *Avian Medicine and Surgery*, pp. 475–488. WB Saunders, Philadelphia.

Pass DA, Wylie SL, Forshaw D (1986) Acute pancreatic necrosis of galah (*Cacatua roseicapilla*). *Australian Veterinary Journal* **63**: 340–341.

Petrak ML, Gilmore CE (1982) Neoplasms. In: Petrak ML (ed.) *Diseases of Cage and Aviary Birds*, pp. 606–637. Lea & Febiger, Philadelphia.

Quesenberry KE, Liu SK (1986) Pancreatic atrophy in a blue and gold macaw. *Journal of the American Veterinary Medical Association* **189**: 1107–1108.

Ratcliffe HL (1933) Incidence and nature of tumors in captive wild mammals and birds. *American Journal of Cancer* **17**: 116–135.

Reece RL (1992) Observations on naturally occurring neoplasms in birds in the State of Victoria, Australia. *Avian Pathology* **21**: 3–32.

Rewell RE (1948) Seminoma of the testis in a collared dove (*Streptopelia risoria*). *Journal of Pathology and Bacteriology* **60**: 155.

Richkind M, Gendron AP, Howard EB et al. (1982) Pseudomonas septicemia associated with autoimmune endocrinopathy in a red-vented cockatoo. *Veterinary Medicine Small Animal Clinician* **77**: 1548–1554.

Ritchey JW (1997) Exocrine pancreatic insufficiency in a yellow-napped Amazon (*Amazona ochrocephala*) with pancreatic adenocarcinoma. *Veterinary Pathology*, **34**: 55–57.

Ritzman TK (2000) Pancreatic hypoplasia in an eclectus parrot (*Eclectus roratus polychloros*). *Proceedings of the Association of Avian Veterinarians*, Portland, pp. 83–87.

Romagnano A, Mashima TY, Barnes HJ et al. (1995) Pituitary adenoma in an Amazon parrot. *Journal of Avian Medicine and Surgery* **9**: 263–270.

Ryan CP, Walder EJ, Howard EB (1982) Diabetes mellitus and islet cell carcinoma in a parakeet. *Journal of the American Animal Hospital Association* **18**: 139–142.

Samour JH, Naldo JL (2002) Pancreatic atrophy in a peregrine falcon (*Falco peregrinus*). *Veterinary Record* **151**: 124–125.

Samour JH, Naldo JL, Wernery U, Kinne J (2001) Thyroid cystadenocarcinoma in a saker falcon (*Falco cherrug*). *Veterinary Record* **149**: 277–278.

Sasipreeyajan J, Newman JA (1988) Goiter in a cockatiel (*Nymphicus hollandicus*). *Avian Diseases* **32**: 169–172.

Schlumberger HG (1954) Neoplasia in the parakeet. I. Spontaneous chromophobe pituitary tumors. *Cancer Research* **14**: 237–245.

Schlumberger HG (1955) Spontaneous goiter and cancer of the thyroid in animals. *Ohio Journal of Science* **55**: 23–43.

Schlumberger HG (1957) Tumors characteristic for certain animal species. A review. *Cancer Research* **17**: 823–832.

Schlumberger HG (1959) Polyostotic hyperostosis in the female parakeet. *American Journal of Pathology* **35**: 1–23.

Schmidt RE (1997) Neoplastic diseases. In: Altman RB, Clubb SL, Dorrestein GM, Quesenberry K (eds) *Avian Medicine and Surgery*, pp. 590–600. WB Saunders, Philadelphia.

Schmidt RE, Reavill DR (2002) Thyroid hyperplasia in birds. *Journal of Avian Medicine and Surgery* **16**: 111–114.

Shöne R, Arnold P (1980) *Der Wellensittich. Heimtier und Patient*. VEB Gustav Fischer, Jena.

Speer BL (1997) Diseases of the urogenital system. In: Altman RB, Clubb SL, Dorrestein GM, Quesenberry K (eds) *Avian Medicine and Surgery*, pp. 625–644. WB Saunders, Philadelphia.

Speer BL (2001) A clinical look at the avian pancreas in health and disease. *Proceedings of the European Association of Avian Veterinarians*, Munich, pp. 134–140.

Stauber E, Papageorges M, Sande R, Ward L (1990) Polyostotic hyperostosis associated with oviductal tumor in a cockatiel. *Journal of the American Veterinary Medical Association* **196**: 939–940.

Stogdale L (1986) Definition of diabetes mellitus. *Cornell Veterinarian* **76**: 156–174.

Stoica G, Russo E, Hoffman JR (1989) Abdominal tumor in a military macaw (diagnosis: metastatic ovarian carcinoma). *Laboratory Animals* **18**(5): 17–20.

Turk RJ, Kim J, Gallina AM (1981) Seminoma in a pigeon. *Avian Diseases* **25**: 752–755.

Von Zipper J, Tamasohke CH (1972) Pathologische Schilddrüsenbefunde bei Vögeln. In: *Diseases of Zoo Animals, 14th International Symposium*, Wroclaw, pp. 113–122. Akademie Verlag, Berlin.

Wadsworth PF, Jones DM (1979) Some abnormalities of the thyroid gland in non-domesticated birds. *Avian Pathology* **8**: 279–284.

Wadsworth PF, Jones DM, Pugsley SL (1985) A survey of mammalian and avian neoplasms at the Zoological Society of London. *Journal of Zoo Animal Medicine* **16**: 73–80.

Waller-Pendleton E, Rogers D, Epple A (1993) Diabetes mellitus in a red-tailed hawk (*Buteo jamaicensis*). *Avian Pathology* **22**: 631–635.

Wheler C (1992) Pituitary tumors in cockatiels. *Journal of the Association of Avian Veterinarians* **6**(2): 92.

Wight PAL (1986) Hemiagenesis of the thyroid gland in the quail (*Coturnix coturnix japonica*). *Journal of Comparative Pathology* **96**: 235–236.

Wilson RB, Holscher MA, Fullerton JR, Johnson MD (1988) Pineoblastoma in a cockatiel. *Avian Diseases* **32**: 591–593.

Woerpel RW, Rosskopf WJ (1984) Clinical experience with avian laboratory diagnostics. *Veterinary Clinics of North America* **14**: 249–286.

Zenoble RD, Kemppainen RJ, Young DW, Clubb SL (1985) Endocrine responses of healthy parrots to ACTH and thyroid stimulating hormone. *Journal of the American Veterinary Medical Association* **187**: 1116–1118.

Infectious diseases

8

Conservation biology of parasites

Paolo Zucca, Mauro Delogu

Omne vivum ex ovo [All life from an egg].
William Harvey, Exercitationes de generatione animalium,
1651

It may seem contradictory to start a manuscript on parasitology with a section devoted to the conservation of parasites. For decades veterinary parasitology books described parasites as plagues to be removed from every single animal. This is because veterinarians and wildlife managers understandably tend to focus on individual sick animals rather than on population aspects of infections (May, 1988). However, parasites represent a substantial aspect of biodiversity that has not yet been studied in detail (Windsor, 1995; Hoberg *et al.*, 1997). Many species of bird host diverse parasite fauna; some species are host-specific and some others spend their entire life cycle on the host. However, not all parasites are pathogenic to the host and the difference between parasitism, symbiosis, mutualism, commensalism and phoresis is not well defined for each parasite species and its hosts. For example, most of the parasites identified from wild birds cause no clinical diseases (Friend and Franson, 2002) and some parasites, such as avian mites, might even be beneficial for the host (Proctor and Owens, 2000).

When the population size of a host is reduced, the population size of host-specific parasites may also be reduced (Gompper and Williams, 1998) and the extinction of the parasitic species may happen before the extinction of the specific host. Although many of the arguments for conserving biodiversity or saving individual species also apply to parasite species (Gompper and Williams, 1988), the perception of parasites among the public is negative and it could be very difficult to justify expenditure for protecting an endangered parasite species (Gompper and Williams, 1988; Kellert, 1993; Aznar *et al.*, 2001).

It is important to emphasize that protecting populations of host-specific parasites may be essential for the health or survival of the host population involved in any conservation program (Gompper and Williams, 1988). The disappearance of one parasite species can strongly alter the balance and interaction among remaining parasite species within the host. In fact, the evolutionary destiny of parasites is linked to that of their hosts (Stork and Lyal, 1993). Conservation of endangered avian species requires the evaluation of several parameters, such as population dynamics, community ecology, breeding rate and environmental patterns. Monitoring and understanding the health status of a population should be another factor to be included in each conservation project (Deem *et al.*, 2001). Furthermore, veterinary involvement in conservation projects should start with a preliminary phase and not when the situation has already reached the crisis point. On the other hand, wildlife veterinarians should be prepared to work at an avian population level, where, for example, parasites and their biodiversity become useful indicators of the health status of the population.

The next time you found parasites on an avian patient belonging to an endangered species please remember that, from a biological point of view, the parasite may be more endangered than the host you are trying to save.

Arthropods

Paolo Zucca, Mauro Delogu

Arthropods comprise more than a million species and make up the largest and most varied phylum of the Animal Kingdom. We will focus our attention to those groups that are pathogenic to birds. Many of the species that affect birds are ectoparasites inhabiting the integument, although some are also found at a subcutaneous level, in the respiratory organs (trachea, airsacs) and in the viscera (Table 8.1).

Cooper (2002) advises, in the case of small birds, putting a piece of cotton wool soaked in ether or chloroform inside a plastic bag and keeping the bird in it for about 5 min, making sure that its head remains outside. The parasites are anesthetized and fall off the bird into the bottom of the bag (see also Ch. 9).

TABLE 8.1 Major groups of external parasites (ectoparasites) that affect birds

Type of parasite	Clinical signs	Diagnosis, differential diagnosis (DD) and post-mortem changes (PM)	Treatment/prevention
Bugs (Hemiptera – Cimicidae)	Poor appearance, irritability, restlessness especially at night, swelling and irritation of the derma	The discovery of parasites on the birds (especially at night) DD: other nocturnal bloodsucking parasites	Disinfestation of the environment, treatment of the birds with pyrethrin powder
Chewing lice (Phthiraptera – Mallophaga)	Scratching, itching, irritability, dull opaque plumage, ruffled damaged feathers	The presence of eggs attached to the feathers and of nymphs and adult parasites on the feathers PM: dull damaged feathers, the presence of eggs and dead adults on the plumage	Pyrethrin based powder insecticides, rotenone spray. Treatment, once a week, 2–3 times using also the plastic bag technique (Ccoper, 2002)
Dipterous (Diptera): mosquitoes (Culicidae); biting midges (Ceratopogonidae); blackflies (Simuliidae); blowflies (Calliphoridae); hippoboscid flies (Hippoboscidae)	Anemia, irritation, dermatitis on the parts of the body uncovered by the feathers, the presence of eggs or larvae around the natural orifices or on skin wounds	The presence of biting insects in aviaries or shelters or on the birds PM: skin swellings, weight loss, the presence in some cases of eggs and/or larvae; immediately after death the parasites abandon the corpse	*Mosquito*: mosquito nets, pyrethrins *Other flies*: very difficult to eradicate *Blowflies*: removal by hand of the larvae from wounds, disinfection with warm water containing disinfectant
Fleas (Siphonaptera)	Skin irritation, preening and ruffling of feathers, loss of blood through the skin, dirty and matted plumage	Identification of eggs and larvae, which can be found mostly in nests and on nestlings. *Echidnophaga* attaches itself to the head of the bird	Disinfestation of the environment, treatment of the birds with pyrethrin powder
Ticks (Ixodida)	Anemia, irritation, itching and lesions of the tissues, poor growth, death	The discovery of larvae, nymphs or adults on the body of the bird	Removal by hand of the parasites, treatment of the environment
Mites (Acari)	See Table 8.2		
Beetles (Coleoptera)	Irritation, itching and lesions of the tissues	The presence of *Dermestes* sp. or other species in nests or on the birds	As for ticks

Bugs (Hemiptera – Cimicidae)

All the species belonging to the Family Cimicidae are obligate hematophagous ectoparasites of vertebrates. They are not regarded as disease carriers but their blood-feeding activity frequently causes loss of blood and irritation to their hosts. Cimicids are dorsoventrally flattened and brownish or yellowish in color according to the species; females are larger than males and their life cycle requires 28–120 d from egg to adult according to the environmental conditions. All avian species are susceptible, in that the bugs are rarely host-specific. Poultry and cage and aviary birds are usually more likely to be affected than free-living birds because these parasites hide in the cracks of walls near bird shelters. The most common species that feed on avian hosts are *Cimex lectularius* in North America, Europe and the former Soviet Union, *Haematosiphon inodorus* in Central America and *Ornithocoris toledoi* in Brazil (Krinsky, 2002). Several other cimicid species, such as the pigeon bug (*C. columbarius*) or the house martin bug (*Oeciacus hirundinis*), live in bird nests and feed on them but can also feed on humans. Adult blood-suckers can survive long periods of fasting, both in the nests of free-living birds (who may act as direct vectors) and in the vicinity of cages and aviaries. See also Table 8.1 for clinical and pathological features.

Chewing lice (Phthiraptera – Mallophaga)

The mallophaga are among the most common external parasites of birds. There are about 2250 known species associated with birds all over the world. The long coevolutionary history between chewing lice and birds, confirmed by fossil records (Fig. 8.1), points to an early origin for lice. It is possible that the ancestral host of parasitic lice was not a modern bird or mammal, as is generally accepted, but an early feathered dinosaur (Wappler *et al.*, 2004), although all the available evidence indicates that the original blood-feeding insects, and the plague of dinosaurs, were the Diptera (Grimaldi and Engel, 2005). Although few species imbibe blood, they usually feed on host feathers, skin or skin products. They have a dorsoventrally flattened body of small size (a few millimeters), a rather large head with a pair of

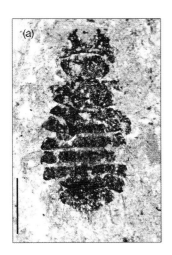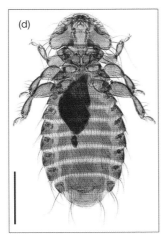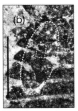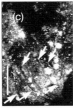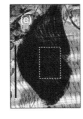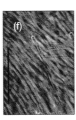

Fig. 8.1 *Megamenopon rasnitsyni* gen. et sp. nov. and its extant close relative *Holomenopon brevithoracicum*. (a) Complete exoskeleton of *Megamenopon rasnitsyni*. (b) Enlargement of the crop (encircled), part of the foregut visible within the abdomen. (c) Enlargement of the rectangular section highlighted in (b) showing feather barbules preserved within the crop. Examples are highlighted with arrows. (d) *Holomenopon brevithoracicum* from a mute swan (*Cygnus olor*). (e) Enlargement of the *Holomenopon* crop. (f) Enlargement of the section highlighted in (e) showing feather barbules within the *Holomenopon* crop. Scale bars: (a, b) 2 mm, (c) 0.125 mm, (d) 0.5 mm, (e) 0.3 mm, (f) 0.1 mm. (Courtesy of the Royal Society of London, Dr. T. Wappler and Dr. V. Smith; reproduced with permission from Wappler *et al.*, 2004).

rudimentary eyes (sometimes absent), short antennae and a masticatory system with robust mandibles. They have no wings and their legs, which are rather short, have strong nails as hooks at the end (Fig. 8.2). The females lay their eggs on the feathers of the bird on which they live. They usually exhibit strong host specificity and some species also site specificity, inhabiting different regions of the body of the host (Durden, 2002). The entire life cycle takes place on the host and they can survive for only a few days away from it. Because of the importance of maintaining a continuous association with their host, *Mallophaga* evolved several host-attachment mechanisms to resist the preening activities of infested birds. On the other hand, as reported by Clayton *et al.* (2005), the adaptive radiation of avian beak morphology has also been strongly influenced by preening, which is the first line of defense against harmful ectoparasites such as feather lice.

They are frequently found on free-living birds and also on cage and aviary birds such as passerines, psittacines, raptors and poultry (Figs 8.3–8.5). The most common lice of poultry are the chicken body louse (*Menacanthus*

stramineus), the shaft louse (*Menopon gallinae*) and the wing louse (*Lipeurus caponis*). The heaviest infestations are usually found on sick or injured birds. The reduction of preening activity in sick birds can result in an increased louse population. Direct exchange from bird to bird is usually the primary transmission mechanism for lice, but there are also some new phoresis mechanisms. See also Table 8.1 for clinical and pathological features.

Dipterous (Diptera)

God in His wisdom
Made the fly
And then forgot
To tell us why
Ogden Nash (cited by Grimaldi and Engel, 2005)

The insects of this Order are significant not only because of the lesions they can cause to the host but above all because they are important vectors of infectious and parasitic diseases. They are usually cosmopolitan and attack practically all bird species. The families that most often affect birds are:

- Mosquitoes (Culicidae): the blood-sucking females cause irritation, anemia and are vectors of serious infectious diseases (malaria, trypanosomiasis and viral diseases)
- Biting midges (Ceratopogonidae): minute blood-sucking flies; only the females are blood-sucking; vectors for several viruses and hemosporidians (blood protozoa of birds); intermediate hosts for filarial roundworms
- Blackflies (Simuliidae) – small, powerful fliers; blood-sucking females transmit *Leucocytozoon*, some avian trypanosomes, filariasis and several viral diseases
- Blowflies (Calliphoridae) – agent of myiasis of the skin and internal organs; nesting or injured birds are most often affected
- Hippoboscid flies (Hippoboscidae) – quite large (7–9 mm); adapted morphologically to attach themselves to the feathers of the bird; cause anemia and are carriers of infectious and parasitic diseases such as avian trypanosomiasis and hemosporidians. They are frequent on free-living birds, especially juvenile raptors, pigeons, swifts and passerines. See also Figs 8.6 and 8.7 and Table 8.1 for clinical and pathological features.

Fleas (Siphonaptera)

There are hundreds of flea species and as a group they have principally evolved as parasites of mammals (Durden and Traub, 2002). However, about 6% (five families and 25 genera) of the known species affect birds. Adult fleas are small (1–8 mm), laterally flattened ecto-

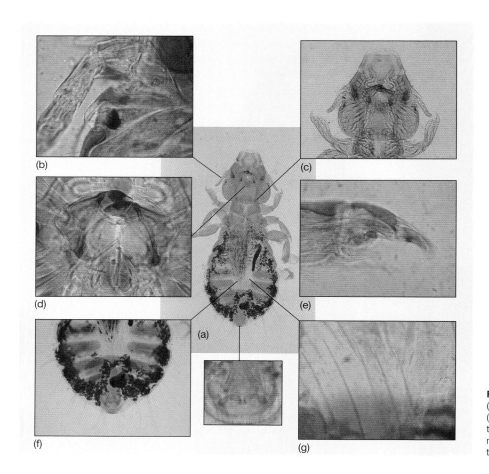

Fig. 8.2 Louse from a long eared owl (*Asio otus*). (a) Complete exoskeleton. (a–g) Enlargements of respectively (b) the eye and antennae (c) the head (d) the mandible (e) the hook (f) the abdomen (g) the fur.

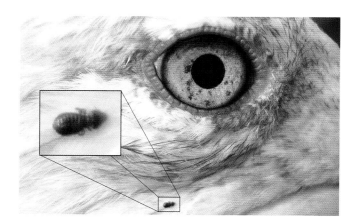

Fig. 8.3 Louse from a Mediterranean herring gull (*Larus cachinnans*).

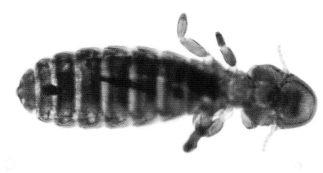

Fig. 8.4 *Degeeriella rufa* is probably the most common ectoparasite found in captive Falconiformes.

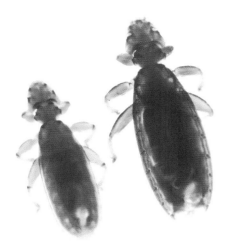

Fig. 8.5 *Laemobothrion tinnuculi* is a louse species frequently found in captive falcons in the Middle East.

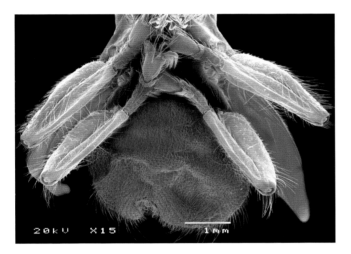

Fig. 8.6 Hippoboscidae, *Craterina pallida* from a common swift (*Apus apus*) dorsal view, scanning electron microscopy (SEM). (Courtesy of Professor M. Trentini).

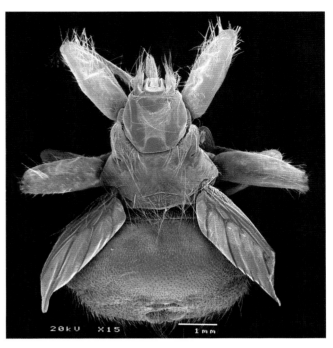

Fig. 8.7 Hippoboscidae, *Craterina pallida* from a common swift, ventral view, SEM. Note the long, sharp hooks. (Courtesy of Professor M. Trentini).

Ticks and mites

The arthropods belonging to the suborder Metastigmata are characterized by their relatively large size and are called ticks, while those of the other suborders (characterized by their very small size) are called mites. They both have a rounded body divided into an upper part of reduced size called the capitulum (false head) and a trunk called the podosome, with four pairs of legs in the adults and nymphs and three pairs in the larvae. They have the following characteristics: separate sexes and sexual dimorphism (the male is smaller than the female), mostly oviparous, adapted to temporary, periodic or continuous ectoparasitism.

Ticks (Ixodida)

These are quite large arthropods (Figs 8.8 and 8.9) and have an oval, flattened body when fasting, but it becomes rounded after eating. They are obligatory, temporary or periodic parasites of reptiles, birds and mammals. Ticks transmit a greater variety of infectious organisms than any other group of blood-sucking arthropods and they are of great importance from the zoonotic point of view (Sonenshine *et al.*, 2002). The suborder Ixodida contains three families: the Ixodidae, Argasidae and Nuttalliellidae. The last family has only one known species, which shares common features with the other two families but has no veterinary

parasites. Although the adults have no wings, they are fast runners and can jump long distances. The mouth apparatus is able to fix on to the skin and suck blood. Because of their need to locate the host, fleas have developed a complex host-finding behavior that is influenced by several host stimuli such as body warmth, vibrations, air movement, odor of host organic fluids, etc. (Durden and Traub, 2002). The most representative species of avian veterinary importance are the stick-tight flea (*Echidnophaga gallinacea*) and the European chick flea (*Ceratophyllus gallinae*). Cage and aviary birds are rarely affected by these parasites, which are, however, frequent in domestic fowl and nesting free-living birds. It is often difficult to completely eradicate them from breeding facilities. See also Table 8.1 for clinical and pathological features.

importance. Of the family Ixodidae, *Ixodes ricinus* has a hard dorsal shield (hard tick) that covers the whole back of the males and only the upper part of the body of the larvae, nymphs and adult females. Hard ticks have an accentuated sexual dimorphism, the body of the female being soft and very elastic while that of the male is hard and not very extensible. The life cycle includes four stages – egg, larva, nymph and adult – and requires about 3 years to be completed. Usually, each instar feed once on the host and more than 90% of the life cycle is spent off the host. This life-cycle pattern is termed a three-host life cycle. However, males remain on the hosts and feed repeatedly while inseminating several females.

Of the family Argasidae, *Argas persicus* (Fig. 8.10), *A. reflexus* and *Ornithodoros* spp. are commonly called soft ticks since they have no dorsal shield or chitinous plates. The rostrum is laid out in an anteroventral position and therefore is not visible when looking at the parasite from above. The Argasidae are temporary parasites of birds and mammals; they suck blood mostly at night and then abandon the host and hide in the crevices and cracks of the ground or building. They are able to survive long periods of fasting. Compared to *Ixodes* spp. they have two or more nymphal instars in their 'multihost' life cycle. Ticks have a worldwide distribution. The most significant tick from the point of view of avian parasitology is *A. persicus*, which is mostly found in tropical and temperate regions. *I. ricinus*, on the other hand, is widely distributed in North America, Europe and Asia.

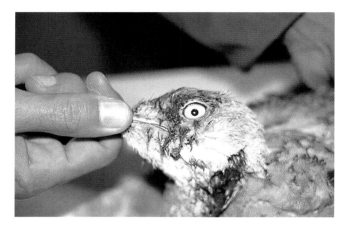

Fig. 8.8 *Ixodes* sp. around the eyes of a houbara bustard (*Chlamydotis undulata*). (Courtesy of Dr. J. Samour).

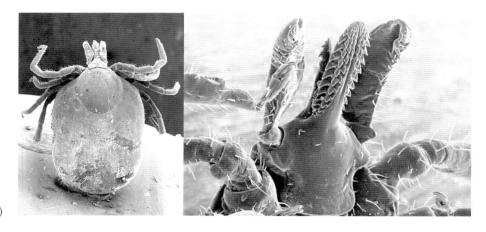

(a)

(b) Fig. 8.9 *Ixodes ricinus*. (a) Female, dorsal view. (b) Ventral view of capitulum. (Courtesy of Professor L. De Vos).

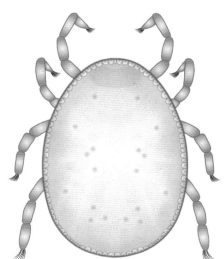

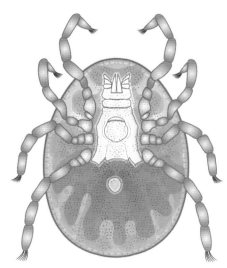

Fig. 8.10 *Argas persicus* – female, dorsal and ventral view.

Birds are usually affected mostly by soft-ticks and all species of bird in captivity are likely to be infested. Even if many ticks exhibit strong host specificity, over than 300 species of vertebrates have been recorded as hosts for *I. ricinus* (Sonenshine *et al.*, 2002). Because of the host-seeking behavior of the different instars, birds are more often attacked by larvae and nymphs (host I and II). Transmission is usually direct, indirect in the environment. Hard ticks should be gently removed from the avian host using a tick-remover device (Fig. 8.11), to avoid squeezing and thus injecting the midgut tick content into the host. For the same reason, it is not recommended before removal to put any solution on the tick that might induce regurgitation of saliva and its content inside the avian host to minimizing the risk of transmitting tick-borne diseases. See also Table 8.1 for clinical and pathological features.

Mites (Acari)

The mites are among the most common ectoparasites to affect cage and aviary and free-living birds. They rarely exceed 2 mm in size and the types of problem they cause include:

- Temporary or chronic dermatitis due to bites or feeding on the host skin and feathers
- Chronic dermatitis due to invasion of the skin
- Feather loss
- Transmission of pathogenic microorganisms and metazoan parasites
- Intermediate hosting of tapeworms
- Invasion of respiratory tract and sometimes internal organs. According to the different mite species and to the parasitic burden, chronic or heavy infections might result in debilitation, anemia, reduced growth and death.

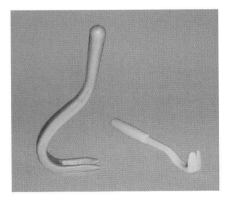

Fig. 8.11 A patented tick remover device, the O'Tom hook (H3D Company, France), which has proved useful for removing ticks from birds.

There are more than 250 species of mite recognized as pathogenic and given the great number of taxa involved it is quite difficult to identify and to give detail about the behavior and ecology of each species, especially for the mites inhabiting free-living birds (Mullen and O'Connor, 2002). Instead they are considered in relation to the different anatomical areas they affect. See also Table 8.2 for clinical and pathological features.

Skin mites

Red mite (*Dermanyssus gallinae*)

Synonyms: *Chicken mite, red poultry mite, pigeon mite.* The body of this mite is small and oval (600–700 µm); it is whitish when fasting and becomes reddish after eating (Fig. 8.12). It has a worldwide distribution and it parasitized virtually all species of bird although poultry, canaries, pigeons and some species of free-living birds are the most often affected. It is found less frequently on raptors and parrots (Keymer, 1982; Cooper, 2002). This mite lives in nesting materials or around the cages and it visits birds during the night to feed on their blood. It lays its eggs in the cracks of walls around cages or aviaries or inside nests. The female is able to lay eggs 12–14 h after the first meal of blood, and in high temperatures the eggs can hatch in 48–72 h. In optimal environmental conditions the cycle can be completed in 5–7 d and the adults can survive many months without feeding. St Luis encephalitis (SLE), eastern equine encephalitis (EEE) and western equine encephalitis (WEE) viruses have been isolated from *D. gallinae*; however there is conflicting evidence that these mites are able to spread these viruses among birds or transmit them to humans (Mullen and O'Connor, 2002).

Northern mite (*Ornithonyssus sylviarum*)

Synonym: *Northern fowl mite.* Together with the preceding mite, this is one of the most widespread ectoparasites of domestic ducks and free-living birds. The life cycle of this mite differs from that of the red mite in that it takes place entirely on the host; it can survive only for a few days away from its host. It has a wide distribution: it has been reported mainly in North America, Europe and some subtropical countries. It is less frequent in cage and aviary birds than *D. gallinae*. Many species are susceptible, including poultry, passerines, crows, pigeons, canaries and mynah birds and transmission is usually direct. It has been proved that *O. sylviarum* can transmit WEE virus from one bird to another but, as reported for *D. gallinae*, it seems that this mite does not play any role in transmitting these arboviruses to humans.

TABLE 8.2 Major groups of mites that affect birds

Parasite	Clinical signs	Diagnosis, differential diagnosis (DD) and post-mortem changes (PM)	Treatment and prevention
SKIN MITES			
Red mite, *Dermanyssus gallinae*	Anemia, itching, weakness, nocturnal agitation, dull plumage	Identification of parasites on the birds; it is better to look for them in the night hours using the method of putting a white cloth over the cage* PM: anemic birds, the presence of ingested mites in the crop and esophagus	Treatment of the environment and treatment of the birds with pyrethroids and piperonilbutoxide
Northern mite, *Ornithonyssus sylviarum*	Similar to the preceding with the difference that, since they always remain on the bird, the irritation is continuous	Identification of the parasite on the bird. In this case they are always present PM: as red mite	Treatment as for lice
FEATHER MITES			
Megninia spp., *Pterolichus* spp.	Occasionally cause dermatitis and debilitation in avian hosts	Identification of the mites on the bird	Topical acaricides such as rotenone, pyrethroids or other
Quill mites: *Syringophilus* spp., *Dermatoglyphus* spp.	Loss of feathers, mainly on the tail and wings	Identification of the mites found inside the quills	Difficult to eradicate because not very host specific
MANGE MITES			
Epidermoptid mites: *Epidermoptes* spp., *Microlichus* spp.	Itching, pityriasis, superficial dermatitis and other clinical signs similar to those caused by other skin mites	Identification of the mites on the bird	Treatment as for cnemidocoptic mites
Knemidocoptid mites: *Knemidocoptes pilae*, *Knemidocoptes mutans*	The presence of scabs and sometimes deforming crusty lesions on the beak and legs	Identification of the mites by means of an examination of the skin scarification previously put in a 10% potassium hydroxide solution DD: carcinoma of the beak in budgerigars; lesions caused by other mites	Topical acaricides such as rotenone, pyrethroids or other. Topical ivermectin
RESPIRATORY MITES			
Rhinonyssid mites, *Sternostoma tracheacolum*	Pneumonia, ruffled feathers, respiratory wheezing and whistling, frequent coughing, gasping for breath and attempts to clear the throat	Pulmonary congestion, tracheitis, thickening and accumulation of a yellowish liquid around the airsacs DD: other forms of pneumonia such as aspergillosis, syngamiasis, passerine pox	Topical ivermectin, pyrethrin and rotenone spray via aerosol

* It is a common practice for many breeders to place a white cloth over the cage during the night. The following morning many mites that have attacked the birds during the night take refuge in the cloth.

Feather mites

About 440 species belonging to 33 families of mite live on or in the feathers of birds. Their extreme morphological biodiversity is related to the great number of different hosts and microhabitats provided by feathers, in which they are adapted to live (Fig. 8.13). Species such as *Megninia* spp. and *Pterolichus* spp. usually live on the surface of the feathers, where they feed as saprophages. Occasionally they can cause dermatitis and debilitation in poultry.

Quill mites

These are small mites that are morphologically adapted to live inside the quills of feathers. Their body is narrow and elongated. They are distributed worldwide and they affect many species of bird, particularly gallinaceous birds, passerines, pigeons, psittacines and canaries. Little is known of their life cycle, although it has been suggested that the whole cycle takes place inside the quills of feathers (Keymer, 1982) and that they rarely cause any harm to the host. *Syringophilus bipectinatus* can cause feather loss only when there is a heavy infection.

Mange mites

Epidermoptid mites (*Epidermoptes bilobatus* and *Michrolichus avus*)

Although described as skin or feather mites, these are more appropriately grouped with mange mites because

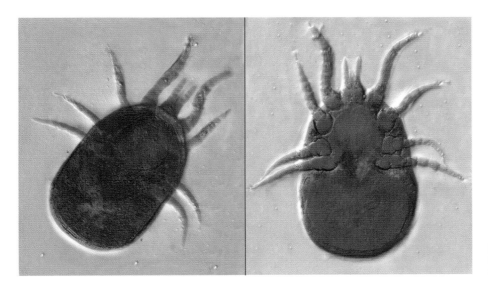

Fig. 8.12 *Dermanyssus gallinae* from a canary (*Serinus canaria*), ventral and dorsal view.

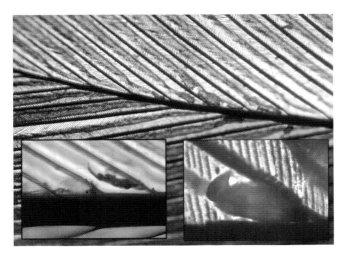

Fig. 8.13 Feather mites, mixed infection, budgerigar (*Melopsittacus undulatus*).

of the scabby dermatitis they can cause on their hosts. Mites of the epidermis do not exceed 0.4 mm and have a soft, rounded body. They are widely distributed in many countries of the world (Europe, North and South America, etc.) and they affect many species of bird, living on the skin surface or in feather follicles, where their feeding can cause itching, pityriasis and other superficial dermatitis. *M. avus* can cause severe mange and crateriform skin lesions in several avian species.

Knemidocoptic mites (*Knemidocoptes pilae* and *K. mutans*)

These are the etiological agents of beak and leg mange, known also, respectively, as scaly face mite and scaly leg mite. *K. pilae*, although it usually affects the budgerigar, has also been reported in other species such as canaries and parakeets. It causes crusty lesions around the beak that may evolve into a chronic distortion of the beak.

K. mutans is located under the epidermal scales of the bird's legs, causing irritation, hyperkeratosis and crusts that may cover the entire limb. Transmission, which is usually direct, may be also environmental.

Respiratory mites

These are endoparasites of the nasal passages, trachea and occasionally the lung and airsacs of several species of bird. Heavy mite infestation can cause rhinitis or sinusitis even if, in most cases, infested birds do not show any respiratory symptoms.

Rhinonyssid mites (*Sternostoma tracheacolum*)

Synonym: *Canary lung mite*. This mite has a higher pathogenicity than other species of respiratory mite and parasitizes the trachea, bronchi, parenchymal lung tissues and airsacs. Canaries would seem to be the species most commonly affected and the mite is widely distributed. Its life cycle is not known, although it appears that it is not influenced to a great extent by external environmental conditions; it is probably transmitted directly, especially when adult birds feed their nestlings. Chronic heavy infestation usually results in severe respiratory distress, difficult breathing, emaciation and death (Figs 8.14 and 8.15).

Beetles (Coleoptera)

Although not generally considered of great importance in avian medicine, beetles are vectors of pathogens, an intermediate host for helminths and nematodes such as *Serratospiculum* spp. and can cause direct injury to young birds, especially when they infect nests. Larder beetles (*Dermestes* spp.) can attack also adult birds, as reported by several authors (Samour and Naldo, 2003; Merkl *et al.*, 2004). See Table 8.1 for clinical and pathological features.

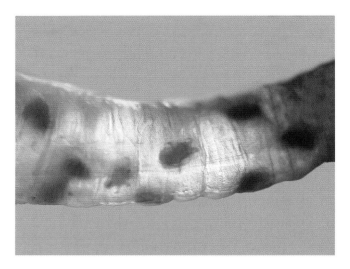

Fig. 8.14 *Sternostoma tracheacolum*, trachea from a canary (*Serinus canaria*). It is possible to see several mites inside the tracheal lumen. Necropsy finding.

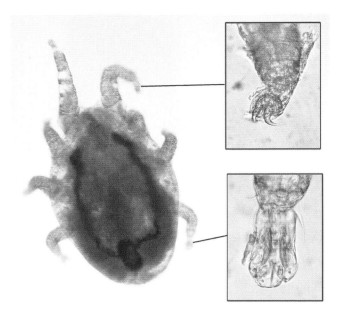

Fig. 8.15 *Sternostoma tracheacolum* from a canary. Full body of the mite and enlargement of the sharp leg hooks.

Protozoa

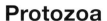

Paolo Zucca, Mauro Delogu

The protozoa are microorganisms made up of a single cell containing one or more nuclei visible only under the microscope. They are considered to be the first animals that appeared on earth and some species cause serious diseases in humans and animals.

Trichomonas species

Trichomonas spp. (Figs 8.16–8.28) have one nucleus, a blepharoplast, an axostyle, four flagella and an undulating membrane. In the field of avian medicine, two of the most important protozoa of this family are *Trichomonas gallinae*, which affects the upper digestive and respiratory systems, and *T. gallinarum*, which is found in the lower part of the digestive system. *T. gallinae* affects many species of cage and aviary bird such as budgerigars, pigeons (causing so-called canker) and especially falcons (causing the so-called frounce, which has been known to falconers for centuries), whereas *T. gallinarum* seems to limit its pathogenic activity to gallinaceous birds and turkeys. Infection of psittacines is rare. Pigeons can be carriers and transmit the infection to raptors when fed live or freshly killed. *T. gallinae* is widely distributed and has been reported in America, Europe, Asia and Africa. The clinical signs are variable and infections are sometimes asymptomatic. Affected birds usually show sensory depression, ruffled feathers, anorexia, weight loss and regurgitation or vomiting. The infection produces yellowish caseous growths. According to the species attacked there can be lesions of the oral and nasal cavities, infraorbital sinuses, ear,

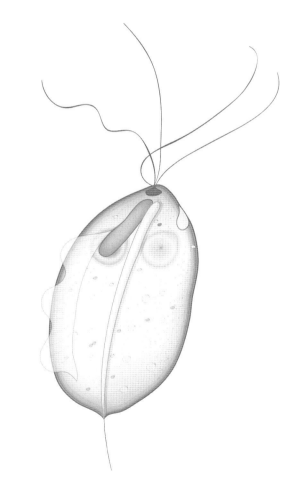

Fig. 8.16 *Trichomonas gallinae*.

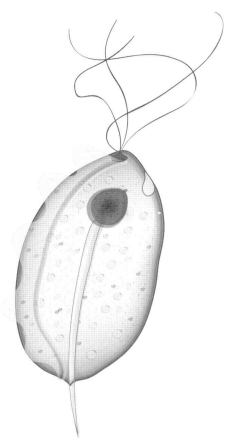

Fig. 8.17 *Trichomonas gallinarum*.

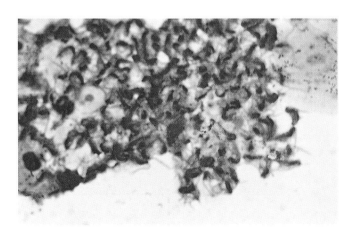

Fig. 8.18 *T. gallinae* in an oropharyngeal aspirate from a domestic pigeon (*Columba livia*). This protozoon is commonly found in the upper respiratory and digestive systems of pigeons and doves. The preparation was stained using cotton blue stain. (Courtesy of Mr. C. Silvanose).

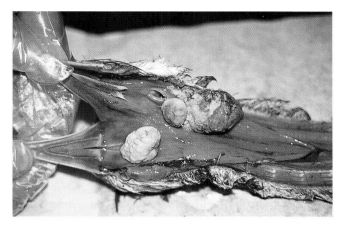

Fig. 8.19 Large caseous trichomoniasis masses around the oropharynx of a houbara bustard. Bustards are very susceptible to infections produced by *Trichomonas gallinae*. (Courtesy of Dr. J. Samour).

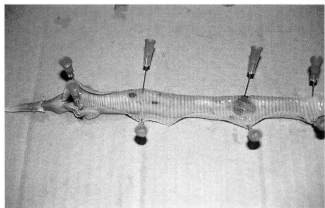

Fig. 8.20 Small nodular trichomoniasis growths in the trachea of a houbara bustard. This type of lesion is atypical of trichomoniasis. Other atypical trichomoniasis lesions include those in the nasal cavity, infraorbital sinuses, trachea and celomic cavity. Such lesion are very frequently overlooked by clinicians. (Courtesy of Dr. J. Samour).

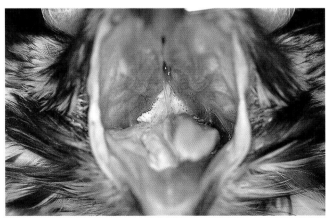

Fig. 8.21 Large trichomoniasis mass on the oropharynx and base of the tongue of a saker falcon (*Falco cherrug*). Large masses such as this require surgical removal under anesthesia 5–7 d after treatment. Very often, cleaning, disinfection and mild curetting is necessary every 3–5 d before healing is completed. (Courtesy of Dr. J. Samour).

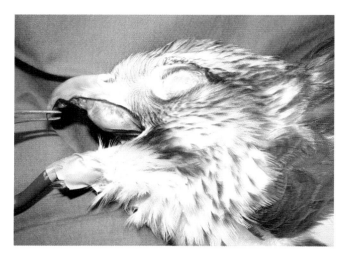

Fig. 8.22 Large trichomoniasis growth in the nasal cavity of a saker falcon protruding through the hard palate. There is also a fistula just cranially to the choana. (Courtesy of Dr. J. Samour).

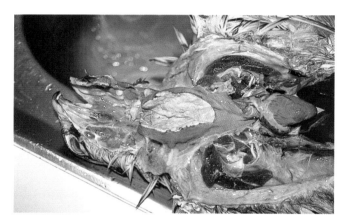

Fig. 8.23 Chronic trichomoniasis infection in the oral cavity and crop of a falcon. Falcons in the Middle East are very commonly infected with *T. gallinae* by feeding on live or freshly killed pigeons. (Courtesy of Dr. U. Wernery).

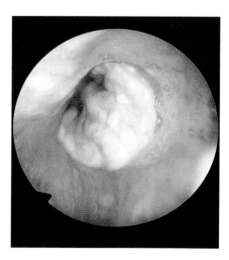

Fig. 8.24 Large nodular, caseous trichomoniasis growth observed during an endoscopy examination at the cervical esophagus of a gyrfalcon (*Falco rusticolus*). (Courtesy of Dr. J. Samour).

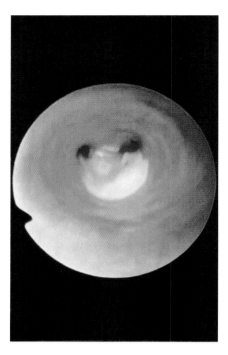

Fig. 8.25 Bilateral trichomoniasis caseous growths obstructing the tracheobronchial syrinx of a peregrine falcon (*Falco peregrinus*). The treatment of such infections very often necessitates the surgical removal of the growths after completing the antiprotozoal treatment. (Courtesy of Dr. J. Samour).

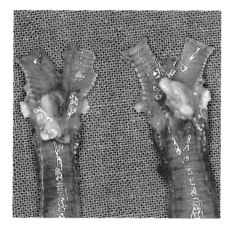

Fig. 8.26 Trichomoniasis growths on the tracheobronchial syrinx of a saker falcon. The lesions were chronic and had penetrated the walls of the syrinx. The bird was presented with laborious breathing and pronounced wet rale. (Courtesy of Dr. J. Samour).

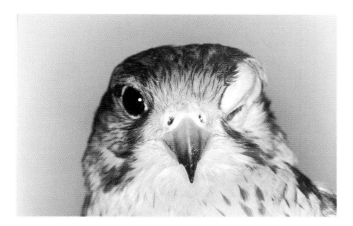

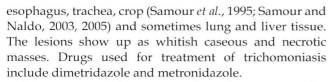

Fig. 8.27 Saker falcon showing a large supraorbital swelling caused by a medium-sized caseous trichomoniasis growth. The infection was located in the supraorbital diverticulum of the infraorbital sinus. Courtesy of Dr. J. Samour.

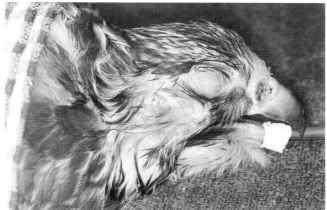

Fig. 8.28 Saker falcon affected with intra-auricular trichomoniasis. Note the presence of a large amount of caseous material within the vestibule of the external ear. In this case, the infection could have spread from the oropharynx to the middle ear through the infundibular cleft. Courtesy of Dr. J. Samour.

esophagus, trachea, crop (Samour *et al.*, 1995; Samour and Naldo, 2003, 2005) and sometimes lung and liver tissue. The lesions show up as whitish caseous and necrotic masses. Drugs used for treatment of trichomoniasis include dimetridazole and metronidazole.

Direct transmission occurs through contact or by the ingestion of contaminated food or water. There is no cystic form of resistance and only the adult protozoan form has been described. Feeding raptors in captivity with live pigeons carries a risk of *T. gallinae* transmission. A useful precaution to avoid the diffusion of this protozoan disease in captive raptors is to freeze the pigeons for a minimum of 24 h; it would seem that this procedure kills the parasite or renders it innocuous (Greiner and Ritchie, 1994; Cooper, 2002).

Giardia species

In this genus, contrary to what happens with *Trichomonas* spp., there is formation of cysts, which are eliminated by the host in its feces (Fig. 8.29). They can stay alive for 3 weeks in damp surroundings. After having been ingested by a new host, the cysts free trophozoites into the small intestine, where they attach themselves to the surface of the villus. Birds are subject to reinfestation, which would suggest that a long-term immunity response after infection does not occur (Greiner and Ritchie, 1994). Many psittacines, herons, raptors, toucans and Anseriformes are susceptible to this protozoon. The transmission is usually direct, through the feces. Often these protozoa are found in the feces of asymptomatic psittacines, which would suggest the existence of healthy carriers. Clinical signs have included debilitation, chronic and recurrent mucoid diarrhea, feces of variable color and consistency, anorexia, lethargy and weight loss. Rate of mortality is up to 50%. Diagnosis

requires identification of the parasite in the intestine or the discovery of cysts in the feces. The cystic form is eliminated intermittently so it is necessary to carry out repeated examinations. Preventions require an environmental hygiene. Keeping aviaries as dry as possible it helps reducing the burden of infectious cysts. Treatment of giardiasis has included dimetridazole and metronidazole.

Hexamita species

The most significant pathogenic protozoa of this genus in avian species are *Hexamita meleagridis*, which affects turkeys, and *H. columbae*, which affects pigeons. *Hexamita* spp. have been isolated in various psittacine species, even in some cases when there were no clinical signs. The parasite is mostly found in the upper intestinal tract and the cysts are probably the infectious form. The differential diagnosis should be made with giardiasis and trichomoniasis. Under microscope the parasites differ from *Trichomonas* in that they have six anterior flagella and their movements are rapid (Fig. 8.30).

Histomonas species

Histomoniasis is a common disease in gallinaceous birds, especially the turkey, while its occurrence in other species of bird is sporadic (Keymer, 1982; Greiner and Ritchie, 1994). *Histomonas meleagridis* has an amebic body of 5–30 μm, with one or two flagella (Fig. 8.31); it does not produce cysts but is transmitted through the eggs and then the larvae of the nematode *Heterakis gallinarum*, which can keep the protozoa alive for a year or more. Clinical signs include a weakened state and sensory depression, with a high mortality rate in

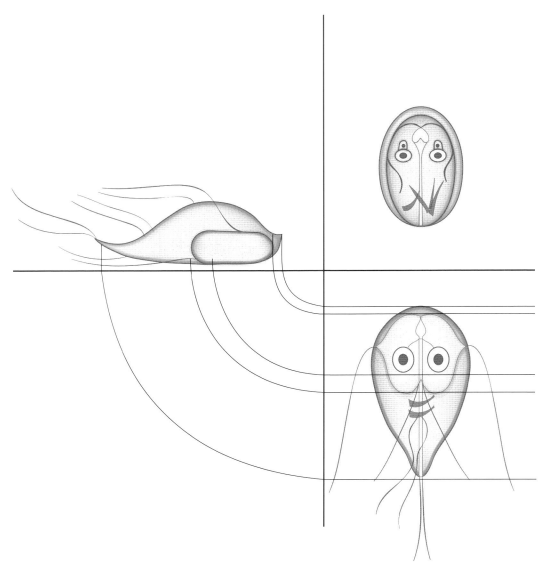

Fig. 8.29 *Giardia intestinalis* – top left and bottom right: trophozoite, orthogonal view (lateral and ventral view); top right: cyst.

the young. Post-mortem findings frequently report ulceration and necrosis of the mucosa of the ceca with the formation of nodules and sometimes of typical liver lesions with yellowish areas of necrosis surrounded by a gray halo and ascites. The characteristic sulfur-yellow color of the feces and the discovery of parasites in the feces are useful diagnostic signs.

Coccidia

This group comprises a notable number of species and represents one of the most serious diseases in poultry. Only some families of cage and aviary bird are particularly subject to this parasite. The life cycle takes place on one host with a phase of resistance and maturation (sporulation) in the external environment

(oocysts). Coccidia are largely intracellular parasites of the epithelial cells of the intestine of vertebrates and enter their host orally. They are rather common in finches, canaries, some species of psittacines and especially in Falconiformes, Galliformes and Columbiformes, in which they are one of the main causes of enteric disorders.

Eimeria and *Isospora* species

The protozoa belonging to the *Eimeria* and *Isospora* genera (Figs 8.32 and 8.33) represent the real coccidia and with few exceptions they are endocellular parasites of the epithelial cells of the intestine of vertebrates. They have only one host, in which they reproduce asexually (schizogony) and sexually (gametogony) with the formation of a zygote, which then becomes

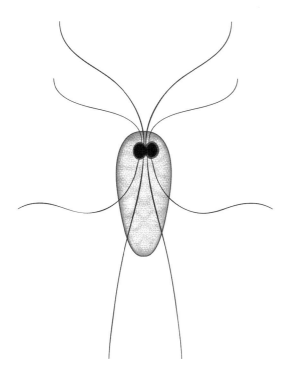

Fig. 8.30 *Hexamita meleagridis* – trophozoite.

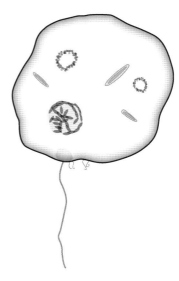

Fig. 8.31 *Histomonas meleagridis*.

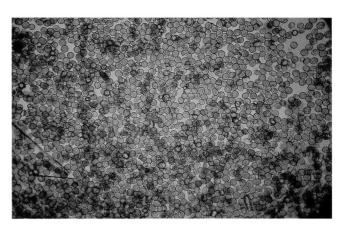

Fig. 8.32 Severe *Isospora* sp. infection in a South American finch (*Carduelis atrata*).

an oocyst and will later mature in the external environment after having been eliminated in the feces (sporogony). During the process of maturation within the oocyst, the sporocysts differ (four in *Eimeria*, two in *Isospora*); they in turn enclose the sporozoites (two in *Eimeria*, four in *Isospora*). At this point the oocysts are infectious if ingested by the definitive host. Sometimes, finches can host an enormous number of coccidia and yet be asymptomatic. Clinical signs have included mucoid or bloody diarrhea, ruffled plumage, inappetence, sensory depression and death. At post-mortem a frequent finding is the presence of hemorrhages in the small intestine, which is congested and dilated. Diagnosis is made by microscopical examination of the feces; *Isospora* in passerines is excreted mostly in the evening when the birds are getting ready to sleep.

They have a worldwide distribution and the infection has been reported in many species of bird and especially in Galliformes, pigeons, finches and psittacines. It has been observed that *Isospora* is less host-specific than *Eimeria*. Direct transmission occurs through the ingestion of the oocysts in food or water contaminated with fecal material.

Caryospora species

Parasites of this genus (Figs 8.34–8.36) affect mainly juvenile and subadult Falconiformes in captivity. Adults are believed to develop a certain degree of

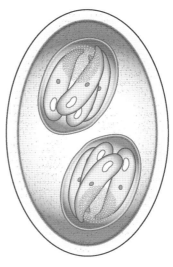

Fig. 8.33 *Isospora* sp., sporulated ococysts.

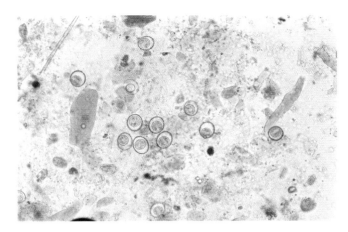

Fig. 8.34 A sporulated *Caryospora megafalconis* oocyst in a fecal sample from a saker falcon. Direct smear. (Courtesy of Mr. S. K. John).

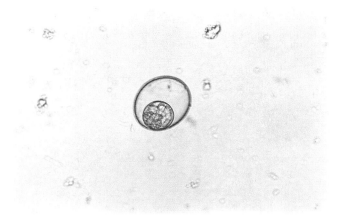

Fig. 8.36 *Caryospora megafalconis* in a fecal sample from a saker falcon. Direct smear. (Courtesy of Mr. S. K. John).

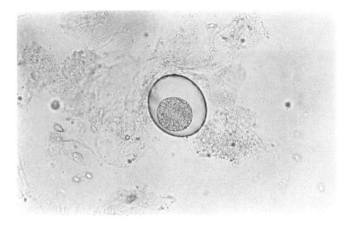

Fig. 8.35 *Caryospora falconis* in a fecal sample from a saker falcon. Direct smear. (Courtesy of Mr. S. K. John).

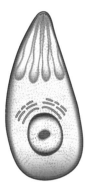

Fig. 8.37 *Toxoplasma gondii* – cystozoite.

immunity. There are at least seven species of *Caryospora* reported in the literature affecting birds of prey (Heidenreich, 1997). The most commonly diagnosed species in the Middle East include *Caryospora falconis*, *C. neofalconis*, *C. megafalconis* and *C. kutzeri* (J. Samour, personal communication). Forbes and Simpson (1997) described coccidiosis in 16 juvenile merlins (*Falco columbarius*) and one juvenile snowy owl (*Nyctea scandiacea*) produced by *Caryospora neofalconis* at breeding facilities in the UK.

Toxoplasma species

Toxoplasma gondii (Fig. 8.37) is the cause of disease in a wide range of species of mammals and birds and is considered to be a cosmopolitan microorganism. Nonetheless, there are very few reports of toxoplasmosis affecting pigeons, domestic fowl, penguins, mynah birds, canaries, crows or parrots. Symptomatology is not pathognomonic. Frequent post-mortem findings are vasculitis and necrotic foci in the lungs, liver and heart, and hepatomegaly. Infection is difficult to diagnose without using laboratory methods. The cysts in the heart or muscles are often confused with those of *Sarcocystis*.

Sarcocystis species

This is a parasite that may produce various pathological disorders depending on the host; the infection has been diagnosed in more than 60 different species of bird, including Passeriformes and psittacines. It is assumed that the life cycle includes sexual multiplication in the intestine of the definitive host and a second phase (extraintestinal) in an intermediate host (birds), in which there is a phase of schizogony with the formation of cysts, usually in the muscular masses. Usually, infection is asymptomatic even in cases of heavy infestation. The presence of small, yellowish cysts (4 × 0.5 mm) in the leg and pectoral muscles is pathognomonic; cardiac

Parasite	Life cycle	Main features of the group
Trematodes (flukes)	Indirect	Flattened, nonsegmented body with a cuticle covering Attachment by suckers Relatively simple digestive system All hermaphroditic except for the blood flukes (Schistosomatidae) Eggs are opercular (except for those of the Schistosomatidae) Complex life cycle in one or two hosts Can be found especially in the digestive, respiratory, reproductive and excretory systems
Cestodes (tapeworms)	Indirect	Flattened, segmented bodies with a scolex (the upper extremity), a neck (area of growth) and strobila (a chain of segments called proglottids) Lacking a digestive system, they absorb nourishment through the cuticle Most are hermaphrodites Attached to the wall of the small intestine by the scolex Size varies from a few centimeters to more than 35 cm
Nematodes (roundworms)	Indirect and direct	Cylindrical unsegmented body, covered by a flexible cuticle Separate sexes and a complete digestive system Generally four larval stages Affect almost all the districts of the avian body Size can vary from a few millimeters to many centimeters The most important group according to the number of species infecting birds and to their pathogenicity
Acanthocephalans (thorny-headed worms)	Indirect	Elongated worms with an armed, retractile, oval or cylindrical proboscis used to attach themselves to the intestinal mucosa Separate sexes Lacking alimentary tract: feed by absorption through the body wall Found in the intestinal tract of birds

TABLE 8.3 Main features of major groups of internal parasites (endoparasites) that affect birds

cysts show up only under microscope. Most frequent post-mortem findings are lung edema, splenomegaly, hepatomegaly and the presence of merozoites in the capillary endothelium. Diagnosis is possible only at post-mortem. Suggested treatment includes trimethoprim and sulfadiazine.

Cryptosporidium species

These are protozoa of small diameter (5–6 µm) and oval shape with a cosmopolitan distribution, and are capable of causing lesions in the respiratory, digestive and urinary tracts of birds. *Cryptosporidium* develop intercellularly at an extracytoplasmic location on the apical surface of epithelial cells (Greiner and Ritchie, 1994). The life cycle of the parasite is direct and it can be transmitted by the ingestion or inhalation of sporulated oocysts. Infestation with this parasite has been reported in Galliformes, Anseriformes, Psittaciformes, ostriches, canaries and finches.

Helminths

Paolo Zucca, Mauro Delogu

The term 'helminths' refers to a heterogeneous group of animals that, although they have similar superficial characteristics, such as the elongated shape of the body and creeping movements, are in fact very different with respect to their taxonomic position, structure and behavior (Table 8.3).

Trematodes (flukes)

The main features of the group are described in Table 8.3. Of note are the family Collyriclidae (which encyst in the skin of birds); the family Schistosomatidae (which live in the blood) and its genera *Trichobilharzia*, *Gigantobilharzia* and *Austrobilharzia*; the family Prostogonimidae and the family Psilostomatidae (parasites of the intestine and of the alimentary canal respectively of birds). They have a worldwide distribution but, although they affect many species of bird in the wild, they are not frequent in cage and aviary birds because it is difficult for them to find all the intermediate hosts necessary for their development in such surroundings. They have been found, however, in many species of Passeriformes, psittacines, Anseriformes and poultry. With regard to transmission, the life cycle of many species of trematode is often unknown but in general they need one to two intermediate hosts in order to complete their development; birds can become infested by eating arthropods, snails and the larvae of dragonflies, which serve as a second host for the trematodes. For this reason most cases of trematode

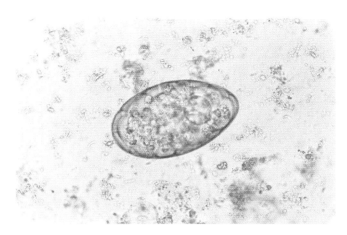

Fig. 8.38 Trematode ovum, probably *Strigea falconis*, from a peregrine falcon. (Courtesy of S. K. John).

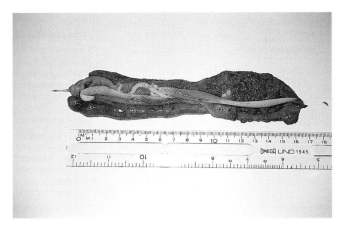

Fig. 8.39 Tapeworms (*Otiditaenia macqueenii*) in the small intestine of a wild-caught houbara bustard. Free-living houbara bustards are known to harbor large numbers of this parasite. (Courtesy of Dr. J. Samour).

infestation occur in Anseriformes and other aquatic birds. Clinical features are not specific: they vary according to the localization of a determined species of nematode in the body of the bird. Diagnosis is usually difficult in life and it requires identification of the eggs in the feces (Fig. 8.38).

Cestodes (tapeworms)

The main features of the group are described in Table 8.3. There are hundreds of different species that affect birds and new species are still being discovered. For example, the following are of note: family Dilepididae (especially in Passeriformes) – *Dilepus* and *Biuterina*; family Davaineidae (passerines, psittacines) – *Davainea*, *Raillietina* and *Cotugna*; family Hymenolepididae (Anseriformes, passerines, other groups) – *Hymenolepis*; and family Anoplocephalidae (Figs 8.39–8.54). Tapeworms have a worldwide distribution and affect many different species of bird but, because they need an intermediate host to complete their life cycle, they affect granivores and frugivores and, less frequently, insectivores and carnivores (Keymer, 1982). Tapeworms have a life cycle with an intermediate host: birds become infected by feeding on the intermediate host, for example arthropods, molluscs and annelids containing the cysticercus (bladder worm stage). Often, infestation is moderate apathogenic; in other cases there can be diarrhea, depression, debilitation and death. In any case the symptomatology is similar to that of many other parasitic diseases. Diagnosis is made by identification of eggs or proglottis in the feces. Heavy infestations can cause enteritis, sometimes with hemorrhaging and intestinal obstruction. Suggested therapy includes niclosamide, praziquantel and rafoxanide.

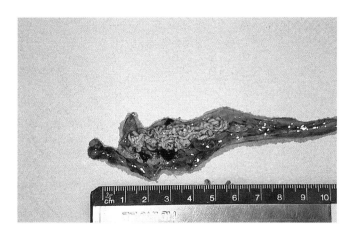

Fig. 8.40 Large number of tapeworms (*Cladotaenia globifera*) in the large intestine of a peregrine falcon (*Falco peregrinus*). The bird died from severe enteritis associated with the tapeworm infestation. (Courtesy of Dr. J. Samour).

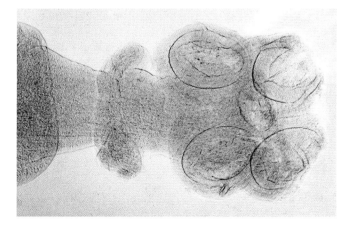

Fig. 8.41 *Otiditaenia conoides* – scolex. (Courtesy of Dr. A. Jones, International Institute of Parasitology, St. Albans).

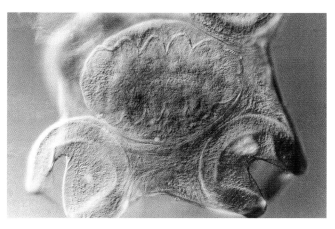

Fig. 8.42 *Otiditaenia macqueenii*. Rostellum with undulating crown of hooks. (Courtesy of Dr. A. Jones, International Institute of Parasitology, St. Albans).

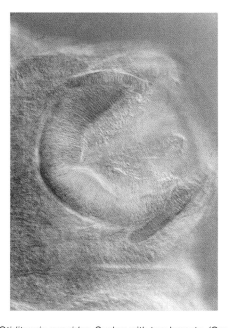

Fig. 8.43 *Otiditaenia conoides*. Sucker with two lappets. (Courtesy of Dr. A. Jones, International Institute of Parasitology, St. Albans).

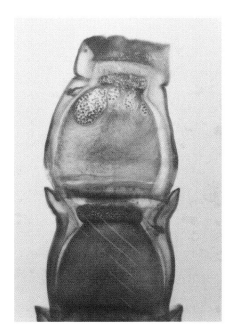

Fig. 8.44 *Otiditaenia conoides*. Mature proglottids. (Courtesy of Dr. A. Jones, International Institute of Parasitology, St. Albans).

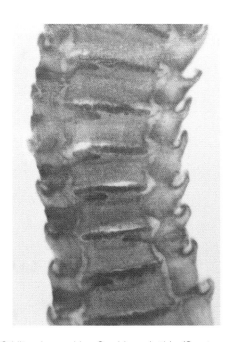

Fig. 8.45 *Otiditaenia conoides*. Gravid proglottids. (Courtesy of Dr. A. Jones, International Institute of Parasitology, St. Albans).

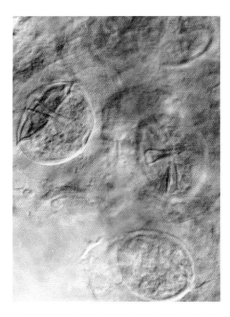

Fig. 8.46 *Otiditaenia conoides*. Eggs. (Courtesy of Dr. A. Jones, International Institute of Parasitology, St. Albans).

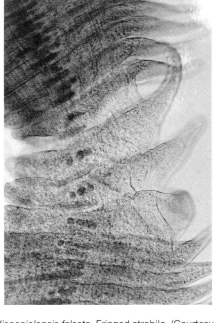

Fig. 8.48 *Hispaniolepsis falsata*. Fringed strobila. (Courtesy of Dr. A. Jones, International Institute of Parasitology, St. Albans).

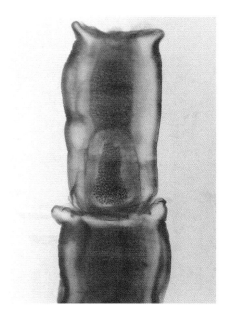

Fig. 8.47 *Ascometra choriotidis*. Gravid proglottids. (Courtesy of Dr. A. Jones, International Institute of Parasitology, St. Albans).

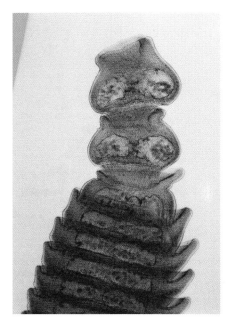

Fig. 8.49 *Hispaniolepsis falsata*. Gravid proglottids. (Courtesy of Dr. A. Jones, International Institute of Parasitology, St. Albans).

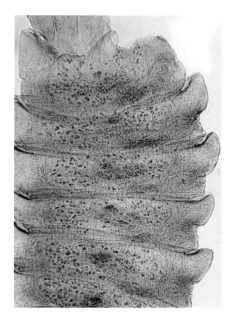

Fig. 8.50 *Raillietina neyrai*. Rostellum and suckers armed. (Courtesy of Dr. A. Jones, International Institute of Parasitology, St. Albans).

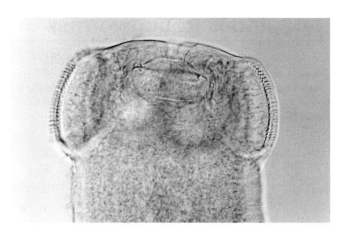

Fig. 8.52 *Raillietina neyrai*. Gravid proglottids. (Courtesy of Dr. A. Jones, International Institute of Parasitology, St. Albans).

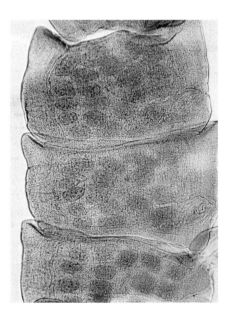

Fig. 8.51 *Raillietina neyrai*. Mature proglottids. (Courtesy of Dr. A. Jones, International Institute of Parasitology, St. Albans).

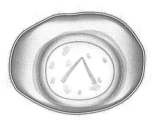

Fig. 8.53 Tapeworm egg.

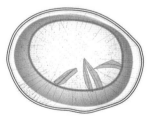

Fig. 8.54 *Raillietina* sp. egg.

Nematodes (roundworms)

The main features of the group are described in Table 8.3. They are usually found in the intestine but many species show a predilection for other parts of the body. For this reason the main representatives of this class are described according to the part of the body they affect rather than their taxonomic order (Figs 8.55–8.77).

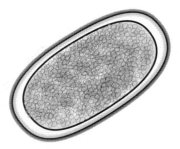

Fig. 8.58 *Heterakis gallinarum* egg.

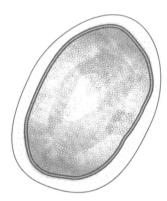

Fig. 8.55 *Ascaridia* sp. egg (macaw).

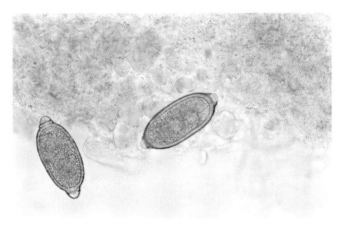

Fig. 8.59 *Capillaria* sp. ova observed in a direct fecal examination from a peregrine falcon. (Courtesy of S. K. John).

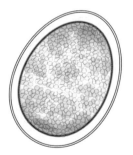

Fig. 8.56 *Ascaridia* sp. egg (pigeon).

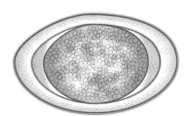

Fig. 8.57 *Porrocaecum* sp. egg.

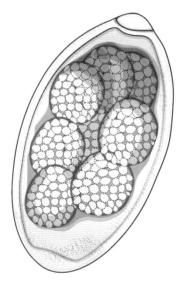

Fig. 8.60 *Syngamus trachea* ovum.

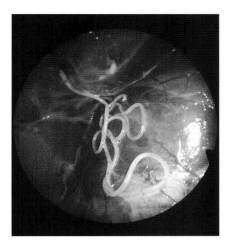

Fig. 8.61 Endoscopic view of *Serratospiculum seurati* adult worms on the abdominal airsac wall of an adult saker falcon. *S. seurati* was recently identified from specimens collected in the Middle East by The International Institute of Parasitology, UK. Serratospiculiasis is a very common parasitic disease in Falconiformes throughout the Middle East. (Courtesy of Dr. J. Samour).

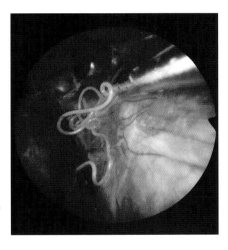

Fig. 8.62 Endoscopy-assisted removal of adult filarial worms is a common procedure carried out by some clinicians, particularly in the Middle East. This procedure is now considered unnecessary as modern therapeutic regimens have made it obsolete. (Courtesy of Dr. J. Samour).

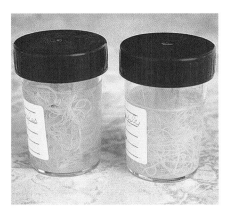

Fig. 8.63 Large numbers of *Serratospiculum seurati* adult filarial worms removed surgically from the celomic cavity of one saker and one gyrfalcon (*Falco rusticolus*). (Courtesy of Dr. J. Samour).

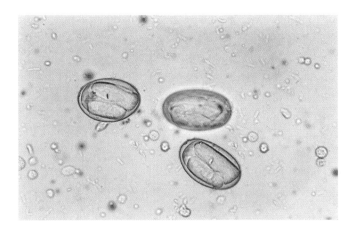

Fig. 8.64 *Serratospiculum seurati* ova in a direct smear from a saker falcon. (Courtesy of Mr. S. K. John).

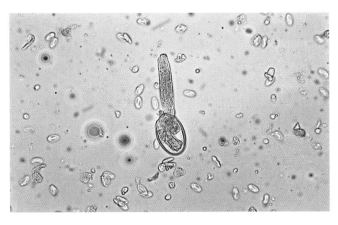

Fig. 8.65 Larvae of *Serratospiculum seurati* at the moment of emerging from the ovum. Methylene blue stain. (Courtesy of Mr. C. Silvanose).

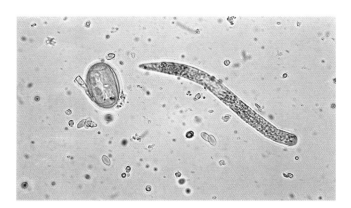

Fig. 8.66 Embryonated ovum and a larva of *Serratospiculum seurati* obtained from an airsac swab collected from a post-mortem examination of a saker falcon. Methylene blue stain. (Courtesy of Mr. C. Silvanose).

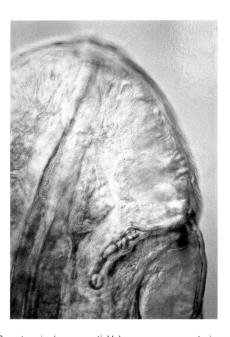

Fig. 8.68 *Serratospiculum seurati*. Vulva opens near anterior region of esophagus. (Courtesy of Dr. L. Gibbons, International Institute of Parasitology, St. Albans).

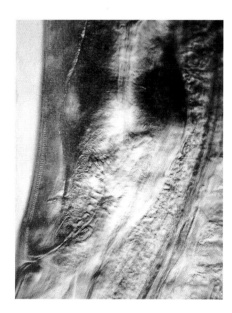

Fig. 8.67 *Serratospiculum seurati*. Vulva and proximal end of ovejector. (Courtesy of Dr. L. Gibbons, International Institute of Parasitology, St. Albans).

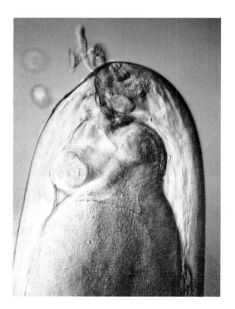

Fig. 8.69 *Serratospiculum seurati*. Anus subterminal, tail bluntly rounded, pair of phasmids present. (Courtesy of Dr. L. Gibbons, International Institute of Parasitology, St. Albans).

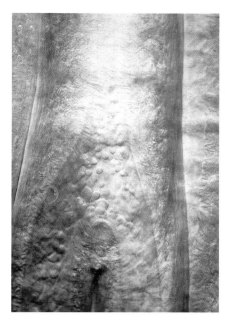

Fig. 8.70 *Serratospiculum seurati*. Ovejector divides posteriorly. (Courtesy of Dr. L. Gibbons, International Institute of Parasitology, St. Albans).

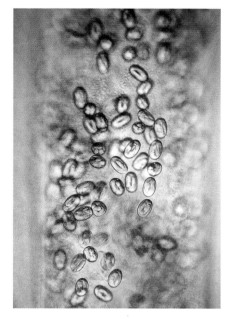

Fig. 8.72 *Serratospiculum seurati*. Thick-shelled embryonated eggs. (Courtesy of Dr. L. Gibbons, International Institute of Parasitology, St. Albans).

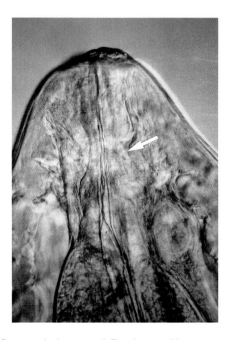

Fig. 8.71 *Serratospiculum seurati*. Esophagus with narrow anterior part and long broader posterior part. Nerve ring arrowed. (Courtesy of Dr. L. Gibbons, International Institute of Parasitology, St. Albans).

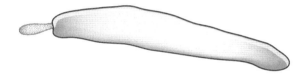

Fig. 8.73 Acanthocephalid worm *Plagiorhynchus cylindraceus*. Adult worm, lateral view.

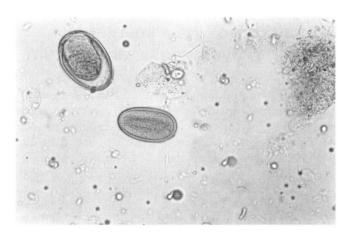

Fig. 8.74 One slightly disrupted ovum and one entire ovum of *Acanthocephalan* sp. in a direct smear from a saker falcon. (Courtesy of Mr. S. K. John).

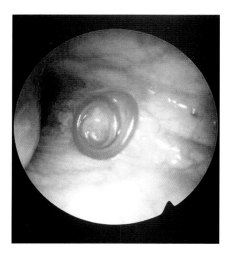

Fig. 8.75 *Physaloptera alata alata* adult worm on the esophageal wall of a saker falcon. The parasite was observed during a routine endoscopy examination of the gastrointestinal tract. (Courtesy of Dr. J. Samour).

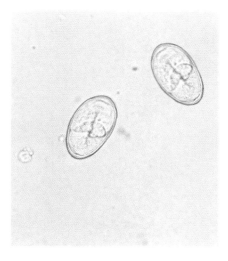

Fig. 8.77 *Paraspiralatus sakeri* ova in a wet preparation from the oropharynx of a saker falcon. This parasite is a new species recently described from the upper digestive tract from a saker falcon in Saudi Arabia. (Courtesy of Mr. S. K. John).

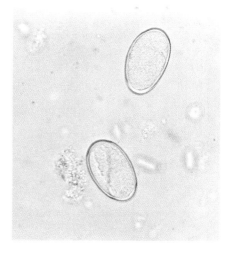

Fig. 8.76 *Physaloptera alata alata* ova observed in a wet preparation from the oropharynx of a saker falcon. (Courtesy of Mr. S. K. John).

Nematodes of the alimentary system: proventriculus and gizzard

Dispharinx nasuta and *Spiroptera incerta* are two spiruroid nematodes that are found in the stomach and sometimes in the esophagus of many species of birds. These nematodes have been recorded in North and South America, Europe, Asia, Africa and Australia but information about the prevalence of this parasite is scarce. Many species belonging to various groups, such as Psittaciformes, Passeriformes, poultry and other gallinaceous birds, are susceptible. With regard to transmission, the life cycle of *D. nasuta* is indirect and the intermediate hosts are arthropods. The life cycle of *S. incerta* is not known: it may have intermediate hosts represented by beetles and ants. Diagnosis requires identification of eggs in the feces or of adults

during the post-mortem examination. The differential diagnosis is important in cases of contemporaneous infestation with filaroids. At post-mortem thickening of the proventriculus, where they may also cause ulcers, inflammation and nodules, is a frequent finding.

Nematodes of esophagus, crop, intestine, cecum

Ascaridia spp. are relatively large nematodes that are found in the small intestine or proventriculus of birds. They have a worldwide distribution and the susceptible species include Psittaciformes, Columbiformes and Galliformes. With regard to transmission, members of the ascarids have a direct life cycle and the infectious larva develops in the egg after a few weeks. Following ingestion, the larva passes into the mucosa of the small intestine and then returns to the gut lumen, where it completes its development. The eggs remain infectious for many months in the ground. Diarrhea, sensory depression, constipation, lethargy, anemia and paralysis of the legs are the most frequent clinical signs, which in any case are not specific. Birds can die as a result of worms obstructing the duodenum and the small intestine, while the larvae can cause lesions to the intestinal mucosa.

Porrocaecum spp. is another ascarid with a worldwide distribution that is commonly found in the intestine of many species of bird. It mainly parasitizes free-living birds and Passeriformes. Unlike *Ascaridia*, these species need an intermediate host (which varies according to the species – usually an insect or annelid) to complete their life cycle.

Heterakis gallinarum is a typical cecal nematode of gallinaceous birds. This parasite is usually not a significant parasite of cage and aviary birds and raptors. It is a miniature version of a typical ascarid and is found in the ceca. It does not usually cause much harm to the host but is important in that it transmits histomoniasis.

Capillaria spp. (Fig. 8.59) is a very small nematode that is found in the crop, the esophagus and the small intestine. Its localization depends on the species of *Capillaria* and on the species of its host. Many cases of capillariasis have been reported in many species of bird throughout the world, but little is known of its prevalence in cage and aviary birds. It frequently infests poultry, pigeons and many species of psittacine, such as macaws and budgerigars, and it has also been reported in canaries. It would seem to be a frequent parasite of raptors (Smith, 1993). With regards to transmission, the life cycle is usually direct and, after the eggs have passed in the feces, an infectious larva develops within 2 weeks. Environmental conditions such as high humidity and moderate temperatures allow the eggs to be infectious for many months. Animals become infested by ingesting eggs, which originate from the fecal material of infected animals. According to some sources, certain species of *Capillaria* use intermediate hosts such as earthworms (Ward, 1978). The most frequent clinical signs are regurgitation, diarrhea, dysphagia, anorexia, cachexy, melena and weight loss due to the fact that it attaches itself to the mucosa of the digestive system. Diagnosis is made by inspection of the oral cavity and parasitological examination of the oral mucus and of the feces to look for eggs. *Capillaria* fixes on to the mucosa and causes areas of necrosis in various tracts of the digestive system – the oral cavity, the esophagus, the small intestine. The carcass is anemic and dehydrated with slight intestinal hemorrhaging. It is often necessary to use the microscope in order to identify adults in the intestinal material. Treatment includes mebendazole, fenbendazole, ivermectin, moxidectin and levamisole.

Trichostrongylids spp. are gastrointestinal nematodes that infest many species of cage and aviary birds and free-living birds. Despite their small size they are capable of causing serious lesions. Their life cycle is direct and, after the elimination of eggs in the feces, the larva needs 2 weeks to become infectious. Transmission takes place through ingestion of the larva. Ulceration and necrosis of the intestinal mucosa and catarrhal enteritis are frequent findings.

Nematodes of the respiratory system

Syngamus trachea (Fig. 8.60) is a nematode of the respiratory system that is distributed worldwide and is usually found in the trachea and bronchi. It is bright red in color and attaches itself to the mucosa. The males are very small, about 5 mm long, and live permanently attached to the vulva of the females, which can reach a length of 40 mm. Although it has been reported in many species of cage and aviary birds and free-living birds such as Passeriformes, Piciformes, Apodiformes, pigeons, raptors, etc., infestation is more common in Galliformes and Anseriformes. With regards to transmission, eggs are laid in the trachea of the host, which then usually ingests them and expels them in its feces. They can sometimes be directly expelled orally through coughing. After a few weeks of incubation on the ground, a larva emerges, which is then ingested by a new host. After having been ingested, the larvae pass through the intestinal wall of the host and reach the lungs by means of the blood vessels. After a period of maturation, the nematodes migrate into the trachea, where the cycle is repeated. Partial or total obstruction of the tracheal lumen with dyspnea, coughing, head shaking and the presence of coagulated blood in the beak are the most frequent clinical signs. Diagnosis is based on clinical symptomology and the identification of eggs in the feces. Differential diagnosis is made with respiratory acariasis, aspergillosis. Post mortem findings include tracheitis, accumulation of mucus, bronchitis, areas of lung congestion. Treatment is carried out with fenbendazole, mebendazole, thiabendazole, ivermectin and physical removal.

Serratospiculum (Figs 8.61–8.72) is a common nematode often found in the airsacs of falcons and other birds of prey. Opinions as to its pathogenicity vary from author to author. Cooper (1985) does not consider it pathogenic, while others report cases of presumed death in raptors as a result of this parasite (Kocan and Gordon, 1976). It seems to be widely distributed throughout the world, although not uniformly. It has been reported in North America and some European countries but appears to be more widely distributed in tropical and subtropical countries. *Serratospiculum amaculata* has been described from several species of North American bird of prey (Bigland *et al.*, 1964; Ward and Fairchild, 1972; Kocan and Gordon, 1976; Ackerman *et al.*, 1992). *S. seurati* has been identified in captive gyr, peregrine and saker falcons in the Middle East (Samour and Naldo, 2001).

Only diurnal raptors appear to be susceptible to this parasite and transmission, although there is little information about the life cycle of this parasite, is believed to be indirect, with an arthropod as intermediate host (Wehr, 1971). In the Middle East, several arthropods have been identified as the intermediate host of *S. seurati* (Samour and Naldo, 2001). Usually, infection is apathogenic but sometimes infected birds show different respiratory signs, including moderate to severe sacculitis. Diagnosis is made by identification of eggs in the feces. Being oviparous, the nematodes do not release microfilariae into the blood. Differential diagnosis includes syngamiasis, aspergillosis and other respiratory pathologies. Frequent post-mortem findings include the thickening of the airsacs, and sometimes peritonitis because the parasites migrate into the celomic cavity. The suggested drug is thiabendazole 100 mg/kg, but ivermectin and moxidectin have also been used successfully (Samour and Naldo, 2001).

Filaroids are long, thin nematodes that affect many different species of bird all over the world. The adults are found in the body cavities, airsacs, heart, eye cavities, nasal cavities and subcutaneous tissues of birds. In many cases these nematodes can be considered apathogenic (Greiner and Ritchie, 1994). Among the most frequent in avian genera are the following: *Splendidofilaria, Cardiofilaria, Chandlerella, Aprocta lissonema* (nasal cavities) and *Avioserpens* (subcutaneous tissue). They are reported in many species of bird and especially in Passeriformes, Psittaciformes, Falconiformes and Anseriformes. With regards to transmission, the life cycle is indirect and includes the intervention of an intermediate host, which acts as vector (dipterous hematophagus). The females lay many eggs, which give rise to microfilariae. These enter the blood circulation and are ingested by dipterous hematophagus, which in turn, after a variable period, transmits the larvae to a new host in which they develop and the cycle is repeated. Diagnosis is made searching for microfilariae in the blood. It is necessary to take a series of samples. The differential diagnosis is made with trypanosomiasis under smear test (the microfilariae are larger and more mobile.). At post-mortem the most frequent lesions involve serosa airsacs, thickening fibrosis stegnosis and necrosis of the vessels, lung edema and congestion and subcutaneous abscesses. In cases of subcutaneous lesions, surgical removal of the adults might be indicated. Pharmacological therapy does not always provide good results.

Eyeworms: The nictitating membrane, conjunctival sacs and lachrymal ducts of birds can be affected by various genera of nematodes, among which are *Oxyspirura, Thelazia* and *Ceratospira*. Information about their distribution is scarce but they would seem to be distributed in many continents. Among the species of bird most frequently affected are Anseriformes, Passeriformes, Columbiformes, Psittaciformes and sometimes raptors. Clinical signs include restlessness, scratching of the eyes and constant blinking of the nictitating membrane.

Acanthocephalans (thorny-headed worms)

The main features of the group are described in Table 8.3. See also Figure 8.74. Numerous cases have been reported, in wildfowl, passerines and raptors, but little is known about the prevalence of these parasites in birds. Their life cycle requires an intermediate host, which contains the larval stage; birds become infested

by ingesting this host. Usually infections are asymptomatic although it is reported sometimes an intestinal symptomatology. Diagnosis usually is not possible in the live bird.

Therapy

See Appendix 8. For further details the reader is referred to Clubb, 1986; Coles 1991, 1997; Robertson, 1991; Ritchie and Harrison, 1994; Beynon *et al.*, 1996; Rupley 1997; Cooper, 2002; Carpenter 2005; Plumb, 2005; Marx, 2006.

REFERENCES

Ackerman N, Isaza R, Greiner E, Berry CR (1992) Pneumocoelon associated with *Serratospiculum amaculata* in a bald eagle. *College of Veterinary Medicine Journal* **33**: 351–355.

Aznar JF, Balbuena JA, Fernandez M, Raga JA (2001) Living together: the parasites of marine mammals. In: Evans PGH, Raga JA (eds) *Marine Mammals: Biology and Conservation*, pp. 385–424. Kluwer Academic/Plenum Press, New York.

Beynon P, Forbes N, Harcourt-Brown N (1996) *Manual of Raptors, Pigeons and Waterfowl*. British Small Veterinary Association, Cheltenham.

Bigland CH, Liu S-K, Perry ML (1964) Five cases of *Serratospiculum amaculata* (Nematoda: Filarioidea) infection in prairie falcons (*Falco mexicanus*). *Avian Diseases* **8**: 412–419.

Carpenter JW (2005) *Exotic Animal Formulary*, pp. 178–198. WB Saunders, Philadelphia.

Clayton DH, Moyer BR, Bush SE et al. (2005) Adaptive significance of avian beak morphology for ectoparasite control. *Proceedings of the Royal Society of London B (Suppl.), Biology Letters* **272**: 811–817.

Clubb SL (1986) Therapeutics. In: Harrison GJ, Harrison LR (eds) *Clinical Avian Medicine and Surgery*, pp. 327–355. WB Saunders, Philadelphia.

Coles BH (1991) In: Beynon PH, Cooper JE (eds) *Cage and Aviary Birds. Manual of Exotic Pets*. British Small Veterinary Association, Cheltenham.

Coles BH (1997) *Avian Medicine and Surgery*. Blackwell Science, Oxford.

Cooper JE (1978) *Veterinary Aspects of Captive Birds of Prey*. Standfast Press, Saul, Gloucestershire.

Cooper JE (2002) *Birds of Prey: Health and Disease*. Blackwell Science, Oxford.

Deem SL, Karesh WB, Weisman W (2001) Putting theory into practice: wildlife health in conservation. *Conservation Biology* **15**:1224–1233.

Durden LA (2002) Lice. In: Mullen G, Durden L (eds) *Medical and Veterinary Entomology*, Academic Press, Orlando, FL.

Durden LA, Traub R (2002) Fleas. In Mullen G, Durden L (eds) *Medical and Veterinary Entomology*, Academic Press, Orlando, FL.

Forbes NA, Simpson GN (1997) *Caryospora neofalconis*: an emerging threat to captive-bred raptors in the United Kingdom. *Journal of Avian Medicine and Surgery* **11**: 110–114.

Friend M, Franson C (2002) Introduction to parasitic diseases. In: Friend M, Franson C (eds) *Field Manual of Wildlife Diseases: General Field Procedures and Diseases of Birds*, p. 188. Biological Resources Division, Information and technology report 1999–2001, US Geological Survey, National Wildlife Health Center, Madison, WI.

Gompper ME, Williams ES (1998) Parasite conservation and the Black-Footed Ferret Recovery Program. *Conservation Biology* **12**: 730–732.

Greiner EC, Ritchie BW (1994) Parasites. In: Ritchie BW, Harrison GJ, Harrison LR (eds) *Avian Medicine: Principles and Application*, pp. 1007–1029. Wingers Publishing, Lake Worth, FL.

Grimaldi D, Engel MS (2005) *Evolution of the Insects*. Cambridge University Press, New York.

Heidenreich M (1997) *Birds of Prey: Medicine and Management*, p. 133. Blackwell Science, Oxford.

Hoberg EP, Brooks DR, Siegel-Causey D (1997) Host-parasite conspeciation: history, principles and prospects. In: Clayton D, Moore J (eds) *Host–Parasite Evolution: General Principles and Avian Models*, pp. 212–235, Oxford University Press, Oxford.

Kellert SR (1993) Values and perceptions of invertebrates. *Conservation Biology* 7: 845–855.

Keymer IF (1982) Parasitic diseases. In: Petrak ML (ed.) *Diseases of Cage and Aviary Birds*, 2nd edn, pp. 535–598. Lea & Febiger, Philadelphia.

Kocan AA, Gordon LR (1976) Fatal air sac infection with *Serratospiculum amaculata* in a prairie falcon. *Journal of the American Veterinary Medical Association* 169: 908.

Krinsky WL (2002) True bugs. In: Mullen G, Durden L (eds) *Medical and Veterinary Entomology*, pp. 69–85. Academic Press, Orlando, FL.

Marx KL (2006) Therapeutic agents. In: Harrison GJ, Lighfoot TL (eds) *Clinical Avian Medicine*, pp. 241–342. Spix Publishing, Palm Beach, FL.

May RM (1988) Conservation and Disease. *Conservation Biology* 2: 28–30.

Merkl O, Bagyura J, Rózsa L (2004) Insects inhabiting saker (*Falco cherrug*) nests in Hungary. *Ornis Hungarica* 14.

Mullen GR, O'Connor BM (2002) Mites. In: Mullen G, Durden L (eds) *Medical and Veterinary Entomology*, pp. 449–510. Academic Press, Orlando, FL.

Plumb DC (2005). *Plumb's Veterinary Drug Handbook*, 5th edn. Iowa State University Press, Ames, IA.

Proctor H, Owens I (2000) Mites and birds: diversity, parasitism and coevolution. *TREE* 15: 358–364.

Ritchie BW, Harrison GJ (1994) Formulary. In Ritchie BW, Harrison GJ, Harrison LR (eds) *Avian Medicine: Principles and Application*, pp. 457–478. Wingers Publishing, Lake Worth, FL.

Robertson EL (1991) Antinematode drugs. In: Booth NH, McDonald LE (eds) *Veterinary Pharmacology and Therapeutics*, 6th edn. Iowa State University Press, Ames, IA.

Rupley AE (1997) *Manual of Avian Practice*. WB Saunders, Philadelphia.

Samour JH, Naldo JL (2001) Serratospiculiasis in captive falcons in the Middle East: a review. *Journal of Avian Medicine and Surgery* 15: 2–9.

Samour JH, Naldo JL (2003) Infestation of *Dermestes carnivorus* in a saker falcon (*Falco cherrug*). *Veterinary Record* 153: 658–659.

Samour JH, Naldo JL (2005) Intra-auricular trichomonosis in a saker falcon (*Falco cherrug*) in Saudi Arabia. *Veterinary Record* 156: 384–386.

Samour JH, Bailey TA, Cooper JE (1995) Trichomoniasis in birds of prey (order Falconiformes) in Bahrain. *Veterinary Record* 136: 358–362.

Smith SA (1993) Diagnosis and treatment of helminths in birds of prey. In: Redig PT, Cooper JE, Remple JD *et al.* (eds) *Raptor Biomedicine*, pp. 21–27. University of Minnesota Press, Minneapolis.

Sonenshine DE, Lane RS, Nicholson WL (2002) Ticks. In: Mullen G, Durden L (eds) *Medical and Veterinary Entomology*, pp. 518–556. Academic Press, Orlando, FL.

Stork NE, Lyal HC (1993) Extinction or co-extinction rates? *Nature* 366: 307.

Wappler T, Smith V, Dalgleish RC (2004) Scratching an ancient itch: an Eocene bird louse fossil. *Proceedings of the Royal Society of London B (Suppl), Biology Letters* 271: 255–258.

Ward FP (1978) Parasites and their treatment in birds of prey. In: Fowler ME (ed.) *Zoo and Wild Animal Medicine*, pp. 276–281. WB Saunders, Philadelphia.

Ward FP, Fairchild DG (1972) Air sac parasites of the genus *Serratospiculum* in falcons. *Journal of Wildlife Diseases* 8: 165–168.

Wehr EE (1971) Nematodes. In: Davis JW, Anderson RC, Karstad L, Trainer DO (eds) *Infectious and Parasitic Diseases of Wild Birds*. Iowa State University Press, Ames, IA.

Windsor DA (1995) Equal right for parasites. *Conservation Biology* 9: 1–2.

FURTHER READING

Sloss MW, Kemp RL (1994) *Veterinary Clinical Parasitology*. Iowa State University Press, Ames, IA.

ACKNOWLEDGMENTS

Paolo Zucca and Mauro Delogu would like to thank the Royal Society of London, Dr Torsten Wappler, Department of Geology, Paleontology and Mineralogy, Hessisches Landesmuseum Darmstadt, Darmstadt, Germany and Dr Vince Smith, Natural History Museum, Cromwell Road, London, for the reproduction of Figure 8.1 from the *Proceedings of the Royal Society of London B (Suppl.), Biology Letters* 2004; 271: 255–258; Dr Mauro Giacca

and Dr Raffaella Klima, International Centre for Genetic Engineering and Biotechnology, AREA Science Park, Trieste, Italy for the use of a high-quality microscope/photocamera; Dr Luciano Iob, Istituto Zooprofilattico Sperimentale of Pordenone, Cordenons (PN), Italy for providing us a fresh specimen of *Rhinonyssid* mite; Professor Louis De Vos, Faculté des Sciences Université Libre de Bruxelles, Brussels for permission to reproduce Figures 8.9a and 8.9b; Professor Massimo Trentini, Department of Veterinary Public Health, University of Bologna for providing us with the SEM pictures of *Craterina pallida* and Dr Dino Scaravelli, Ichthyopathology and Aquaculture Centre, University of Bologna, for commenting on the manuscript.

Hemoparasites

Michael A. Peirce

Blood parasites occur in nearly all species of birds, but those living in extreme climatic conditions and in areas where vectors are absent are usually found to be infected only when transferred to other locations as exhibits in zoological collections or captive breeding programs, or as pets. Such birds are frequently totally susceptible to infection by a wide range of parasites, many of which may be pathogenic (Peirce, 1989).

The extent of mortality in wild populations due to hemoparasites is difficult to gauge. Unless there is a noticeable die-off in a specific population where a veterinary diagnosis confirms the involvement of hematozoa either as sole infection or as a component of concomitant infection with other disease agents, most sick or dead birds rapidly become prey to predators and scavengers. Thus, nearly 90% of all records of mortality and pathogenicity due to avian hematozoa have been described from domestic species (chickens, turkeys, ducks and geese) and only 5% from free-living birds (Bennett *et al.*, 1993b).

With the exception of microfilariae (the immature stages of filarial worms) and *Aegyptianella*, most blood parasites are protozoa. Diagnosis is dependent upon Giemsa-stained thin smears of peripheral blood. Although most post-mortem blood smears are of little value taxonomically, they are still valuable in identifying parasites, at least to the generic level, and in correlating endogenous stages that may be found on histopathology examination.

Plasmodium species

The genus *Plasmodium* (Figs 8.78–8.83) is an apicomplexan parasite closely related to *Haemoproteus* and *Leucocytozoon*. There are some 34 species of *Plasmodium* found in birds (Bennett *et al.*, 1993a), which can be grouped into five subgenera (Table 8.4) according to specific morphological characteristics such as size and shape of gametocytes and schizonts.

With the one known exception of *Plasmodioides*, which is transmitted by *Anopheles* spp., all other subgenera and species are transmitted by culicine mosquitoes. When an infected vector bites a new host, parasite sporozoites are passed into the blood, where they eventually reach the liver and undergo development into pre-erythrocytic schizonts. These produce merozoites, which enter the erythrocytes and develop into macro- (female) or micro- (male) gametocytes or segmenters (asexual schizonts). All stages contain melanin pigment granules. The merozoites produced from asexual schizonts repeat the erythrocytic cycle. The intraerythrocytic merogony cycles continue indefinitely unless the host's immune system or death intervenes. Thus there is a potential for persistence of infection with frequent relapses. Second-generation exoerythrocytic schizonts may occur in tissues other than the liver, as also may subsequent generations. In early infections, only trophozoites and schizonts may occur in erythrocytes, so specific diagnosis will be difficult. Likewise, in older established infections only gametocytes may be present and if

these are of a species with an elongated form they can easily be confused with those of *Haemoproteus*.

Some avian species of *Plasmodium* are known to occur only in the type host from which the parasite was originally described. Other *Plasmodium* spp. occur in a wide range of hosts and families and often the morphology differs markedly. This frequently makes a definitive diagnosis to species level difficult unless tissue stages and vectors are also known.

Specific clinical signs of *Plasmodium* infection are lacking, but listlessness, lethargy and anemia may be indicators of the disease. Generally *Plasmodium* spp.

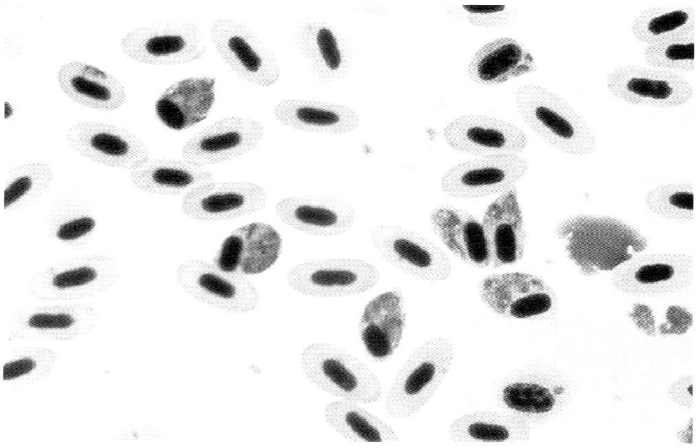

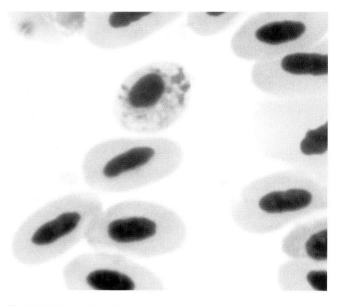

Fig. 8.80 *Plasmodium (Giovannolaia) circumflexum* microgametocyte.

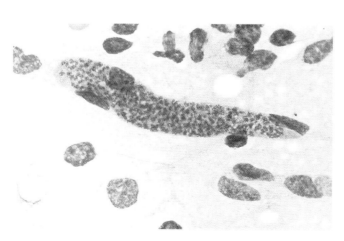

Fig. 8.78 *Plasmodium (Haemamoeba) relictum* from a house sparrow (*Passer domesticus*).

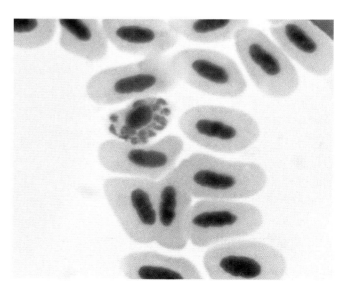

Fig. 8.81 *Plasmodium (Giovannolaia) circumflexum* schizont.

Fig. 8.79 *Plasmodium (Haemamoeba) gallinaceum* schizont in a brain smear from a chicken (*Gallus domesticus*).

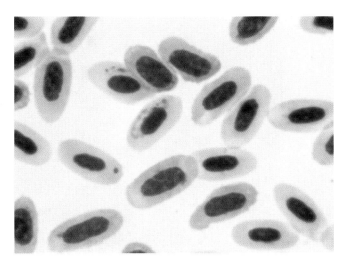

Fig. 8.82 *Plasmodium (Novyella) rouxi* microgametocyte.

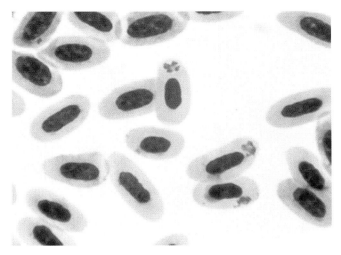

Fig. 8.83 *Plasmodium (Novyella) rouxi* schizont.

TABLE 8.4 Key to the avian subgenera of *Plasmodium*

1a	Parasites lacking pigment; gametocytes and schizonts large; mature parasites displace host cell nucleus; present only in circulating leukocytes	*Plasmodioides*
1b	Parasites with pigment	2
2a	Gametocytes round or nearly so; mature parasites typically displace host cell nucleus towards pole	*Haemamoeba*
2b	Gametocytes elongate; mature forms do not displace host cell nucleus towards pole	3
3a	Schizonts present in circulating erythrocyte precursors, not in mature erythrocytes	*Huffia*
3b	Schizonts in mature erythrocytes, not in erythrocyte precursors	4
4a	Erythrocytic schizonts generally larger than erythrocyte nucleus and contain noticeable amount of cytoplasm	*Giovannolaia*
4b	Erythrocytic schizonts smaller than erythrocyte nucleus; without noticeable cytoplasm	*Novyella*

are more pathogenic in domestic birds: *P. gallinaceum* in chickens (frequent involvement of brain schizonts), *P. durae* in turkeys, and *P. circumflexum* in ducks and geese. The species that occurs most in free-living birds is *P. relictum*, which has been recorded from over 360 hosts from 70 families. This parasite and *P. elongatum* are frequent causes of mortality in penguins in zoological collections.

P. vaughani has been recorded from 265 hosts and is particularly common in passerine species, and *P. circumflexum* occurs in about 140 avian hosts. Other species of *Plasmodium* are less common and are considered to be of little clinical significance, with the possible exception of *P. juxtanucleare* in chickens.

Mixed infections with two species of *Plasmodium* are not uncommon, complicating diagnosis even further. Xenodiagnosis, by blood inoculation into laboratory birds such as canaries, is possible for many *Plasmodium* spp. Color illustrations of most species can be found in Garnham, (1966).

Haemoproteus species

Species of *Haemoproteus* (Figs 8.84–8.89) differ from those of *Plasmodium* in that the erythrocytic stages produce only gametocytes. Macro- and microgametocytes can be differentiated in Giemsa-stained thin blood smears. Generally, the nucleus of macrogametocytes is more compact and the cytoplasm denser. Melanin pigment granules tend to be evenly distributed in macrogametocytes but more clustered in polar positions in microgametocytes. The pigment granules are similar to those of *Plasmodium* but are frequently larger. There are some 128 species of *Haemoproteus* (Bennett *et al.*, 1994), all of which are host-specific to the family level and can be divided into five distinct morphological forms (Bennett and Peirce, 1988). These are microhalteridial, halteridial, circumnuclear, rhabdosomal and discosomal. Halteridial species are most common and account for the largest group (65%). The vectors are known for only 10 species, and eight of these are

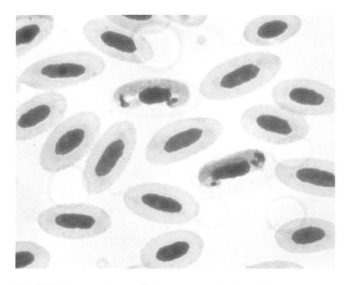

Fig. 8.84 *Haemoproteus psittaci* macrogametocyte and microgametocyte (microhalteridial haemoproteid) from African gray parrot (*Psittacus erithacus*).

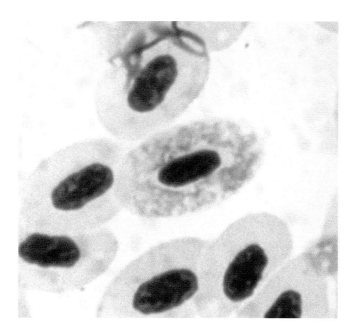

Fig. 8.86 *Haemoproteus handai* macrogametocyte (circumnuclear haemoproteid). Parasite of psittacines.

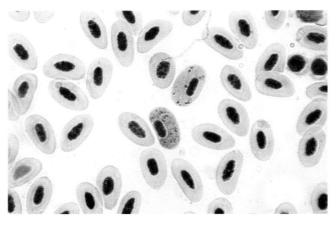

Fig. 8.85 *Haemoproteus syrnii* macrogametocyte and microgametocyte (halteridial haemoproteid). Parasite of Strigidae.

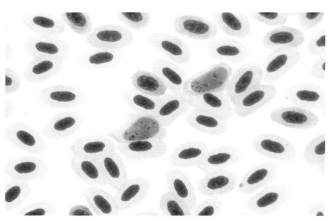

Fig. 8.87 *Haemoproteus enucleator*. Two macrogametocytes (rhabdosomal haemoproteid), from pygmy kingfisher (*Ispidina picta*).

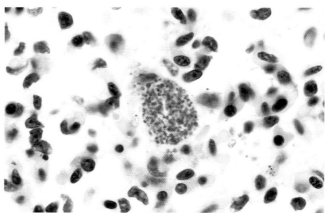

Fig. 8.88 Post-mortem section of lung from a crowned crane (*Balearica pavonina gibbericeps*) showing schizont of the microhalteridial haemoproteid *Haemoproteus balearicae*.

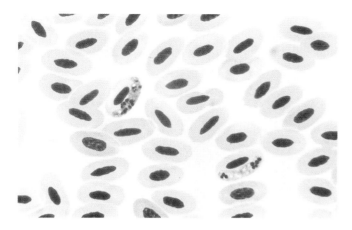

Fig. 8.89 Immature macrogametocyte and microgametocyte of *Haemoproteus columbae* showing distinctive large, purple volutin granules. Cape turtle dove (*Streptopelia capicola*).

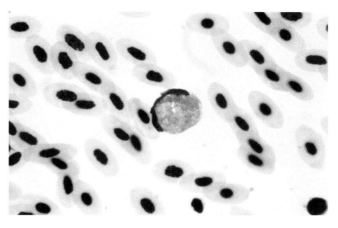

Fig. 8.90 *Leucocytozoon neavei* macrogametocyte (round morph) from yellow-necked spurfowl (*Francolinus leucoscepus*).

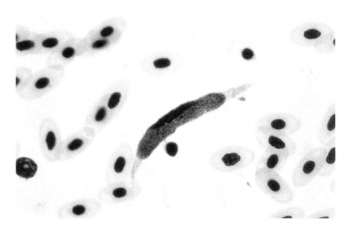

Fig. 8.91 *Leucocytozoon neavei* macrogametocyte (fusiform morph) from yellow-necked spurfowl.

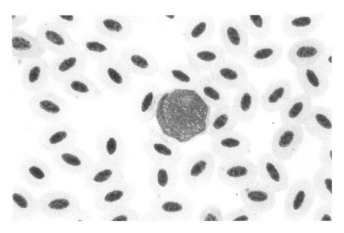

Fig. 8.92 *Leucocytozoon marchouxi* macrogametocyte from pink pigeon (*Columba mayeri*).

transmitted by *Culicoides* spp. Only two are transmitted by hippoboscids. Schizonts of *Haemoproteus* occur in a wide range of organs but are usually most frequent in the lung and liver tissue. Few species of *Haemoproteus* are known to be pathogenic; *H. meleagridis* in turkeys, *H. nettionis* in ducks and geese, and *H. columbae* in pigeons and doves are the general exceptions. No definitive clinical signs of haemoproteid infection are applicable but the general observations pertaining to *Plasmodium* infections can be considered also to apply to *Haemoproteus*. A clinically sick emerald-spotted wood dove in Zambia with mixed infection with *H. columbae* and *Leucocytozoon marchouxi* was 25% under average weight (Peirce 1984).

Mixed infections with *Haemoproteus* and *Plasmodium* are common and multiple invasion of erythrocytes occurs. Differential diagnosis is required but may not always be possible when parasitemias are low. Some species of *Haemoproteus* (e.g. *H. enucleator*) may completely expel the host cell (erythrocyte) nucleus, similar to some *Plasmodium* spp. (e.g. *P. relictum*). Some species of *Haemoproteus* contain reddish-purple volutin granules, which can often be quite large. The exact significance of these granules is not clear but they may represent strain differences. They have often been mistaken for schizonts of *Plasmodium*, from which differential diagnosis is required.

Leucocytozoon species

Species of *Leucocytozoon* (Figs 8.90–8.94) have a life cycle similar to that of *Haemoproteus*. In some species, the gametocytes develop in erythrocytes, in others in monocytes and lymphocytes. Although the macro- and microgametocytes of *Leucocytozoon* can be differentiated on similar characteristics from those of *Plasmodium*

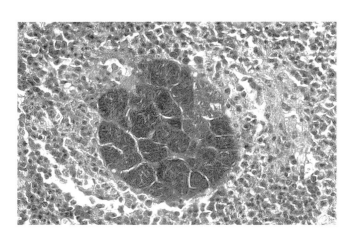

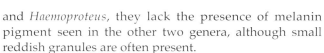

Fig. 8.93 *Leucocytozoon marchouxi* megaloschizont in spleen of pink pigeon.

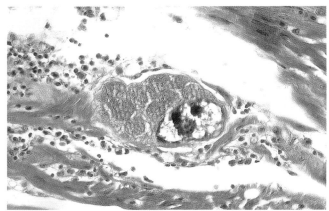

Fig. 8.94 *Leucocytozoon marchouxi* megaloschizont in heart muscle of pink pigeon.

and *Haemoproteus*, they lack the presence of melanin pigment seen in the other two genera, although small reddish granules are often present.

As the gametocytes develop they cause considerable distortion of the host cell. Two distinct morphological forms occur: round and elongated (fusiform) morphs. In some species, only one type of morph occurs, but in others both may occur. In species with both morphs, the round ones arise from the first-generation hepatic schizonts and the fusiform morphs from second-generation megaloschizonts (Fallis *et al.*, 1974). The precise significance of megaloschizonts is not known, since they also occur in species with only round morphs.

There are some 60 species of *Leucocytozoon* (Bennett *et al.*, 1994), all of which are host-specific at least to the family level and, with the exception of *L. (Akiba) caulleryi*, which is transmitted by *Culicoides*, the vectors are all simuliids. Pathogenicity due to *Leucocytozoon* is generally more common than with *Haemoproteus*. High levels of mortality have been recorded with *L. (Akiba) caulleryi* in chickens, *L. smithi* in turkeys and *L. simmondi* in both domestic and free-living ducks and geese. Until recently, there was little evidence of pathogenicity with *L. marchouxi* in pigeons and doves (Peirce, 1984) but recent studies have shown this species to be pathogenic in the endangered pink pigeon (*Columba mayeri*) in Mauritius, with recorded mortality in squabs. It has also been shown to be a species producing megaloschizonts, although only round morphs occur. There is also some evidence that *L. danilewskyi* may be pathogenic in certain species of owl.

The endogenous stages (schizonts) occur in nearly all organs and muscle, causing severe damage and necrosis (Peirce *et al.*, 2004). It is the degree of tissue damage that causes mortality rather than the gametocyte parasitemia. Very high levels of parasitemia have been observed in some hosts without any obvious clinical signs of disease. Outward clinical signs of the disease are similar to those of *Plasmodium*, together with weight loss as birds become too sick to feed.

Mixed infections with *Plasmodium* and/or *Haemoproteus* are common and differential diagnosis is required. It is often in cases of concomitant infection that the usually benign single infections may become pathogenic.

Trypanosoma species

Trypanosomes (Figs 8.95–8.97) are very pleomorphic and of the 98 or so species described from birds probably no more than eight to ten are valid. They are transmitted by a variety of vectors, including mosquitoes, hippoboscids, simuliids and mites. Very high parasitemias are not uncommon but there is no evidence to indicate that any species is pathogenic. There is very little evidence of host specificity. Detection by examination of Giemsa-stained thin blood smears will only illustrate trypanosomes when present in the host at reasonable levels. A more reliable method is by use of the microhematocrit tube and preparing a smear from the buffy coat formed after centrifuging. Trypanosomes are frequently observed in mixed infections with other hematozoa.

Hepatozoon species

There are 15 species of *Hepatozoon* (Figs 8.98 and 8.99) described from birds (Bennett *et al.*, 1992). The parasites normally invade monocytes but occasionally lymphocytes may be targeted. The full life cycle is unknown for any of the avian species but an argasid tick and a flea have been shown as probable vectors for *H. atticorae* of swallows. Ixodid ticks and mites as well as other arthropods may also be involved in transmission.

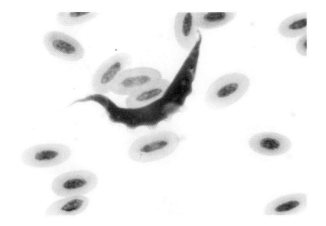

Fig. 8.95 *Trypanosoma corvi.*

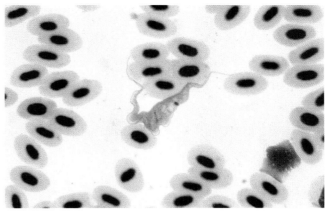

Fig. 8.96 *Trypanosoma bouffardi.*

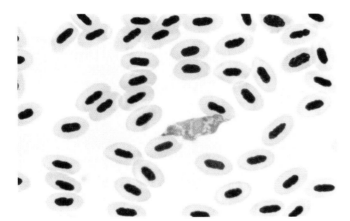

Fig. 8.97 *Trypanosoma everetti.*

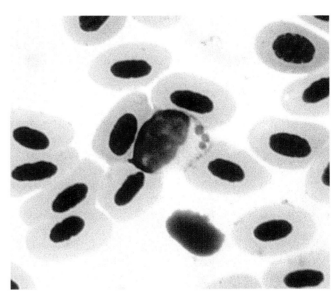

Fig. 8.98 *Hepatozoon estrildus* (early stage) from blue waxbill (*Uraeginthus angolensis*).

None of the avian species is known to be pathogenic. The genus probably has a far more common distribution than current records suggest but is most likely overlooked in screening blood smears. Known hosts range from the tropics to Antarctica.

Babesia species

There are some 14 species described of the avian piroplasm *Babesia* (Fig. 8.100). The group was reviewed by Peirce (2000). The parasites invade erythrocytes, where the trophozoites multiply by binary fission forming pairs or by schizogony forming tetrads. Until recently only *Babesia shortti* occurring in Falconiformes was thought to be pathogenic (Samour and Peirce, 1996), but *B. kiwiensis* from *Apterygidae* also is pathogenic in

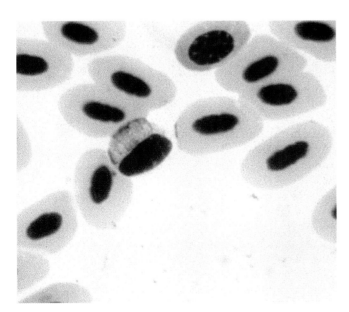

Fig. 8.99 *Hepatozoon estrildus* mature parasite from blue waxbill (*Uraeginthus angolensis*).

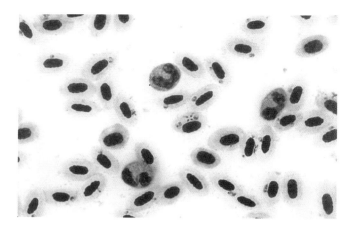

Fig. 8.100 *Babesia shortti* from kestrel (*Falco tinnunculus*).

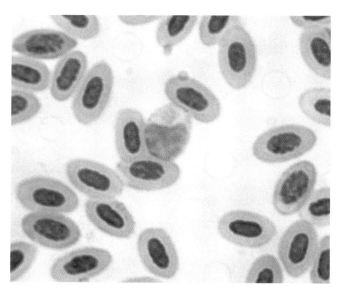

Fig. 8.101 *Atoxoplasma* from willow warbler (*Phylloscopus trochillis*).

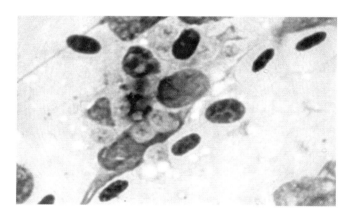

Fig. 8.102 *Atoxoplasma* in spleen impression smear from superb starling (*Spreo superbus*).

kiwi chicks (Peirce *et al.*, 2003). The disease in birds follows a similar pattern to that in mammals, where multiple invasion of erythrocytes leads to destruction of cells, anemia, jaundice and death.

None of the vectors of avian *Babesia* spp. are known but they are assumed to be ixodid ticks, although an argasid tick of the genus *Ornithodoros* has been suggested as a possible vector of *B. shortti* in prairie falcons.

Removal of ticks from birds and prevention of reinfestation is required to control *Babesia* infections. Differential diagnosis between *Babesia* and the trophozoite stages of *Plasmodium* and early gametocytes of *Haemoproteus* is required. The tetrads of *Babesia* are morphologically similar to the small schizonts of some *Plasmodium* spp. (e.g. *P. rouxi*). The main differential characteristics of *Babesia* are the absence of melanin pigment granules and the distinctive white vacuole.

The prevalence of *Babesia* in birds is probably greater than records would suggest. The small number of records is no doubt due to misdiagnosis of *Plasmodium* or *Haemoproteus*. The occurrence of mixed infections should also be considered. Experience with *B. shortti* infections in falcons indicates that an early diagnosis is required if appropriate chemotherapy is to be successful.

Atoxoplasma species

The life cycle and taxonomic position of *Atoxoplasma* parasites (Fig. 8.101) have been the subject of much discussion and confusion. It is now generally accepted that the genus is a member of the Eimeriidae and is closely related to *Isospora*. Separation of the two genera requires molecular techniques. Extraintestinal stages result from the ingestion of *Isospora*-like oocysts, where the parasites invade mononuclear leukocytes. The parasites are particularly common in passerine birds and about 19 species have been described.

High parasitemias are common in nestlings and young birds but are rarely pathogenic; most infections being subclinical. Recent studies, however, have shown that, with some species, mortality can occur in adult birds, particularly when kept in captivity. Post-mortem Giemsa-stained impression smears of liver and spleen (Fig. 8.102) frequently reveal large numbers of parasites. There are a few reports attributed to *Atoxoplasma* sp. where specific clinical signs have been described. The parasite has been implicated as a cause of 'going light' in greenfinches (Cooper *et al.*, 1989) and as a cause of inappetence and 'fluffed-up feathering' in 4–8-week-old bullfinches. Histopathology of one bird with enlarged liver and spleen revealed various pathological changes including encapsulated granulomata with necrotic areas and general hepatic congestion (McNamee *et al.*, 1995). Preventive measures recommended are good aviary hygiene and especially frequent replacement of drinking water and bathing bowls to prevent ingestion of sporulated oocysts.

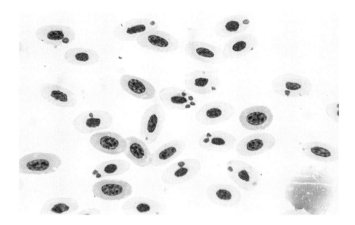

Fig. 8.103 *Aegyptianella pullorum*.

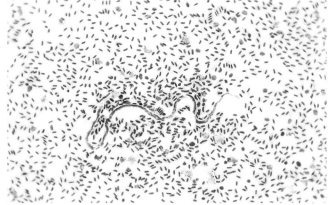

Fig. 8.104 Microfilaria from Senegal parakeet (*Psittacula krameri*).

Aegyptianella species

Parasites of the genus *Aegyptianella* (Fig. 8.103) are rickettsias with close affinities to *Anaplasma*, *Eperythrozoon*, etc., all of which are grouped in the family Anaplasmataceae.

In domestic poultry *A. pullorum* is pathogenic. The intraerythrocytic parasites cause severe anemia, jaundice and frequently death. The vector of *A. pullorum* is the argasid tick *Argas persicus* and the control of this tick is essential in preventing exposure of chickens to the disease. Parasites resembling *A. pullorum* have been recorded from turkeys, ducks, geese and in other hosts, including psittacines from South America and East Africa. Many of these records are probably of closely related species. *Aegyptianella botuliformis* has been described from guinea fowl in South Africa (Huchzermeyer *et al.*, 1992) and more recently *A. minutus* from passerine birds in Malaysia (Peirce, 1999).

Differential diagnosis is required to separate *Aegyptianella* from early trophozoites and gametocytes of *Plasmodium* and *Haemoproteus* respectively. The absence of melanin pigment is usually indicative of *Aegyptianella* and in higher parasitemias the morphology is more varied.

Microfilariae

Microfilariae are the larval stages of filarial worms, of which there are many genera and species occurring in birds. The morphology varies considerably from short and stumpy to long and thin (Fig. 8.104). The larvae usually demonstrate a circadian rhythm coinciding with vector activity. During this time large numbers may be present in peripheral blood. The majority of species appear to be benign but, where concomitant infection with other parasites or diseases prevails, large numbers of larvae may cause some degree of morbidity.

Discussion

The accurate diagnosis of blood parasites requires good-quality, Giemsa-stained, thin blood smears. Smears prepared post-mortem are useful in indicating the presence of parasites, even if this is restricted to the generic level only because of the morphological distortion that rapidly occurs following death. If a bird has been dead for a few hours, it is still possible to produce slides by opening up the heart (usually the last area to clot) and scraping the blood clot with the edge of a microscope slide, which will release sufficient blood cells to make a reasonable thin smear. Without the back-up of blood smears it is often difficult to correlate tissue stages of parasites present on histopathology examination.

Prevention and control of many blood parasites is difficult and in some cases is almost impossible. Parasites such as *Babesia*, *Aegyptianella* and probably *Hepatozoon* can be controlled to some degree by eliminating tick vectors by use of safe acaricides. However, those parasites transmitted by flying insects, especially hemosporidia, are more difficult to control unless the birds are maintained in fly-proof cages or aviaries, which is both costly and inconvenient. An added problem is that this approach results in birds reared under such conditions being totally susceptible to infection if released into the wild as part of a captive breeding or rehabilitation program.

No specific recommendations for chemotherapy of infections have been included, for several reasons. First, there are few, if any, drugs licensed for use in exotic avian hosts. Many birds can react severely to certain drugs and the treatment often causes more problems than the disease itself. A misdiagnosis can result in the administration of a drug that has no effect on the disease present. In cases where drug therapy is deemed necessary, appropriate chemotherapy and dose rates are at the discretion of the veterinarian responsible.

As seen from available evidence, the more pathogenic parasites generally occur in domestic species, and treatment of whole flocks is usually undertaken with established prophylactics for specific disease entities.

In birds exposed to infections not encountered in their normal host range, the resulting disease picture can be totally different. For example, penguins may die from *Plasmodium* infection without the detectable presence of any erythrocytic stages, the damage being caused by exoerythrocytic schizonts in the tissues.

The majority of hemoparasites occurring in birds within their normal host range are usually benign and it is not exceptional to find infections with six or more different parasites in a single host without any signs of ill effects. Many parasites cause seasonal relapses, often associated with the onset of breeding in the avian host and an increase in vector availability. Such relapses in free-living birds do not appear to cause any significant problems. When such birds are suffering with other concomitant disease agents or are under stress, normally benign parasites may become pathogenic. These factors are particularly important in monitoring the disease status of endangered species as part of a captive breeding program, and in pet or collection birds not bred in captivity.

The spectrum of blood parasites to which both domestic and free-living birds can be exposed is wide and varied. Traditionally, textbooks of avian medicine have concentrated on the post-mortem histopathology changes often associated with specific parasitic diseases, and their prevention and treatment. The emphasis in this chapter has been to present pointers to differential diagnosis of the peripheral blood forms in order to aid in the correct identification and subsequent treatment when necessary.

REFERENCES

Bennett GF, Peirce MA (1988) Morphological form in the avian haemoproteidae and annotated checklist of the genus *Haemoproteus* Kruse 1890. *Journal of Natural History* **22**: 1683–1696.

Bennett GF, Earle RA, Peirce MA (1992) New species of avian *Hepatozoon* (Apicomplexa: Hemogregarinidae) and a re-description of *Hepatozoon neophrontis* (Todd and Wolbach, 1912) Wenyon, 1926. *Systematic Parasitology* **23**: 183–193.

Bennett GF, Bishop MA, Peirce MA (1993a) Checklist of avian species of *Plasmodium* Marchiafava and Celli, 1885 (Apicomplexa) and their distribution by avian family and Wallacean life zones. *Systematic Parasitology* **26**: 171–179.

Bennett GF, Peirce MA, Ashford RW (1993b) Avian haematozoa: mortality and pathogenicity. *Journal of Natural History* **27**: 993–1001.

Bennett GF, Peirce MA, Earle RA (1994) An annotated checklist of the valid avian species of *Haemoproteus*, *Leucocytozoon* (Apicomplex: Haemosporida) and *Hepatozoon* (Apicomplexa: Hemogregarinidae). *Systematic Parasitology* **29**: 61–73.

Cooper JE, Gschmeissner S, Greenwood AG (1989) Atoxoplasma in greenfinches (*Carduelis chloris*) as a possible cause of 'going light'. *Veterinary Record* **124**: 343–344.

Fallis AM, Desser SS, Khan RA (1974) On species of *Leucocytozoon*. *Advances in Parasitology* **12**: 1–67.

Garnham PCC (1966) *Malaria Parasites and other Haemosporidia*, Blackwell Science, Oxford.

Huchzermeyer FW, Horak IG, Putterill JF, Earle RA (1992) Description of *Aegyptianella botuliformis* n. sp. (Rickettsiales: Anaplasmataceae) from the helmeted guineafowl, *Numida meleagris*. *Onderstepoort Journal of Veterinary Research* **59**: 97–101.

McNamee P, Pennycott T, McConnell S (1995) Clinical and pathological changes associated with *Atoxoplasma* in a captive bullfinch (*Pyrrhula pyrrhula*). *Veterinary Record* **136**: 221–222.

Peirce MA (1984) Weights of birds from Balmoral, Zambia. *Bulletin of the British Ornithologists Club* **104**: 84–85.

Peirce MA (1989) The significance of avian haematozoa in conservation strategies. In: Cooper JE (ed.) *Disease and Threatened Birds*. ICBP Technical Publication, **10**: 69–76.

Peirce MA (1999) A new species of *Aegyptianella* from south-east Asia. *Veterinary Record* **145**: 288.

Peirce MA (2000) A taxonomic review of avian piroplasms of the genus *Babesia* Starcovici, 1893 (Apicomplexa: Piroplasmorida: Babesiidae). *Journal of Natural History* **34**: 317–332.

Peirce MA, Jakob-Hoff RM, Twentyman C (2003) New species of haematozoa from Apterygidae in New Zealand. *Journal of Natural History* **37**: 1797–1804.

Peirce MA, Lederer R, Adlard RD, O'Donoghue PJ (2004) Pathology associated with endogenous development of haematozoa in birds from southeast Queensland. *Avian Pathology* **33**: 445–450.

Samour JH, Peirce MA (1996) *Babesia shortti* infection in a saker falcon. *Veterinary Record* **139**: 167–168.

Bacterial diseases

Peernel Zwart

Chlamydophilosis

Definition

Chlamydophilosis is an infectious disease, caused by a Gram-negative obligate intracellular organism (Figs 8.105–8.107 and Table 8.5).

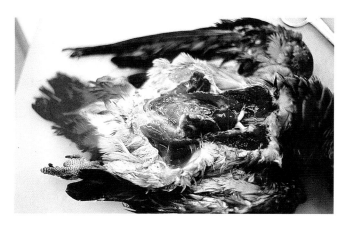

Fig. 8.105 Chlamydophilosis in an African gray parrot (*Psittacus erithacus*). Typical post-mortem findings include peritonitis and serositis, as observed in this photograph. (Courtesy of Dr. U. Wernery).

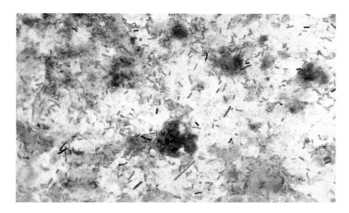

Fig. 8.106 Intestinal contents contain larger aggregates of *Chlamydophila* sp. Mealy amazon (*Amazona farinosa*). Stamp, ×1000.

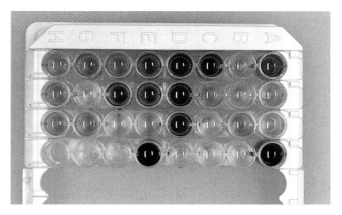

Fig. 8.107 Enzyme-linked immunosorbent assay test for *Chlamydophila* sp. antigen detection (Ideia™ Chlamydophila, Dako, Denmark) widely used in birds. The photograph shows the results from a group of birds tested. The positive reactions are seen as red-magenta, negative reactions as clear. Pale pink reactions should be read with the aid of a colorimeter or the patient should be re-tested. (Courtesy of Dr. U. Wernery).

TABLE 8.5 Chlamydophilosis: clinical signs, post-mortem changes and differential diagnosis

Clinical sign	Post-mortem changes	Differential diagnosis
Conjunctivitis	Swelling of eyelids	Pox, irritation, vitamin A deficiency
Keratitis	Hyperemia. Exudation leads to adhesion of eyelids	
Nasal exudation	Hyperemia, exudation	Bacterial and mycotic nasal infections
Respiratory distress	Pneumonia, airsacculitis	Aspergillosis
Fluffy feathers		General infections
Inappetence	Gastroenteritis	General infections
Diarrhea (green-gray)	Enteritis, swollen liver and spleen	Parasitic infections, intestinal mycosis
Polydipsia (pigeon)		Enteritis

Etiological agent

Chlamydophila psittaci. The species is divided in serotypes (genotypes).

Distribution

The infection occurs worldwide.

Species susceptible

Psittacines: Genotype A (It is considered as the major source for human psittacosis)
Fera pigeons: Genotype B (It is considered endemic in European non-psittacine birds)
Ducks: Genotype C
Poultry, Turkeys: Genotype D
Various birds: Genotypes E and F (both are rare)

Transmission

Respiratory infections are of special importance in the spread of the disease, as nasal secretion may be rich in organisms. The feces, however, may also contain large numbers of organisms. Other infective materials include tears, ocular exudate and crop food or crop milk. Direct infection from bird to bird is accomplished through crop milk in the case of pigeons. Indirect infection occurs via inhalation of droplets of nasal secretion or dried fecal particles. The new host is infected via the epithelia of either the respiratory or the digestive tract. Especially when birds are caught in an aviary, whirling dust mixed with dried feces and feather particles is inhaled deeply both by birds and humans. The additional stress can evoke a manifest disease in latent carriers.

Diagnosis

Impression smears of organs (spleen, lung, liver, intestinal contents) and lesions, stained with Stamp give a first impression. Cultivation methods are laborious, time consuming and replaced by serological techniques. Serological tests are available. An ELISA test is fairly sensitive, although it only indicates previous contact with the agent and false negatives are possible. The prevalent method is the outer membrane protein A (ompA) genotype-specific real-time PCR.

Materials to be sent (before treatment with antimicrobial agents) for testing are:

1. Whole blood submitted in a heparin or EDTA containing tube (0.2 cc minimum)
2. Cloacal swab (collected on cotton-tipped wooden sticks and shipped in a specific transport medium)
3. Feces sample submitted in a sterile container.

Treatment/prevention

The therapeutic regimen should be meticulously and conscientiously followed to reach a favorable result.

- Enrofloxacin 10 mg/kg bodyweight
- Doxycycline 75 mg/kg IM in the breast musculature, 9 injections at 5 d intervals
- Chlortetracycline (CTC) 10 mg/kg daily over 45 d. CTC can also be dosed orally with specific medicated food or as a self-made prescription of a boiled mixture of seeds, rice and water (2:2:3), to which 5% CTC is added
- Stress must be minimized in the infected bird or flock. Breeding must be stopped. Any concurrent disease must be treated. If medicated pellets are to be used, the bird should be gradually converted to a pelleted diet. Supportive therapy, especially with multivitamins, is indicated.
- Prevention in the clinic or laboratory, is with 1:1000 dilution of quaternary ammonium compounds (alkyldimethylbenzylammonium chloride, e.g. Roccal® or Zephiran®) is effective, as well as 70% isopropyl alcohol, 1% Lysol®, 1:100 dilution of household bleach (2¹/₂ tablespoons per gallon) or chlorophenols.

Avian tuberculosis

Definition

Generalized chronic disseminated granulomatous infectious disease caused by acid-fast bacteria (Figs 8.108–8.115 and Table 8.6).

Etiological agent

Mycobacterium avium complex (MAC); i.e. *M. avium, M. intracellulare* and other poorly identified strains. Various serotypes of *M. avium* occur. Geographic differences in the distribution of serotypes exists. In Europe, especially, serotype 2 has been found (Baumgartner and Isenbügel, 1995). In psittacines and wood pigeons (*Columba palumbis*) a specific enteric infection occurs that resembles paratuberculosis. On the basis of DNA analysis the 'wood pigeon' mycobacteria are classified as *Mycobacterium avium* subsp. *columbae* (Saxegaard and Baess, 1988).

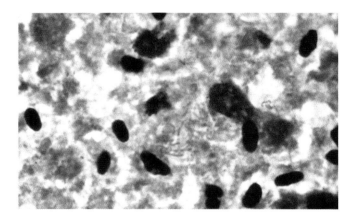

Fig. 8.108 Acid-fast bacilli (Ziehl–Neelsen stain) in the feces of a gyrfalcon (*Falco rusticolus*), showing pink rods of bacteria characteristic of *Mycobacterium* sp. ×1000. (Courtesy of Dr. U. Wernery).

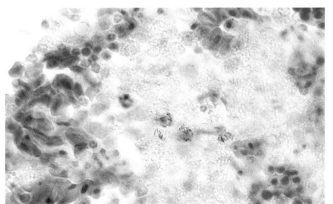

Fig. 8.109 Bone marrow with acid-fast organisms located in macrophages. Green-cheeked amazon parrot (*Amazona viridigenalis*). Ziehl–Neelsen stain, ×1000.

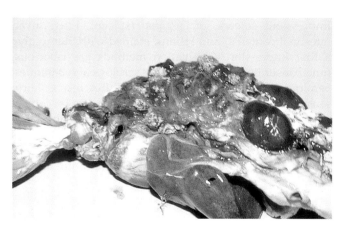

Fig. 8.110 Lung dotted with tubercles – most probably due to secondary hematogenous spread. Goshawk (*Accipiter gentilis*).

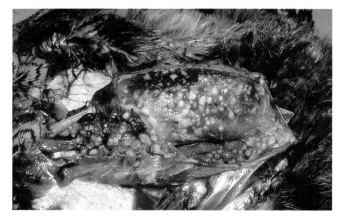

Fig. 8.111 Tubercles in the liver. Ring-necked pheasant (*Phasianus colchicus*).

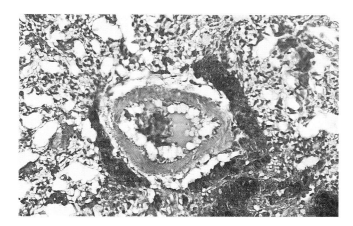

Fig. 8.112 Localization of *Mycobacterium avium/intracellulare* in a lymph vessel in lung tissue surrounding an artery. Canary (*Serinus canaria*). Ziehl–Neelsen stain, ×250.

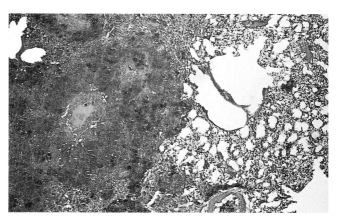

Fig. 8.113 Lung with a larger area of consolidation caused by *Mycobacterium avium/intracellulare*. Canary. Ziehl–Neelsen stain, ×100.

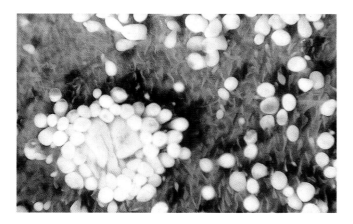

Fig. 8.114 Small intestine. Enlargement of villi due to accumulations of acid-fast mycobacteria (*M. avium* subsp. *columbae*) in macrophages. Wood pigeon (*Columba palumbus*).

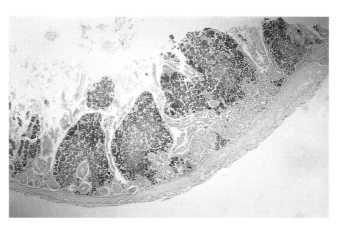

Fig. 8.115 Small intestine, revealing enlargement of villi due to massive accumulation of acid-fast mycobacteria (*M. avium* subsp. *columbae*) in macrophages. Orange winged amazon parrot (*Amazona amazonica*). Ziehl–Neelsen stain, ×250.

TABLE 8.6 Avian tuberculosis: clinical signs, post-mortem changes and differential diagnosis

Clinical sign	Post-mortem changes	Differential diagnosis
Chronic emaciation		Coligranulomas, yersiniosis, listeriosis, mycosis
Ruffled feathers, slow molting	Tubercles in organs	Chronic pathology of parenchymatous organs
Subcutaneous granulomata	Tubercles	Coligranulomas
Diarrhea	Tuberculous ulcerating granulomata Enlargement of intestinal villi (Psittaciformes, pigeon)	*Macrorhabdus ornithogaster* infection Candidiasis
Dyspnea (Passeriformes)	Larger areas of consolidation	Aspergillosis, chronic interstitial pneumonia
Paralysis	Tubercles in bone marrow of tibia and femur (Psittaciformes) Adenocarcinoma	Salmonellosis, renal adenocarcinoma (budgerigar), tumor of testicle (budgerigar)

Distribution

The infection occurs worldwide.

Species susceptible

In principle all birds are susceptible to *M. avium/intracellulare*. However, the disease is rare in budgerigars and psittacines. *M. avium/intracellulare* reveals a characteristic ingestion infection. The tubercles are located in the intestinal tract, the liver and spleen, to be distributed to all organs in a later stage. In canaries and in particular gouldian finches the lesions are located especially in the lungs. Woodpeckers showing an enlarged abdomen revealed an even distribution of acid-fast organisms accumulated in large numbers in macrophages. *M. avium* subsp. *columbae* is found in wood pigeons and psittacines, located in the intestinal villi.

Transmission

Mainly by oral uptake, especially in the case of open tuberculosis (shedding via feces). Infection by aspiration is extremely rare in birds.

Diagnosis

Radiological examination (Psittaciformes) reveals enlarged liver, spleen and/or small intestine. Endoscopic examination of parenchymatous organs, with biopsy of foci and examination for acid-fast organisms. Fecal examination for acid-fast organisms (episodes of non-shedding may occur). Examination of blood reveals leukocytosis and heterophilia. Blood test with ELISA (not very reliable in the individual but suitable for flock diagnosis). At post-mortem: impression smears of lesions stained with Hemacolor, Giemsa or comparable stain may reveal macrophages with rod-shaped blank spaces in the protoplasm, representing the unstained mycobacteria.

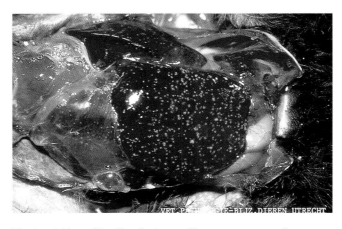

Fig. 8.116 Liver with miliary foci caused by enormous spread of *Yersinia pseudotuberculosis* bacteria. Ornate umbrella bird (*Cephalopterus ornatus*).

TABLE 8.7 Pseudotuberculosis: clinical signs, post-mortem changes and differential diagnosis (concerns especially Passeriformes)

Clinical sign	Post-mortem changes	Differential diagnosis
High mortality (acute cases)		Inhalation of PTFE fumes
Apathy	Foci in liver and spleen	Salmonellosis, tuberculosis
Anorexia	Inflammation caeca (lymphoid)	Salmonellosis, tuberculosis
Respiratory distress	Foci in lungs (in toucans peracute catarrhal pneumonia)	Salmonellosis, colibacillosis, atoxoplasmosis, mycosis (aspergillosis)

Treatment/prevention

In view of the zoonotic capacities of the infection, therapy is not applied. Prevention is by quarantine of long duration (3–5 months) for birds to be introduced to a colony.

Pseudotuberculosis (yersiniosis)

Definition

Generalized disseminated infectious disease caused by Gram-negative bacteria (Figs 8.116 and 8.117 and Table 8.7).

Etiological agent

Yersinia pseudotuberculosis (serotypes 1 and 2).

Distribution

The infection occurs worldwide.

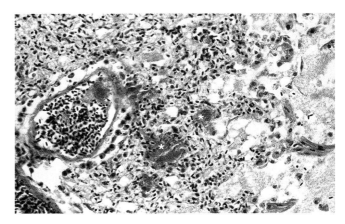

Fig. 8.117 Lung with accumulations of *Yersinia pseudotuberculosis* bacteria in pulmonary blood-capillaries and hyperemia. Crimson rosella (*Platycercus elegans*). Hematoxylin and eosin, ×250.

Species susceptible

A wide variety of passeriform species are especially susceptible, in particular arassaris and toucans. The disease is rare in budgerigars, Psittaciformes and pigeons.

Transmission

By fecal contact – also if food is contaminated by feces of small rodents.

Treatment/prevention

Antibiotic (bactericidal, e.g. ampicillin 1000–2000 mg or amoxicillin 200–400 mg per liter of water) over a period of 14 d, eventually longer. In canaries, enrofloxacin offers promising results (Haesebrouck *et al.*, 1995). Hygiene. Prevent contacts with free-living birds. Stores for seeds used as food should be rodent-proof. Larger birds (toucans) can be vaccinated with a killed vaccine (Zwart *et al.*, 1981).

Salmonellosis

Definition

Salmonellosis (Figs 8.118–8.122 and Table 8.8) is a contagious infection caused by a Gram-negative bacterium.

Etiological agent

Salmonella spp. In general *S. typhimurium* (Sato and Wada, 1995). In racing pigeons, *Salmonella typhimurium* var. *Copenhagen*, which lacks the antigen O5.

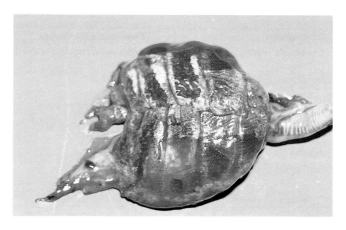

Fig. 8.120 Catarrhal pneumonia due to infection with *Salmonella typhimurium* var. *Copenhagen*. Pigeon.

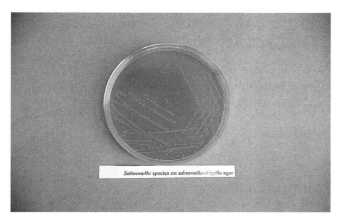

Fig. 8.118 *Salmonella* sp. in salmonella and shigella agar after 24 h of incubation at 37°C (98.6°F). Colonies are 2–3 mm in diameter and pale yellow in color. (Courtesy of Mr. C. Silvanose).

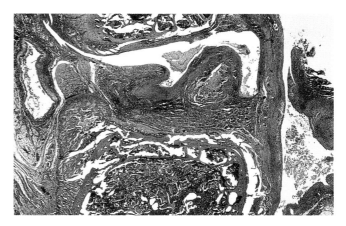

Fig. 8.121 Arthritis and osteomyelitis in adjacent bone, due to *Salmonella typhimurium* var. *Copenhagen*. Pigeon. Hematoxylin and eosin, ×10.

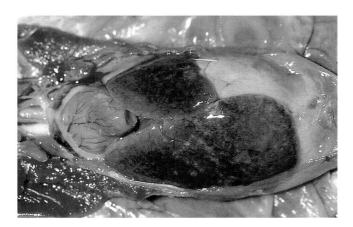

Fig. 8.119 Salmonellosis with inflammation of the liver. Turtle dove (*Streptopelia turtur*). (Courtesy of Dr. G. M. Dorrestein).

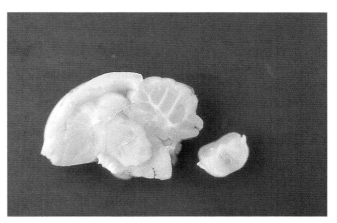

Fig. 8.122 Abscessation of the brain due to *Salmonella typhimurium* infection. Canary.

TABLE 8.8 Salmonellosis: clinical signs, post-mortem changes and differential diagnosis

Clinical sign	Post-mortem changes	Differential diagnosis
General distress	Septicemia, hepatitis with inflammatory foci	Yersiniosis, colibacillosis, psittacosis, adenovirus, paramyxovirus
Polydipsia, polyuria, diarrhea	Enteritis	Candida–mycosis, helminths, coccidia, hexamites, cochlosomiasis
Respiratory distress	Pneumonia	Aspergillosis
Conjunctivitis	Inflammation	Toxoplasmosis
Panophthalmia	Inflammation	Toxoplasmosis
Arthritis	Inflammation	
CNS symptoms	Brain abscess	Paramyxovirus, deltamethrin intoxication

Distribution

Salmonellosis occurs worldwide, especially in outdoor aviaries. Newly arrived individuals can introduce the disease.

Species susceptible

Especially racing pigeons and Passeriformes; occasional infections in Psittaciformes (the budgerigar included). Young pigeons and weakened birds in general are susceptible. Deficient feeding (old seeds, rancid vitamin preparations on an oil base), overcrowding and a cold, humid climate are predisposing factors.

Transmission

The infection is most often transmitted by oral uptake, either during crop feeding or via contaminated foods, or by birds roosting on the aviary. Aerogenic transmission is known. Birds may become infected by carrier birds and occasionally by humans.

Diagnosis

Clinical signs (especially arthritis (pigeon)), post-mortem findings and bacteriological examination (use enrichment media).

Treatment/prevention

Clinically ill animals are separated and eventually euthanized (Passeriformes, budgerigar, pigeon). According to the resistance-test, antibiotics are used over a period of 14–21 d. The result of the therapy is checked by culture between 3 and 6 weeks after the treatment is finished. Occasionally the therapy must be repeated. Hygiene is essential, especially in caged and aviary birds (Passeriformes, budgerigar, pigeon).

In order to prevent spread from other infected flocks, owners should be warned not to participate in bird exhibitions during the season because of the risk of carriers.

Escherichia coli infections

Definition

Colibacillosis (Figs 8.123–8.125 and Table 8.9) is a contagious infectious disease caused by a Gram-negative bacterium.

Etiological agent

Escherichia coli (various serotypes), eventually in association with other Enterobacteriaceae or *Candida* spp. infections (Prattis *et al.*, 1990).

Distribution

The infection occurs worldwide.

Species susceptible

Almost all species of bird may at a given time suffer from colibacillosis.

Transmission

The infection is transmitted by oral uptake of *E. coli* from the environment and excreters. Poor hygiene, overcrowding, stress factors, nutritional deficiencies and concomitant infections are important factors in outbreaks.

Diagnosis

Post-mortem and bacteriological examination. If possible serotyping of the *E. coli*. In seed-eating Passeriformes, budgerigars and other Psittaciformes, a fecal smear stained with Hemacolor will reveal large numbers of rod-shaped bacteria. Healthy birds of the groups mentioned that have little contact with feces harbor only minimal numbers of bacteria in the intestinal tract.

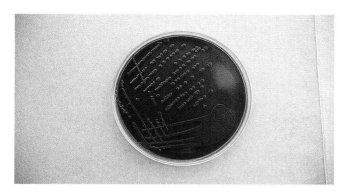

Fig. 8.123 *Escherichia coli* on MacConkey agar after 24h of incubation at 37°C (98.6°F). The lactose fermented colonies are pink in color. (Courtesy of Mr. C. Silvanose).

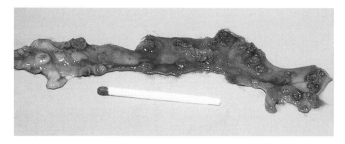

Fig. 8.124 Multiple granulomata along the intestinal tract, due to infection with *Escherichia coli*. African gray parrot (*Psittacus erithacus*).

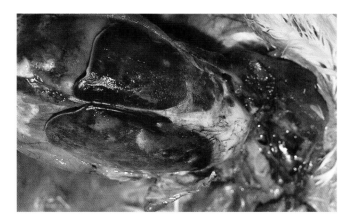

Fig. 8.125 Colibacillosis in a domestic chicken (*Gallus domesticus*). (Courtesy of Dr. U. Wernery).

Treatment/prevention

Under the guidance of sensitivity tests, antibiotics are applied over periods of 2–3 weeks. Hygiene is of utmost importance. In cage birds, the floor can be covered with paper, which is removed on a daily basis to minimize fecal contact.

TABLE 8.9 *Escherichia coli* infections: clinical signs, post-mortem changes and differential diagnosis

Clinical sign	Post-mortem changes	Differential diagnosis
ADULT BIRDS		
Enzootic General malaise, emaciation Apathy, conjunctivitis, rhinitis		Salmonellas, aeromonads, pseudomonads, staphylococci
Diarrhea (Psittaciformes, pigeon)	Enteritis	Capillariasis (pigeon)
Dyspnea	Pneumonia, airsacculitis	Aspergillosis
Swollen joints	Arthritis	Salmonellosis
CNS symptoms		Paramyxovirus infection (pigeon)
NESTLINGS		
Sudden death		
Poor growth		Cochlosoma (Passeriformes) *Macrorhabdus ornithogaster*
Diarrhea		
Omphalitis (pigeon)		
Distended abdomen	Retained yolk sac	
Wet skin		
Dirty, humid nest		

Pasteurellosis

Definition

Pasteurellosis (Table 8.10) is a contagious infectious disease caused by a Gram-negative bacterium.

Etiological agent

Pasteurella multocida (several serotypes); occasionally *P. gallinarum*.

Distribution

The infection occurs worldwide.

Species susceptible

The disease occurs with low frequency in canaries and budgerigars and is very rare in pigeons. Weakened young and old individuals develop the disease.

Transmission

The disease is transmitted by bites of cats and rats. Contact with contaminated rodent feces is also considered in the transmission of the disease.

Clinical sign	Post-mortem changes	Differential diagnosis
General malaise	Enlarged liver and spleen	Infections leading to septicemia (enteric), streptococci (*Streptococcus bovis*), *E. coli* infection, etc.
Respiratory distress	Edema of the lungs	Hyperthermia, aspergillosis
Nasal exudate	Rhinitis	Chlamydophilosis
Conjunctivitis		Chlamydophilosis
Overfilling of nasal sinuses		
Anorexia, diarrhea	Petechiae in intestinal wall	Coccidiosis, capillariasis

TABLE 8.10 Pasteurellosis: clinical signs, post-mortem changes and differential diagnosis

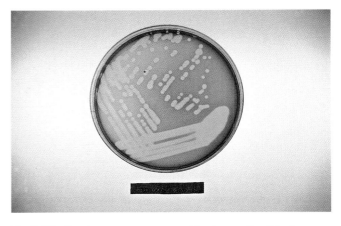

Fig. 8.126 *Streptococcus pyogenes* on blood agar after 48 h of incubation at 37°C (98.6°F). The colonies are surrounded by a clear halo (beta hemolysis). (Courtesy of Mr. C. Silvanose).

Diagnosis

Clinical signs, bite wounds, bacteriological examination of secretions and post-mortem examination. Blood smear reveals large numbers of bipolar bacteria.

Treatment/prevention

Wound-care. Antibiotics are dosed according to sensitivity test. If such a test is not (yet) available, then doxycycline (75–100 mg/kg IM every second day over a period of 6–8 d) may prove to be effective. Prevention is by hygiene and cat- and rat-proof construction of aviaries.

Other bacterial diseases

Definition

Different species of bacteria may cause small epidemics or disease among the birds under consideration (Figs 8.126–8.137 and Table 8.11).

Etiological agents

- *Erysipelothrix rhusiopathiae*
- *Listeria monocytogenes*
- *Streptococcus* spp. and *Staphylococcus* spp.; in pigeons, especially *Streptococcus bovis* (Devriese *et al.*, 1990)
- *Helicobacter jejuni*
- *Macrorhabdus ornithogaster*
- *Klebsiella* spp.
- *Pseudomonas*/*Aeromonas* spp.

Distribution

These infections are widespread.

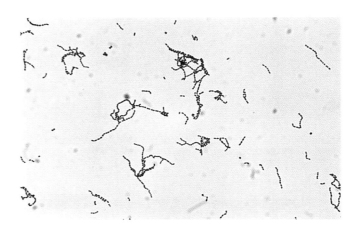

Fig. 8.127 Microscopic appearance of *Streptococcus* sp. in Gram stain showing Gram-positive, chain-forming cocci. ×1000. (Courtesy of Mr. C. Silvanose).

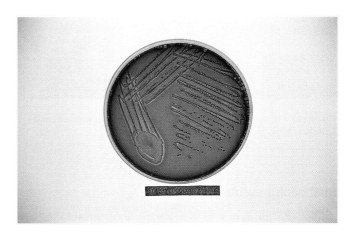

Fig. 8.128 *Staphylococcus aureus* on blood agar after 24 h of incubation at 37°C (98.6°F). The colonies are golden-yellow in color, 1–2 mm in size and surrounded by a clear halo (bêta hemolysis). (Courtesy of Mr. C. Silvanose).

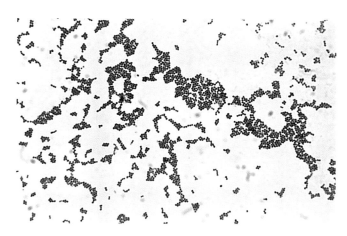

Fig. 8.129 Microscopic appearance of *Staphylococcus* sp. in Gram stain showing Gram-positive cluster-forming cocci. ×1000. (Courtesy of Mr. C. Silvanose).

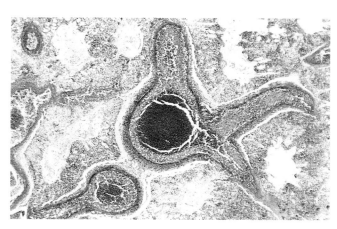

Fig. 8.132 Lung with diffuse pneumonia and accumulations of *Pseudomonas aeruginosa* in lymph vessels situated around the blood vessels, a consequence of nebulizing water containing the microorganism. Canary. Hematoxylin and eosin, ×400.

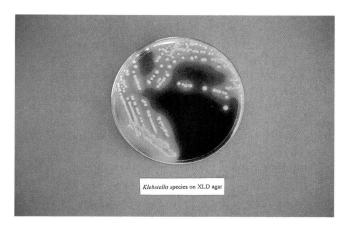

Fig. 8.130 *Klebsiella pneumoniae* in xylose lysine deoxycholate agar after 24 h of incubation at 37°C (98.6°F). The colonies are raised, yellow in color, mucoid in appearance and 2–4 mm in size. (Courtesy of Mr. C. Silvanose).

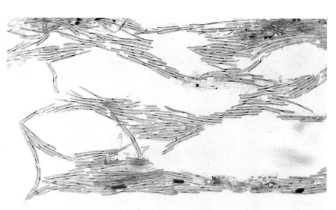

Fig. 8.133 *Macrorhabdus ornithogaster* in a smear of the mucus covering the proventriculus. Canary. Hemacolor, ×400.

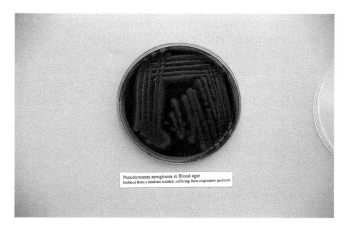

Fig. 8.131 *Pseudomonas aeruginosa* in blood agar after 24 h of incubation at 37°C (98.6°F). The colonies are flat and pigmented in appearance, measuring 2–4 mm in size. Cultures of *P. aeruginosa* have a distinctive, earthy smell. (Courtesy of Mr. C. Silvanose).

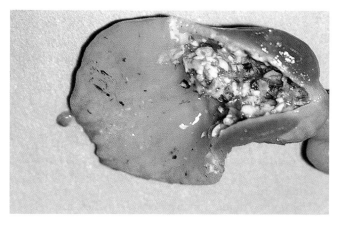

Fig. 8.134 The inner mucosa of the proventriculus is thickened, as a result of chronic infection with *Macrorhabdus ornithogaster*. Canary.

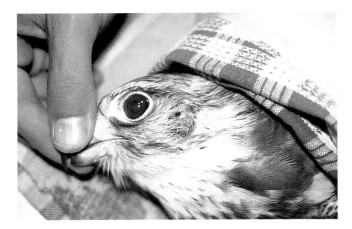

Fig. 8.135 Otitis is not commonly observed in falcons but is usually the result of a localized reaction triggered by ectoparasites and foreign objects and mixed bacterial invasion. Clinical signs include purulent discharges, bad smell, tilting of the head and sometimes loss of balance. (Courtesy of Dr. J. Samour).

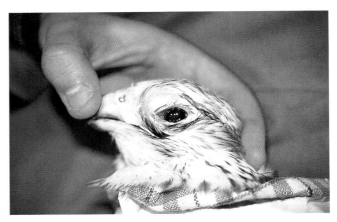

Fig. 8.136 Sinusitis is often diagnosed in falcons in the Middle East. The condition is usually caused by mechanical obstruction with dust and sand but may be the result of intrasinal or intranasal infection with *Trichomonas gallinae* and mixed bacterial infections. (Courtesy of Dr. J. Samour).

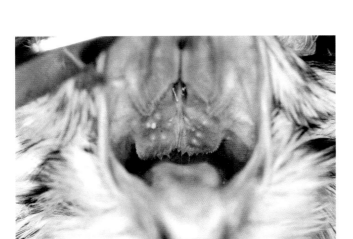

Fig. 8.137 Stomatitis produced by *Pseudomonas aeruginosa* as a sequel of trichomoniasis in a saker falcon. This condition was recently reported in Saudi Arabia.

Species susceptible to etiological agents listed above

- *E. rhusiopathiae* is very rare in Passeriformes, budgerigars, Psittaciformes and pigeons
- Canaries, pigeons and parrots are susceptible to *L. monocytogenes*
- Streptococci and staphylococci are frequent in Passeriformes, budgerigars (especially birds in poor condition) and Psittaciformes; in pigeon especially enteric infections with *S. bovis*
- *H. jejuni* is frequent in ornamental finches, much less in canaries. Rare in budgerigars, Psittaciformes and pigeons
- *M. ornithogaster* is frequent in canaries, rare in other Passeriformes. Frequent in budgerigars and agapornids, much less in neophemas; rare in other Psittaciformes and in pigeons
- *Klebsiella* spp. occur occasionally in canaries, frequently in ornamental finches and other Passeriformes; very rare in budgerigars, Psittaciformes and pigeons
- *Pseudomonas/Aeromonas* spp. occur occasionally in Passeriformes and in immunosuppressed (antibiotic treatment) budgerigars and Psittaciformes; rare in pigeons.

Transmission

- *E. rhusiopathiae* is transmitted orally by contact with contaminated food or water; trauma will occasionally provide an entry
- *L. monocytogenes* is believed to be transmitted by contact with rats
- Streptococci and staphylococci enter via lesions of the mucosa in the oral cavity, digestive tract, respiratory tract and/or conjunctiva
- *H. jejuni* is likely to be transmitted by oral contact. Birds with diminished resistance are especially susceptible. This is generally due to poor-quality food (lack of animal protein, vitamins and minerals) or poor management (overcrowding, humid, cold environment)
- *M. ornithogaster* is transmitted by oral contact (feeding of nestlings with crop-food)
- *Klebsiella* spp. invade after oral contact
- *Pseudomonas/Aeromonas* spp. originate from a humid environment (water) containing some protein. Oral infection predominates. Severe respiratory infections are known after spraying water containing *Pseudomonas* spp.

TABLE 8.11 Other bacterial diseases: clinical signs, post-mortem changes and differential diagnosis

Clinical sign	Post-mortem changes	Differential diagnosis
ERYSIPELOTHRIX RHUSIOPATHIAE		
Sudden death	Septicemia, intoxication	Bacterial infections
LISTERIA MONOCYTOGENES		
Sudden death	Septicemia, intoxication	Bacterial infections
STREPTOCOCCI AND STAPHYLOCOCCI		
Abscessation, omphalitis	Septicemia, abscess	*E. coli* infections, other respiratory distress such as tracheitis (Passeriformes) and pneumonia (budgerigar), bacterial infections
Bumblefoot	Swollen foot, abscessation (Psittaciformes)	Intoxication
Diarrhea	Enteritis (pigeon)	
HELICOBACTER JEJUNI (PASSERIFORMES)		
General malaise, whitish feces	Voluminous intestinal convolute, undigested starch in small intestine	Subchronic cochlosomosis
MACRORHABDUS ORNITHOGASTER		
General malaise, incidental death case	Stomach dilated, mucus rich in rod-shaped fungi, thick mucosa of proventriculus	Lambliasis (budgerigar)
KLEBSIELLA SPP. (BUDGERIGAR)		
Respiratory distress	Pneumonia	Other bacterial infections
CNS symptoms	Meningoencephalitis, hepatitis, nephritis	Adenovirus infection
PSEUDOMONAS AND *AEROMONAS* SPP.		
Diarrhea, dehydration	Enteritis	Other bacterial infections
Pneumonia (Passeriformes)	Airsacculitis, pneumonia	

Diagnosis

- *E. rhusiopathiae:* bacteriological examination
- *L. monocytogenes:* bacteriological examination
- Streptococci and staphylococci : bacteriological examination
- *H. jejuni:* bacteriological examination (special medium); fecal smear stained with Hemacolor reveals numerous undulated bacteria
- *M. ornithogaster:* wet mount of mucus in proventriculus; fecal examination (wet mount)
- *Klebsiella* spp.: bacteriological examination
- *Pseudomonas/Aeromonas* spp.: bacteriological examination.

Treatment/prevention

- *E. rhusiopathiae:* ampicillin, amoxicillin orally via food and water
- *L. monocytogenes:* ampicillin, amoxicillin orally via food and water
- Streptococci and staphylococci : ampicillin, amoxicillin orally via food and water
- *H. jejuni:* antibiotics; improvement of general condition (food, management)
- *M. ornithogaster:* acidification of the drinking water (6 ml HCl 1 N/l results in a pH of 2.4–2.6). Add 30% of

a good concentrated food to the seeds. The use of a cereal product makes the concentrate adhere to the seeds
- *Klebsiella* spp.: antibiotics under the guidance of sensitivity tests
- *Pseudomonas/Aeromonas*: antibiotics under the guidance of sensitivity tests.

REFERENCES

Baumgartner R, Isenbügel E (1995) Wellensittiche. In: Gabrisch K, Zwart P (eds) *Krankheiten der Heimtiere*, vol. I, pp. 449–450. Schlütersche Verlag, Hannover.

Devriese LA, Uyttebroek E, Gevaert D *et al.* (1990) *Streptococcus bovis* infections in pigeons. *Avian Pathology* 19: 429–434.

Haesebrouck F, Vanrompay M, de Herdt P, Ducatelle R (1995) Effect of antimicrobial treatment on the course of an experimental *Yersinia pseudotuberculosis* infection in canaries. *Avian Pathology* 24: 273–283.

Prattis SM, Cioffee CJ, Reinhard G, Zaoutis TE (1990) A retrospective study of disease and mortality in Zebra finches. *Laboratory Animal Science* 40: 402–405.

Sato Y, Wada K (1995) Isolation of *Salmonella typhimurium* from zebra finches (*Poephila guttata*). *Journal of Veterinary Medical Science* 57: 137–138.

Saxegaard F, Baess I (1988) Relationship between *Mycobacterium avium*, *Mycobacterium paratuberculosis* and 'wood pigeon mycobacteria'. Determinations by DNA–DNA hybridization. *Acta Pathologica, Microbiologica et Immunologica* 96: 37–42.

Zwart P, Wiesner H, Göltenboth R (1981) Erfahrungen mit dem Einsatz einer Pseudotuberkulose-Totvakzine bei Vögeln. *Verhandlungsbericht des XIII Internationalen Symposiums über die Erkrankungen der Zootiere* 23: 73–76.

Viral diseases

Ulrich Wernery

Influenza

Etiology

The influenza virus belongs to the family *Orthomyxoviridae*, which is divided into three types (A, B and C). The pleomorphic viruses are enveloped and measure 60–120 μm in diameter. The genome consists of a single-stranded ribonucleic acid (RNA). Influenza A virus is the only type that is of veterinary significance. Influenza viruses possess two surface antigens that are of importance in their identification and control. The more important is hemagglutinin (H), which is responsible for the virus's ability to agglutinate erythrocytes and to attach and penetrate host cells. The other surface antigen is neuraminidase (N), which is involved in the release of newly formed viral particles from host cells. To date, 16 H (H1–H16) and nine N (N1–N9) subtypes have been detected in wild birds and poultry throughout the world (World Health Organization, 1980; Spielman *et al.*, 2004). Subtypes H5, H7 and H9 possess a high pandemic potential (Webster and Hulse, 2004).

Influenza viruses are relatively stable when outside the host, particularly in pond or lake water. In a cool environment, the virus remains infectious in feces for over a month. The viruses can be destroyed in minutes by extremes in pH, heating to 56°C, exposure to sunlight and by most detergents and disinfectants.

Distribution

The best known disease caused by an avian influenza virus (AIV) is fowl plague. Fowl plague was first reported in 1878 and in 1901, causing severe losses in poultry, and in 1955 it was identified as AIV. From the 1970s onward surveillance indicated the ubiquitous presence of AIV in waterfowl and the risk these birds posed to commercial chicken industries. In 1983 there was a large epidemic in the broiler industry of Pennsylvania, which cost US$60 million to control and in 1990 there was a severe outbreak in the Mexican broiler industry. In 1997 a highly pathogenic avian influenza virus (HPAIV) emerged in Hong Kong that had killed close to 150 million birds in Asia up to the beginning of 2005. The loss of their chickens has left many farmers deep in debt and the Asian poultry industry had lost US$15 billion by the end of 2004. The virus spread westward and reached Russia, where it had killed 120000 birds by mid 2005. In April 2005, this H5N1 strain also transferred to pigs and killed 147 out of a total of 418 tigers in Thailand in 2002 through the medium of raw chicken meat.

Since its detection in 1997, more than 17 reassortments have occurred, which have claimed so far more than 70 human lives in Asia. An avian influenza outbreak caused by another HPAI virus, type H7N7, occurred in 2003 in the Netherlands. This virus was considerably less pathogenic for humans than AH5N1 and killed only one person, but millions of chickens were killed to contain the disease.

Epizootiology

Severe acute respiratory syndrome (SARS) exploded into the world's consciousness in March 2003 and made us aware that zoonotic diseases will continue to increase because of closer interactions between people and animals. Human beings have a great impact on their emergence, through the tremendous increase in global travel, intensification of agriculture, changes in the world trade patterns, and global warming. Influenza originates in aquatic birds and is carried by migratory ducks, geese and herons, usually without harming them. Not only are wild birds playing a significant role in spreading the disease but trade through live bird markets and movement of domestic waterfowl are also very influential in the spread of the virus (Sinus *et al.*, 2005). It is estimated that, twice a year, 50 billion birds migrate around the globe, carrying viruses to any corner of the world. As the birds migrate, they can pass the viruses on to domestic birds such as chickens via feces or during competitions for food, territory and water (Garrett, 2005). The influenza virus does not undergo any significant genetic change in these migratory birds (Osterholm, 2005) but when the virus is transmitted from wild to domesticated birds it undergoes changes that allows it to infect humans, pigs and potentially other mammals. Once in the lung cells of a mammalian host, the virus can 'reassort', or mix genes with influenza viruses that are already present. This process can lead to an entirely new viral strain capable of sustained human-to-human transmission.

Whether or not this particular H5N1 influenza strain will mutate into a human-to-human pandemic form is not clear but scientific evidence points to the likelihood that such an event will take place, perhaps soon. H5N1 has now reached the Urals and migratory birds have transported it to Europe. Influenza virus has not only been isolated from aquatic birds, which serve as a reservoir of the virus but also from companions in aviaries and zoological parks. The virus is transmitted through direct contact with feces and aerosol from infected birds but contaminated water in overcrowded ponds or lakes is also considered to be an important source of virus (Ritchie, 1995).

Scientists have observed that influenza viruses can switch from the low-pathogenicity avian influenza (LPAI) phenotype, which is common in wild birds and poultry, to HPAI phenotypes. This is achieved by the introduction of basic amino acid residues into the HAO cleavage site (Munster *et al.*, 2005). Because HPAI outbreaks in poultry originate with LPAI viruses present in waterfowl, influenza A virus surveillance in wild birds could function as an early warning system for HPAI outbreaks. Minor antigenic and genetic diversity were observed among H genes of mallard influenza A isolates and those of HPAI viral strains. These new findings indicate that influenza A surveillance in wild birds provides an excellent opportunity for pandemic preparation, production of vaccines and development of valid diagnostic tests.

Clinical features

The virus may cause high mortality in some avian species and no clinical signs in others. The morbidity and mortality vary widely with the species of bird and strain of infecting virus, and therefore the World Organisation for Animal Health (OIE) differentiates between HPAIV and LPAIV. HPAIV is an OIE list A disease. When clinical changes are present, they may include mild to severe respiratory signs, anorexia, depression, decreased egg production and diarrhea (Figs 8.138–8.141). Highly virulent strains such as H5N1 damage the endothelial cells, resulting in bleeding disorders. It is fatal to domestic poultry. In two different bustard species the clinical signs were dyspnea, lethargy, discharge from eyes and nares, severe tracheitis, pneumonia and pancreatitis (Wernery *et al.*, 2004).

A H7N3 influenza A strain that was isolated from a healthy peregrine falcon (*Falco peregrinus*) induced severe disease in 6-week-old chickens (Fig. 8.141).

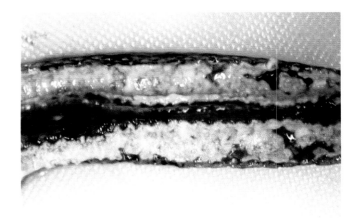

Fig. 8.139 Severe tracheitis with pus production in a houbara bustard with influenza A infection.

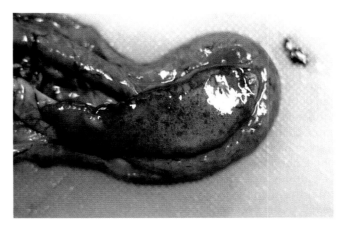

Fig. 8.140 Pancreatitis in a houbara bustard caused by influenza A infection. H7N1 was identified from all these cases. (Courtesy of Dr. J. Kinne).

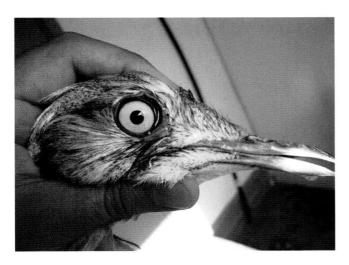

Fig. 8.138 Clear discharge from eyes and nostrils of a houbara bustard with influenza A infection. (Courtesy of Dr. L. Molnar).

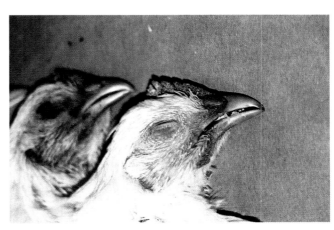

(a)

Fig. 8.141a, b See overleaf for caption.

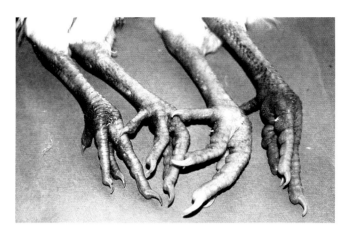

(b)

Fig. 141a, b Acute cyanosis of wattles, comb and legs, 3 d after infection of chickens with a falcon H7N3 strain. (Courtesy of Ms. R. Manvell).

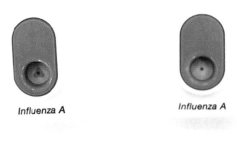

Fig. 8.142 Positive Flu A ELISA from an oropharyngeal swab taken from a quail with H9N2 infection.

Diagnosis

Virus isolation is essential not only to establish the cause of an outbreak but also to assess objectively the virulence of the causative virus. Virus is best isolated from cloacal swabs but ground tissue specimens may also be inoculated into the allantoic cavity of 10–12-day-old embryonated chicken eggs and on to monolayers of cultures of chicken embryo fibroblasts (CEF). Fluid from the allantoic cavity and from cell cultures are subjected to hemagglutination and neuraminidase inhibition testing using reference influenza A antisera. An influenza A antigen ELISA (Directigen Flu A, Becton Dickinson, France) has also been successfully used to diagnose the disease (Fig. 8.142).

Prevention and control

Avian influenza is not eradicable and prevention and control are the only realistic goals. The following recommendations should be put in place:

- Monitor movement of poultry between farms and markets
- Monitor birds in live markets and exports/imports
- Improve biosecurity measures (e.g. prevent contact with wild aquatic birds)
- Separate land-based poultry, pigs and aquatic avian species in farms and markets
- Close live bird markets and keep all poultry indoors while HPAIV is circulating in the region
- Conduct serological and other epidemiological studies in wild birds to determine whether HPAIV has become established in wild populations
- Only allow controlled effective vaccination in response to virulent outbreaks.

Attenuated subtype-specific vaccines are used in domestic fowls. However, these vaccines have limited application because of the speed of antigenic drift and reassortment.

REFERENCES

Garrett L (2005) The next pandemic? *Foreign Affairs* **84**(4): 3–23.

Munster VJ, Wallensten A, Baas C *et al.* (2005) Mallards and highly pathogenic avian influenza ancestral viruses, northern Europe. *Emerging Infectious Diseases* **11**: 1545–1551.

Osterholm MT (2005) Preparing for the next pandemic. *Foreign Affairs* **84**(4): 24–37.

Ritchie W (1995) *Avian Viruses*, pp. 351–364, Wingers Publishing, Lake Worth, FL.

Sinus LD, Domenech J, Benigno C *et al.* (2005) Origin and evolution of highly pathogenic H5N1 avian influenza in Asia. *Veterinary Record* **157**: 159–164.

Spielman D, Mauroo N, Kinoshita R *et al.* (2004) Wild bird species and the ecology of virulent avian influenza. *Proceedings of the American Association of Zoo Veterinarians, American Association of Wildlife Veterinarians and Wildlife Disease Association*, pp. 40–45, San Diego, CA.

Webster RG, Hulse DJ (2004) Microbial adaptation and change: avian influenza. *Revue Scientifique et Technique de l'Office International des Epizooties* **23**: 453–465.

Wernery R, Wernery U, Kinne J, Samour J (2004) *Colour Atlas of Falcon Medicine*, pp. 56–57. Schlütersche, Hannover.

World Health Organization (1980) A revision of the system of nomenclature for influenza viruses: a WHO memorandum. *Bulletin of the World Health Organization* **58**: 585–591.

Newcastle disease

Etiology

The family *Paramyxoviridae* contains three genera: paramyxovirus, morbillivirus and pneumovirus. They include some of the most important pathogens of domestic animals and humans. The Newcastle Disease virus (NDV) (Figs 8.143–8.149) belongs to the genus paramyxovirus and is recognized as serotype paramyxovirus 1 (PMV 1). Nine serotypes of avian paramyxovirus have been differentiated so far (Box 8.1), and few strains have been isolated that could not be grouped (Telbis *et al.*, 1989).

The virions of members of the family *Paramyxoviridae* are pleomorphic, roughly spherical enveloped particles with one large molecule of single-stranded RNA. Two glycoproteins from the surface projections possess both hemagglutinin and neuraminidase activities. NDV is relatively heat stable. It remains infectious in bone marrow and muscles of slaughtered chickens for at least 6 months at –20°C (–4°F) and up to 134 d at 1°C (33.8°F). It can survive for several years in dried mutes. Quaternary ammonium compounds, 1–2% Lysol®, 0.1% cresol and 2% formalin, are used for disinfection (Fenner *et al.*, 1987).

Newcastle disease infects most avian species, producing inapparent or mild disease in many and severe

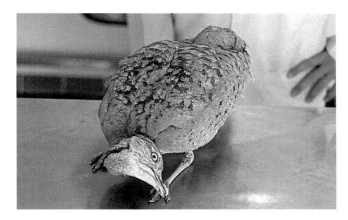

Fig. 8.145 Houbara bustard (*Chlamydotis undulata*) affected with Newcastle disease showing typical CNS signs of incoordination and torticollis. Large numbers of this species are affected with Newcastle disease when houbara bustards are kept in close proximity or are transported to Middle Eastern markets together with pigeons and domestic fowl.

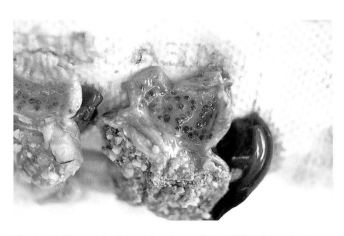

Fig. 8.143 Newcastle disease in a domestic fowl. Note the typical petechial hemorrhages within the gizzard.

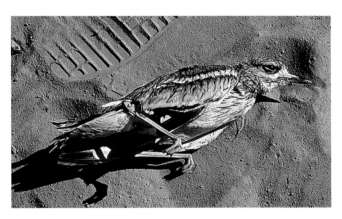

Fig. 8.146 Stone curlew (*Burhinus oedicnemus*) affected with Newcastle disease. Efforts have been made in the Middle East to breed this species in captivity; therefore, preventive medicine programs would have to target this disease through adequate vaccination. Newcastle disease has seldom been reported in this species.

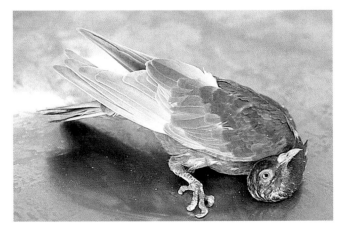

Fig. 8.144 Domestic pigeon (*Columba livia*) affected with Newcastle disease, showing typical central nervous system (CNS) signs of incoordination and torticollis. This is a seasonal disease affecting large flocks of pigeons in many parts of the world.

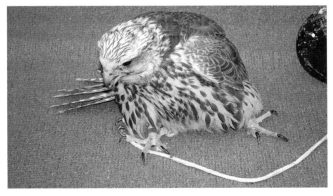

Fig. 8.147 Saker falcon (*Falco cherrug*) displaying clinical signs consistent with the neurotrophic form of Newcastle disease. In the Middle East, falcons are commonly infected with the virus after eating infected pigeons. (Courtesy of Dr. J. Samour).

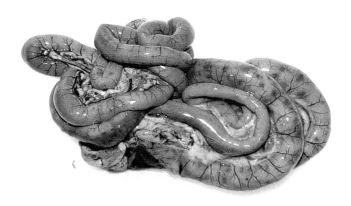

Fig. 8.148 Newcastle disease in a saker falcon. Note the typical petechial hemorrhages throughout the gastrointestinal tract clearly seen through the intestinal wall. (Courtesy of Dr. J. Samour).

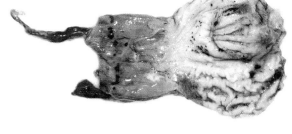

Fig. 8.149 Newcastle disease in a saker falcon. Note the typical petechial hemorrhages within the proventriculus and ventriculus. The vomiting of semidigested blood is a common finding in falcons affected with Newcastle disease when such lesions are present in these organs. (Courtesy of Dr. J. Samour).

Box 8.1 Avian paramyxovirus: the nine classified serotypes (Ritchie, 1995)

- PMV1 Newcastle disease virus
- PMV2 Chicken/California/Yucaipa/56
- PMV3 Turkey/Wisconsin/68
- PMV4 Duck/Hong Kong/D3/75
- PMV5 Budgerigar/Japan/Kunitachi/75
- PMV6 Duck/Hong Kong/199/77
- PMV7 Dove/Tennessee/4/75
- PMV8 Goose/Delaware/1053/76
- PMV9 Duck/New York/22/78

---

and lethal disease in others, indicating a great variety in its virulence. Virulence is measured as a 'neuropathic index' (NI) determined by intracerebral inoculation of day-old chicks. Lentogenic (NI 0.25: avirulent or mildly virulent), mesogenic (NI 0.6–1.8: intermediate virulence) and velogenic (NI 2.0: highly virulent) strains are differentiated.

Paramyxovirus type 2 and 3 infections have been described in Passeriformes and parakeets with respiratory, enteric and central nervous signs similar to those seen with PMV1.

Distribution

Panzootics of Newcastle disease occurred throughout the world between 1940 and 1948, between 1968 and 1972 and during the 1980s, primarily involving racing pigeons (Kaleta and Hettels-Resmann, 1992).

Clinical features

The clinical signs seen in birds infected with NDV vary widely and are dependent on many different factors (Alexander, 1995). One important factor is the variability of the virus's virulence. Newcastle disease ranges from inapparent to severe, fatal illness. Although none of the clinical signs can be regarded as pathognomonic, certain symptoms do appear to be associated with particular Newcastle disease isolates. This has resulted in the grouping of NDV into five pathotypes on the basis of the predominant signs in affected chickens (Alexander, 1995). These are:

- *Viscerotropic velogenic*: high mortality with swelling of tissues around the eyes, bloody diarrhea and hemorrhagic lesions in proventriculus and intestines
- *Neurotropic velogenic*: high mortality followed by respiratory and nervous signs, characterized by paresis of limbs, wings, ataxia, torticollis, circling movements and tremors
- *Mesogenic*: respiratory signs, occasional nervous signs, head tics (falcon), mortality moderate to low
- *Respiratory lentogenic*: mild or subclinical respiratory infection
- *Asymptomatic enteric*: subclinical enteric infection.

These five groupings are by no means clear cut. In all bird species overlapping does occur. Acute and subacute disease associated with mesogenic and lentogenic virus strains are most common in developed countries with modern poultry industries (Fenner *et al.*, 1987).

Disease in chickens may consist of signs of depression, diarrhea and nervous signs such as paralysis and torticollis. In layers a drop in egg production to complete cessation of egg-laying may follow the disease (Mayr, 1993).

In pigeons, quails and houbara bustards PMV1 produces diarrhea and nervous signs (Wernery *et al.*, 1995, Wernery and Manvell, 2003).

Falcons suffering from PMV1 infections initially show gastrointestinal symptoms such as anorexia, vomiting and paralytic ileus. Later in the course of the disease central nervous system signs develop. These signs are associated with ataxia, head tics, tremors, wing and leg paralysis and, very rarely, torticollis (Wernery *et al.*, 1992).

It is known that virulent strains may still replicate in vaccinated birds but the clinical symptoms will be greatly diminished in relation to the antibody level achieved (Alexander, 1995).

Pathological features

Lesions are highly variable, reflecting the variation in tropism and pathogenicity of NDV. As with clinical signs, no gross or microscopic changes are pathognomonic for any form of Newcastle disease. Gross pathological findings include hemorrhagic lesions throughout the intestines with typical petechiae in the proventriculus. Hemorrhagic changes and congestion are seen in the respiratory tract when respiratory signs are present. In birds showing neurological signs prior to death there is no evidence of lesions in the brain. In falcons with clinically reported gastrointestinal symptoms, the crop, proventriculus, ventriculus and enteral tract are usually empty, apart from a considerable amount of bile, which stains parts of the duodenal and jejunal mucosa. In falcons with head tics and paralysis no gross lesions are detected.

Microscopic lesions have no diagnostic significance. In most tissues and organs where changes occur, hyperemia, necrosis and edema are found. In the central nervous system nonpurulent encephalomyelitis may occur. In many birds mild to severe demyelinization in the cerebrum is observed.

Diagnosis

Since clinical symptoms and pathological lesions are relatively nonspecific, diagnosis must be confirmed by virus isolation and to a lesser extent by serology. It is necessary to isolate NDV from infected birds and characterize the virus to exclude viruses of low virulence, which are ubiquitous in feral birds throughout the world, and live vaccines. The virus may be isolated from spleen, brain or lung by allantoic inoculation of 10–12-day-old embryonated eggs or through infection of tissue culture (CEF). NDV is differentiated from other viruses by hemagglutination and hemagglutination inhibition tests using polyclonal antisera. NDV strains can be differentiated by a series of tests and the intracerebral pathogenicity test distinguishes strains within pathotypes (Hitchner *et al.*, 1980).

Prevention and control

Airborne infections are an increasingly important factor in veterinary centers, quarantine units and breeding facilities. People who work in these centers are also susceptible to some airborne infections that can develop within them. Aspergillosis, mycoplasmosis, chlamydophilosis, Newcastle disease and influenza are the common airborne infections, the source of which may be the birds themselves, the facility's staff, the facility itself and built-in air-conditioning systems. A new mobile air-cleaning device/infection control unit is available that significantly reduces and even eliminates airborne pollution (Mattei *et al.*, 2002).

Newcastle disease is a notifiable disease in most countries. Where the disease is enzootic, control can be achieved by proper hygiene combined with immunization. Live virus vaccines of naturally occurring lentogenic strains with an intracerebral pathogenicity index (ICPI) of less than 0.4 are commonly used. They are administered via drinking water, which must not contain chlorine or disinfectants, and via spraying. Vaccinated birds may shed the vaccine virus up to 15 days after vaccination.

Immunization of exotic birds with live vaccines via drinking water is not useful because of the poor serological response. Inactivated vaccines administered subcutaneously are usually used for pigeons, houbara bustards, pheasants, quails and falcons. It might be more effective to use vaccines from locally derived strains (Wernery *et al.*, 1995).

A new vaccine, manufactured specifically against Newcastle disease in falcons and containing strains from four different avian species, has been produced by the Central Veterinary Research Laboratory, Dubai, United Arab Emirates in collaboration with the Veterinary Faculty, University of Munich. The vaccine is widely used in falcons and has dramatically reduced PMV1 in hunting falcons.

Pneumovirus infections

Pneumovirus infections have been observed with severe rhinotracheitis in turkeys and decreased egg production and 'swollen head syndrome' in chickens. Pheasants, guinea fowl and ostriches exhibit mild disease. Infections in turkeys and chickens are associated with sneezing, swelling of infraorbital sinuses and conjunctivitis. The disease resembles mycoplasmosis. For the diagnosis of this disease, a commercial avian pneumovirus antibody ELISA (Flock Chek APV Testkit) is available from IDEXX Laboratories containing the three serotypes A, B and C.

REFERENCES

Alexander DJ (1995) Newcastle disease. *State Veterinary Journal* **5**: 21–24.

Fenner F, Bachmann PA, Gibbs EPJ *et al.* (1987) *Veterinary Virology*, pp. 493–496. Academic Press, New York.

Hitchner SB, Domermuth CH, Purchase HG, Williams JE (1980) *Isolation and Identification of Avian Pathogens*, pp. 63–66a, American Association of Avian Pathologists, Philadelphia.

Kaleta EF, Hettels-Resmann U (1992) Workshop on avian paramyxoviruses, Rauischholzhausen. Germany, CEC, Giessen.

Mattei D, Mordini N, Lonigro C *et al.* (2002) MedicCleanAir® devices for air filtration, a low cost very effective method of managing ambiental *Aspergillus* spp. colonization. *Bone Marrow Transplantation* **29**(suppl. 2): 5245.

Mayr A (1993) *Rolle/Mayr Medizinische Mikrobiologie, Infektions- und Seuchenlehre*, pp. 407–411. Ferdinand Enke, Stuttgart.

Ritchie BW (1995) *Avian Viruses, Function and Control*. Wingers Publishing, Lake Worth, FL.

Telbis C, Neumann U, Siegmann D (1989) Vorkommen von Paramyxoviren bei Wildvögeln: epizootiologische Aspekte, Eigenschaften *in vivo* und *in vitro. Journal of Veterinary Medicine B* **36**: 203–216.

Wernery U, Alexander DJ, Neumann U *et al.* (1995) Newcastle disease in captive falcons. *Middle East Falcon Research Group Specialist Workshop*, Abu Dhabi, pp. 24–32.

Wernery U, Manvell R (2003) Avian viral diseases in the United Arab Emirates (UAE). *Proceedings of the European Association of Avian Veterinarians*, Tenerife, pp. 72–77.

Wernery U. Remple JD, Newmann U *et al.* (1992) Avian Paramyxovirus serotype 1 (Newcastle disease virus) – infections in falcons. *Journal of Veterinary Medicine* **39**: 153–158.

FURTHER READING

Cornelissen H (1993) Vaccination of over 200 bird species against Newcastle disease: Methods and vaccination reactions. *Proceedings of the European Association of Avian Veterinarians*, Utrecht, pp. 275–287.

Wernery R, Wernery U, Kinne J, Samour J (2004) *Colour Atlas of Falcon Medicine*. Schlütersche, Hannover.

Avian pox

Etiology

The Family *Poxviridae* is subdivided into two subfamilies: *Chordopoxvirinae* (poxviruses of vertebrates, Figs 8.150–8.165) and *Entomopoxvirinae* (poxviruses of insects). The subfamily *Chordopoxvirinae* is subdivided into eight named genera.

- Family: *Poxviridae*
- Subfamily: *Chordopoxvirinae*
- Genera: orthopoxvirus, avipoxvirus, capripoxvirus, eporipoxvirus, suipoxvirus, molluscipoxvirus, yatapoxvirus, parapoxvirus.

Although the genus avipoxvirus (APV) is divided into 10 defined species (Box 8.2), many avian pox isolates are not clearly classified and their status within the genus is unclear or not known. It is, for example, not yet clear whether the turkeypox virus and eventually also the pigeonpox virus are only variants or serotypes of the fowlpox virus (Mayr, 1993), which is the prototype of the avian poxviruses.

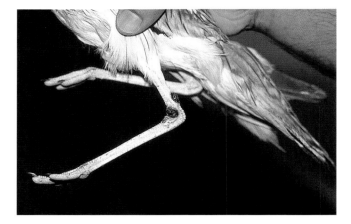

Fig. 8.150 A dried scab on the anterior aspect of the hock joint in a stone curlew produced by avian poxvirus.

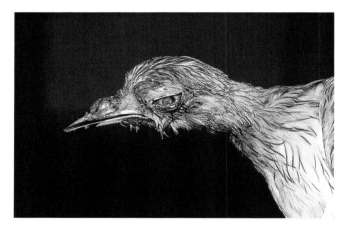

Fig. 8.151 Typical pox lesions on the cere of a stone curlew.

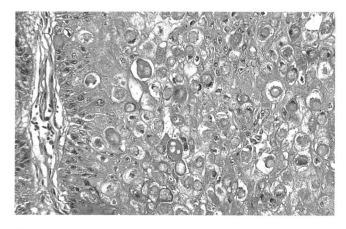

Fig. 8.152 Bollinger's intracytoplasmic bodies in a histological preparation of the stratum spinosum of the skin in a peregrine falcon (*Falco peregrinus*). The presence of Bollinger's bodies at microscopical examination is characteristic of avian pox infection. Hematoxylin and eosin stain. (Courtesy of Dr. J. Kinne).

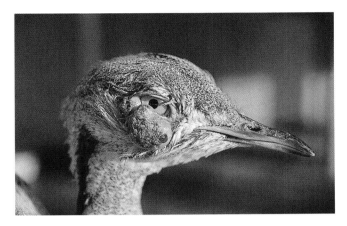

Fig. 8.153 A houbara bustard with a large scab on the lower eyelid. The lesions were produced by avian poxvirus. (Courtesy of Dr. J. Samour).

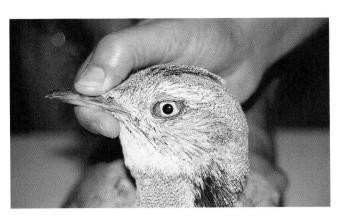

Fig. 8.154 Early atypical poxvirus lesions on the third eyelid of a houbara bustard. (Courtesy of Dr. J. Samour).

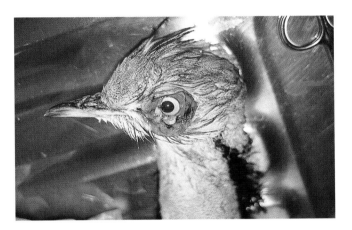

Fig. 8.155 Post-mortem examination of the same bird as in Fig. 8.154, 1 week after the onset of the disease. Note the 'cauliflower' appearance of the lesions on the third eyelid and conjunctiva. (Courtesy of Dr. J. Samour).

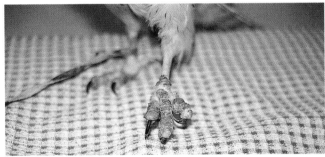

Fig. 8.156 Extensive dried pox scabbing on the feet of a common kestrel (*Falco tinnunculus*). Avian pox is seldom reported in this species. (Courtesy of Dr. J. Samour).

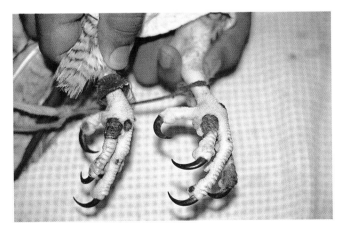

Fig. 8.157 Typical pox scabs on the feet of a peregrine falcon (*Falco peregrinus*). The most dangerous scabs on the feet are those developing around the last phalanx. Severe scabbing on this area may result in the loss of the last phalanx as a result of distal necrosis or self-mutilation. (Courtesy of Dr. J. Samour).

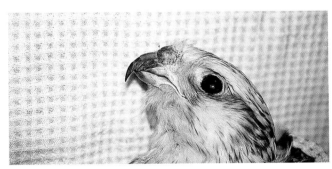

Fig. 8.158 Large pox lesion on the cere of a saker falcon (*Falco cherrug*). (Courtesy of Dr. J. Samour).

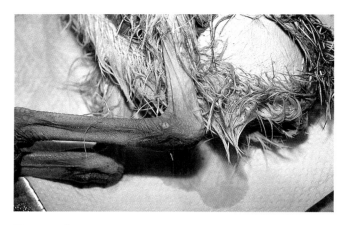

Fig. 8.159 Small pox lesions on the hock joint of an ostrich (*Struthio camelus*) chick.

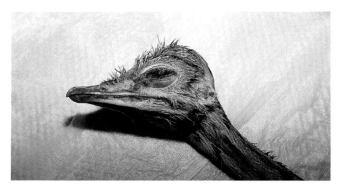

Fig. 8.160 Pox lesions on the lower eyelid and cere of the same ostrich chick as in Fig. 8.159.

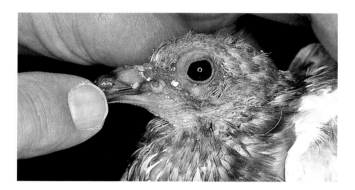

Fig. 8.161 Early proliferative pox lesions around the cere of an immature domestic pigeon.

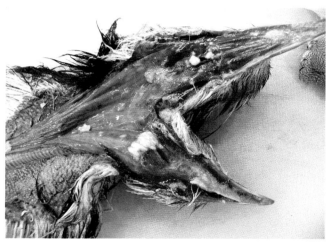

Fig. 8.162 Diphtheroid pharyngitis in a houbara bustard with wet pox.

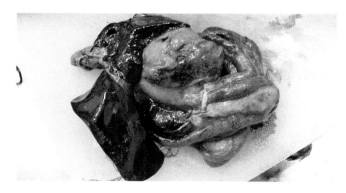

Fig. 8.163 Pancreatitis and hepatomegaly in a houbara bustard with systemic pox.

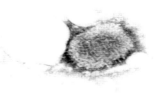

Fig. 8.164 Electron microscopic image of a houbara bustard pox virus. (Courtesy of Ms. R. Manvell).

The poxviruses are the largest and the most complex of all viruses. Avian poxviruses are only distantly related at the antigenic level to other poxvirus genera (Binns and Smith, 1992). Under natural conditions they produce a disease in avians only, and their virions are larger than those of other poxviruses. The virions are typically brick-shaped with dimensions of about 330×280×200 nm. The genome consists of a linear, nonsegmented, covalently closed, double-stranded DNA, which encodes for about 150–300 different proteins. Avian poxviruses are antigenically and immunologically distinguishable from each other to an extent, but various degrees of

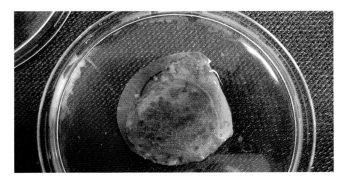

Fig. 8.165 A pock-lesion caused by the systemic poxvirus on the chorioallantoic membrane of an 11-day-old chicken embryo.

cross-relationships exist. The genetic profiles of fowlpox, pigeonpox and juncopox viruses appear similar but the genetic profiles of quailpox, canarypox and mynapox viruses are fairly different from that of fowlpox.

Poxviruses are resistant to ambient temperatures and may survive many years in dried scabs. Orthopoxviruses and most avipoxviruses are ether-resistant but parapoxvirus, capripoxviruses and leporipoxviruses are ether-sensitive (Fenner *et al.*, 1987). Fowlpox virus is inactivated by 1% caustic potash. It withstands 1% phenol and 1:1000 formalin for 9 d.

Distribution

Avian pox is a common viral disease of domestic and free-living birds that occurs worldwide. The disease has been reported in more than 70 species of free-living birds representing 20 families (Castro and Heuschele, 1992).

Clinical features

Avian pox is a relatively slowly spreading viral disease that is characterized by the development of three different forms. The cutaneous or dry pox form is characterized by the appearance of nodular scabs on various parts of unfeathered skin. The lesions vary in size and appearance. Removal of lesions leaves a hemorrhagic moist surface. When the crusts are dry they drop off, leaving scars. Mechanical transmission of the avian poxvirus by arthropods, especially mosquitoes, provides a mechanism for transfer of the virus between a variety of different bird species. The cutaneous form, which is most common, probably results from infection by biting arthropods or by direct contact with infected birds or their fomites. Poxviruses cannot pass intact skin and must enter the body through abrasions or cuts.

In the diphtheritic or wet pox form, the lesions occur on the mucous membranes of the mouth, nares, pharynx, larynx, esophagus or trachea. This form is probably due to aerosol infection. Tracheal lesions can cause difficulties in breathing and symptoms can resemble those of infectious laryngotracheitis in chickens and vitamin A deficiency. The diphtheric form often turns into a septicemic or systemic form, as recently reported in waterfowl (Anonymous, 2004) and houbara bustards (Oliveros *et al.*, 2007).

During the septicemic form of the disease only general symptoms such as somnolence, cyanosis and fatigue are observed in infected birds (canaries) without any cutaneous lesions. In these cases the virus may be found in the lungs. Areas of necrosis in the myocardium are also described (Mayr, 1993).

Pathological features

Pox lesions in the skin follow a typical developmental sequence. They commence as erythematous macules and become papular and then vesicular. The vesicles develop into pustules with a depressed center and raised, often erythematous edges. These lesions are the so-called pocks. The pustules rupture and a crust forms on the surface. Dry crusts fall off and leave residual scars. Histologically, pox lesions start as epidermal cytoplasmic swelling, vacuolation, ballooning degeneration and production of intraepithelial vesicles affecting the cells of the outer stratum spinosum. Further dermal lesions include edema, vascular dilatation and at a later date perivascular mononuclear and neutrophilic cell infiltration. Mucosal lesions are briefly vesicular and develop into ulcers rather than pustules.

During a recent outbreak of avian wet and systemic pox in houbara bustards and waterfowl, multiple discrete, pale yellow/cream-colored, raised necrotic lesions were irregularly distributed across the oropharyngeal mucosa, which can be easily confused with trichomonosis. Mucoid rhinitis and tracheitis were also observed. Additionally, the birds had a focal bronchopneumonia with miliary necroses, a swollen, hemorrhagic and enlarged pancreas and hepatomegaly.

Diagnosis

Although pox lesions are easy to recognize, laboratory tests should be carried out to confirm the diagnosis. Because of the large size and distinctive structure of poxvirus virions, electron microscopic examination of scab material or other lesions is the preferred method of laboratory diagnosis. Avian poxviruses produce pocks on the chorioallantoic membrane of embryonated hen's eggs, and viruses grow productively, but also abortively, in avian cell lines (Samour *et al.*, 1996). The virus multiplies in the cytoplasm of infected cells with the formation of inclusion bodies (Bollinger bodies) or elementary bodies (Borrel bodies), which can be stained with different staining methods. The specificity of the viral inclusions can be determined by fluorescent-antibody and immunoperoxidase methods.

Prevention and control

The vaccinia virus has become famous as a vector for expressing heterologous genes into its genome, using it for the production of recombinant vaccines. This is a relatively new approach with a potentially wide application in veterinary medicine. Avian poxviruses are not yet being produced by this new method.

For prophylactic immunization against avian pox, live attenuated vaccines are commercially available. Chickenpox, pigeonpox and turkeypox virus strains are used to protect many different avian species with varying degrees of success. Pigeonpox vaccines are less immunogenic and their immunity does not last very long. Pigeonpox vaccines and turkeypox vaccines are used in falcons with varying degrees of success. An attenuated falconpox vaccine has been successfully used in the Middle East for several years (Kaaden *et al.*, 1995, Wernery and Manvell, 2003). A canarypox vaccine has also been established for the vaccination of pet birds and an attenuated houbara bustard pox vaccine is currently being tested (Wernery *et al.*, 2007).

Vaccination procedures are often used in combination with insecticide spraying to reduce the number of arthropods. The live attenuated vaccines are administered either subcutaneously (wing web method) or intramuscularly (canarypox).

REFERENCES

Anonymous (2004) Fowlpox. *Veterinary Record* **155**: 728.

Binns MM, Smith GL (1992) *Recombinant Poxviruses*, p. 299. CRC Press, Boca Raton, FL.

Castro AE, Heuschele WP (1992) *Veterinary Diagnostic Virology*, pp. 60–62. Mosby Year Book, St Louis.

Fenner F, Bachmann PA, Gibbs EPJ *et al.* (1987) *Veterinary Virology*, pp. 403–404. Academic Press, New York.

Kaaden OR, Riddle KE, Wernery U (1995) Falcon pox in the Middle East. *Middle East Falcon Research Group Specialist Workshop*, Abu Dhabi.

Mayr A (1993) *Rolle/Mayr Medizinische Mikrobiologie, Infektions- und Seuchenlehre*, pp. 296–298. Ferdinand Enke, Stuttgart.

Kinne J, Oliveros S, Joseph S et al. (2007) Severe outbreak of pox in captive houbara bustards (*Chlamydotis undulata undulata*) in Morocco. *Proceedings of the European Association of Avian Veterinarians*, Zürich, pp. 78–85.

Samour J, Kaaden OR, Wernery U, Bailey TA (1996) An epornitic of avian pox in houbara bustards (*Chlamydotis undulata*). *Journal of Veterinary Medicine B* **43**: 287–292.

Wernery U, Manvell R (2003) Avian viral diseases in the United Arab Emirates (UAE). *Proceedings of the European Association of Avian Veterinarians*, Tenerife, pp. 72–78.

Wernery U, Basker VJ, Joseph S et al. (2007) An attenuated vaccine protects houbara bustards from systemic pox. *Proceedings of the European Association of Avian Veterinarians*, Zürich, pp. 86–93.

Herpesvirus infections

Etiology

More than 100 herpesviruses have been characterized, and they have been found in reptiles, insects and amphibia, as well as in virtually every species of bird and mammal that has been investigated (Figs 8.166–8.168). The classification of viruses within the family *Herpesviridae* is complex and not yet fully resolved. Three subfamilies have been created: *Alphaherpesvirinae*, *Betaherpesvirinae* and *Gammaherpesvirinae* (Table 8.12).

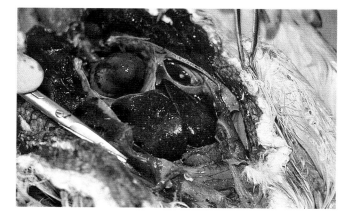

Fig. 8.166 Herpesvirus infection in a gyrfalcon (*Falco rusticolus*). Note the multiple miliary necrotic lesions in the liver. An attenuated herpesvirus vaccine for falcons has been produced by CVRL, Dubai.

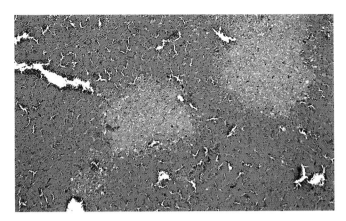

Fig. 8.167 Multiple miliary necrotic lesions in the liver of the same gyrfalcon as in Fig. 8.166. Hematoxylin and eosin stain. (Courtesy of Dr. J. Kinne).

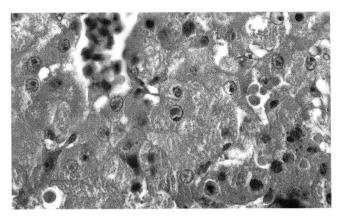

Fig. 8.168 Herpesvirus inclusion body (center) in a liver section of the same gyrfalcon as in Fig. 8.166. Hematoxylin and eosin stain. (Courtesy of Dr. J. Kinne.)

TABLE 8.12 Avian herpesvirus infections

Serogroup	Disease	Virus	Subfamily
1	Marek's disease of chickens	Gallid HV2	Gammaherpesvirinae
2	Duck plague – duck viral enteritis	Anatid HV1	Alphaherpesvirinae
3	Infectious laryngotracheitis of chicken	Gallid HV1	Alphaherpesvirinae
4	Pacheco's disease of psittacines	Psittacid HV1	NC
5	Pacheco's disease of psittacines	Psittacid HV2	NC
6	Pacheco's disease of psittacines	Psittacid HV3	NC
7	Inclusion body hepatitis of pigeons	Columbid HV1	NC
8	Inclusion body hepatitis of pigeons	Columbid HV2	NC
9	None? HV of cormorants	Phalacrocoracid HV1	NC
10	Inclusion body hepatitis of cranes	Gruid HV1	NC
11	Inclusion body hepatitis of storks	Ciconiid HV1	NC
–	Inclusion body hepatitis of falcons	Falconid HV1	NC
–	Inclusion body hepatitis of eagles	Accipitrid HV1	NC
–	Inclusion body hepatitis of owls	Strigid HV1	NC
–	Inclusion body hepatitis of quails	Perdicid HV1	NC
–	None? HV of turkeys	Meleagrid HV1	Gammaherpesvirinae
–	None? HV of penguins	Spheniscid HV1	NC

NC, not classified.

Classification into genera on the basis of the genome arrangement and serological reactivity has just begun. The characteristic property of all herpesviruses is their lifelong persistence in the organism. They survive from generation to generation by establishing latent infections from which virus is periodically reactivated and shed.

Many of the avian herpesviruses are not classified into subfamilies. Their characteristics, pathogenicity and host-specificity, and the antigenic relationship between them are poorly understood (Mayr, 1993). Avian herpesviruses are only pathogenic to birds and vary widely in their virulence.

The herpesvirus virion is enveloped by an icosa-hedral capsid consisting of 162 capsomers. Within the core of the nucleocapsid lies the genome, a single molecule of linear double-stranded DNA.

Herpesviruses are readily grown in cell cultures derived from their natural host species. Alphaherpes-virinae produce a rapid cytopathic effect whereas Betaherpesvirinae and Gammaherpesvirinae are slowly cytopathogenic in cell culture but produce similar intranuclear inclusion bodies. Intranuclear inclusion bodies are characteristic of herpesvirus infections and can usually be found in tissues from herpesvirus-infected birds and in appropriately fixed and stained cell cultures.

Free herpesviruses are very sensitive to all disinfectants with virucidal properties and a temperature of 55°C (131°F) inactivates herpesviruses within seconds (Fenner et al., 1987).

Avian herpesviruses of the first three groups (Table 8.12) cause diseases of hemorrhagic or neoplastic nature (gallid HV1 and 2, anatid HV1) and are of great importance to the commercial poultry industry. These three diseases are discussed separately from diseases causing hepatosplenitis. For completeness, herpesviruses that do not cause disease are mentioned at the end of the chapter.

Marek's disease

In 1907 the Hungarian physician–pathologist Marek described paralysis associated with a polyneuritis affecting some domestic fowl kept in his backyard. For about 50 years Marek's disease was considered to be part of a large group of diseases referred to as the avian leukosis complex. The specific herpesvirus etiology of Marek's disease, however, was established in 1967.

Marek's disease is a contagious, lymphoproliferative disease of chickens caused by Marek's disease virus (MDV) and is prevalent wherever the domestic poultry industry is found. It is occasionally detected in pheasants, turkeys, quails and francolins (Mayr, 1993). The virus is slowly cytopathic and remains highly cell-associated, so that cell-free infectious virus is virtually impossible to obtain. The virus is immunologically unique and is closely related to herpesvirus of turkeys (HVT). Virus strains of different virulence exist.

Marek's disease is a progressive disease with variable signs. Four overlapping syndromes are described (Fenner *et al.*, 1987):

- *Neurolymphomatosis* (classical Marek's disease) is an asymmetric paralysis of one or both legs or wings: one leg is held forward and the other backward
- *Acute Marek's disease* occurs in explosive outbreaks in which a large proportion of birds in a flock show depression followed after a few days by ataxia and paralysis; there are no localizing neurological signs
- *Ocular lymphomatosis*: the iris of one or both eyes is gray in color because of lymphoblastoid cell infiltration; there may be partial or total blindness
- *Cutaneous Marek's disease* is readily recognized after plucking, when round nodular lesions up to 1 cm in diameter are observed, particularly at feather follicles.

Marek's disease is characterized by a mononuclear infiltrate within peripheral nerves and other tissues and organs. In the vast majority of cases a diagnosis can be made if the celiac, cranial, intercostal, mesenteric, brachial, sciatic and greater splanchnic nerves are examined. In diseased birds, the nerves are up to three times their normal diameter.

Lymphomatous lesions, indistinguishable from those of avian leukosis, appear in the gonads, heart, proventriculus and lungs, but are seldom found in the bursa of Fabricius, which in cases of avian leukosis is the site of most tumor development.

Many apparently healthy birds are lifelong carriers and shedders of the virus. The virus is not transmitted *in ovo*.

Marek's disease and avian leukosis (Figs 8.169 and 8.170) are usually present in the same flock and both diseases may also occur even in the same bird. The two diseases were long confused but can be differentiated by clinical and pathological features (Table 8.13) as well as by specific viral and antibody tests.

Congenital infection does not occur and chicks are protected by maternal antibodies for the first few weeks of life. They then become infected by inhaling virus dust. Epizootics of Marek's disease usually involve adult birds 2–5 months old and there is a high mortality rate of about 80%.

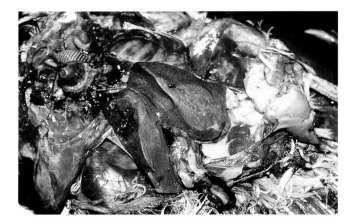

Fig. 8.169 An unusual record of lymphoid leukosis in a female houbara bustard. Note the grossly enlarged liver. Until recently it was believed that lymphoid leukosis was confined to domestic poultry. During post-mortem examinations affected chickens usually display diffuse or nodular lymphoid growths involving mainly the liver, spleen and bursa of Fabricius, but occasionally lesions can also be observed in the kidneys, gonads and mesenterium.

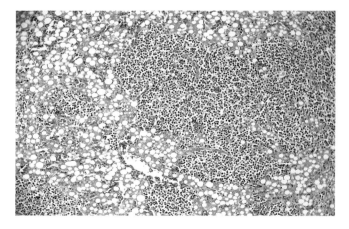

Fig. 8.170 Histological preparation of the liver from the same houbara bustard as in Fig. 8.169, showing diffuse lymphocytic infiltration. The neoplastic cell types are lymphoblasts and lymphocytes. (Courtesy of Dr. J. Kinne).

Disease parameter	Marek's disease	Avian leukosis
Etiology	Herpesvirus	Retrovirus
Target cells	T lymphocytes	Various hematopoietic cells
Age of onset of clinical signs	4 weeks	16 weeks
Gross lesions:		
Liver, spleen, kidney	+	+
Gonads, lung, heart	+	Rare
Nerve trunks	+	Rare
Iris	+	Rare
Skin	+	Rare
Bursa	Rare	+ (nodular)
Histology:		
Size of affected lymphoblasts	Varied	Uniform
Intranuclear inclusion bodies	Yes	No

TABLE 8.13 Marek's disease and avian leukosis: clinical and histological differentiation

The current vaccination programs for Marek's disease have effectively decreased its natural incidence but the eradication of Marek's disease from flocks of chickens is impossible. The vaccination prevents the development of the disease but not MDV infection. It is certain that there are no chicken flocks in the field that are completely free of MDV. Therefore, neither isolation of MDV nor antibody detection in such flocks is a valid criterion for a diagnosis (Castro and Heuschele, 1992).

Day-old chicks are vaccinated parenterally. Avirulent strains of MDV are used as vaccines, but the antigenically related turkey Gammaherpesvirus is the preferred vaccine strain, because it infects cells productively.

The production of chickens on the 'all-in, all-out' principle would improve the efficacy of vaccination as a control measure and a combination of three methods is used to control Marek's disease: vaccination; isolation and sanitation procedures; and breeding for resistant stock.

Duck plague (duck enteritis)

This Alphaherpesvirus infection was first recognized in 1923 in the Netherlands, where it was initially diagnosed as influenza. Subsequently it was recognized as a major disease in North America, China, India and Europe. In addition to domestic ducks, free-living ducks, geese, swans and other waterfowl are equally susceptible (Fenner *et al.*, 1987). Major epizootics occur worldwide and migratory waterfowl may contribute to outbreaks within and between continents.

Virus strains vary in their virulence, although only a single antigenic type has been recognized. The virus grows on the chorioallantoic membrane of embryonated duck eggs and in duck embryo fibroblasts but poorly or not at all in chicken cells. As with members of this family, there is evidence that this virus can establish a latent infection.

Clinical signs of duck enteritis include depression, a drop in egg production, ruffled and dull feathers, ocular and nasal discharge, anorexia, labored breathing, watery diarrhea, extreme thirst and ataxia followed by death. Morbidity and mortality vary from 5–100%. Lesions seen at necropsy are typical of vascular damage. Blood is present in the body cavities including gizzard and intestinal lumens. Petechial hemorrhages and focal necrosis are present in many tissues. Herpesvirus inclusions are most readily demonstrated in hepatocytes, intestinal epithelium and lymphoid tissues.

Ingestion of contaminated water is thought to be the major mode of transmission, although the virus may also be transmitted by contact.

Chicken or duck embryo attenuated strains are used for immunization in combination with hygiene measures.

Avian infectious laryngotracheitis

This viral disease of domestic fowl was first observed in the USA in 1926. It occurs among chickens worldwide and it is rarely recognized as a cause of disease in other avian species (Fig. 8.171). Strains of the virus vary considerably in virulence. Infectious laryngotracheitis is an acute, highly contagious respiratory disease of domestic fowl that is characterized by distressed breathing with loud gasping, coughing and expectoration of bloody mucus. However, signs and lesions can vary from peracute to mild. Birds of all ages are susceptible but disease is most common in those aged 4–18 months. In peracute infectious laryngotracheitis

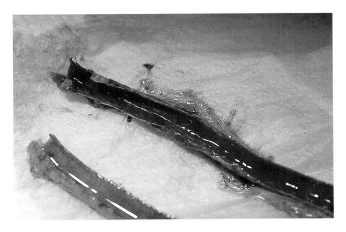

Fig. 8.171 Diffuse hemorrhage in the trachea of a peacock (*Pavo cristatus*) with infectious laryngotracheitis.

the mortality can exceed 50% of the flock, and in acute infectious laryngotracheitis the mortality is reduced to 10–15%, although the morbidity is as high as in the per-acute form. Chronic or mild infectious laryngotrache-itis forms are of low morbidity and mortality (2–5%). The disease is always accompanied by lowered egg production. In infectious laryngotracheitis there is a severe laryngotracheitis characterized by necrosis, hem-orrhage, ulceration and the formation of diphtheritic membranes. Bloody mucoid pseudomembranes (casts) along the trachea lead to death through asphyxiation. The extensive diphtheritic membrane formation and death from asphyxia prompted the designation 'fowl diphtheria'. Infections of infectious laryngotracheitis virus are transmitted by direct or indirect contact but are not transmitted within eggs from infected chickens. The virus is shed through conjunctival excretions, tracheal mucus and feces.

Clinical and necropsy findings are characteristic for infectious laryngotracheitis. Fluorescent antibody staining of smears and tissues and isolation of the virus from tracheal mucus, either by inoculation on the chorioallantoic membrane of embryonated eggs or cell cultures, confirm the diagnosis. Giemsa staining for infectious laryngotracheitis intranuclear inclusion bodies in virus-infected syncytial cells of the tracheal epithelium is another method of diagnosing infectious laryngotracheitis.

For control, site quarantine and hygiene measures should be the first approach. Immunization with attenuated live-virus vaccine via instillation of eyedrops, spray or drinking water protects birds against clinical disease but does not protect against infection with virulent virus or the development of a latent carrier status for either the virulent or the vaccine viruses. Despite a proper vaccination program it is to be expected that virulent virus persists in flocks and that some losses due to infectious laryngotracheitis, either alone or in combination with other pathogens, will continue.

Raptor herpesvirus causing hepatosplenitis

Three distinct herpesviruses causing hepatosplenitis have been isolated from raptors:

- Inclusion body hepatitis of falcons: falconid HV1 (FHV1)
- Inclusion body hepatitis of owls: strigid HV1 (SHV1)
- Inclusion body hepatitis of eagles: accipitrid HV1 (AHV1).

Raptor herpesviruses cause a fatal disease in birds of prey that is characterized by multifocal necrosis of the liver and spleen (Wheler, 1993). Clinical signs are nonspecific and range from sudden death to severe depression, anorexia, regurgitation and weakness fol-lowed by death (Remple, 1995). Very typical of the disease is the appearance of lime-green urates in the feces. Microscopic lesions in liver and spleen reveal necrotic foci without any inflammatory response.

The epizootiology of these viruses is unknown. It is believed that the infection in falcons might be caused by feeding on infected pigeons. Diagnosis of this disease is confirmed by typical necropsy findings and by virus isolation from liver and spleen in CEF followed by serological identification. A cytopathic effect develops after 3–4 d that is characterized by foci of round refractile cells in the monolayer with subsequent formation of syncytia.

Herpesvirus infections in falcons are a constant threat to falconry (Fig. 8.172). The majority of herpesvirus infections occur in gyrfalcons and hybrids of this species, and it seems that this species has a greater susceptibility to the virus than other falcon species.

Preliminary investigations have shown that falcons do not contract the infection orally but most probably ocularly and/or nasally (Wernery and Kinne, 2004).

No commercial vaccine is available but scientists at the Central Veterinary Research Laboratory, Dubai, have developed an attenuated herpesvirus vaccine the efficacy and safety of which have been proved in different vaccination trials (Remple, 1995; Wernery et al., 2001, 2003; Wernery and Manvell, 2003).

A lesser spotted eagle was subcutaneously infected with a pathogenic herpesvirus that had killed falcons. The eagle did not show any clinical signs nor did it seroconvert. It seems that eagles may be refractory to FHV1 (Wernery and Kinne, 2004).

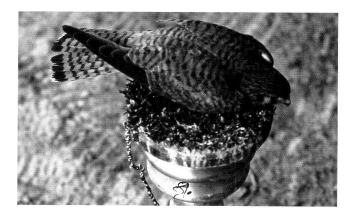

Fig. 8.172 A common kestrel (*Falco tinnunculus*) with FHV1 infection. The kestrel was very weak and anorectic and excreted green mutes due to the destruction of the liver parenchyma by the virus. The source of this infection is mainly pigeons that are fed to hunting falcons.

Nonraptor herpesvirus causing hepatosplenitis

Several distinct herpesviruses causing hepatosplenitis have been isolated from different avian species (Table 8.12). The predominant lesions are focal necrosis in liver and spleen, although other lesions are often seen. The clinical symptoms of nonraptor herpesvirus infection vary. In Pacheco's disease nasal discharge, anorexia, sneezing, coughing, weight loss and neurological signs are observed. Sudden death without any obvious signs may also occur. In pigeons the herpesvirus infection can cause conjunctivitis, rhinitis, weakness, ataxia and tremoring wings, but occasionally no clinical signs are observed prior to death (Wheler, 1993). Commercial vaccines are available against pigeon herpesvirus and psittacine herpesvirus infections.

Avian herpesvirus infections causing no disease

These viruses include herpesviruses of cormorants, turkeys and penguins. The phalacrocoracid HV1 was isolated in 1951 from a single nesting cormorant on Lake Victoria, Australia. It is unrelated serologically to any of the other avian herpesviruses. No clinical, gross or microscopic lesions have been associated with natural infections with turkey herpesvirus, which is serologically related to MDV. In two adult black-footed penguins that suffered from loss of condition and respiratory distress with microscopic lesions resembling infectious laryngotracheitis, inclusion bodies were detected in syncytial cells of the sinuses, trachea and bronchi (Ritchie, 1995). A herpesvirus has been recently isolated from the liver of a houbara bustard but when the virus was subcutaneously injected into the same species no sickness was detected.

REFERENCES

Castro AE, Heuschele WP (1992) *Veterinary Diagnostic Virology*, pp. 26–31. Mosby Year Book, St Louis.

Fenner F, Bachmann PA, Gibbs EPJ et al. (1987) *Veterinary Virology*, pp. 339–373. Academic Press, New York.

Mayr A (1993) *Rolle/Mayr Medizinische Mikrobiologie, Infektions- und Seuchenlehre*, pp. 277–282. Ferdinand Enke, Stuttgart.

Remple JD (1995) Falcon herpesvirus and immune consideration for the production of a vaccine. Presented at the Middle East Falcon Research Group Specialist Workshop, Abu Dhabi.

Ritchie BW (1995) *Avian Viruses, Function and Control*, pp. 171–222. Wingers Publishing, Lake Worth, FL.

Wernery U, Kinne J (2004) How do falcons contract a herpesvirus infection? Preliminary findings. *Falco* 23: 16–17.

Wernery U, Manvell R (2003) Avian viral diseases in the United Arab Emirates (UAE). *Proceedings of the European Association of Avian Veterinarians*, Tenerife, pp. 72–78.

Wernery U, Joseph S, Kinne J (2001) Attenuated herpesvirus may protect gyr hybrids from fatal inclusion body hepatitis. A preliminary report. *Journal of Veterinary Medicine* B 48: 727–732.

Wernery U, Sanchez AL, Joseph S, Wernery R (2003) Falconid response to the attenuated herpesvirus vaccine DuFaHe. *Proceedings of the European Association of Avian Veterinarians*, Tenerife, pp. 72–78.

Wheler CL (1993) Herpesvirus disease in raptors. A review of the literature. In: Redig PT, Cooper JE, Remple JD et al. (eds) *Raptor Biomedicine*, pp. 103–107. University of Minnesota Press, Minneapolis.

Other viral diseases

Other viral diseases are set out in Table 8.14.

Fungal diseases – aspergillosis

Patrick Redig

General description

This fungal disease of the respiratory system (Figs 8.173–8.199) is the most commonly occurring disease among wild birds held in captivity and is an occasional, but always possible, problem in companion birds. Rarely, it occurs among free-living birds that have become otherwise debilitated through injury or inanition. Although it may occur in individuals of virtually any species, there are clearly species predilections. Among North American raptors, goshawks (*Accipter gentilis*), gyrfalcons (*Falco rusticolus*), immature red-tailed hawks (*Buteo jamaicensis*), golden eagles (*Aquila chrysaetos*) and snowy owls (*Nyctea scandiacea*) are more likely to develop the disease. There is a tendency for raptors originating from arctic or subarctic climates to be more susceptible.

Several species of *Aspergillus* (*A. nigricans*, *A. terreus*, *A. nidulans*, *A. glaucus* and *A. flavus*) may be involved in any of the common forms of this disease. In most clinical presentations among captive companion and falconry birds, *A. fumigatus* is by far the most commonly encountered organism. However, the occurrence of these others can lead to some of the variations seen in pathogenesis and response to treatment. Additionally, available serological tests are highly specific for *A. fumigatus* and do not necessarily detect antibodies formed in response to one of the other species.

The route of infection is inhalation, thereby rendering the respiratory system the main target organ. Direct deposition of spores in the air on exposed vulnerable surfaces may also occur. Among parrots, and occasionally raptors, the upper respiratory system is often affected (sinuses, larynx and syrinx). The most serious disease occurs with infection of the lower respiratory system (lungs and airsacs). Spores in the lower respiratory system can migrate widely throughout

TABLE 8.14 Diseases caused by families of viruses that infect avian species

Family	Subfamily	Genus	Disease
Papovaviridae	Papillomavirinae	Papillomavirus	Benign skin tumors (papillomas), generalized infection, budgerigar fledgling disease and other psittacines, French molt
	Polyomavirinae	Polyomavirus	
Circoviridae		Circovirus	Psittacine beak and feather disease, chicken anemia virus (CAV)?
Adenoviridae		Adenovirus I (aviadenovirus)	12 serologically distinct adenoviruses – quail bronchitis; inclusion body hepatitis of chickens; turkey viral hepatitis; disease in pigeons, budgerigars, ducks, geese, guinea fowl; hemorrhagic enteritis of turkeys; splenomegaly of chickens; marble spleen disease of pheasants
		Adenovirus II Adenovirus III	Egg-drop syndrome virus (EDS-76)
Reoviridae (respiratory, enteric, orphan)		Orthoreovirus	11 serotypes – Psittaciformes, pheasants, pigeons, raptors, geese, ducks, chickens, turkeys, quails: arthritis, tenosynovitis, respiratory disease, hepatic necrosis, pericarditis, feather abnormalities, bursal atrophy, diarrhea
		Orbivirus	Transmitted by ticks but clinical signs of disease not described except in cockatiels and budgerigars: enlarged liver and spleen, diarrhea
		Rotavirus	Enteritis in pheasants, ducks, pigeons, lovebirds, guinea fowl and partridges
Retroviridae		Retrovirus (type C retroviruses)	Avian leukosis sarcoma (Rous sarcoma) virus (ALSV) – chicken, pheasant, partridge, quail, fowl, turkeys: lymphoid leukosis (most common), erythroblastosis, myeloblastosis, nephroblastomas, hemangiomas, osteopetrosis
		Reticuloendotheliosis virus	Ducks, geese, pheasants, quails, turkeys, chickens: stunting, anemia, runting, formation of neoplasias, immunodepression
Togaviridae		Alphaviruses and eastern equine encephalitis virus	Arthropod vectors (arboviruses), all avian species are considered susceptible: severe enteritis or neurological disease
		Western equine encephalitis virus	Pheasants, emus, chukars, English sparrows, chickens, turkeys: ruffled feathers, somnolence, depression, weakness, incoordination, torticollis, paresis and paralysis
		Species-specific encephalitic disease	Avian viral serositis in macaws and ring-necked parakeets: enlarged, yellowish liver, congested edematous lungs and fluid in abdomen
Coronaviridae		Coronavirus	Infectious bronchitis virus
Picornaviridae		Picornavirus	Cockatoo enteritis virus, avian encephalomyelitis virus, duck hepatitis virus, turkey hepatitis virus
Birnaviridae		Birnavirus	Infectious bursal disease virus in ostriches, ducks, pheasants, chickens, turkeys
Flaviviridae		Flavivirus	Turkey meningoencephalitis virus: causes paralysis and decreased egg production
Astroviridae		Astrovirus	Fatal hepatitis in ducks
Parvoviridae		Parvovirus	Derzsy's disease, hepatitis in goslings
Rhabdoviridae		Lyssavirus	No clinical changes associated with rabies have been seen in naturally infected birds

the celomic cavity by means of the ramifying and interconnecting airsac system that reaches into every part of the body. Consequently, lesions may be found in the pericardium, on the kidneys, in the mesenteries and among the vertebral bodies of the spinal column.

While the respiratory system provides an ideal environment in which the thermophylic, oxyphilic *Aspergillus* fungus can grow, the organism is an opportunist and may colonize superficial damaged epithelial and mucosal tissues. Mycotic keratitis and intraocular infections due to *A. fumigatus* have

been reported and I have on several occasions found *A. fumigatus* colonizing skin wounds covered by a bandage.

Factors implicated in causality

The disease occurs typically as a result of inhalation of the ubiquitously available spores. Multiple infections in a single facility imply common exposure rather than bird-to-bird spread. Infection can be overwhelming

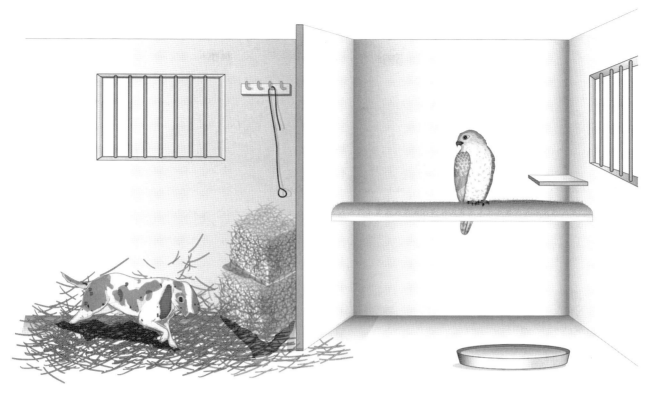

Fig. 8.173 In one actual case of acute aspergillosis, a gyrfalcon (*Falco rusticolus*) was housed in a chamber adjacent to another in which a pointer dog was kept, separated by a short divider. A few days after straw was spread on the floor for the dog, the falcon succumbed to acute aspergillosis.

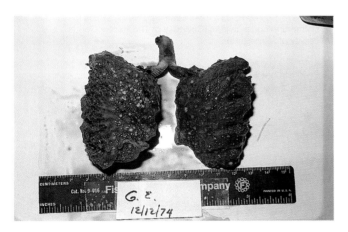

Fig. 8.174 This pair of lungs was removed from a juvenile golden eagle (*Aquila chrysaetos*) that was admitted in severe respiratory distress and showing signs of an encounter with a porcupine. It was speculated that, in attempting to subdue the quilled prey item, the eagle inhaled a large number of spores that were present in leaf litter or other ground detritus. (Courtesy of The Raptor Center, University of Minnesota).

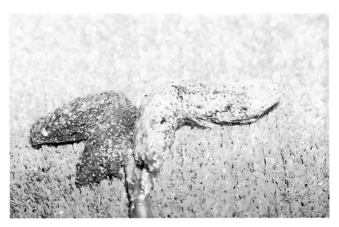

Fig. 8.175 These lungs were removed from a gyrfalcon that was housed in a mews adjacent to a hayfield. The hay had been cut, but was rained on before being baled. After a week, the hay was turned with a hay rake and baled. A few days later the gyrfalcon succumbed acutely to aspergillosis. The lungs were hard and studded with thousands of miliary granulomas from which *Aspergillus fumigatus* was cultured. (Courtesy of The Raptor Center, University of Minnesota).

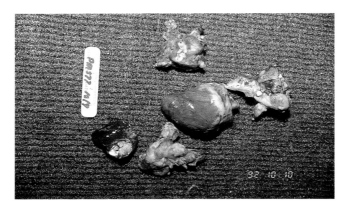

Fig. 8.176 Chronic aspergillosis lesions removed from the airsacs of a gyrfalcon and displayed as they appeared *in situ*. The large mass anterior to the heart was found in the interclavicular airsac, a site that is more often affected in gyrfalcons than in other raptors. (Courtesy of The Raptor Center, University of Minnesota).

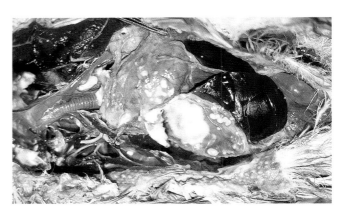

Fig. 8.177 Lesions of aspergillosis may occur in just about any location throughout the body, including the pericardial sac, as shown here. This lesion occurred in a gyrfalcon. (Courtesy of Dr. J. Samour).

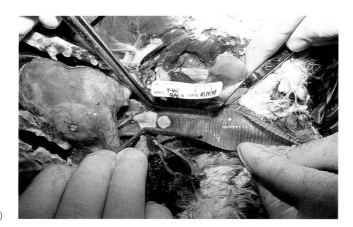

(a)

(b)

Fig. 8.178 Lesions may occur in the main lumen of the trachea (a) or, more commonly, in the narrowed air passages of the syrinx (b). Such cases exhibit rapid onset of progressively severe dyspnea but little debilitation. (Courtesy of The Raptor Center, University of Minnesota).

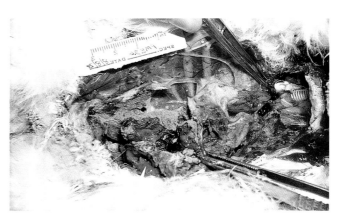

Fig. 8.179 Free-growing mold (*A. fumigatus*) in the airsacs of a juvenile red-tailed hawk (*Buteo jamaicensis*). This case may represent gross immunological failure. (Courtesy of The Raptor Center, University of Minnesota).

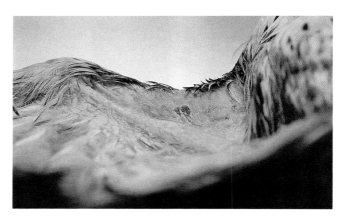

Fig. 8.180 Cutaneous aspergillosis affecting the propatagium of the wing of a goshawk (*Accipiter gentilis*). The exudative lesion was secondary to an extensive lacerating wound, which had previously been treated with a hydroactive vapor seal dressing. The lesion eventually responded to daily application of enilconazole (dilution 10:1). Marked improvement occurred after 7 d and complete resolution within 12 d. It was necessary to debride the lesion extensively before each application. (Courtesy of Mr. N. A. Forbes).

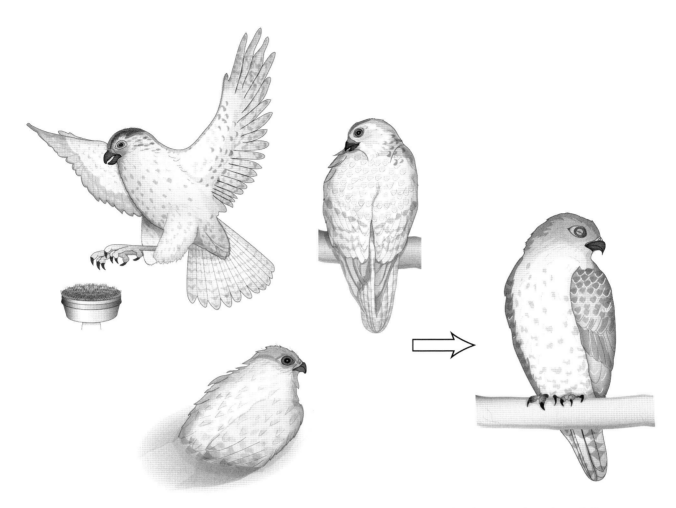

Fig. 8.181 Subtle changes in behavior such as a decrease in preening activity, failure to bathe or otherwise engage in routine activities are sometimes the first signs of the development of aspergillosis.

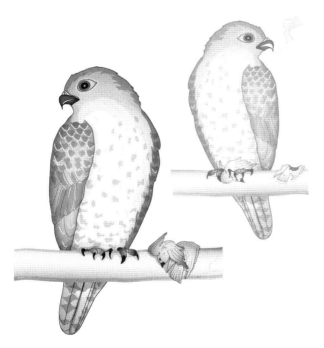

Fig. 8.182 Another early sign of developing aspergillosis is partial anorexia. Affected birds may vigorously grasp a food item, pluck a few feathers from it, then sit with it clenched in their talons. If offered small pieces of meat by hand, they will take them in their beak and fling them away. Such behavior may reflect gastrointestinal disease of other etiologies also.

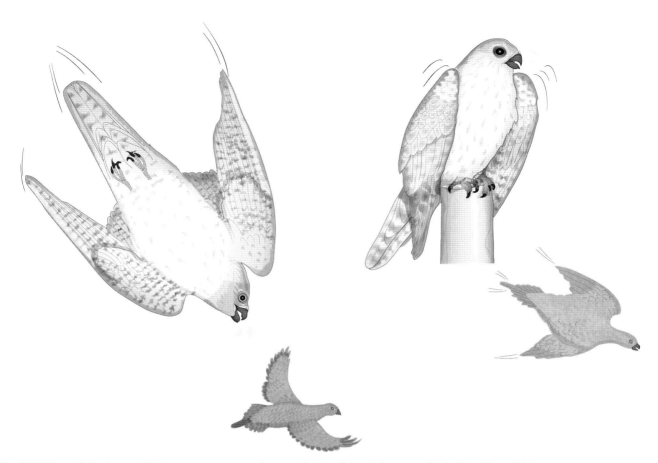

Fig. 8.183 Loss of stamina or ability to pursue quarry may be an early sign of developing aspergillosis. The affected bird may mount to a regular pitch and begin its stoop when quarry is flushed, but quickly give up the chase and alight on the ground or an elevated perch, clearly out of breath.

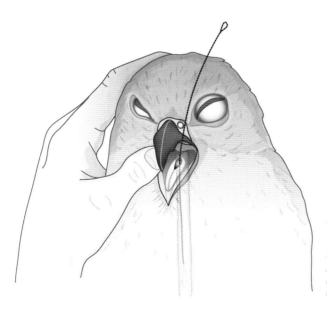

Fig. 8.184 Tracheal culturing is conducted by passing a small nasopharyngeal swab deep into the trachea. This may be done with or without anesthesia. The material recovered on the swab is transferred immediately to Sabouraud's dextrose agar and cultured at 37°C (98.6°F). Growth is typically apparent in 48 h, but may require up to a week. Alternatively saline, at the rate of 3 cc/kg, may be flushed into the trachea, recovered by aspiration and cultured in similar fashion. Cytological examination may also be conducted on recovered material.

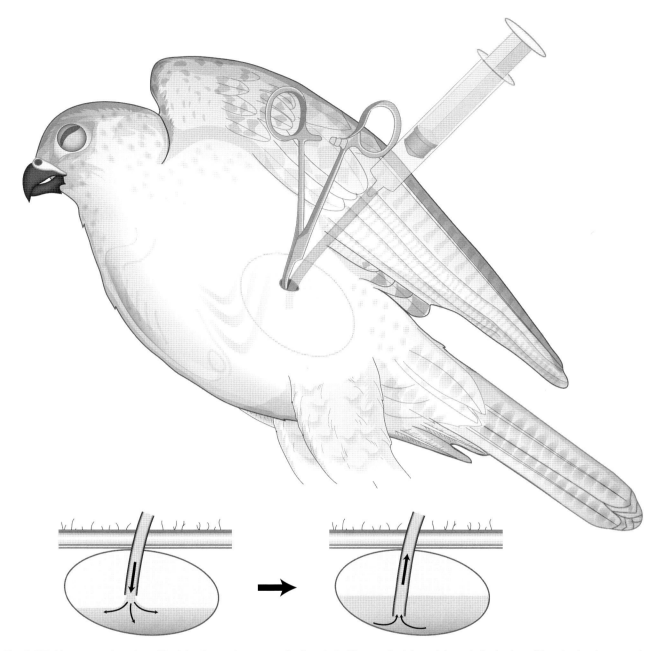

Fig. 8.185 Airsacs may be cultured by irrigation and recovery of saline: 3–5 ml/kg may be injected through the body wall into the last intercostal space and recovered by aspiration with a urinary catheter or similar device. The recovered material is cultured and/or examined cytologically.

and acute, as when a bird is exposed to a point source of heavy spore contamination, or it can occur as a result of low-level ambient exposure coupled with compromised immune function in the host. Some factors that have been implicated as causal in the development of aspergillosis include:

- Recent capture
- Change of ownership
- Poor ventilation

- Neonatal and geriatric conditions
- Birds subjected to multiple doses of corticosteroids, especially dexametasone
- Exposure to respiratory irritants such as cigarette smoke or ammonia
- Lead poisoning.

However, aspergillosis is also seen to occur, but with much lower frequency, in apparently well adjusted, trained birds for inapparent or undetermined reasons.

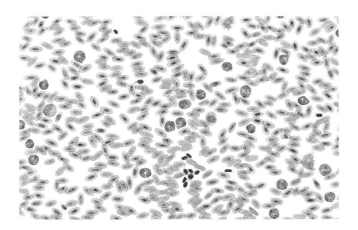

Fig. 8.186 Elevated white cell counts characterized by heterophilia and monocytosis are characteristically seen with aspergillosis. Heterophils often exhibit toxic signs such as degranulation. Gyrfalcons have a less brisk response in the white cell compartment compared with other raptors, often exhibiting total white cell counts in the range of 12–15000 cells/mm³ while other raptors exhibit counts of 30000–100000 cells/mm³. ×500. (Courtesy of Dr. B. Aird).

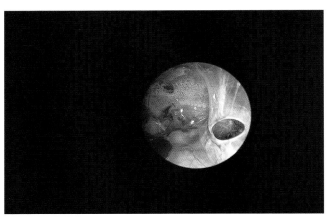

Fig. 8.187 Endoscopic view of normal anatomy as seen at the level of the last intercostal space in a red-tailed hawk (*Buteo jamaicensis*). Note the clear, nonvascularized, membranous nature of the airsac wall. The hole in the airsac was created with the endoscope to gain visual access to the anterior thoracic airsac). This effectively creates a communication between the two normally separate anterior and posterior portions of the avian respiratory system and should be avoided in a hunting falcon. (Courtesy of Dr. M. Taylor).

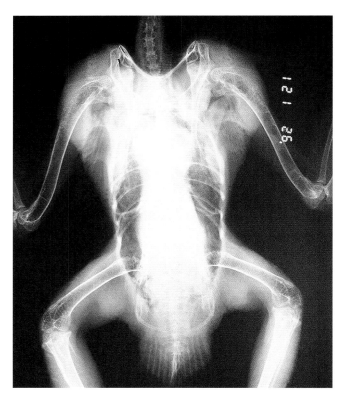

Fig. 8.188 Radiograph of a gyrfalcon with well developed chronic aspergillosis. There is evidence of radiographically dense material anterior and lateral to the heart and in the lower abdomen on either side of the gastrointestinal mass. (Courtesy of The Raptor Center, University of Minnesota).

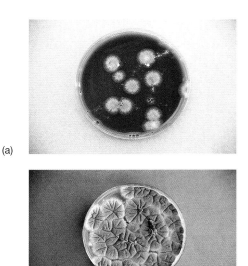

(a)

(b)

Fig. 8.189 Cultural appearance of *A. fumigatus* on (a) blood agar and (b) Sabouraud's dextrose agar after 4 d of incubation at 37°C (98.6°F). The colonies are a blue-green color with a powdery surface after 3–5 d of incubation. (Courtesy of Mr. C. Silvanose).

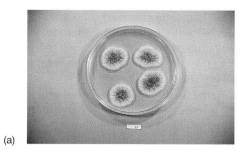

(a)

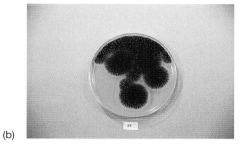

(b)

Fig. 8.190 Cultural appearance of (a) *A. flavus* and (b) *A. niger* in Sabouraud's dextrose agar after incubation for 3 d at 37°C (98.6°F). *A. flavus* is granular in appearance and green in color with a yellowish shade; *A. niger* is black-brown in color with a 'black pepper' effect due to the profuse proliferation of black spores. On rare occasions, these two may cause a disease similar to that caused by *A. fumigatus*. (Courtesy of Mr. C. Silvanose).

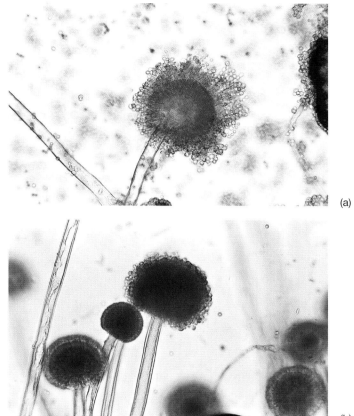

(a)

(b)

Fig. 8.192 Microscopic appearance of (a) *A. flavus* and (b) *A. niger* in lactophenol–aniline blue stain. In both cases, the vesicle head is covered by two rows of sterigmata crowned by abundant conidiospores. ×400. (Courtesy of Mr. C. Silvanose).

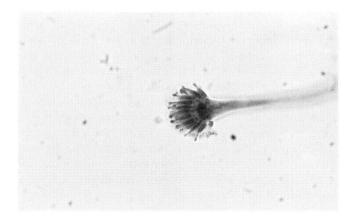

Fig. 8.191 Microscopic appearance of *A. fumigatus* in lactophenol–aniline blue stain showing a conidiophore, vesicle head and one row of close-packed sterigmata crowned by conidiospores. ×400. (Courtesy of Mr. C. Silvanose).

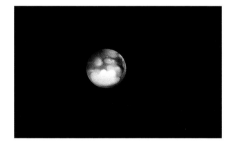

Fig. 8.193 Endoscopic view of a plaque on an airsac caused by *A. fumigatus*. In early stages of growth the surface of the plaque has a fuzzy, white appearance but it will later turn blue-green. Spores borne on these plaques can cause development of secondary sites of infection within the respiratory system. Finding such lesions yields a definitive diagnosis. (Courtesy of Dr. M. Taylor).

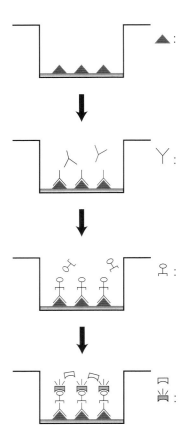

Fig. 8.194 The indirect ELISA is a useful aid for detecting antibodies to *A. fumigatus*. The enzyme-labeled second antibody (conjugate) detects antibodies bound to antigen, which is attached to a solid phase such as the well of a microtiter plate. A commercially available goat antiturkey conjugate adequately recognized immunoglobulins from *Buteo* species of raptors; however, specific conjugates must be made for use in falcons, accipiters, owls or psittacines. (Courtesy of The Raptor Center, University of Minnesota).

Respiratory system forms of the disease

Acute, chronic, and localized forms of the disease are recognized. An acute form occurs when a bird is exposed to a large number of spores from a point source. Hundreds of miliary foci of inflammation develop, mostly in the lung. This form is known as 'brooder pneumonia' when it affects neonatal poultry and it arises as a result of environmental contamination in the hatcher or brooder. In adult birds, it occurs from exposure to clouds of spores in poorly kept food or bedding, or other environmental sources. Moldy silage, leaf piles, bales of straw or shavings, and eucalyptus bark have been implicated as sources. In one situation, it was felt that the source of the spores was a mown field of alfalfa, adjacent to and downwind of the weathering yard in which a gyrfalcon was housed, which had been rained on before it was finally raked and baled. The affected falcon became ill within a few days of the harvesting activity and died acutely with lungs studded with miliary granulomas. Other similar occurrences have been encountered when breeding chambers of falcons were cleaned without the birds being removed from the chamber.

Other forms of aspergillosis are more chronic and include focal lesions in the lungs and airsacs, pericardium, trachea or syrinx, and occasionally the brain or anterior chamber of the eye. In all the chronic forms, host immunosuppression is implicated in the pathogenesis. Localized forms involve granuloma formation in the syrinx or the sinuses.

Aspergillosis in gyrfalcons is a serious problem for falconers. In the history of the use of the gyrfalcon for falconry, it is well established that this species is highly impacted by this disease. With the large-scale production of gyrfalcons and gyr hybrids through captive breeding and use in falconry, the numbers of encounters of birds with this disease have increased markedly in the last two decades. The disease most often becomes apparent at about the time the birds are becoming hard-penned, at approximately 10 weeks of age. Post-mortem examination reveals extensive involvement of the airsacs and lungs, suggesting that the process has been ongoing for several weeks. The premise of immunosuppression or exposure to large numbers of spores from a point source does not appear to apply, as affected birds are typically raised in carefully monitored and managed facilities, provided with an abundance of nutritional food and raised without overt evidence of stress. It is possible that the juvenile gyrfalcon is constitutionally unable to defend itself against ambient exposure to *Aspergillus* spores. Other possibilities may include immunosuppression by exposure to high ambient temperatures occurring in temperate zones (where the majority of propagation occurs) in late July and early August when the greatest number of cases are seen, or exposure to some immunosuppressive, clinically inapparent viral agent. A further possibility is that the captive-raised gyrfalcon is affected by unrecognized psychological stresses arising from a mismatch between the normal development it would experience in the wild in an Arctic environment and containment, relocation or other artifacts of rearing in captivity. Research into these issues is necessary to reduce the incidence of this disease in young gyrfalcons.

Diagnosis and management

The management and diagnosis of aspergillosis is challenging because of:

● The variability and subtleness of the signs of the disease at onset
● The advanced state of the disease when clearly recognizable signs become apparent.

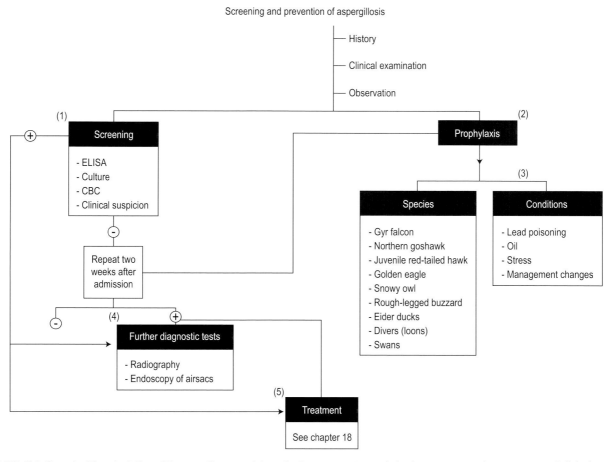

Fig. 8.195 This flow chart is a depiction of the overall approach to patient assessment, prophylactic treatment and management of clinical cases of aspergillosis. Prophylaxis and early detection of subclinical cases are essential for favorable outcomes. Once overt clinical signs of weight loss, dyspnea and general debilitation are present, the prognosis is poor. (Modified with permission from Redig, 1996).

Immunologically suppressed birds may elicit a poor antibody response, rendering antibody-based diagnostic tests less useful

- The role played by immunosuppression in the pathogenesis: the host often puts up little defense and gives little help in the treatment, and in many instances the apparent causes of the immunosuppression appear to be very small and relatively innocuous events, such as a change of management of the bird.

Clinical appearance

The disease is typically seated in the respiratory system, although lesions may occur in other parts of the body. However, the early clinical signs of the chronic forms do not necessarily, and most often do not, result in expression of respiratory signs. Rather the early signs are subtle and nonspecific, such as:

- Change in behavior, especially a reduction in overall or expected levels of activity
- Change in voice
- Food flicking or anorexia
- Slight loss of stamina or willingness to chase quarry
- At the point at which respiratory signs or weight loss are apparent, the disease is extensively developed.

Diagnosis

In general

The battery of tools to be used in establishing a diagnosis include:

- Clinical suspicion (signs, species, sex, time of year, present and recent circumstances)
- Antibody detection with a high level sensitivity test such as an ELISA[a] or an antigen capture test[b]
- Tracheal culture and/or washes

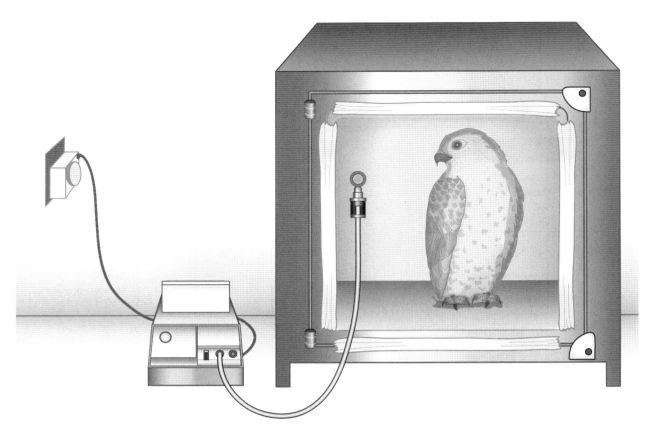

Fig. 8.196 Illustration of a typical nebulization set-up. The chamber should be just large enough to comfortably contain the bird during periods of nebulization in order to eliminate material loss from dead space effects. A wall timer is useful for controlling the nebulizer cycle.

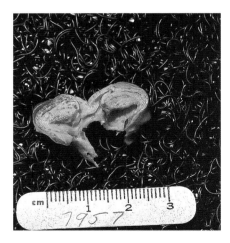

Fig. 8.197 An aspergillosis granuloma recovered from the syrinx of a golden eagle. Where the lesion is localized, surgical removal through a tracheostomy may yield immediate relief of dyspnea. Presence of the granuloma was detected endoscopically. (Courtesy of The Raptor Center, University of Minnesota).

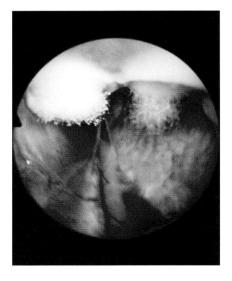

Fig. 8.198 Early aspergillosis granulomas in the thoracic airsac wall of a peregrine falcon (*Falco peregrinus*). Diagnosis of early aspergillosis lesions is commonly carried out through endoscopy examination, as such lesions are not visible on conventional survey radiographs. (Courtesy of Dr. J. Samour).

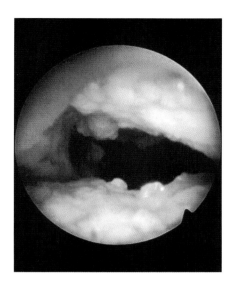

Fig. 8.199 Chronic aspergillosis in a hybrid gyr/saker falcon (*Falco rusticolus–Falco cherrug*). The infection was characterized by the formation of large caseous plaques occupying most of the thoracic airsac space. Infections such as this are difficult to treat, since it is very often necessary to debride and remove the masses surgically after specific antifungal treatment. In many cases, surgery proves impossible because of the close association of such masses with the airsac wall and other organs such as the lungs. (Courtesy of Dr. J. Samour).

- Airsac washes
- Hematology analysis characterized by heterophilic leukocytosis, toxic heterophils and varying degrees of monocytosis. Protein electrophoresis may exhibit a characteristic increase in β and γ globulins that is strongly associated with aspergillosis or other granulomatous disease
- Endoscopy – this is the single most useful tool in establishing a diagnosis of aspergillosis in clinically suspected cases
- Radiology is generally of limited value as a diagnostic tool during stages of development at which treatment is a reasonable possibility, but may yield useful information.

Organisms recovered from swabs or washes are cultured on Sabouraud's dextrose agar. Identity can be readily confirmed from wet mounts prepared with lactophenol–aniline blue stain or other methylene-blue-based stain.

Specifically

Clinical suspicion coupled with positive tracheal culture (taken from deep within the trachea with a nasopharyngeal swab[c]) and an elevated white cell count (25000–100000 cells/mm³+) is taken as circumstantial evidence of occurrence of aspergillosis and the basis upon which to commence treatment. Endoscopy is invaluable as it allows examination of the trachea and the airsacs for lesions referable to aspergillosis. Whereas well developed granulomas or lesions that are

sprouting fungal hyphae leave little doubt, in many early cases one sees vascularized airsacs only. These should be regarded as strong evidence of an inflammatory response by the airsacs.

High sensitivity serological tests specifically for aspergillosis have limited global availability. However, where used they have been very useful for assessing a patient's status with regard to aspergillosis. The indirect ELISA measures the presence of antibody. A positive result indicates active infection, long-term exposure or an elevated antibody level resulting from a previous infection. A negative result indicates no antibodies, either as a result of lack of disease or inability to produce them. As used at The Raptor Center, University of Minnesota, three categories of response are used:

- *Below cut-off*, which implies no detectable antibodies, and is a category in which false negatives have been encountered only in circumstances where the patient, in addition to having aspergillosis, had another debilitating condition such as tuberculosis or lead poisoning
- *Mid-range* (gray zone), which implies exposure and low-level antibody production due to either 1) ongoing exposure with no clinical disease, 2) low-level or early stage disease development, or 3) poor immune response to severe disease
- *High-range*, which is associated with vigorous immune response and may bode well for recovery. An affected bird often yields a mid-range response early in the disease that increases into the high range during the second to fourth week of treatment. Failure to show increasing optical density readings during treatment may imply lack of antibody response and be indicative of a guarded prognosis.

The ELISA is a good screening test and, when used in conjunction with other parameters, aids the clinician in establishing a diagnosis. Its availability is presently limited and it is species- or group-specific, depending on immunoprotein recognition by antibodies produced in goats or rabbits. As such, a specific custom-made conjugate-labeled antibody is needed specifically each for psittacines, falcons and accipiters, while immunoglobulins of other species of diurnal raptor cross-react well with a commercially available goat or rabbit anti-turkey conjugate. A conjugate antibody has not been made for owls and the other conjugates do not have sufficient cross-reactivity with owl serum to render them effective in antibody detection with this test.

The need for species-specific conjugates may be circumvented by the development of antigen capture tests, which detect molecular elements of the *Aspergillus* organism itself that may be present in the blood stream. While the extent to which antigen may be present from non-disease-causing exposure as compared with active infection is not yet clear, these tests nevertheless represent another potentially valuable means of assessing a patient's status with regard to this disease. There is one polymerase chain reaction (PCR)-based test available in the USA, which is useful when used on aspirates/washes taken from the trachea or airsacs or on serum (Dalhausen, personal communication).

Treatment

The treatment options for aspergillosis are limited. Drugs used have included 5-fluorocytosine (5FC),[d] itraconazole,[e] fluconazole,[f] clotrimazole,[g] enilconazole,[h] voriconazole,[i] terbinafine HCl[j] and amphotericin B.[k] The last two are fungicidal. Amphotericin B is the gold standard against which other antifungal agents are compared *in vitro*. Amphotericin B, along with 5FC, itraconazole and clotrimazole, and particularly the last two in combination, is efficacious in treating known cases of aspergillosis; fluconazole appears to be ineffective. Enilconazole and ketoconazole have also been used with a modicum of success by individual clinicians. Itraconazole is the most widely used antifungal agent at present, but work done in 2004 with voriconazole indicates that this recently available compound may have greater clinical utility than other forms of treatment (Di Somma *et al.*, 2004). This drug was found to be effective in treating clinical cases of aspergillosis in falcons when dosed at 12.5 mg/kg, although further work has suggested that multiple doses may need to be given to maintain inhibitory concentrations throughout the day (Scope *et al.*, 2005). Much more research is needed, first to establish a means of assessing the antifungal sensitivity of recovered strains of *Aspergillus* spp. at the beginning and during courses of clinical treatment, and second to assess the efficacy of different drugs and treatment protocols in a laboratory-controlled infection model.

A representative treatment regime for aspergillosis consists of amphotericin B administered intratracheally (1.5 mg/kg in a 1 cc volume of sterile water, bid.) and intravenously (1 mg/kg given by bolus injections every 8–12 h) for the first 3–4 d. Itraconazole is administered at 5–15 mg/kg b.i.d for the first five days, then once daily thereafter for the duration of treatment, usually 3–4 months. Amphotericin B is replaced by nebulized clotrimazole (5–10% solution in polyethylene glycol with 5% DMSO, obtained from a compounding pharmacy). Nebulization schedules vary widely, however, we typically provide two 1 h sessions per day separated by a 12 h interval. Most recently, voriconazole has come to the fore as a clearly improved agent for treating aspergillosis (Di Somma *et al* 2004, Scope 2005). Dosed at 12.5 mg/kg PO, b.i.d. for 4 days, followed by s.i.d, the drug is best absorbed with no or little food in the gastrointestinal

tract. A liquid form is also available that can be concurrently nebulized. Because of the varying sensitivities of various strains of A. *fumigatus* to these agents, and uncertainties regarding pharmacokinetics in various species, combination therapies are recommended. Nebulization therapy should be undertaken in the realization that it will deliver material only to those areas of the respiratory system where there is airflow, and that its utility may be therefore limited.

Aggressive treatment of severe aspergillosis may be undertaken by a method of endoscopic laser ablation of granulomas and direct installation of antifungal agents into accessible granulomas. Methods for more expansive access to the thoracic cavity and respiratory system for such ablative procedures have been described (Hernandez-Divers, 2002).

From a prognostic and treatment perspective, aspergillosis can be categorized into four levels:

- *Class I*: A patient in this category may express vague signs of illness such as reduction in appetite, slight weight loss, decreased activity such as not flapping its wings as vigorously as usual when bating, or loss of stamina. In the absence of endoscopic confirmation, or where endoscopic results are inconclusive, if two other indicators are positive (e.g. elevated white cell count and vague signs of illness, especially in a high incidence species), initiate treatment with a 2–3 week course of itraconazole (5–10 mg/kg twice daily for 5 d, followed by once daily at the same dose) or voriconazole (12.5 mg/kg once or twice daily). Some individual birds may exhibit anorexia and vomiting after a few days at the higher dosages of itraconazole. Monitor white cell picture, tracheal culture and patient condition. Typically, the prognosis is excellent
- *Class II*: A patient in this category has discrete clinical signs referable to aspergillosis (respiratory difficulty), positive tracheal culture and endoscopic confirmation of lesions or at least vascularized airsacs. Full-scale treatment should be undertaken as described above. Prognosis is fair to good
- *Class III*: In this category the patient will present with severe clinical signs (dyspnea, anorexia, vomiting, notable weight loss), radiographically visible lesions, endoscopically visible lesions and, often, a low antibody response. In this case, aggressive treatment is aided by surgical debulking of masses in airsacs through an exploratory surgery. Prognosis is poor in goshawks and red-tailed hawks and guarded in large falcons
- *Class IV*: This category is syringeal aspergillosis as detected by endoscopic evaluation of the trachea. In some, but not all cases the lesion can be removed through an incision in the lower trachea, proximal to the syrinx. An airsac cannula is very helpful for administering anesthesia during such surgery. Following removal, the patient is treated with

intratracheal amphotericin B for 5 d and itraconazole or voriconazole by mouth for about 3 weeks. The patient parameters of white cell count and distribution and its antibody status (ELISA) are monitored. If there is no further involvement of the respiratory system, the prognosis is excellent.

Depending on the site of the lesions and the severity of the disease, there are many aspects to treatment. The total treatment program typically extends over 3 months but if recovery is likely an initial favorable response to treatment is seen within 7–10 d.

Prevention and prophylaxis

Clearly aspergillosis is to be prevented. Protection from exposure to aerosols that may contain spores is paramount. Prophylactic treatment with 5FC or itraconazole/voriconazole is recommended for newly captured or newly admitted birds of species that have an established track record of susceptibility, especially gyrfalcons. The recommended protocol is to administer an antifungal (itraconazole or voriconazole) for 3 weeks. Gyrfalcons will tolerate itraconazole only up to a dose of 8 mg/kg. The course of treatment may be extended if clinical indications warrant. This approach should extend also to individuals of highly susceptible species that are undergoing a change of management (e.g. transfer to new owner or new enclosure), regardless of age or other circumstance. Treatment for 1 week prior to the move and 2 weeks after is recommended. Domestically reared gyrfalcons and gyr hybrids should be provided with this prophylactic regimen from a period beginning at 45 d of age through 75–90 d of age. If extreme heat conditions prevail during the months of August and September in any given locale, young gyrfalcons should be provided with extended prophylactic treatment during this time. The tendency for these prophylactic regimens to induce drug-resistant strains of Aspergillus is unknown.

Aspergillosis is the most challenging medical problem affecting avian species. There are many tools available for diagnosis and treatment but no formulaic protocols that will guarantee success. Each case must be evaluated on its own merits and it is up to the clinician to select the proper tools and apply them effectively in order to achieve success. Prevention and prophylaxis are vital.

REFERENCES

Di Somma, A., Bailey, T. A., Silvanose, C., Garcia-Martinez, C. 2004 The use of voriconazole for the treatment of aspergillosis in falcons. Proceedings of SIVEA, Rome, Italy.

Hernandez-Divers S (2002) Endosurgical debridement and diode laser ablation of lung and air sac granulomas in psittacine birds. Journal of Avian Medicine and Surgery 16: 138–145.

Redig PT (1996) Avian emergencies. In: Beynon PH, Forbes NA, Harcourt-Brown NH (eds) Manual of Raptors, Pigeons and Waterfowl, pp. 30–41. British Small Animal Veterinary Association, Cheltenham.

Scope A, et al. (2005) Pharmacokinetics and pharmacodynamics of the new antifungal agent voriconazole in birds. Proceedings of the Association of Avian Veterinarians, Arles, pp. 217–221.

Product reference list

[a]Aspergillus ELISA testing. The Raptor Center, 1920 Fitch Avenue, St. Paul, MN 55108, USA.

[b]Antigen Capture testing for Aspergillus sp. University of Miami, School of Medicine, PO Box 016960 (R-46), Miami, FL 33101, USA.

[c]Nasopharyngeal calcium alginate tipped applicators. Hardwood Products, Guilford, ME 04443–0149, USA.

[d]Ancobon®. Hoffman-LaRoche Laboratories, Nutley, NJ 17110, USA.

[e]Sporanox®. Janssen Pharmaceutica, Piscataway, NJ 08854, USA.

[f]Diflucan®. Pfizer Inc., New York, NY 10017, USA.

[g]Lotrimin®. Schering-Plough Health Care Products Inc., Memphis, TN 38151, USA (1% clotrimazole product – obtain 5% clotrimazole in propylene glycol with 5% DMSO from compounding pharmacy).

[h]Imaverol®. Janssen Pharmaceutica, Piscataway, NJ 08854, USA.

[i]Vfend®. Pfizer Island Pharmaceuticals, Ringaskiddy, Ireland.

[j]Lamasil®. Novartis International AG, Basel, Switzerland.

[k]Fungizone®. ER Squibb & Sons, Princeton, NJ, USA.

FURTHER READING

Aguilar RF, Redig PT (1995) Diagnosis and treatment of avian aspergillosis. In: Bonagura JD (ed.) Current Veterinary Therapy XI, pp. 1294–1299. WB Saunders, Philadelphia.

Arca-Ruibal, B, U Wernery, R Zachariah, TA Bailey, A Di Somma, C Silvanose, P McKinney. Assessment of a commercial sandwich ELISA in the diagnosis of aspergillosis in falcons. Vet. Rec. 158: 442–444. 2006

Bauck L (1994) Mycoses. In: Ritchie BW, Harrison GJ, Harrison LR (eds) Avian Medicine: Principles and Application, pp. 997–1006. Wingers Publishing, Lake Worth, FL.

Bennett RA (1999) Approach to the thoracic cavity of birds. Exotic DVM 1(3): 55–58.

Espinel-Ingroff A (1998) In vitro activity of the new triazole voriconazole (UK-109,496) against opportunistic filamentous dimorphic fungi and common and emerging yeast pathogens. Journal of Clinical Microbiology 36: 198–202.

Jones, M, Orosz SE (2000) The diagnosis of aspergillosis in birds. Seminars in Avian and Exotic Pet Medicine 9: 52–58.

Joseph, V (2000) Aspergillosis in raptors. Seminars in Avian and Exotic Pet Medicine 9: 66–74.

Langhofer B (2004) Emerging antifungals and the use of voriconazole with amphotericin to treat Aspergillus. Proceedings of the Association of Avian Veterinarians, New Orleans, pp. 21–24.

Orosz SE (2000) Overview of aspergillosis: pathogenesis and treatment options. Seminars in Avian and Exotic Pet Medicine 9(2): 59–65.

Orosz SE, Frazier DL (1995) Antifungal agents: a review of their pharmacology and therapeutic indications. Journal of Avian Medicine and Surgery 9: 8–18.

Pacetti SA (2003) Caspofungin acetate for treatment of invasive fungal infections. Annals of Pharmacotherapy 37: 90–98.

Redig PT, Post GS, Concannon TM (1986) Development of an ELISA test for the diagnosis of aspergillosis in avian species. Proceedings of the Association of Avian Veterinarians, Miami, pp. 165–178.

Silvanose CD, TA Bailey, and A Di Somma. Susceptibility of fungi isolated from the respiratory tract of falcons to amphotericin B, itraconazole, and voriconazole. Vet. Rec. 159:282-284. 2006.

Yamakami YA, Hashimoto IT, Nasu M (1996) PCR detection of DNA specific for Aspergillus species in serum of patients with invasive aspergillosis. Journal of Clinical Microbiology 34: 2464–2468.

Fungal diseases – candidiasis

Christudas Silvanose

Candidiasis (Figs 8.200–8.206) is one of the most common fungal diseases in birds. It is usually confined to the upper alimentary tract but can also invade the nasal cavity and sinuses. This disease is caused by fungi of the genus *Candida*. *Candida albicans* is the most common pathogenic species isolated from clinical specimens. *C. krusei* and *C. tropicalis* have also been reported from clinical cases. Candidiasis has been reported in several avian species including falcons, pigeons, parrots, pheasants, chickens and turkeys. This disease is usually associated with malnutrition, inhibition of normal bacterial flora caused by prolonged use of broad-spectrum antibiotics, and poor husbandry.

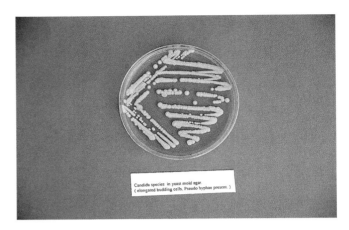

Fig. 8.202 *C. krusei* culture on yeast and mold agar. The colonies of *C. krusei* are also white, but larger than those of *C. albicans*.

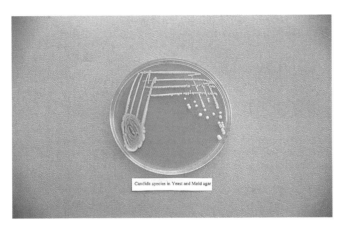

Fig. 8.200 *Candida albicans* on yeast and mold agar. The colonies are white in color and 2–3 mm in size after 48 h of incubation at 37°C (98.6°F).

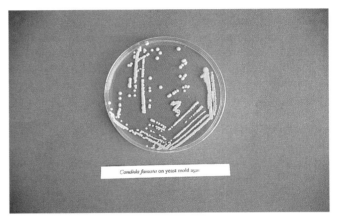

Fig. 8.203 *C. famata* on yeast and mold agar. The cultural appearance of *C. famata* and *C. albicans* is similar and they can only be differentiated by biochemical and germ tube tests.

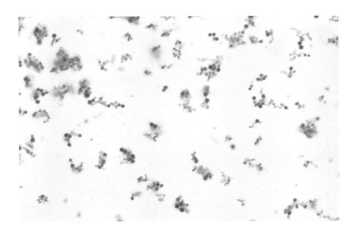

Fig. 8.201 Microscopic appearance of *C. albicans* in methylene blue stain, illustrating budding yeast cells. ×200.

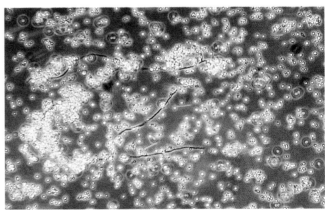

Fig. 8.204 Microscopic appearance of *C. tropicalis*. Note the chlamydospore with the pseudohyphae. ×400.

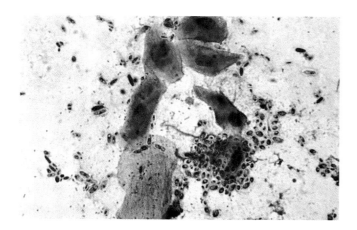

Fig. 8.205 Oropharyngeal smear from a houbara bustard (*Chlamydotis undulata*) with candidiasis. The smear shows exfoliated epithelial cells and oval-elongated *C. albicans*. ×1000.

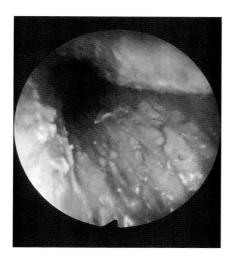

Fig. 8.206 Early *C. albicans* infection in a saker falcon (*Falco cherrug*) presented with a history of regurgitation and reduced appetite. On endoscopy examination the mucosal membrane of affected areas had a typical 'Turkish towel' appearance. Courtesy of Dr. J. Samour.

Clinical signs and lesions

Clinical signs are nonspecific and varied. Infected fowl chicks show inadequate and retarded growth, are apathetic and their feathers are ruffled. In young turkeys, the symptoms include listlessness and diminished appetite, but especially noticeable is the way in which the head drops backwards between the shoulder blades and the sunken breast. The eyes sink deep into their sockets and the head of the bird has a disheveled appearance. *Candida* spp. infection in birds is usually manifested by the presence of lesions in the oropharynx and crop, characterized by white, circular ulcers with raised surface scabs causing thickening of the mucosa. In most cases, pseudomembrane and inflammatory changes, such as exfoliation of epithelial cells, are common. In certain chronic cases,

beak rot, tongue rot and enteritis are also observed. If the infection invades the intestinal mucosa, a malabsorption syndrome may develop. Affected falcons commonly showed amorphous diphtheritic membranes, from white-gray to gray-green in color, affecting the crop (Fig. 8.206). On endoscopy examination the mucosal membrane of affected areas has a typical 'Turkish towel' appearance. On external examination, through palpation, the affected areas appeared thicker to the touch (Samour and Naldo, 2002). Clinical signs include reduced appetite, anorexia, regurgitation, shredding and flicking of the food and subsequent progressive weight loss.

Laboratory diagnosis

Direct phase-contrast microscopic examination of sample suspension in normal saline is a quick and easy method of detecting the presence of *Candida* spp. The sample can also be examined by direct light microscopy with the help of lactophenol–aniline blue stain. *C. albicans* is an oval, budding yeast that produces pseudohyphae, both in tissue and exudates and in broth culture. Eosin and methylene blue stain (Neat stain, Rapi-Diff®) is also used for the detection of exfoliated epithelial cells and *Candida* spp. in the smear. In Gram-stained smears, *Candida* spp. appear as a Gram-positive, oval, budding yeast measuring $2–3 \times 4–6\,\mu m$, and elongated budding cells resembling hyphae called pseudohyphae. Culture or serological studies are necessary for the species identification.

Culture studies are the most widely used diagnostic method for detecting *Candida* spp. These fungi grow well in yeast mold agar (Oxoid, UK) after 48–72 h of incubation at 37°C (98.6°F). Media used for the primary isolation and identification of *Candida* spp. include *Candida* BCG agar, corn meal peptone yeast agar and Sabouraud's agar; corn meal agar, LIU Newton agar, Rice infusion Oxgall Tween 80 agar and Rice Tween agar are used to detect the production of chlamydospores of *C. albicans*. BIGGY agar (Nickerson medium) is used for the selective isolation, differentiation and presumptive identification of *C. albicans* and *C. tropicalis*.

The identification of *Candida* spp. is based on morphological appearance by microscopic examination, cultural characteristics on primary and selective media and biochemical reactions, which include assimilation and fermentation of carbohydrates. API 20 C Aux, MUAG Candi test and Flow Uni-Yeast-Tek wheel are commercially available kits used for the identification of yeast from clinical specimens by assimilation and fermentation reactions. Germ tube test is used for the detection of pseudohyphae production of *C. albicans*. Serological testing by agglutination reaction with specific antisera is also used for the diagnosis of *Candida* spp.

Treatment

The treatment for candidiasis in the upper digestive tract of birds includes the use of nystatin at 200 000–300 000 units/kg PO every 12 h for 7–10 d (Bauck, 1994; Boydell and Forbes, 1996; Oglesbee, 1997; Redig and Ackermann, 2000), ketoconazole at 10–30 mg/kg PO every 12 h for 7 d (Bauck, 1994; Boydell and Forbes, 1996; Oglesbee, 1997), itraconazole at 5–10 mg/kg PO every 12 h for 7–21 d (Bauck, 1994; Boydell and Forbes, 1996) and fluconazole at 2–5 mg/kg PO every 24 h for 7 d (Bauck, 1994; Oglesbee, 1997). The latter is being postulated as the most effective antifungal agent for the treatment of tissue-based yeast infections in birds (Flammer, 1993). Nystatin suspension, 2–5 ml (100 000 IU/ml)/kg (weight of the bird) has also been used, applied directly to the mucosal membranes of the mouth of raptors (Redig, personal communication). Recently, the use of a miconazole gel preparation (Daktarin oral gel, Janssen-Cilag Ltd, UK) was successfully used in the treatment of upper digestive tract candidiasis infections in falcons (Samour and Naldo, 2002). This gel may prove useful for similar infections in other avian species.

REFERENCES

Bauck L (1994) Mycoses. In: Ritchie BW, Harrison GJ, Harrison LR (eds) *Avian Medicine: Principles and Application*, pp. 997–1006. Wingers Publishing, Lake Worth, FL.

Boydell IP, Forbes NA (1996) Diseases of the head (including the eyes). In: Beynon PH, Forbes NA, Harcourt-Brown N (eds) *Manual of Raptors, Pigeons and Waterfowl*, pp. 140–146. British Small Animal Veterinary Association, Cheltenham.

Flammer K (1993) An overview of antifungal therapy in birds. *Proceedings of the Association of Avian Veterinarians*, Nashville, pp. 1–4.

Jones MP, Orosz SE, Cox SK, Frazier DL (2000) Pharmacokinetic disposition of itraconazole in red-tailed hawks (*Buteo jamaicensis*). *Journal of Avian Medicine and Surgery* **14**:15–22.

Oglesbee BL (1997) Mycotic diseases. In: Altman RB, Clubb SL, Dorrestein GM, Quesenberry K (eds) *Avian Medicine and Surgery*, pp. 323–331. WB Saunders, Philadelphia.

Redig PT, Ackermann J (2000) Raptors. In: Tully TN, Lawton MPC, Dorrestein GM (eds) *Avian Medicine*, pp. 180–214. Butterworth-Heinemann, Oxford.

Samour JH, Naldo JL (2002) Diagnosis and therapeutic management of candidiasis in falcons in Saudi Arabia. *Journal of Avian Medicine and Surgery* **16**: 129–132.

FURTHER READING

Biberstein EL (1990) *Candida*. In: Biberstein EL, Zee YC (eds) *Veterinary Microbiology*, pp. 141–145. Blackwell Science, Oxford.

McCluggage DM (1996) Zoonotic disorders. In: Rosskopf WJ Jr, Woerpel RW (eds) *Diseases of Cage and Aviary Birds*, 3rd edn, pp. 535–547. Williams & Wilkins, Baltimore.

Quinn PJ, Carter ME, Markey B, Carter GR (1994) The pathogenic yeasts. In: *Clinical Veterinary Microbiology*, pp. 395–401. Wolfe Publishing, London.

Richard JL, Beneke ESA (1989) Mycoses and mycotoxicoses. In: Purchase HG, Arp LH, Domermuth CH, Pearson JE (eds) *A Laboratory Manual for the Isolation and Identification of Avian Pathogens*, pp. 70–76. American Association of Avian Pathologists, Athens, GA.

Van Cutsem J, Rochette F (1991) *Poultry: Candidiasis: Mycoses in Domestic Animals*, pp. 122–125. Janssen Research Foundation, Beerse, Belgium.

Fungal diseases – dermatophytosis, favus or ringworm infection

Ian F. Keymer

This relatively rare disease of birds (Figs 8.207–8.209), which is caused by invasion of the keratinized layers of the skin and appendages by dermatophytes or ringworm fungi, was reviewed by Keymer (1982). Since then there have been a limited number of other reports. Pathogenic dermatophytes appear to be worldwide in distribution.

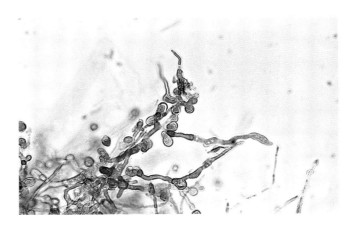

Fig. 8.207 Microscopic appearance of *Trichophyton verrucosum* in lactophenol–aniline blue stain. The main characteristics of this fungus are septate hyphae and half empty chlamydospores. × 400. (Courtesy of Mr. C. Silvanose). This image is for the purpose of differentiation with *T. mentagrophytes*.

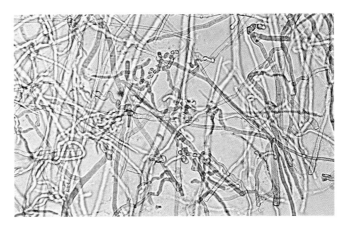

Fig. 8.208 Microscopic appearance of *T. mentagrophytes* in lactophenol–aniline blue stain. The hyphae of this fungus are spiral or tangled in shape. × 400. (Courtesy of Mr. C. Silvanose).

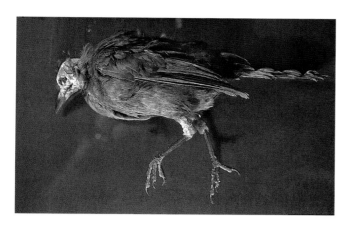

Fig. 8.209 Favus-like lesions affecting the head and legs of a free-living European blackbird (*Turdus merula*). Dermatitis of this type appears to be multifactorial in origin and may be associated with fungal infections such as *Trichophyton* and *Cladosporium* spp. as well as mite infestations (Keymer, 1982); also bacteria (e.g. *Staphylococcus* spp. and *Escherichia coli*). Frequently it is difficult to isolate and identify the fungi involved.

Host range

The infection occurs occasionally in free-living passerines, being reported mostly in the UK (Blackmore and Keymer, 1969). In captivity, the disease is relatively uncommon. It is mostly seen in Psittaciformes, Columbiformes and Passeriformes. Other orders of birds in which the infection has been recorded include Struthioniformes, Anseriformes, Falconiformes and Galliformes.

Cause

According to Perry (1987) there are more than 20 species of pathogenic dermatophytic fungi. Those most commonly reported are *Trichophyton* and *Microsporum* spp. Less frequently, other fungi (e.g. *Aspergillus*, *Candida*, *Cladosporium*, *Helminthosporum*, *Mucor*, *Malassezia* (also called *Pityrosporon*) and *Paecilomyces* spp.) may be involved.

Clinical signs

Most commonly affected are the unfeathered areas of the skin of the head and, when present, also the comb and wattles. Less frequently, lesions affect other parts of the body such as the neck, the legs and the leading edge of the wings. However, Baker (1996) recorded unilateral feather loss of the body caused by a *Trichophyton* sp. in a budgerigar (*Melopsittacus undulatus*). In most cases partial or complete alopecia is present and the skin becomes thickened and corrugated, grayish-white or yellowish in color, sometimes with the formation of encrustations and scabs. Crusty exudates may occur around the feather follicles. Sometimes the skin lesions are rough and porous in appearance. Usually there is little evidence of pruritus. Tudor (1983) isolated a *Paecilomyces* sp. and *Mucor circinelloides* from the feather shafts of pigeons (*Columba livia*) and various psittacines, which he regarded as the cause of pruritus and feather pulling. Some mycotic infections were associated with bacteria.

Hine *et al.* (1990) recorded candidiasis of the uropygial gland of chinstrap penguins (*Pygoscelis antarctica*). N. A. Forbes (personal communication, 1997) has also encountered *Malassezia* sp. (a yeast-like fungus) associated with feather loss and greasy skin in Harris hawks (*Parabuteo unicinctus*) and has found *Candida* and *Aspergillus* spp. to be relatively common secondary infective agents in chronic bumblefoot, especially when the foot remains bandaged for long periods with infrequent dressing changes. Sartory (1942) recorded *Aspergillus fumisalordes* var. *roseus* n. sp. as pathogenic to the feathers of pigeons (*Columba livia*). Krautwald (1990) has also described favus in parrots (*Amazona* spp.) associated with *Aspergillus* spp., namely *A. fumigatus* and *A. niger*. She also described pruritus caused by *Mucor* spp. in African gray parrots (*Psittacus erithacus*), small parakeets and other species. She said that in these infections the fungi may spread to the respiratory system and cause death. According to Perry (1987) *Helminthosporium* spp. infection of the skin and feathers in psittacines can cause extensive feather loss.

Pathology

Lesions are usually superficial and confined to the epidermis, dermis and base of the feathers. Hyperkeratosis is associated with infiltration of the keratinized layers of the skin and feather follicles by fungal hyphae; acanthosis, acantholysis and hydropic degeneration of cells in the stratum spinosum may also occur with infiltration of the underlying dermis by mononuclear cells (Droual *et al.*, 1991).

Diagnosis

The disease can be suspected from the macroscopic appearance of the lesions. The presence of septate hyphae on microscopical examination of skin scrapings, softened and cleared by crushing and soaking in aqueous potassium hydroxide (10–20% KOH w/v) for about 30 min, confirms the diagnosis when associated with histopathological lesions. Frequently, the fungi prove difficult to isolate and identify, even when using special culture media. Some species of normally saprophytic fungi may be found in association with the lesions, making it difficult to determine their significance. It is believed that sometimes mycotic infections may be secondary to immunosuppressive disorders. Perry (1994) stated that dermatophytes of birds do not fluoresce under ultraviolet light.

Differential diagnosis

The disease is most likely to be confused with skin lesions caused by epidermoptic, cnemidocoptic or *Neocheyletiella* mites. Malnutrition, especially hypovitaminosis A, affecting the health of the skin, may be a predisposing cause in some cases. Perry (1987) described 'pseudofavus' as a non-specific disorder of unknown etiology affecting birds in late summer and early autumn. It closely resembles favus but microscopic examination reveals no evidence of fungal involvement.

Control and treatment

A good standard of hygiene and avoidance of malnutrition are essential prophylactic measures. Tudor (1983) recommended STA (salicylic acid, 3 g; tannic acid, 3 g; and ethyl alcohol, qs 100 ml) or copper sulfate (1:2000 dilution) applied to affected areas of the skin as being safe and effective for fungal infections. However, since then, several other fungicidal agents have been developed. For example, Broadbent (1994) reported the successful treatment of *Trichophyton mentographytes* infection of an ostrich (*Struthio camelus*) using three treatments with natamycin (Mycophyt®, Mycofarm) at 4 d intervals followed by 'three soakings' with an enilconazole emulsion (Imaverol®, Janssen) at 3 d intervals. The natamycin only reduced the scabbing, but subsequent use of enilconazole produced total resolution. Forbes (personal communication, 1997) described treatment of cutaneous aspergillosis in a goshawk (*Accipter gentilis*; Fig. 8.149). Hine *et al.* (1990) satisfactorily treated candidiasis of the uropygial gland of penguins by feeding fish containing itraconazole (Sporanox®, Janssen) at a dosage rate of 10 mg/kg/d for 20 d. For the treatment of favus caused by

Microsporum gallinae, Bradley *et al.* (1995) recommended miconazole nitrate 2% (Micatin®, Advanced Care Products).

It should be remembered that oil/lipid-based products for topical application are contraindicated in birds because they mat the plumage and lead to excessive preening.

REFERENCES

Baker JR (1996) Survey of feather diseases of exhibition budgerigars in the United Kingdom. *Veterinary Record* **139**: 590–594.

Blackmore DK, Keymer IF (1969) Cutaneous diseases of wild birds in Britain. *British Birds* **62**: 316–331.

Bradley FA, Bickford AA, Walker RL (1995) Efficacy of miconazole nitrate against favus in oriental breed chickens. *Avian Diseases* **39**: 900–901.

Broadbent RS (1994) Favus in ostrich. *Veterinary Record* **135**: 536.

Droual R, Bickford AA, Walker RL *et al.* (1991) Favus in a backyard flock of game chickens. *Avian Disease* **35**: 625–630.

Hine S, Sharkey P, Friday RB (1990) Itraconazole treatment of pulmonary, ocular and uropygeal (*sic*) aspergillosis and candidiasis in birds – data from five clinical cases and controls. *Proceedings of the American Association of Zoo Veterinarians*, South Padre Island, pp. 322–327.

Keymer IF (1982) Mycoses. In: Petrak ML (ed.) *Diseases of Cage and Aviary Birds*, 2nd edn, pp. 599–605. Lea & Febiger, Philadelphia.

Krautwald ME (1990) Befiederungsstörungen bei Ziervögeln. *Praktische Tierarzt* **71**: 5–14.

Perry RA (1987) Avian dermatology. In: Burr EW (ed.) *Companion Bird Medicine*, pp. 40–50. Iowa State University Press, Ames, IA.

Perry RA (1994) A diagnostic approach to avian self-mutilation syndromes. In: Cross GM (ed.) *Proceedings of the Australian Association of the Avian Veterinarians*, Currumbin, pp. 159–178.

Sartory A (1942) *Aspergillus fumisalordes* var. *roseus* n. sp., pathogenic to pigeon feathers. *Comptes Rendues* **214**: p. 565. Académie des Sciences Colon, Paris.

Tudor DC (1983) Mycotic infections of feathers as a cause of feather pulling in pigeons and psittacine birds. *Veterinary Medicine/Small Animal Clinician* **78**: 249–253.

FURTHER READING

Fonseca E, Mendoza L (1984) Favus in a fighting cock caused by *Microsporum gallinae*. *Avian Diseases* **28**: 737–741.

Perry RA, Gill J, Cross GM (1991) Disorders of the avian integument. In: Rosskopf WJ Jr, Woerpel RW (eds) *Veterinary Clinics of North America, Small Animal Pet Avian Medicine*. WB Saunders, Philadelphia.

Reavill D (1996) Fungal diseases. In: Rosskopf WJ Jr, Woerpel RW (eds) *Diseases of Cage and Aviary Birds*, 3rd edn, pp. 586–595. Williams & Wilkins, Baltimore.

Post-mortem examination, with anatomical notes

Ian F. Keymer

9

It is important to remember that a comprehensive necropsy is time-consuming and expensive. It may not always be necessary to deal with every detail as outlined below. Much depends on the circumstances of the death. If there is any chance of legal proceedings or the bird is a rare species, then it is essential to carry out as detailed an examination as possible and keep full records. After the necropsy is finished, all remains of the carcass should be suitably preserved in case further examinations of tissue prove necessary.

No attempt has been made to give complete anatomical details for each order or other taxonomic group. Only salient features are included and those of special interest.

Carcasses destined for laboratory examination should, without delay, be thoroughly chilled in a refrigerator before packing and dispatch. Soaking bird carcasses in cold detergent at this stage is not recommended because it can damage the skin and hamper examination. Ectoparasites may also be lost and the skin will be unsuitable for taxonomic studies or taxidermy (Figs 9.1 and 9.2).

Carcasses should never be deep frozen unless the examinations are to be entirely of a toxicological nature or there is likely to be delay of over a week before necropsy, because when the carcasses thaw, artifacts are produced. The freezing and thawing causes hemolysis of red blood cells and alters the microscopic appearance of many tissues by damaging cell structure, thus hindering histopathological examination. The gross appearance of the organs is also altered by the exudation of fluid.

Packing material should be light in weight, waterproof and have good insulating properties. A full history should be provided and enclosed in the parcel in a sealed plastic bag separate from the carcass, so that it does not become contaminated with body fluids. The history should state the name and address of the sender/owner, date of death and method of euthanasia if applicable. The name of the species (including the scientific name if possible) should also be given, as well as the age, sex and reference number. It is also important to describe any clinical signs noted prior to death and details of treatment.

It is essential that local postage and customs regulations are strictly adhered to and that there is no risk of any leakage from the parcel. When endangered species are involved, special CITES (Convention on International Trade in Endangered Species of Wild Fauna and Flora) legislation may be applicable (see Appendix 6). Fresh tissues must not be dispatched to some countries (e.g. the UK) without a special license. Immediately beneath the first layer of packing there should be a clear message indicating the nature of the contents. If there is any risk that the carcass may be contaminated with a zoonotic infection, such as psittacosis (*Chlamydophila psittaci* infection), this should be clearly stated. This is very important, because the person who opens the parcel may not be a veterinarian or somebody who appreciates the potential risk of contracting a disease.

Carcasses not destined for another laboratory should be examined with the minimum of delay and kept as cool as possible, preferably by storing them temporarily in a refrigerator at 4°C (39.2°F). Most carcasses will keep satisfactorily at this temperature for at least 4 d. If carcasses are too large to go into a standard refrigerator, they can be placed in a deep freezer for a short time if one is available, taking care not to actually freeze them. A moderately autolyzed carcass is usually preferable to one that has been deep frozen.

Preparations for necropsy

1. Read the history if there is one! Ascertain whether the bird died naturally or was killed. If euthanasia was carried out, it is infrequently not recorded in the history. When injections of pentobarbital sodium have been given, this sometimes results in the deposition of whitish deposits on the surfaces of some internal organs or may cause brownish discoloration of the liver. These artifacts can easily be confused with genuine lesions of disease, especially visceral gout.
2. Assemble equipment, including sterile instruments of an appropriate size for the carcass being examined (Fig. 9.3). For very small specimens, ophthalmic

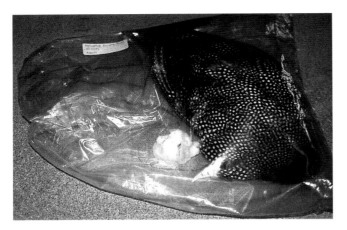

Fig. 9.1 Before opening the carcass, place it in a plastic bag to collect ectoparasites that may be in the plumage. Inclusion of a wad of cotton wool soaked in chloroform will facilitate collection of live parasites.

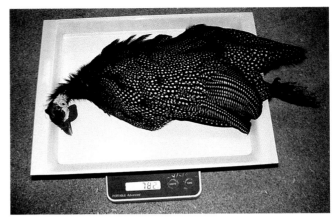

Fig. 9.2 Helmeted guinea fowl (*Numida meleagris*) after removal from plastic bag and prior to examination. Collection of bodyweights of specimens is an integral part of a post-mortem examination.

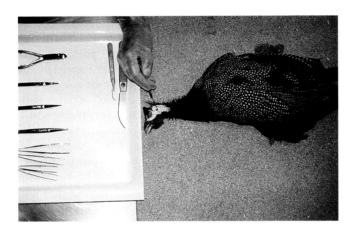

Fig. 9.3 Carcass with assembled instruments. including bone forceps, scissors, scalpels, forceps and seekers for probing into orifices such as the auditory meatus.

instruments may be most suitable. Assign a necropsy reference number to the specimen and record in the laboratory or practice daybook the date and the time that the necropsy was carried out.

3. While carrying out stage 2, think about the history, clinical signs, management and environment. If there is any reason to suspect a zoonotic infection, prepare to examine the carcass in a safety cabinet if this is available. If the carcass is too large or no cabinet is available, then in addition to wearing standard protective clothing, including disposable surgical gloves, it is essential to wear a face-mask and eye shields.

4. If the carcass is deep frozen, allow it to thaw out for a few hours before attempting examination. At room temperature this may take 48 h for a large bird.

5. Before commencing the necropsy, check 'Supplementary diagnostic procedures' at the end of this chapter in order to be fully prepared.

6. When performing a necropsy it is extremely important to *record all lesions as they are found* on to the necropsy forms (Tables 9.1 and 9.2). Preferably, record findings by dictation to an assistant or by using a tape recorder. Do not wait until the necropsy has been completed before recording the findings. By this time the appearance of some of the lesions will have been forgotten (especially if interruptions have occurred) or lesions will have been destroyed either by accident or during subsequent dissection. If for some reason a body system (e.g. the central nervous system or part thereof) or some organs have not been examined, because of damage or decomposition, be sure to record the fact that they have not been examined; (see 'NE' – Not examined – on the Necropsy sheet; Table 9.1).

External examination

Skin and appendages (reproductive system)

Closely examine the carcass (Fig. 9.4). If it is very small use a magnifying lamp or magnifying spectacles or a dissecting microscope. At this and every subsequent stage of the examination, be prepared to take photographs. Look for any evidence of trauma; search for ectoparasites and collect; examine cloaca; and look for lesions on feet and skin by parting feathers. Examine the plumage: normal molting must be differentiated from molting due to pathological causes.

TABLE 9.1 Necropsy sheet

Necropsy sheet _____ **Clinical reference number** _____

Pathology reference number _____

Name of species: _____ **Scientific name:** _____

Age: _____ **Sex:** _____

Identity number: _____ **Pet name:** _____

Owner's name: _____

Address: _____

Contact No: _____ **E-mail:** _____

Veterinarian's name: _____

Address: _____

Contact No: _____ **E-mail:** _____

Date of death: _____ **Date of necropsy:** _____

POST-MORTEM FINDINGS*

Body weight _____ (g). **Physical condition:** Normal ☐ Fat ☐ Thin ☐ Emaciated ☐ Other ☐

State of carcass: Fresh ☐ Refrigerated ☐ Deep frozen ☐ Decomposed ☐ Incomplete ☐

Systems

1. Skin/appendages	NLD ☐ NE ☐	8. Liver	NLD ☐ NE ☐
2. Skeletal	NLD ☐ NE ☐	9. Digestive	NLD ☐ NE ☐
3. Sensory	NLD ☐ NE ☐	10. Lymphoreticular	NLD ☐ NE ☐
4. Muscular	NLD ☐ NE ☐	11. Urinary	NLD ☐ NE ☐
5. Respiratory	NLD ☐ NE ☐	12. Reproductive	NLD ☐ NE ☐
6. Cardiovascular	NLD ☐ NE ☐	13. Nervous	NLD ☐ NE ☐
7. Endocrine	NLD ☐ NE ☐	14. Others:	

Post-mortem findings/lesions

_____

_____

_____

_____

_____

_____

_____

_____

_____

_____

_____

_____

_____

_____

_____

_____ _(continue over)_

DIAGNOSIS: PROVISIONAL ☐ FINAL ☐

_____

_____

_____

*Tick boxes and describe in the space provided. Under 'Systems', if no lesions of skin/appendages, etc. are detected tick 'NLD' box. If a system is not examined tick 'NE'. When lesions are found use the number given for the system and describe in the space beneath 'Post-mortem findings/lesions', continuing on back of sheet if necessary.

TABLE 9.2 Necropsy sheet *(cont'd)*

Necropsy sheet

Clinical reference number _____

Pathology reference number _____

SPECIMENS TAKEN			IDENTIFICATION/RESULTS

☐ **Parasitology**　　Arthropods ☐　　_____

　　　　　　　　　　　Helminths ☐　　_____

　　　　　　　　　　　Protozoa ☐　　_____

☐ **Microbiology**　　Bacteria ☐　　_____

　　　　　　　　　　　Fungi ☐　　_____

　　　　　　　　　　　Viral/other ☐　　_____

☐ **Hematology**　　Blood smear ☐ Blood sample (EDTA) ☐ Blood sample (Heparin) ☐

☐ **Tissue impression smears**　　Spleen ☐　　_____

　　　　　　　　　　　　　　　　Bone marrow ☐　　_____

　　　　　　　　　　　　　　　　Liver ☐　　_____

☐ **Histology**

Skin	☐	Tongue ☐	Bursa of Fabricius	☐	
Bone	☐	Esophagus ☐	Thymus	☐	
Eye	☐	Crop ☐	Kidney	☐	
Skeletal muscle	☐	Stomach ☐	Testis/ovary	☐	
Lung/airsac	☐	Proventriculus ☐	Oviduct	☐	
Heart	☐	Gizzard ☐	Cerebrum	☐	
Anterior/posterior aorta	☐	Duodenum ☐	Cerebellum	☐	
Thyroid	☐	Pancreas ☐	Spinal cord	☐	
Parathyroid	☐	Small intestine ☐	Peripheral nerve	☐	
Adrenal	☐	Cecum ☐	Other: _____		
Pituitary	☐	Large intestine ☐	Other: _____		
Liver	☐	Spleen ☐	Other: _____		

☐ Biochemistry _____

☐ Toxicology _____

☐ Electron microscopy _____

☐ Radiology _____

☐ Photography _____

*Tick boxes as applicable and complete details in spaces provided

_____

Veterinary surgeon

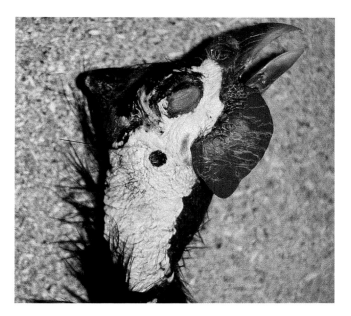

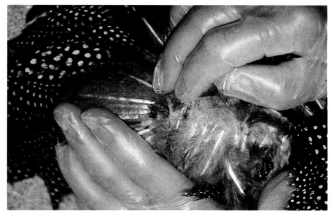

Fig. 9.5 The uropygial gland can be examined by parting the feathers over the last vertebra.

Fig. 9.4 Head of helmeted guinea fowl showing normal horny protuberance, 'comb' or 'crown' (dorsal aspect of head), red fleshy wattles and bare skin (normal for the species) on lateral aspects of cheeks and neck. In most birds the auditory meatus, visible here as a dark, round structure, is covered by feathers (the ear coverts).

Examine the uropygial or preen gland by parting the feathers over the last vertebra situated at the base of the tail (Fig. 9.5). It is absent in the following groups: Struthioniformes, Rheiformes, Casuariiformes and bustards (Otididae). The gland is either absent or very small in some members of the Caprimulgiformes, Columbiformes, Psittaciformes and Piciformes. It is especially well developed in most aquatic species, such as Sphenisciformes, Podicipediformes and gulls (Laridae).

Search for brood or incubation patches. These develop only during egg laying and are present throughout incubation. In some species they occur in both sexes, in others they are confined to females, in others to males and in some species they are absent. They are situated on the skin of the breast and appear as thickened, highly vascular areas of alopecia involving the dermis. There may be a single median patch or lateral patches. They must be differentiated from pathological lesions.

It is also necessary to examine the oral cavity and the beak closely for lesions such as deformities (Fig. 9.6). A horny layer, known as the rhamphotheca, covers the beak. This is a keratinized thickening of the stratified corneum of the epidermis. Histologically, the horny part of the beak resembles skin. Beneath the epidermis lies the dermis, which is closely attached to the periosteum of the underlying bone of the mandibles. The rhamphotheca of the upper mandible grows from the dermis that covers the premaxilla, there being a vascular layer between it and the dermis. The growth rate varies

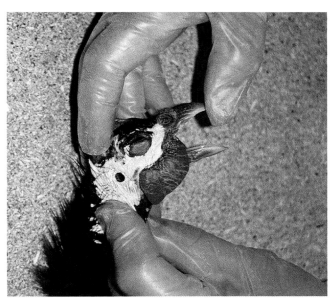

Fig. 9.6 Examination of the oral cavity and the beak.

according to the anatomical position of the germinal layer and also according to the degree of wear and tear on the beak. It is not known what actually controls the rate of growth. Beaks vary considerably in shape depending on feeding habits and diet. It is therefore necessary to be conversant with the normal appearance of the species being examined (see, for instance Arnall and Keymer, 1975; King and McLelland, 1984 for illustrations). In gannets (*Morus* spp.) for example, the external nares are closed and not visible at the normal site for most species (i.e. at the base of the upper mandible). These birds breathe through the commissures of the mouth.

Look for artificial methods of identity (e.g. sub-cutaneous ID microchips, leg rings (bands), tattoos, wing tags or rubber stamping of wing feathers (remiges)). Record any identification numbers on the necropsy record sheet.

If any skin lesions suggestive of dermatophytosis (ringworm) are found, then examine (whole bird if possible) in a darkened room under a Wood's lamp, parting the feathers at frequent intervals and looking for the presence of fluorescing infected skin or feathers. However, many avian dermatophytes may not fluoresce. Collect specimens for microscopy and culture. If any ectoparasites are found, collect all of them or alternatively a large representative sample and transfer to a bottle of 70% ethyl alcohol, which can be firmly sealed. Label the specimen immediately using a waterproof pen or pencil with the relevant reference number, both on a piece of card placed in the bottle and on the outside of the container – not on the lid, because this can be accidentally transferred to another container.

Weigh the carcass and record whether it is wet or dry. Record and describe any skin lesions. If the specimen is a free-living rare species, measure wing, beak and tail length (Bibby, 1985), or consult an ornithologist for instructions. It may be necessary to remove the skin for taxonomic studies or taxidermy. However, this is best carried out by an expert taxidermist. Examine the subcutaneous tissues carefully for any signs of trauma or other lesions.

Skeletal system

The avian skeleton shows a moderate degree of variation. It may be necessary therefore when examining an unfamiliar species to check for descriptions of the skeletal anatomy in advance.

Radiograph the entire carcass of small birds if there is any reason to suspect skeletal lesions such as minor fractures, which are not immediately obvious, nutritional bone disease and foreign bodies such as lead shot in the gizzard or gunshot wounds. If foreign bodies of this kind are located, they should be collected as they become available, labeled and put in a safe place. This should be done in the presence of a witness (who should initial the label) if there is any possibility of legal proceedings.

Open the major limb joints and examine the articular surfaces. Note the appearance of the synovial fluid and take swabs for bacteriological examination if considered necessary.

Sensory system

In birds the openings of the external auditory meatuses are not immediately obvious, because they are covered

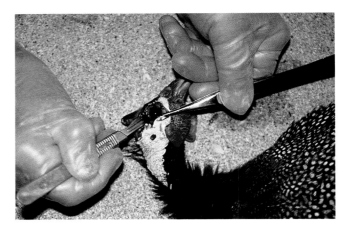

Fig. 9.7 The eyes should be examined by deflecting the eyelids for evidence of macroscopic lesions and by indirect ophthalmoscopy (if mydriasis is present and the carcass is very fresh) for microscopic internal lesions.

by feathers (the ear coverts). These therefore need to be raised in order to make an examination. A meatus is situated caudal to and slightly below each eye. In owls, unlike other species, the positions of the auditory meatuses are not quite symmetrical and the openings are relatively large.

Examine the external nares. In some marine species these are absent (see Skin and appendages, above). Examine the eyes initially by deflecting the eyelids for evidence of macroscopic lesions, ideally followed by indirect ophthalmoscopy (if mydriasis is present and the carcass is very fresh) for microscopic internal lesions; remove the eyes and examine the orbits (Fig. 9.7). If required for histopathological examination, fix the eyes without delay.

Internal examination

At this stage the carcass can be positioned for examination of the internal organs. Small carcasses should be placed on a board or post-mortem room table and fixed securely in position with the ventral surface uppermost. They may either be nailed on a board through the feet and wings or secured with strings or ropes to cleats on the post-mortem room table as appropriate. This is facilitated by dislocating the hip joints using both hands to grip the upper part of each leg and deflecting the legs dorsally to the body (i.e. downwards towards the surface of the table). The carcass will then lie flat. In the case of small birds the wings can be fixed in position by inserting pins between the ulna and radius at the distal end of these bones, or through the carpal joint, in larger birds, using nails. If the skin is not required for taxonomic studies or taxidermy, dip the carcass in disinfectant

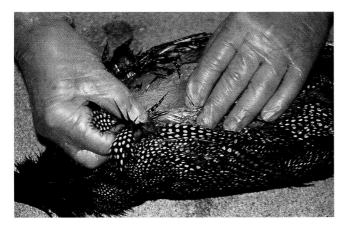

Fig. 9.8 The feathers of the ventral surface of the body should be carefully plucked, using the other hand to tense the skin to avoid tearing.

solution and pluck the feathers from the neck, breast and abdomen (Fig. 9.8). This lessens the dispersal of feathers and feather 'dust' (powder down) into the atmosphere and helps to prevent contamination of the internal organs. Large carcasses such as ostriches (*Struthio camelus*) may require no method of stabilization and stay in position on most surfaces.

Muscular system

A good time to make the initial examination of the muscles is soon after the carcass has been skinned or partly skinned (Figs 9.9 and 9.10). At this stage

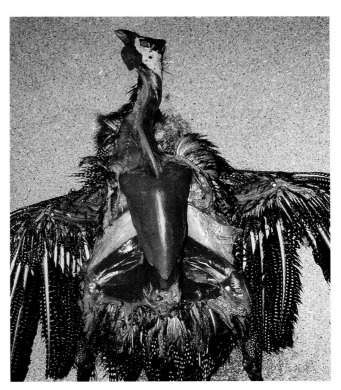

Fig. 9.10 Deflect the skin by blunt dissection to expose the subcutaneous tissues of the neck, pectoral muscles, rib cage, and abdominal and leg muscles.

muscles can be incised and examined for lesions. The final examination can be completed at the end of the necropsy.

Respiratory and cardiovascular systems

If the skull is not needed, expose and examine the nasal passages, sinuses (including the infraorbital sinus) and internal nares, using bone forceps. Do not expose the brain (see later).

Open the carcass in the midline by starting the incision at the base of the throat and extending it caudally to the region of the cloaca. Deflect the skin by blunt dissection to expose the subcutaneous tissues of the neck, pectoral muscles, rib cage and abdominal and leg muscles. Make a small incision in the abdominal wall near the cloaca using fine scissors to expose the abdominal viscera (Fig. 9.11). Enlarge it forwards to the sternum and open the abdomen.

This exposes the internal organs intact, including the liver, which should be carefully removed, partly by blunt dissection, for examination later. Unless the intact skeleton is required, expose the thoracic cavity by cutting through the rib cage and the coracoid and clavicle bones on both sides. Then deflect to one side the sternum with the pectoral muscles attached

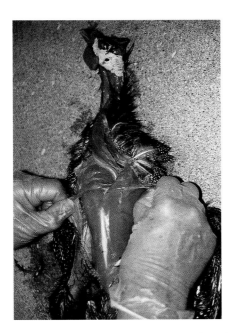

Fig. 9.9 The skin is carefully removed by blunt dissection using the hands, after the initial incision has been made using a scalpel. Removal of skin and subcutaneous tissues exposes the ventral surface of the pectoral muscles.

(Figs 9.12 and 9.13). Figures 9.14 and 9.15 illustrate exposure of the spleen by deflection of the liver and of the ventral surface of the neck by removal of the sternum.

A true diaphragm is absent in birds. However, a pulmonary fold is present, situated ventral to the lungs, separating the pulmonary area of the celom from the peritoneal area.

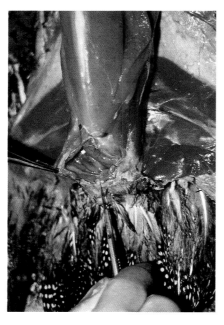

Fig. 9.11 Make a small incision in the abdominal wall near the cloaca using fine scissors to expose the abdominal viscera. Enlarge it forwards to the sternum and open the abdomen.

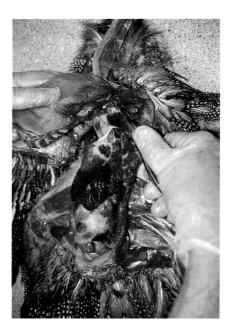

Fig. 9.13 The sternum is deflected to the right side of the bird to expose the left lung, heart, liver, left kidney, gizzard and part of the gut.

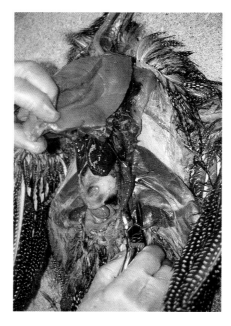

Fig. 9.12 The celomic cavity has been exposed and the sternum partly deflected cranially to expose part of the lung on one side, the liver overlapping part of the gizzard, the duodenal loop surrounding the pancreas and a small part of the lower intestinal tract.

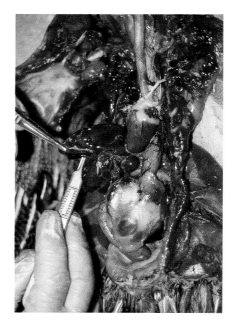

Fig. 9.14 The liver has been carefully partly removed and deflected to one side, exposing the oval-shaped spleen, which is situated between the proventriculus and the liver and gallbladder. The heart is situated cranially and the gizzard caudally to the spleen.

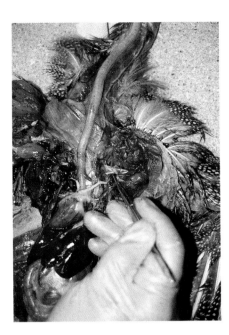

Fig. 9.15 Ventral surface of neck exposed by removal of sternum, showing left brachial plexus (above tip of forceps), trachea overlying esophagus, empty crop on the right side of the bird, heart with great vessels and liver.

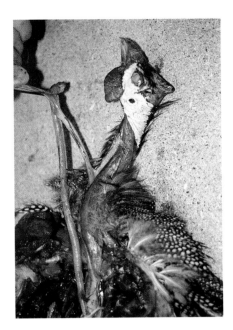

Fig. 9.17 The esophagus has been severed at the base of the buccal cavity and the larynx (both held by forceps), together with the trachea, and separated from their attachments.

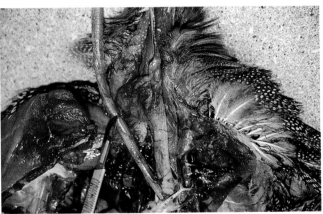

Fig. 9.16 The trachea has been deflected to expose the cervical esophagus, the crop (on the right side of the bird) and the thoracic esophagus.

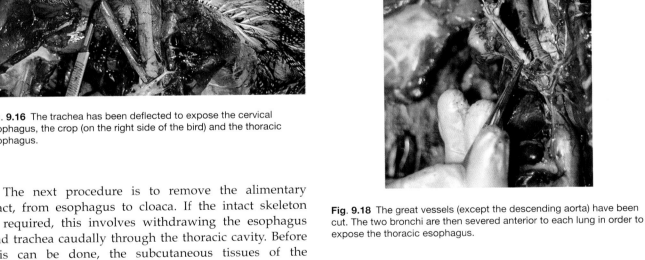

Fig. 9.18 The great vessels (except the descending aorta) have been cut. The two bronchi are then severed anterior to each lung in order to expose the thoracic esophagus.

The next procedure is to remove the alimentary tract, from esophagus to cloaca. If the intact skeleton is required, this involves withdrawing the esophagus and trachea caudally through the thoracic cavity. Before this can be done, the subcutaneous tissues of the neck must be excised, and the trachea and esophagus exposed and separated from their attachments (Figs 9.16 and 9.17), taking care to identify and collect the thymus and thyroids (see Endocrine system, below). Next, cut with fine scissors the great vessels (except the descending aorta), which overlie the ventral aspect of the esophagus (Fig. 9.18) a short distance from their cardiac origins. The esophagus is then severed immediately posterior to the pharynx so that the alimentary tract from pharynx to cloaca can be removed in one piece (Fig. 9.19). This is examined

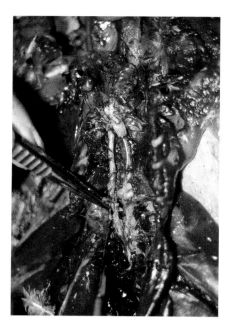

Fig. 9.19 The alimentary tract has been removed, the heart has been opened and all the great vessels severed except the descending aorta. The aorta has been dissected from its attachments to below the gonads. Part of the right kidney is visible below the forceps.

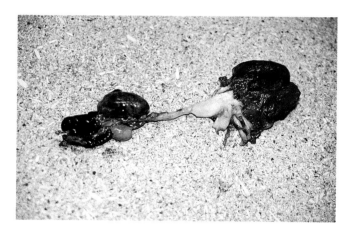

Fig. 9.20 Opened heart and aorta showing intima of proximal descending aorta and the right brachiocephalic artery. The kidney and testes are also visible. The right testis is cream-colored and normal in appearance. The left testis is unusually hypertrophied in comparison.

Examine the heart, both internally and externally, and the cardiac blood vessels. If the carcass is fresh (especially free-living or recently captured birds) make blood smears from the heart blood and peripheral blood vessels to examine blood cells and look for hematozoa.

In most species the trachea terminates in a swollen structure known as the syrinx, formed by the lowest rings of the trachea being fused into a cylindrical tympanum. However, there are other variations and sometimes the organ can be a very large and complex structure. In male ducks (smaller species of Anatidae), for example, a cartilaginous enlargement (bulla) surrounds the syrinx. In most species the trachea is a simple, straight tube. However, in some it is an elongated, coiled structure that in some species emerges from the sternum and lies between the skin and the pectoral muscles, for example in curassows (large species of Cracidae; Galliformes) (King and McLelland, 1984). In birds, the lungs (Fig. 9.21) are

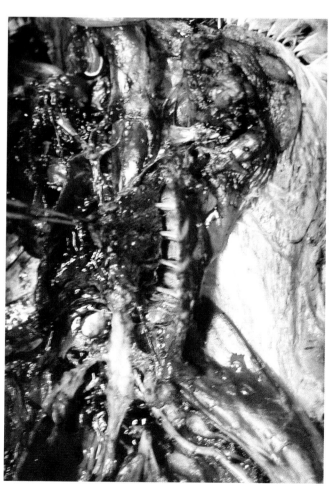

Fig. 9.21 Ventral aspect of body with viscera removed, with the exception of the lungs. The left lung has been partly detached from its attachments to the rib cage.

later (see Digestive system). The heart and great vessels can now be removed, the descending aorta being carefully dissected at least as far as it becomes the terminal aorta and divides into the iliac arteries. The descending aorta and great vessels, which leave and enter the heart, can then be opened using fine scissors and the intima examined for lesions such as arterio-sclerosis (Fig. 9.20).

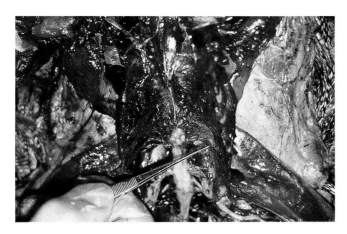

Fig. 9.22 The forceps point to the left caudal thoracic airsac. The abdominal airsacs have been removed.

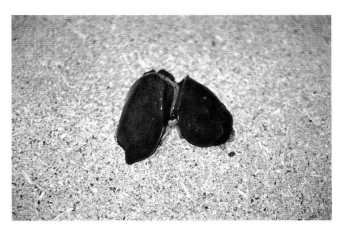

Fig. 9.23 Ventral surface of the liver. The right lobe is normally larger than the left.

closely attached to the wall of the thoracic cavity by fibrous strands, greatly reducing the extent of the visceral and parietal pleura. Birds also have well-developed airsacs (Fig. 9.22), which are extensions of the lungs. They are transparent and sometimes difficult to detect when normal. The airsac system involves some bones and replaces the marrow.

Examine the lungs (remove by blunt dissection) and the airsacs. In addition to lesions of septicemia, these organs are frequently the site of mycosis and sometimes mycoplasmosis.

Endocrine system (lymphoreticular system)

The thyroids are paired, dark-red, ovoid structures at the base of the neck on each side of the trachea in close association with the jugular veins. In Figure 9.14, the left thyroid is visible immediately to the left of the jugular vein and anterior to the left carotid artery.

The parathyroids are often difficult to find but can usually be detected associated with the thyroid by using a magnifying glass or on histological examination. They are small, yellowish structures just caudal to the thyroids. Enlargement may occur with metabolic bone disease.

The thymus glands are bilateral, pale pinkish, multi-lobular structures situated on each side of the neck close to the jugular vein. It may be necessary to take suspected glandular tissue for histopathological examination in order to make a definite identification, because in small species these glands can be difficult to recognize. They involute as the bird reaches maturity but in some species may re-enlarge after the breeding season. Under some circumstances the thyroids and thymus may need to be weighed and/or measured.

In most birds, the adrenal glands are yellowish and paired, situated at the anterior end of each kidney. (Fig. 9.19 shows an adrenal immediately caudal to the right testis.) The pituitary gland is situated on the ventral surface of the brain and it is therefore necessary to remove the brain in order to examine it.

Liver

Examine the surface of the liver, which has already been removed (Fig. 9.23). Before making any incisions, weigh and measure the organ. If psittacosis is suspected, make 'touch' impression smears of the intact surface for *Chlamydophila psittaci* elementary bodies. Examine by slicing and make impression smears of the cut surface to examine for *Plasmodium* parasites or for *Chlamydophila* if indicated. Air dry 'touch' impression smears and place others in a suitable fixative.

A gallbladder is present in many species, but is absent in most Columbidae, many psittacines and the ostrich.

Examine the gallbladder and check for patency of the bile duct and contents of the bladder. If gallstones are found, these should be collected for analysis and stored by refrigeration or deep frozen.

Digestive system (lymphoreticular system and endocrine system)

The buccal cavity and pharynx can be exposed by using scissors to cut through the commissures of the mouth on one side and bone forceps to cut the hyoid apparatus on both sides, enabling the head to be deflected. Do not overlook examination of the mouth and buccal cavity, because these are common sites for lesions caused by a variety of agents. Tongues vary

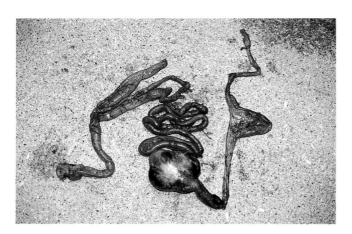

Fig. **9.24** Alimentary tract of helmeted guinea fowl showing cervical esophagus (top right hand corner) leading to crop, thoracic esophagus, proventriculus, muscular gizzard, duodenum forming loop round the pancreas, small intestine, two well-developed ceca, and large intestine (colorectum) terminating in the cloaca.

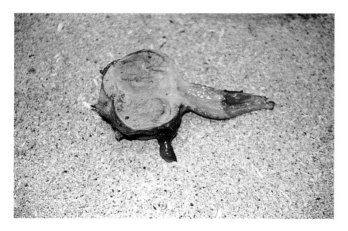

Fig. **9.25** The opened proventriculus or glandular stomach (right) showing the mucosa, and the muscular gizzard showing the hardened cuticle of the koilin layer. This type of 'stomach' is typical of a graminivorous bird.

in shape, size and mobility in different species, so it is important to be aware of their normal appearance and that of the entire alimentary tract before proceeding with the dissection (King and McLelland, 1984; McLelland, 1991).

The esophagus leads directly into the glandular stomach, known as the proventriculus (Figs 9.24 and 9.25). However, in some species a diverticulum of the esophagus occurs to form a crop. This is large in gallinaceous species, psittacines and many seed-eating passerines. In pigeons (Columbiformes), the crop is divided into two large, lateral glandular sacs, which secrete crop 'milk' for feeding the young. The crop wall is highly vascular in pigeons, especially when producing this secretion. In psittacines it stretches transversely across the base of the neck. The crop is

also fairly well developed in some birds of prey. However, in some of these species and some passerines, and in Anseriformes, it is less well developed, being a spindle-shaped swelling of the esophagus near the thoracic inlet. In predominantly insectivorous or frugivorous passerines, the crop is also fusiform in shape. It is absent in some birds, such as penguins (Sphenisciformes), gulls (Laridae) and Caprimulgiformes. The males of some breeds of domestic pigeon (*Columba livia*), the ostrich, sage grouse (*Centrocercus urophasianus*) and great bustard (*Otis tarda*) have inflatable esophageal diverticula that act as resonating chambers when displaying.

The proventriculus precedes the gizzard or ventriculus. In non-seed-eating birds the gizzard is thin-walled with little muscular tissue, and the junction with the proventriculus is difficult to detect externally; in such cases the two portions are frequently referred to as the 'stomach'. The degree of glandular and muscular tissue is related to the nature of the diet. The orifices of the gastric glands are easily visible to the naked eye where they open into the lumen. A well-developed sphincter separates the organ from the entrance to the gizzard. Tall, columnar, mucous cells line the ducts of the unilobular and multilobular glands and discharge mucus after feeding. Parietal, acid-secreting and peptic-enzyme-secreting cells are also present and similar to those in the mammalian stomach. In predominantly seed-eating birds the gizzard has a thick muscular wall and is lined by a hardened cuticle (the koilin layer). In the Sphenisciformes the distensible stomach extends caudally into the lower abdomen almost as far as the cloaca. However, in fruit eaters such as lories (many species of the subfamily Psittacinae of the family Psittacidae, e.g. *Domicella* spp.) it is lightly muscled and flaccid.

The intestinal tract is divided into small and large intestines, although these areas are not always immediately obvious. The duodenum is a U-shaped loop of the gut with a proximal descending part and a distal ascending part enclosing the pancreas. The duodenum then merges into the jejunum. This is separated from the ileum by the vitelline or Meckel's diverticulum, which is the small blind remnant of the yolk sac and yolk duct. Except in young birds, it is very difficult to locate this diverticulum. For detailed descriptions of the appearance and positioning of the intestinal tract the reader should consult King and McLelland, 1984. The small intestine is typically divided into the duodenum, jejunum and ileum. In nectar-feeding species such as humming birds (Trochilidae) the small intestine is unusually short. The duodenum is the most anterior part and is associated with the pancreas, around which it forms a loop. In most species of bird the various parts of the small intestine are not well differentiated and merge imperceptibly.

The ceca, when present, are regarded as part of the large intestine and mark the junction between the small and large intestines. Ceca are absent in some species, including some members of the Coraciiformes, Piciformes and Psittaciformes such as the budgerigar (*Melopsittacus undulatus*). Most birds have two ceca; exceptions include herons (Ardeidae) and Gaviiformes, which have only one. In some species, e.g. Columbiformes, the ceca are vestigial and in some other species, such as small passerines, may be difficult to detect with the naked eye. The largest ceca are seen in the Tetraoninae (grouse and capercaillies). In owls (Strigiformes), the distal extremities of the ceca are expanded, forming saccular structures. In the ostrich the ceca are long and sacculated.

The large intestine in birds (unlike many other vertebrates) is short and probably homologous to the mammalian rectum. It is sometimes referred to as the colorectum. Together with the genital and urinary tracts it empties into the cloaca. In psittacines, and many other families of bird, there is no clear distinction between colon and rectum, this part of the gut being represented by a short colorectum. Its diameter is larger than the preceding small intestine. The cloaca is a chamber into which the terminal parts of both the digestive and urogenital systems open. The cloaca opens to the outside at the vent. The chamber is divided internally by two mucosal folds, which form three compartments: the coprodaeum, urodaeum and proctodaeum.

The alimentary tract (already removed) should be unraveled and examined systematically but, before opening the crop, proventriculus and gizzard, suitable containers should be available for the contents. These may be required for toxicological examination or for identification of the food that has been eaten. Open and examine one area of the tract at a time.

Examine serosal surfaces and look for adhesions. Starting at the esophagus, note the contents and appearance of the mucosa, and similarly of the proventriculus and gizzard, and throughout the gut. Examine beneath the koilin layer of the gizzard. Take scrapings on a microscope slide from various areas, make wet preparations (preferably on a warmed slide to activate motile protozoa) and examine microscopically for *Macrorhabdus ornithogaster*, *Trichomonas* spp., *Giardia* spp. and *Hexamita* spp., coccidia, etc. and helminths. Collect parasites and/or prepare smears. Leave a small area of the tract intact for histopathological and other examinations. Never submit portions of gut that have been scraped with a scalpel for histological, mycological or virological examination, because this damages tissues and causes contamination.

Examine the pancreas and do not delay fixation for histology.

Lymphoreticular system

The spleen is the most important organ in the system. It is situated between the proventriculus and the gizzard on the right side. The shape varies considerably. It is elongated and sausage-shaped in Passeriformes and Columbiformes; almost spherical in Galliformes and Psittaciformes; and roughly triangular in Anseriformes.

Most birds do not have lymph nodes but they are present in Anseriformes. In these birds one pair is situated near the thyroids and the other pair near the kidneys. They are spindle-shaped. The bursa of Fabricius, situated in the dorsal wall of the cloaca, is a lymphatic organ. It is most easily seen in the young, because it involutes with age.

When examining the spleen, it is important to remember that enlargement is not necessarily pathological and can be physiological.

It may be necessary to make impression smears of the spleen (see Liver, above). Using bone forceps, examine the bone marrow (Fig. 9.26), remembering

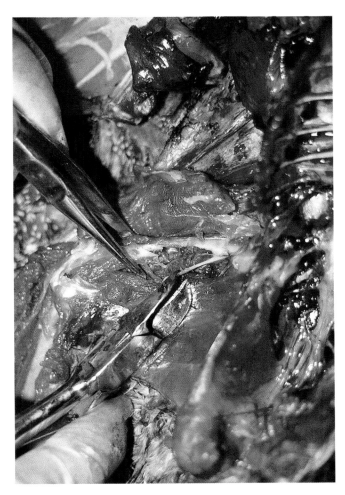

Fig. 9.26 Using bone forceps, the right femur has been cracked open to expose the bone marrow.

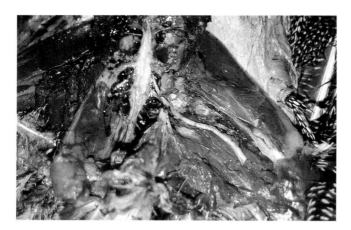

Fig. 9.27 The kidneys have been removed from the synsacrum to expose the lumbosacral plexus on each side. Using bone forceps to cut through the ilium on the left side, the ischiatic nerve has been exposed. This is the largest nerve supplying the leg.

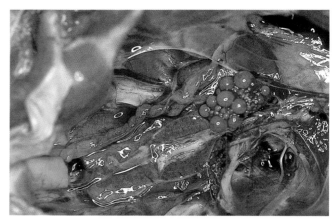

Fig. 9.28 Active ovary and developed oviduct of a mature guinea fowl at the beginning of the breeding season. Most female avian species possess only a functional left ovary with the exception of several species of the Falconiformes and the brown kiwi (*Apteryx australis*).

that this may be replaced by extensions of the airsac system in some of the larger limb bones. Bone marrow can be collected for histological examination by removing a small piece of bone intact, fixing in formol saline and later decalcifying the bone, or by removing the bone marrow and wrapping it in muslin to form a 'sausage' before fixation. Impression smears of the marrow are especially useful but must be made with care to avoid rupturing the cells. This is best carried out by aspirating the marrow using a syringe and hypodermic needle. Bone marrow specimens must be collected as soon after death as possible, because the cells rapidly undergo degeneration.

Urinary system

In birds, the kidneys are lobular and situated in bony depressions of the synsacrum. They extend from the posterior edges of the lungs to the end of the synsacrum. The urinary bladder is absent in all birds.

The appearance and especially the color of the kidneys should be noted. A brownish color, with tubules prominently distended with whitish urates, indicates nephrosis. The kidneys can be removed by cutting through the external iliac and ischiatic blood vessels on the lateral surfaces and carefully lifting them out of the dorsal wall of the synsacrum using a scalpel (Fig. 9.27). This exposes the lumbosacral plexus (see Nervous system, below).

Reproductive system

Females

In most vertebrates the ovaries are paired internal organs but in birds only the left ovary is usually present (Fig. 9.28), exceptions being many Falconiformes of the families Cathartidae, Accipitridae and Falconidae and the brown kiwi (*Apteryx australis*).

Record the appearance of the ovary and look for follicles. Only the left oviduct is normally present. If a fully formed egg is found in the oviduct of an uncommon bird, this should be collected intact, in case it is needed for special studies. If there is any possibility of salmonellosis, then the ova should be taken for bacteriological examination, because some *Salmonella* spp. can be egg-transmitted.

Completely open the oviduct and look for impactions with egg material and other lesions.

Males

The testes are paired, as in mammals, but are internal and situated just anterior to the kidneys. They are usually ovoid and variable in color; whitish gray (Fig. 9.29) or black. The single penile organ (lacking a urethra) is vestigial in most birds, except Ratites and Anseriformes.

Nervous system (endocrine system)

The nervous system, especially the autonomic, is the most difficult to examine. When dysfunction of the autonomic nervous system (dysautonomia) is suspected, the autonomic ganglia need to be located and examined histologically. This disorder occurs in proventricular dilatation disease of psittacines.

The peripheral nerves (especially the brachial and lumbosacral plexuses) can be examined at various stages of the necropsy. The brachial plexus is very obvious in the brachial region but in order to see the lumbosacral plexus it is necessary to remove the kidneys (see Urinary system, above). Nerves taken for histology should be pressed on a piece of card and fixed in formol saline. Pressing

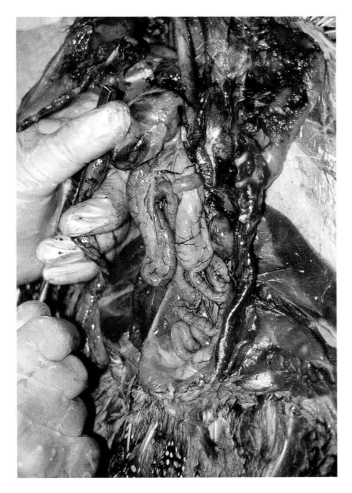

Fig. 9.29 The gizzard is deflected to show where the left bronchus has been cut immediately posterior to the syrinx. The left testis is visible immediately posterior to the left lung. The testis is hypertrophied and mottled grayish white.

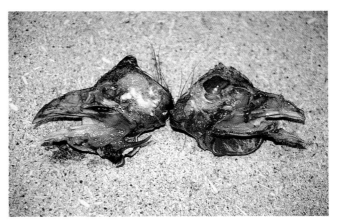

Fig. 9.30 A sagittal section of the head of a helmeted guinea fowl clearly shows on the left hand portion the cerebrum, cerebellum, and below these, the medulla oblongata. The nasal sinuses, tongue and part of the buccal cavity are also visible.

flat on card ensures that the nerve remains straight during fixation and prevents curling.

Frequently when skinning the head of a small bird in preparation for removal of the brain, hemorrhages can be observed in the bony substance of the skull. These are usually agonal and of no pathological significance, unless they are associated with contusions and/or hemorrhages intracranially and/or in the overlying skin of the head. These hemorrhages are also believed to occur in birds following severe terminal activity, such as following fright.

Brains of large species can be exposed by sawing off the top of the cranium using an oscillating or hand saw, so that it can be replaced should the skull be needed for taxidermy. To remove the brain, the skull is held upside down and the brain is gently detached out of the cranium with a scalpel handle, using gravity. If it is suitable for histology and the skull is needed, it may be possible using a curette to scoop out a small piece of hind-brain for histological examination, although this will be of limited value. For the purposes

of bacteriological or virological examinations a sterile swab can be inserted through the foramen magnum.

Brains should always be examined with extra care, because handling and autolysis can cause artifacts, which make histological examination difficult. Large brains should preferably be partly sliced transversely, in order to facilitate penetration of the fixative. It is preferable to keep the brain intact and renew the fixative every 12 h for 3–4 d. To examine small brains, place the entire head in fixative and later decalcify the bone. Alternatively, for larger brains a sagittal section of the skinned head can be made (Fig. 9.30) and fixed intact. The halved brain is removed after fixation. Use bone forceps and/or scalpel to remove the spinal cord. Place it on a piece of card before fixation.

Termination

Re-read the history and check that nothing has been forgotten. Retain all carcass remains and refrigerate for 72 h in case some are needed. In the case of rare species or if legal procedures are expected, retain the carcass in a deep freezer and suitably preserve remains of all organs. In such cases, it may be prudent to have a witness present to confirm that the necropsy findings have been accurately recorded and that specimens, which might be needed for forensic purposes, are correctly labeled and sealed. When deep freezing tissues it is especially important to tie labels very securely to all carcass remains and containers so they do not become detached, and also to use waterproof markers. Even so, labeling often becomes illegible in deep freezers. Color-coded labels are helpful. Enter details and record provisional or final diagnosis on the necropsy sheet (Table 9.1) and elsewhere, for instance in the practice or laboratory daybook.

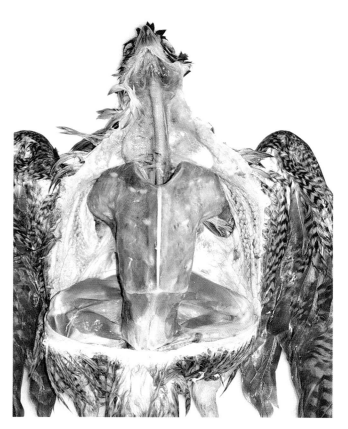

Fig. 9.31 Post-mortem examination of a peregrine falcon (*Falco peregrinus*). The skin has been deflected to expose the body prior to full dissection. Note the well-defined crop on the right side of the neck. (Courtesy of Dr. J. Samour).

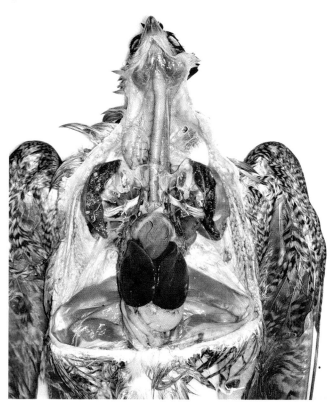

Fig. 9.32 The sternum with the attached pectoral muscles has been removed and the abdominal muscles have been dissected to allow viewing of all major organs. (Courtesy of Dr. J. Samour).

Cleanse and disinfect instruments and area, including external surfaces of specimen containers. When tissues have to be transported to a laboratory for histopathological examination, the overall weight can be reduced by removing fixed tissues from the containers and sending them in formalin-soaked cloth gauze, carefully labeled and sealed in plastic bags. However, if this is done, care must be taken to ensure that the tissues are not crushed when packing and also that they cannot be damaged during transit.

Photographs of the post-mortem examination of a peregrine falcon (*Falco peregrinus*) (Figs 9.31–9.33) have been included for comparative purposes.

Supplementary diagnostic procedures

Only the more common procedures are briefly discussed here. For detailed information specialized texts should be consulted (see Further reading).

If the condition of the carcass is suitable, take specimens for the following.

Histopathological examination

Routinely collect at least the liver, lung, kidney and any tissue showing macroscopic lesions. Do not use rat-tooth forceps for this purpose, because they damage the tissues. Always submit a representative portion of the lesion to include apparently normal tissue from the periphery and also obviously diseased tissue in the center. Do not use tissues that are discolored or autolyzed (e.g. as the result of being in contact with the intestinal tract or exposed for an excessive amount of time to the atmosphere, resulting in desiccation).

Some tissues, such as the alimentary tract, pancreas, bone marrow, brain and kidney decompose more quickly than heart and skeletal muscle. Fix tissues in 10% buffered formol–saline, using at least 6 times (preferably 10–20 times) the volume of the fluid to the volume of the specimens. Ideally tissues should not be more than 1 cm thick.

When specimens are large in diameter and if several are placed in one container, it is important to increase the volume of fixative proportionately and to replace with fresh fixative twice a week. Fixation time varies with different tissues: for example, those containing fibrous

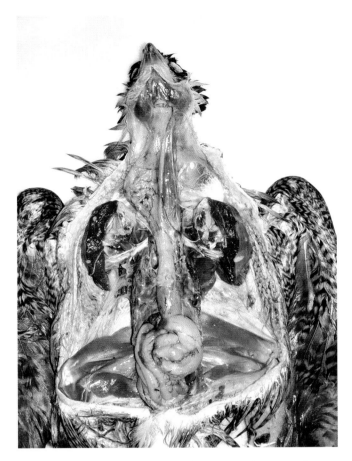

Fig. 9.33 The heart and the liver have been removed to expose the organs underneath. Note the ventriculus and intestinal tract stained with bile because of the proximity of the gallbladder. Courtesy of Dr. J. Samour.

tissue take longest, but it can be hastened by slightly warming the formol–saline fixative. With some tissues it may be necessary for them to remain in the fixative for as long as 2 weeks before they can be processed for histological examination.

Label specimen containers (not the lids) immediately after introducing tissues and keep different areas of the gut in separate containers.

For urgent cases, tissues can be frozen using a cryostat, but the results are usually less satisfactory than when fixed with formalin.

Bacteriological examination

Routinely take swabs of contents of at least two areas of the intestinal tract. If the bird died naturally or was killed because it was sick, routinely culture heart blood, liver and any organ showing macroscopic lesions. Place uncontaminated tissues in sterile Petri dishes (or use sterile swabs), label and submit for subsequent examination in case they are needed (see Virological examination, below).

Mycological examination

Take for culture and other examinations any tissue suspected of being infected, and label container (see Bacteriological examination, above).

Toxicological examination

Routinely take liver, kidneys, skeletal muscle, brain, content of crop and proventriculus and, if present, body fat. Label containers with a waterproof marker and place in deep freezer at –20°C (–4°F) until required.

Virological examination

Remove tissues as applicable and obtain instructions from the virologist who will examine them. Attempt sterile precautions, although under many circumstances some contamination of tissues is almost inevitable. If tissues are not to be pooled, then use separate sterile instruments for each tissue collected. If examination is likely to be delayed, tissues should be frozen at below –60°C (–76°F) and transported packed in dry ice or liquid nitrogen. When taking tissues for electron microscopy they should be cut in very small pieces not exceeding 1 mm square and fixed immediately in freshly prepared cold gluteraldehyde or similar fixative. If an ultracryomicrotome is available for 'cryosectioning', tissues can be stored until required at –70° (–94°F) instead of being fixed.

Parasitological examinations

In addition to collecting parasites as described previously and examining intestinal tract, also tie off and label representative areas of the gut for subsequent examination, and refrigerate.

Polymerase chain reaction (PCR)

This relatively recent test for identification of bacteria and viruses was believed to be more suited for use in research than for routine diagnostic procedures (Grainger and Madden, 1993). However, the last few years have seen significant advances in the development and application of PCR techniques in avian medicine. PCR diagnostic techniques are nowadays widely used by practitioners in the diagnosis of infectious diseases, including chlamydophilosis and psittacine beak and feather disease virus, polyoma virus and herpesvirus infections (Rosenthal, 2001; Greenacre, 2002; Styles *et al.*, 2004). A recent study reported the use of real-time PCR in the diagnosis of *Aspergillus fumigatus* in avian samples (Dahlhausen *et al.*, 2004).

ACKNOWLEDGMENTS

I am grateful to Dr. J. Samour for taking photographs during the post-mortem examination and to Mr. A. D. Malley for reading the text and for his helpful comments.

REFERENCES

Arnall L, Keymer IF (1975) Sampling and necropsy. In: Arnall L, Keymer IF (eds) *Bird Diseases: An Introduction to the Study of Birds in Health and Disease*, pp. 441–450. TFH Publications, Neptune City, NJ.

Bibby CJ (1985) Measurement. In: Campbell B, Lack E (eds) *A Dictionary of Birds*, pp. 342. British Ornithologists Union. T & AD Poyser, Carlton, Staffordshire.

Dahlhausen B, Abbott R, VanOverloop P (2004) Rapid detection of pathogenic *Aspergillus* species in avian samples by real-time PCR assay: a preliminary report. *Proceedings of the Association of Avian Veterinarians*, New Orleans, pp. 37–40.

Grainger J, Madden D (1993) The polymerase chain reaction: turning needles into haystacks. *Biologist* **40**: 197–200.

Greenacre CB (2002) My case work-up for 3 common presentations. *Proceedings of the Association of Avian Veterinarians*, Monterey, pp. 222–241.

King AS, McLelland J (1984) *Birds: Their Structure and Function*. Baillière Tindall, London.

McLelland J (1991) *A Color Atlas of Avian Anatomy*. WB Saunders, Philadelphia.

Rosenthal K (2001) Interpreting clinical pathological results in avian patients. *Proceedings of the Association of Avian Veterinarians*, Orlando, pp. 281–287.

Styles DK, Tomaszewski EK, Phalen DN (2004) Psittacid herpesvirus associated with internal papillomatous disease in psittacine birds. *Proceedings of the Association of Avian Veterinarians*, New Orleans, pp. 79–81.

FURTHER READING

Aughey E, Frye FL (2001) Comparative Veterinary *Histopathology with Clinical Correlates*. Manson Publishing. The Veterinary Press, London.

Evans HE (1982) Anatomy of the budgerigar. In: Petrak ML (ed.) *Diseases of Cage and Aviary Birds*, 2nd edn, pp. 111–187. Lea & Febiger, Philadelphia.

Fowler ME (1986) *Zoo and Wild Animal Medicine*, 2nd edn. WB Saunders, Philadelphia.

Fowler ME (1991) Comparative clinical anatomy of ratites. *Journal of Zoo and Wildlife Medicine* **22**: 204–277.

Fowler ME (1993) Clinical anatomy of ratites. In: Fowler ME (ed.) *Zoo and Wild Animal Medicine, Current Therapy 3*, pp. 194–198. WB Saunders, Philadelphia.

Fowler ME (1993) *Zoo and Wild Animal Medicine, Current Therapy 3*. WB Saunders, Philadelphia.

Latimer KS, Rakich PM (1994) Necropsy examination. In: Ritchie BW, Harrison GJ, Harrison LR (eds) *Avian Medicine: Principles and Application*, pp. 355–379. Wingers Publishing, Lake Worth, FL.

Lowenstine LJ (1986) Necropsy procedures. In: Harrison GJ, Harrison LR (eds) *Clinical Avian Medicine and Surgery*, pp. 298–309. WB Saunders, Philadelphia.

Simpson VR (1996) Post-mortem examination. In: Beynon PH, Forbes NA, Lawton MPC (eds). *Manual of Psittacine Birds*, pp. 69–86. British Small Animal Veterinary Association, Cheltenham.

Veit HP (1981) Mistakes to avoid when submitting tissue for histologic evaluation. *Veterinary Medicine Small Animal Clinician* **76**: 1143–1149.

Waine JC (1996) Post-mortem examination technique. In: Beynon PH, Forbes NA, Harcourt-Brown NH (eds) *Manual of Raptors, Pigeons and Waterfowl*, pp. 98–112. British Small Animal Veterinary Association, Cheltenham.

Appendices

Appendix 1

Sex-linked bodyweights reference table for selected avian species

Merle M. Apo

Order	Species	Scientific name	Male (g)	*n*	Female (g)	*n*
Anseriformes	Magpie goose	*Anseranas semipalmata*	2766		2071	
	Spotted (tree) whistling duck	*Dendrocygna guttata*	800		800	
	Plumed (Eyton's/grass whistle-duck/tree) whistling duck	*Dendrocygna eytoni*	788		792	
	Fulvous (tree) whistling duck	*Dendrocygna bicolor*	675		690	
	Cuban (black-billed tree) whistling duck	*Dendrocygna arborea*	1150		1150	
	Javan (Indian tree) whistling duck	*Dendrocygna javanica*	450–600		450–600	
	White-faced (tree) whistling duck	*Dendrocygna viduata*	686		662	
	Northern black-bellied (red-billed tree) whistling duck	*Dendrocygna autumnalis*	816		839	
	Coscoroba swan	*Coscoroba coscoroba*	4600		3800	
	Black swan	*Cygnus atratus*	6270		5100	
	Mute swan	*Cygnus olor*	12200		8900	
	Black-necked swan	*Cygnus melanocoryphus*	5400		4000	
	Whistling swan	*Cygnus columbianus*	7100		6200	
	Whooper swan	*Cygnus cygnus*	10800		8100	
	Swan (Chinese) goose	*Anser cygnoides*	3500		2850–3450	
	Western (yellow-billed) bean goose	*Anser fabalis*	3198		2843	
	Pink-footed goose	*Anser brachyrhynchus*	2620		2352	
	European white-fronted goose	*Anser albifrons*	2290		2042	
	Lesser white-fronted goose	*Anser erythropus*	1440–2300		1300–2100	
	Western graylag goose	*Anser anser*	3531		3105	
	Bar-headed goose	*Anser indicus*	2000–3000		2000–3000	
	Lesser snow (blue) goose	*Anser coerulescens*	2744		2517	
	Ross's goose	*Anser rossi*	1315		1224	
	Emperor goose	*Anser canagicus*	2812		2766	
	Néné (Hawaiian) goose	*Branta sandvicensis*	2212		1923	
	Canada goose	*Branta canadensis*	3809		3310	
	Barnacle goose	*Branta leucopsis*	1672		1499	
	Brent goose (brant)	*Branta bernicla*	1410		1410	
	Red-breasted goose	*Branta ruficollis*	1315–1625		1150	
	Ruddy shelduck	*Tadorna ferruginea*	1200–1640		950–1500	
	South African (Cape) shelduck	*Tadorna cana*	1785		1417	
	Australian (mountain duck) shelduck	*Tadorna tadornoides*	1559		1291	
	New Zealand (paradise) shelduck	*Tadorna variegata*	–		1260–1340	
	Common shelduck	*Tadorna tadorna*	980–1450		801–1250	

Continued overleaf

Continued

Order	Species	Scientific name	Male (g)	*n*	Female (g)	*n*
	Moluccan (blacked-backed/burdekin) radjah shelduck	*Tadorna radjah*	750		839	
	Egyptian goose	*Alopochen aegyptiacus*	1900–2550		1500–1800	
	Orinoco goose	*Neochen jubatus*	–		1250	
	Abyssinian blue-winged goose	*Cyanochen cyanopterus*	–		1520	
	Andean goose	*Chloephaga melanoptera*	2730–3640		2730–3640	
	Lesser (upland) Magellan goose	*Chloephaga picta*	2834		2721–3200	
	Patagonian lesser kelp goose	*Chloephaga hybrida*	2607		2607	
	Ashy-headed goose	*Chloephaga poliocephala*	2267		2200	
	Ruddy-headed goose	*Chloephaga rubidiceps*	2000		2000	
	Cape barren (cereopsis) goose	*Cereopsis novaehollandiae*	5290		3770	
	Flying steamer duck	*Tachyeres patachonicus*	3073		2616	
	Magellanic flightless steamer duck	*Tachyeres pteneres*	6039		4111	
	Falkland flightless steamer duck	*Tachyeres brachypterus*	4303–4420		3400	
	Patagonian (South American) crested duck	*Anas specularioides*	1070–1180		900	
	Blue mountain duck	*Hymenolaimus malacorhynchos*	887		750	
	Salvadori's duck	*Anas waigiuensis*	462		469	
	South African (Black River) black duck	*Anas sparsa*	–		952–1077	
	European (Eurasian) widgeon	*Anas penelope*	720		640	
	American (baldpate) widgeon	*Anas americana*	770		680	
	Chiloë widgeon	*Anax sibilatrix*	939		828	
	Falcated duck	*Anas falcata*	713		585	
	Gadwall (gray duck)	*Anas strepera*	990		850	
	Baikal (spectacled) teal	*Anas formosa*	437		431	
	European (common) green-winged teal	*Anas crecca*	329		319	
	Chilean (South American green-winged) teal	*Anas flavirostris*	429		394	
	Cape teal	*Anas capensis*	419		380	
	East Indian gray teal	*Anas gibberifrons*	507		474	
	Chestnut (Australian brown) teal	*Anas castanea*	595		539	
	New Zealand brown teal	*Anas aucklandica*	665		600	
	Mallard	*Anas platyrhynchos*	1261		1084	
	Hawaiian duck (koloa)	*Anas platyrhynchos wyvilliana*	670		573	
	Laysan teal	*Anas platyrhynchos laysanensis*	–		450	
	American black duck	*Anas rubripes*	1330		1160	
	South African yellow-billed duck	*Anas undulata*	954–844		817–677	
	Indian spot-billed duck	*Anas poecilorhyncha*	1230–1500		790–1360	
	New Zealand gray duck	*Anas supercilliosa*	765–1275		623–1275	
	Philippine duck	*Anas luzonica*	906		779	
	Bronze-winged (spectacled) duck	*Anas specularis*	1130		990	
	Northern (common/blue-billed) pintail	*Anas acuta*	850		759	
	Georgian (Chilean/brown) pintail	*Anas georgica*	776		705	
	Lesser Bahamas (white-cheeked) pintail	*Anas bahamensis*	–		505–633	
	Red-billed pintail	*Anas erythrorhyncha*	617		566	
	Puna silver (Northern/versicolor) teal	*Anas versicolor*	422		373	
	Hottentot teal	*Anas punctata*	224–253		224–253	
	Garganey	*Anas querquedula*	240–542		220–445	
	Prairie blue-winged teal	*Anas discors*	360		332	
	Northern cinnamon teal	*Anas cyanoptera*	408		362	

Continued

Continued

Order	Species	Scientific name	Male (g)	n	Female (g)	n
	Argentine red shoveler	*Anas platalea*	608		523	
	Cape (South African) shoveler	*Anas smithii*	688		597	
	Australian shoveler	*Anas rhynchotis*	667		665	
	Northern (common) shoveler	*Anas clypeata*	410–1100		420–763	
	Pink-eared (zebra) duck	*Malacorhynchus membranaceus*	404		344	
	Marbled teal	*Marmaronetta angustirostris*	240–600		250–550	
	Freckled (monkey) duck	*Stictonetta naevosa*	969		842	
	Ringed teal	*Anas leucophrys*	190–360		197–310	
	Pink-headed duck	*Rhodonessa caryophyllacea*	935		840	
	Chilean torrent duck	*Merganetta armata*	440		315–340	
	European (common) eider	*Somateria mollissima*	2253		2127	
	King eider	*Somateria spectabilis*	1830		1750	
	Spectacled (Fischer's) eider	*Somateria fischeri*	1630		1630	
	Steller's (Siberian/little) eider	*Polysticta stelleri*	860		860	
	Red-crested pochard	*Netta rufina*	1135		967	
	South American (Red-eyed/Southern) pochard	*Netta erythrophthalma*	600–977		533–1000	
	Rosy-billed (rosybill) pochard	*Netta peposaca*	1181		1154	
	Canvasback	*Aythya valisineria*	1252		1154	
	European (common) pochard	*Aythya ferina*	998		947	
	Redhead	*Aythya americana*	1080		1030	
	Ring-necked duck	*Aythya collaris*	790		690	
	Australian white-eye (hardhead)	*Aythya australis*	902		838	
	Baer's pochard (Eastern white-eye)	*Aythya baeri*	880		680	
	Ferruginous white-eye pochard	*Aythya nycora*	583		520	
	Tufted duck	*Aythya fuligula*	1116		1050	
	New Zealand scaup (black teal)	*Aythya novaeseelandiae*	695		610	
	European (greater) scaup	*Aythya marila*	1250		900–1200	
	Lesser (little blue-billed) scaup	*Aythya affinis*	850		800	
	Greater Brazilian teal	*Amazonetta braziliensis*	380–480		350–390	
	Maned goose (Australian wood duck)	*Chenonetta jubata*	815		800	
	Mandarin duck	*Aix galericulata*	440–550		440–550	
	North American wood duck (Carolina wood duck)	*Aix sponsa*	680		539	
	African pygmy goose (dwarf)	*Nettapus auritus*	285		260	
	Indian pigmy goose (Australian pygmy/cotton teal)	*Nettapus coromandelianus*	403		380	
	Green pygmy goose	*Nettapus pulchellus*	310		304	
	Hartlaub's duck	*Pteronetta hartlaubii*	800–940		800–940	
	White-winged wood duck	*Cairina scutulata*	2495–3855		1925–3050	
	Muscovy duck	*Cairina moschata*	2000–4000		1100–1500	
	Old world comb (knob-billed) duck	*Sarkidiornis melanotos*	1300–2610		1870–2325	
	(Gambian) Spur-winged goose	*Plectropterus gambensis*	5400–6800		4000–5400	
	Eastern (Atlantic) harlequin duck	*Histrionicus histrionicus*	680		540	
	Oldsquaw (long-tailed) duck	*Claagula hyemalis*	800		650	
	European (common) black scoter	*Melanitta nigra*	1108		1006	
	Surf scoter	*Melanitta perspicillata*	1000		900	
	European white-winged (velvet) scoter	*Melanitta fusca*	1727		1492–1658	
	Bufflehead	*Bucephala albeola*	450		330	
	Barrow's goldeneye	*Bucephala islandica*	1110		800	
	European (common) goldeneye	*Bucephala clangula*	990–1158		710–799	
	Smew (white nun)	*Mergus albellus*	540–935		515–650	
	Hooded merganser	*Mergus cucullatus*	680		540	
	Common red-breasted (redhead) merganser	*Mergus serrator*	1133–1209		907–959	

Continued overleaf

Continued

Order	Species	Scientific name	Male (g)	*n*	Female (g)	*n*
	European (common/redhead) goosander	*Mergus merganser*	1670		1535	
	Black-headed duck	*Heteronetta atricapilla*	513		565	
	Masked duck	*Oxyura dominica*	406		339	
	North American ruddy duck	*Oxyura jamaicensis*	550		500	
	White-headed duck	*Oxyura leucocephala*	737		593	
	Maccoa duck	*Oxyura maccoa*	450–700		450–700	
	Argentine ruddy (blue-billed) duck	*Oxyura vittata*	610		560	
	Australian blue-billed duck	*Oxyura australis*	812		852	
	Australian musk duck	*Biziura lobata*	2398		1551	
	African white-backed duck	*Thalassornis leuconotus*	650–790		625–765	
Caprimulgiformes	Tawny frogmouth	*Podargus strigoides*	400	2	–	
Charadriiformes	Stone curlew	*Burhinus oedicnemus*	407.37 ± 13.13 (350–443)	8	403.9 ± 7.3 (299–435)	20
	Oystercatcher	*Haematopus ostralegus*	387.5 ± 12.5 (375–400)	2	400	1
Ciconiiformes	Rosy flamingo (Caribbean, Cuban)	*Phoenicopterus ruber roseus*	3412.25 ± 63.14 (2600–4200)	31	2641.08 ± 68.12 (1800–3200)	23
	Chilean flamingo	*Phoenicopterus chilensis*	2762.30 ± 77.84 (2000–3600)	26	2344.76 ± 74.88 (1750–3250)	21
	Lesser flamingo	*Phoeniconaias minor*	1656.36 ± 31.77 (1500–1900)	11	1306.66 ± 167.46 (1020–1600)	3
	Greater flamingo	*Phoenicopterus ruber ruber*	3600 ± 155.27 (2750–4250)	10	2923.68 ± 102.19 (2150–3750)	18
	White stork	*Ciconia ciconia*	3300 ± 200 (2800–4200)	7	2950 ± 148.32 (2700–3650)	6
	Marabou stork	*Leptoptilos crumeniferus*	7100	1	2300	1
	Maguari stork	*Ciconia maguari*	4500	1	3883.33 ± 174 (3600–4200)	3
	Adjutant stork	*Leptoptilos dubius*	–		6800	2
	Sacred ibis	*Threskiornis aethiopicus*	1130 ± 83.06 (1000–1400)	5	1341.66 ± 101.99 (1000–1750)	6
	Australian white ibis	*Threskiornis molucca*	1560 ± 52.37 (1300–1700)	7	1300	1
	Scarlet ibis	*Eudocimus ruber*	629 ± 21.36 (515–750)	10	640 ± 78.63 (500–800)	4
	Black-crowned night heron	*Nycticorax nycticorax*	787 ± 52.70 (600–1075)	11	660 ± 15.78 (600–750)	10
	Goliath heron	*Ardea goliath*	–		4200	1
Columbiformes	Blue crowned pigeon	*Goura cristata*	2350 ± 15 (2050–2500)	3	1900	1
	Gray imperial pigeon	*Ducula pistrinaria*	75	1	–	
Coraciiformes	Pied hornbill	*Tockus fasciatus*	–		525	1
	Rufous hornbill	*Buceros hydrocorax*	1400	3	1300	1
	Black hornbill	*Anthracoceros malayanus*	–		750 ± 50 (700–800)	2
	Crowned hornbill	*Tockus alboterminatus*	–		212.5 ± 2.5 (210–215)	2
Cuculiformes	Hartlaub's turaco	*Tauraco hartlaubi*	222.5 ± 2.5 (220–225)	2	–	
	Red-crested turaco	*Tauraco erythrolophus*	180	1	210 ± 5 (205–215)	2
	White-cheeked turaco	*Tauraco leucotis*	272.5 ± 47.5 (225–320)	2	288.33 ± 19.22 (260–325)	3
	Violet turaco	*Musophaga violacea*	646	1	583.5 ± 5.5 (578–589)	2
Falconiformes	Secretary bird	*Sagittarius serpentarius*	4400 ± 57.73 (4300–4500)	3	4750	1

Continued

Continued

Order	Species	Scientific name	Male (g)	n	Female (g)	n
	White-headed vulture	Aegypius occipitalis	4700	1	4125 ± 125 (4000–4250)	2
	African white-backed vulture	Gyps africanus	8300	1	–	
	Palm-nut vulture	Gypohierax angolensis	450	1	–	
	Lappet-faced vulture	Aegypius tracheliotus	8800	1	–	
	Ruppell's griffon vulture	Gyps rueppelli	6150 ± 350 (5800–6500)	2	–	
	Egyptian vulture	Neophron percnopterus	1525 ± 25 (1500–1550)	2	1450 ± 50 (1400–1500)	2
	Griffon vulture	Gyps fulvus	9425 ± 875 (8550–10300)	2	–	
	King vulture	Sarcorhamphus papa	–		3700	1
	Golden eagle	Aquila chrysaetos	3800	2	5000	1
	Chinese serpent eagle	Spilornis cheela ricketti	2060	1	–	
	Wedge-tailed eagle	Aquila audax	2350	1	3000	1
	Buzzard	Buteo buteo	860 ± 40 (820–900)	2	1026.66 ± 54.56 (920–1100)	3
	Common caracara	Polyborus plancus	983.33 ± 136.42 (800–1250)	3	1012.5 ± 37.5 (975–1050)	2
	Saker falcon*	Falco cherrug	773.6 ± 9.9 (712–850)	20	1055.08 ± 17.54 (890–1250)	25
	Peregrine falcon*	Falco peregrinus	697.89 ± 5.7 (650–745)	19	930.68 ± 18.68 (750–1150)	30
Galliformes	Vulturine guinea fowl	Acryllium vulturinum	1675 ± 47.87 (1600–1800)	4	1633.33 ± 88.19 (1500–1800)	3
	Helmeted guinea fowl	Numida meleagris	1137.05 ± 37.5 (1100–1750)	2	1000	1
	Crested guan	Penelope purpurascens	–		1700 ± 100 (1600–1800)	2
Gruiformes	Crowned crane	Balearica pavonina	4164.70 ± 137.18 (2800–4900)	17	3540 ± 120.83 (3300–4000)	5
	Sarus crane	Grus antigone	8166.66 ± 527.04 (6000–9500)	6	7400 ± 450.92 (5400–8500)	6
	Demoiselle crane	Anthropoides virgo	2200 ± 155.45 (1500–2750)	6	2228.57 ± 41.17 (2000–2500)	15
	Common crane	Grus grus	4466.66 ± 448.45 (3600–5100)	3	4700	1
	Stanley crane	Anthropoides paradisea	5150 ± 359.39 (4500–6100)	4	4800 ± 150 (4500–4950)	3
	Manchurian crane	Grus japonensis	7750 ± 150 (7600–7900)	2	7200	1
	Sandhill crane	Grus canadensis	4575 ± 225 (4350–4800)	3	4150	1
	Hooded crane	Grus monacha	–		3900 ± 100 (3800–4000)	2
	South African crowned crane	Balearica regulorum	4100 ± 126.49 (3600–4300)	5	3133.33 ± 88.19 (3000–3300)	3
	Brolga crane	Grus rubicunda	–		5300 ± 500 (4800–5800)	2
	Japanese white-naped crane	Grus vipio	5800	1	5066.66 ± 88.19 (4900–5200)	3
	Wattled crane	Bugeranus carunculatus	7300 ± 1300 (6000–8600)	2	6133.33 ± 600.92 (5300–7300)	3
	Water rail	Rallus aquaticus	200	1	–	
	Kori bustard*	Ardeotis kori	9161.09 ± 729.02 (6800–14200)	11	5089.43 ± 123.75 (3181–6363)	30
	Heuglin's bustard*	Neotis heuglinii	–	4	2589.6 ± 92.67 (2250–2750)	

Continued overleaf

Continued

Order	Species	Scientific name	Male (g)	*n*	Female (g)	*n*
	Houbara bustard*	*Chlamydotis undulata*	1534.53 ± 19.08 (1164–2072)	94	1071.57 ± 13.37 (803–1390)	85
	White-bellied bustard*	*Eupodotis senegalensis*	1203.66 ± 99.14 (1006–1316)	3	991 ± 74 (917–1065)	2
	Buff-crested bustard*	*Eupodotis ruficrista*	598.04 ± 21.93 (413–822)	24	580.61 ± 15.74 (426–663)	18
	Black bustard*	*Eupodotis afra*	769.4 ± 13.91 (731–792)	5	–	
	Gray-headed gallinule	*Porphyrio porphyrio poliocephalus*	525	1	625	1
Passeriformes	White-crested laughing thrush	*Garrulas leucolophus*	100	2	100	1
	Red-billed blue magpie	*Urocissa erythrorhyncha*	222.5 ± 32.5 (190–255)	2	172.5 ± 22.5 (150–195)	2
	Greater hill mynah	*Acridotheres grandis*	235 ± 13.22 (215–260)	3	233.33 ± 12.01 (210–250)	3
	Rothschild's mynah	*Leucopsar rothschildi*	96.44 ± 2.93 (80–110)	10	91 ± 3.76 (75–120)	12
	Jackdaw	*Corvus monedula*	198.92 ± 3.71 (170–220)	14	184.54 ± 4.92 (145–210)	11
	San Blas jay	*Cissilopha sanblasiana*	108.33 ± 1.66 (105–110)	3	100	3
	Common raven	*Corvus corax*	1180 ± 48.98 (1100–1300)	5	1112.5 ± 187.5 (925–1300)	2
	Indian house crow	*Corvus splendens*	21.66 ± 10.83 (170–265)	9	192.5 ± 14.59 (140–230)	6
	Laughing kookaburra	*Dacelo novaeguineae*	310 ± 23.61 (275–400)	6	387.5 ± 26.02 (325–450)	5
Pelecaniformes	American white pelican	*Pelecanus erythrorhynchos*	6475 ± 428.90 (5400–7500)	4	–	
	Shag	*Phalacrocorax aristotelis*	1900 ± 152.75 (1700–2200)	3	–	
Piciformes	Citron throated toucan	*Ramphastos vitellinus citreolaemus*	300	1	372.5 ± 47.5 (325–420)	2
	Plate-billed mountain toucan	*Andigena laminirostris*	–		302.5 ± 22.5 (280–325)	2
	Chestnut-mandibled toucan (Swainson's)	*Ramphastos swainsonii*	500 ± 11.54 (480–520)	3	440	1
	Channel-billed toucan	*Ramphastos vitellinus*	435	1	350	2
	Ariel toucan	*Ramphastos vitellinus ariel*	375	1	–	
	Cuvier's toucan	*Ramphastos tucanus cuvieri*	–		650	1
Psittaciformes	Hyacinth macaw	*Anodorhynchus hyacinthinus*	1366.66 ± 72.64 (1250–1500)	7	1308 ± 73.91 (1100–1500)	10
	Scarlet macaw	*Ara macao*	1023.18 ± 43.63 (817.5–1156)	20	984.87 ± 59.00 (792.5–1231)	16
	Green-winged macaw	*Ara chloroptera*	1273 ± 63.84 (1108–1431)	17	1202.755 ± 46.93 (1051–1301)	14
	Buffon's macaw	*Ara ambigua*	–		1100	2
	Severe macaw	*Ara severa*	391.66 ± 8.33 (375–400)	3	310 ± 10 (320–330)	2
	Blue and gold macaw	*Ara ararauna*	1126 ± 76.58 (937.5–1417)	27	1119.5 ± 159.48 (803–1800)	25
	Military macaw	*Ara militaris*	1050 ± 86.60 (900–1300)	4	1100	1
	Red-fronted macaw	*Ara rubrogenys*	297.5 ± 2.5 (295–300)	2	461.425 ± 20.75 (360–500)	7
	Yellow-naped macaw	*Ara auricollis*	237.42 ± 11.22 (200–275)	7	215 ± 13.22 (190–235)	3
	Red-shouldered macaw	*Diopsittaca nobilis*	148.75 ± 4.03 (138.5–157.5)	8	137.08 ± 4.3 (124–153)	12
	Blue winged macaw	*Propyrrhura maracana*	3245 ± 3.05 (318–328)	3	280 ± 8.5 (250–298)	5

Continued

Continued

Order	Species	Scientific name	Male (g)	n	Female (g)	n
	Lesser sulfur-crested cockatoo	*Cacatua sulphurea*	280	1	355 ± 95 (260–450)	2
	Citron sulfur-crested cockatoo	*Cacatua sulphurea citrinocristata*	450	1	–	
	Palm cockatoo	*Probosciger aterrimus*	850 ± 150 (700–1000)	2	600	1
	Salmon-crested cockatoo	*Cacatua moluccensis*	853.75 ± 7.5 (750–765)	4	787.55 ± 20 (855–895)	3
	Sulfur-crested cockatoo	*Cacatua galerita*	485 ± 15 (440–500)	4	450 ± 30 (420–480)	2
	Greater sulfur-crested cockatoo	*Cacatua galerita galerita*	937.5 ± 37.5 (900–975)	2	881.25 ± 69.55 (600–1250)	8
	Roseate cockatoo (galah)	*Eolophus roseicapillus*	433.41 ± 10.50 (300–480)	17	295.5 ± 9.38 (275–370)	10
	Leadbeater's cockatoo (Major Mitchell's)	*Cacatua leadbeateri*	465	1	–	
	Black cockatoo	*Calyptorhynchus funereus*	595	1	665	1
	Long-billed corella	*Cacatua tenuirostris*	687.5 ± 42.5 (645–730)	7	496.25 ± 34.66 (450–595)	4
	Bared-eyed cockatoo (little corella)	*Cacatua sanguinea*	424 ± 21.25 (369–485.5)	10	375 ± 24.79 (346–429)	6
	Yellow-crowned amazon	*Amazona ochrocephala*	400.575 ± 30.33 (252–474)	7	399.335 ± 20.40 (260–496)	7
	Yellow-billed amazon	*Amazona collaria*	243.75 ± 11.25 (225–270)	4	220 ± 5 (215–225)	2
	Festive amazon	*Amazona festiva*	2895 ± 3 (286–298)	2	300.55 ± 10 (191–211)	3
	Vinaceous amazon	*Amazona vinacea*	450	2	–	
	Orange-winged amazon	*Amazona amazonica*	346.78 ± 6.25 (263–440)	33	328.86 ± 6.62 (257–406)	30
	Red-lored amazon	*Amazona autumnalis*	356.83 ± 12.89 (337.5–381)	6	345.16 ± 52.5 (315.5–421.5)	8
	Lilacine amazon	*Amazona autumnalis lilacina*	316.66 ± 8.33 (300–325)	3	300	3
	Blue-cheeked amazon	*Amazona dufresniana*	–		800	1
	Yellow-headed amazon	*Amazona oratrix*	600	1	350	1
	Blue-fronted amazon	*Amazona aestiva*	410.13 ± 14.62 (331–487)	22	260.215 ± 13.74 (229–250)	8
	Cuban amazon	*Amazona leucocephala*	2585 ± 8 (250–266)	2	224 ± 7.07 (202–254)	6
	Mealy amazon	*Amazona farinosa*	–	512	1	
	African gray parrot	*Psittacus erithacus*	425.465 ± 14.65 (376.5–493.5)	31	382.12 ± 20.20 (334–433)	29
	West African gray parrot	*Psittacus erithacus timneh*	335.755 ± 10.5 (296–317)	3	2745 ± 38 (236–312)	2
	Pesquet's parrot	*Psittrichas fulgidus*	406.45 ± 10.60 (378–434)	5	330	1
	Thick-billed parrot	*Rhynchopsitta pachyrhyncha*	350	1	360	1
	Meyer's parrot	*Poicephalus meyeri*	122.5 ± 7.5 (115–130)	2	–	
	Vasa parrot	*Coracopsis nigra*	433	1	273	1
	Black crowned parrot (black-headed caique)	*Pionites melanocephala*	145.25 ± 4.89 (140.5–154)	5	140.50 ± 4.5 (136–145)	2
	Orange-bellied Senegal parrot	*Poicephalus senegalus*	137.83 ± 3.07 (124–150)	16	133.33 ± 3.33 (130–140)	6
	Hawk-headed parrot	*Deroptyus accipitrinus*	268 ± 22.04 (235–310)	3		
	Blue-headed parrot	*Pionus menstruus*	216.5 ± 5.5 (211–222)	2	208.8 ± 8.95 (178–232)	5
	Red fronted parrot (Jardine's parrot)	*Poicephalus gulielmi*	202		1805 ± 4.16 (172–186)	3
	Eastern rosella	*Platycercus eximius*	–	800	1	

Continued overleaf

Continued

Order	Species	Scientific name	Male (g)	n	Female (g)	n
	Dusky lory	*Pseudeos fuscata*	144 ± 9.94 (141.15–155)	5	1465 ± 4 (142–150)	2
	Red lory	*Eos bornea*	169.5 ± 12.61 (154–193.5)	5	1625 ± 2 (160–164)	3
	Yellow-streaked lory	*Chalcopsitta scintillata*	250	1	200	1
	Black lory	*Chalcopsitta atra*	2295 ± 13 (216–242)	2	222.5 ± 4.1 (210–228)	4
	Brown lory	*Chalcopsitta duivenbodei*	212	1	1805 ± 9.4 (154–198)	4
	Black-capped lory	*Lorius lory*	–		192	1
	Chattering lory	*Lorius garrulus*	1705 ± 26 (144–196)	6	1715 ± 8.80 (142–186)	5
	Rainbow lorikeet	*Trichoglossus haematodus*	141 ± 13.68 (118–171)	6	108.33 ± 14.24 (80–125)	3
	Kea	*Nestor notabilis*	820	1	705 ± 5 (700–710)	2
	Sun conure	*Aratinga solstitialis*	103.61 ± 2.51 (90–120)	23	102.70 ± 4.38 (94–115)	15
	Red-fronted conure	*Aratinga wagleri*	275	1	230 ± 10 (220–240)	2
	Blue-crowned conure	*Aratinga acuticaudata*	183 ± 13.53 (155–220)	5	185	1
	Golden conure (Queen of Bavaria conure)	*Aratinga guarouba*	242.08 ± 3.96 (225–250)	7	246.5 ± 16.71 (222–272.5)	5
	Nanday conure	*Nandayus nenday*	135 ± 5 (130–140)	2	120 ± 5 (115–125)	2
	Slender-billed conure	*Enicognathus leptorhynchus*	280 ± 20 (260–300)	2	258.33 ± 8.3 (250–275)	3
	Maroon-tailed conure	*Pyrrhura melanura*	80	2	72.5 ± 7.5 (65–80)	2
	Peach-fronted conure	*Aratinga aurea*	91.5 ± 11.5 (80–103)	2	–	
	Dusky-headed conure	*Aratinga weddellii*	92	1	88 ± 2 (86–90)	2
	Patagonian conure	*Cyanoliseus patagonus*	258 ± 11.78 (215–275)	5	254.23 ± 3.83 (225–275)	13
	Red-masked conure	*Aratinga erythrogenys*	216.66 ± 24.06 (170–250)	3	170	1
	White eyed conure	*Aratinga leucophthalmus*	148.335 ± 5.8 (142–160)	3	130.33 ± 4.25 (122–136)	3
	Yellow fronted conure	*Cyanoramphus auriceps*	645 ± 4.16 (56–70)	3	–	
	Red fronted parakeet	*Cyanoramphus novaezelandiae*	120	1	130	1
	Olive headed lorikeet	*Trichoglossus euteles*	71.335 ± 1.33 (70–74)	3	72	1
Sphenisciformes	Rockhopper penguin	*Eudyptes crestatus*	2588.88 ± 153.15 (1800–3200)	9	2656 ± 128.67 (1800–3100)	10
	Blackfooted penguin	*Spheniscus demersus*	3176.19 ± 137.86 (2400–5200)	21	2952.52 ± 115.92 (2200–4000)	22
	Humboldt penguin	*Spheniscus humboldti*	4600 ± 155.45 (4000–5250)	9	3975 ± 173.56 (3200–4250)	6
	Gentoo penguin	*Pygoscelis papua*	6466.66 ± 291.74 (5600–7500)	6	5733.33 ± 258.19 (4500–6800)	9
	King penguin	*Aptenodytes patagonicus*	11433.33 ± 279.05 (9400–13200)	15	11076.92 ± 337.44 (9100–14100)	13
	Jackass penguin (black-footed)	*Spheniscus demersus*	3741.66 ± 232.88 (3000–4650)	6	3036 ± 249.99 (2500–3900)	5
Strigiformes	European eagle owl	*Bubo bubo bubo*	1933.33 ± 151.47 (1600–2600)	6	2550 ± 222 (1600–3600)	8
	African spotted eagle owl	*Bubo africanus*	–		800	1

Continued

Continued

Order	Species	Scientific name	Male (g)	n	Female (g)	n
	Snowy owl	*Nyctea scandiaca*	700	1	800	1
	Tawny owl	*Strix aluco*	385.14 ± 15.72 (330–451)	7	442.5 ± 10.14 (400–465)	6
	Boobook owl	*Ninox novaeseelandiae*	275	1	268.75 ± 19.40 (230–320)	4
	Little owl	*Athene noctua*	–	150	1	
	Spectacled owl	*Pulsatrix perspicillata*	800	1	825 ± 25	2
	Long-eared owl	*Asio otus*	210	2	325	1
	Turcmenian eagle owl	*Bubo bubo turcomanus*	–		2820 ± 20 (2800–2840)	2
	Brown fish owl	*Bubo zeylonensis*	1400	1	1400	2
	Barn owl	*Tyto alba*	307.5 ± 17.5 (290–325)	2	350 ± 17.07 (310–405)	6
	Tengmalm's owl	*Aegolius funereus*	145 ± 10 (135–155)	2	155	1
	Dusky eagle owl	*Bubo coromandus*	–	1500	1	
	Indian eagle owl	*Bubo bengalensis*	–	1250	1	
	Rusty barred owl	*Strix hylophila*	350	1	350	1
	Great horned owl	*Bubo virginianus*	–		1970 ± 320 (1650–2290)	2
	Fraser's eagle owl	*Bubo poensis vosseleri*	1000	1	1200	1
	Javan fish owl	*Bubo ketupu ketupu*	1200	1	1216.66 ± 116.66 (1100–1400)	3
	Vermiculated fishing owl	*Scotopelia bouvieri*	975	1	975	1
	Abyssinian spotted eagle owl	*Bubo africanus cinerascens*	540	1	700	1
	Short-eared owl	*Asio flammeus*	325	1	340	1
	White-faced scops owl	*Otus leucotis*	180	1	197.5 ± 7.5 (190–205)	2
	African wood owl	*Strix woodfordii*	–		260	1

Mean ± standard error of mean (minimum–maximum).

The bodyweights of most species presented in the above table were obtained mainly at zoological collections in the UK and the Middle East during 1982–2005 after sex determination using endoscopy (J. Samour, unpublished data) with the exception of the following: all **bustards** (Gruiformes), T. A. Bailey and J. Naldo, National Avian Research Centre, Abu Dhabi, United Arab Emirates, unpublished data; the **saker** and **peregrine falcon** (Falconiformes), J. Samour, unpublished data; the **Indian house crow**, Cooper JE (1996) Health studies in the Indian house crow (*Corvus splendens*). *Avian Pathology* **25:** 381–386; and all **Anseriformes**, extracted and modified from: Olsen JH (1994) Anseriformes. In: Ritchie BW, Harrison GJ, Harrison LR (eds) *Avian Medicine: Principles and Application*, pp. 1237–1275. Wingers Publishing, Lake Worth, FL; Coles BH (1985) *Avian Medicine and Surgery*, Blackwell Science, Oxford; Hayes MB (1984) *Rehabilitation Guidebook for Birds and Mammals*. Brukner Nature Center, Dayton, OH; Todd FS (1979) *Waterfowl: Ducks, Geese and Swans of the World*. Sea World Press, San Diego, CA.

All scientific names were obtained from: Howard R, Moore A (1991) *A Complete Checklist of the Birds of the World*, 2nd edn. Academic Press, San Diego, CA.

Appendix 2

Hematology reference values

Merle M. Apo

Hematology values for selected Gruiformes

Species	Kori bustard* n = 28	Houbara bustard† n = 14	Heuglin's bustard‡ n = 5	Black bustard‡ n = 4	Buff-crested bustard§ n = 14	White-bellied bustard‡ n = 3
Scientific name	*Ardeotis kori*	*Chlamydotis undulata*	*Neotis heuglinii*	*Eupodotis afra*	*Eupodotis ruficrista*	*Eupodotis senegalensis*
RBC × 10^{12}/l	2.30 ± 0.06 (1.74–2.95)	2.53 ± 0.09 (1.95–3.15)	2.18 ± 0.05 (2.05–2.35)	2.68 ± 0.18 (2.12–2.9)	2.89 ± 0.19 (2.00–4.27)	2.31 ± 0.08 (2.16–2.47)
HB g/dl	14.10 ± 0.16 (11.9–15.9)	14.72 ± 0.14 (13.7–15.7)	12.48 ± 0.37 (11.1–13.3)	14.62 ± 0.67 (13.6–16.6)	17.62 ± 0.52 (15.50–22.20)	15.23 ± 0.17 (14.9–15.5)
Hct l/l	0.47 ± 0.05 (0.395–0.525)	0.47 ± 0.08 (0.42–0.51)	0.43 ± 0.005 (0.42–0.45)	0.44 ± 0.01 (0.42–0.49)	0.47 ± 0.01 (0.40–0.50)	0.47 ± 0.01 (0.45–0.50)
MCV fl	208.5 ± 5.1 (161.9–275.4)	189.7 ± 8.85 (146.3–259.1)	198.14 ± 3.85 (185.1–206.3)	170.17 ± 14.04 (147.1–207.5)	172.85 ± 9.36 (105.39–220.00)	205.7 ± 8.3 (190.2–218.6)
MCH pg	62.4 ± 1.6 (48.0–84.6)	58.9 ± 2.44 (46.6–74.3)	57.3 ± 2.57 (49.3–64.8)	55.32 ± 4.26 (47.1–65.5)	65.21 ± 4.46 (40.71–97.50)	66.03 ± 3.06 (60.3–70.8)
MCHC g/dl	30.0 ± 0.4 (29.7–34.9)	31.16 ± 0.54 (26.1–34.1)	28.88 ± 1.15 (24.6–31.6)	32.52 ± 0.46 (31.5–33.5)	37.63 ± 1.18 (31.31–47.56)	32.1 ± 1.0 (30.6–34)
WBC × 10^9/l	7.29 ± 0.42 (3.05–12.85)	5.81 ± 0.29 (4.25–7.6)	4.24 ± 0.3 (3.41–5.2)	7.85 ± 2.22 (3.81–13.8)	5.66 ± 0.38 (4.00–9.80)	6.26 ± 0.7 (5.2–7.6)
Heterophils × 10^9/l	3.98 ± 0.32 (0.95–9.25)	3.64 ± 0.24 (1.99–4.82)	1.55 ± 0.17 (1.34–2.25)	2.92 ± 0.53 (1.52–4.21)	3.32 ± 0.32 (1.44–5.88)	2.73 ± 0.75 (1.92–4.25)
Lympho-cytes × 10^9/l	2.21 ± 0.24 (0.41–5.45)	1.84 ± 0.15 (0.97–3.24)	1.91 ± 0.22 (1.33–2.44)	3.66 ± 1.56 (1.48–8.14)	1.11 ± 0.20 (0.31–3.03)	2.51 ± 0.17 (2.18–2.73)
Monocytes × 10^9/l	0.60 ± 0.07 (0.0–1.57)	0.15 ± 0.03 (0.0–0.42)	0.41 ± 0.1 (0.07–0.72)	0.68 ± 0.23 (0.42–1.38)	0.42 ± 0.10 (0.04–1.30)	0.45 ± 0.14 (0.22–0.72)
Eosinophils × 10^9/l	0.35 ± 0.05 (0.0–1.15)	0.07 ± 0.01 (0.0–0.23)	0.12 ± 0.02 (0.04–0.208)	0.17 ± 0.08 (0.07–0.41)	0.24 ± 0.04 (0.00–0.62)	0.24 ± 0.09 (0.06–0.36)
Basophils × 10^9/l	0.20 ± 0.03 (0.0–0.80)	0.07 ± 0.02 (0.0–0.26)	0.13 ± 0.089 (0.0–0.46)	0.4 ± 0.09 (0.26–0.69)	0.44 ± 0.08 (0.10–1.23)	0.31 ± 0.13 (0.07–0.54)
Thrombo-cytes × 10^9/l	5.5 ± 0.7 (1.49–18.0)	6.82 ± 0.59 (2.76–9.88)	5.11 ± 0.45 (3.85–6.57)	10.48 ± 2.99 (4.68–18.49)	8.81 ± 1.04 (4.00–15.00)	5.99 ± 2.9 (3.06–11.8)
Fibrinogen g/l	2.42 ± 0.10 (1.42–4.5)	1.87 ± 0.26 (0.8–4.8)	1.71 ± 0.16 (1.12–2.11)	1.38 ± 0.19 (0.8–1.63)	1.7 ± 0.23 (0.66–4.31)	2.0 ± 0.15 (1.7–2.19)

Mean ± standard error of mean (minimum–maximum)

* Howlett JC, Samour JH, D'Aloia M-A, Bailey TA, Naldo J (1995) Normal haematology of captive adult kori bustards (*Ardeotis kori*). *Comparative Haematology International* **5**: 102–105.

† Samour JH, Howlett JC, Hart MG *et al.* (1994) Normal haematology of the houbara bustard (*Chlamydotis undulata macqueenii*). *Comparative Haematology International* **4**: 198–202.

‡ D'Aloia M-A, Samour JH, Bailey TA *et al.* (1996) Normal haematology of the white-bellied (*Eupodotis senegalensis*), little black (*Eupodotis afra*) and Heuglin's (*Neotis heuglinii*) bustards. *Comparative Haematology International* **6**: 46–49.

§ D'Aloia M-A, Howlett JC, Samour JH *et al.* (1995) Normal haematology and age-related findings in the buff-crested bustard (*Eupodotis ruficrista*). *Comparative Haematology International* **5**: 10–12.

Hematology values for selected Falconiformes

Species	Turkey vulture n = 10	Egyptian vulture n = 4	Buzzard n = 6	Golden eagle n = 4	Caracara n = 9	Secretary bird n = 4
Scientific name	Cathartes aura	Neophron percnopterus	Buteo buteo	Aquila chrysaetos	Polyborus plancus	Sagittarius serpentarius
RBC × 10¹²/l	2.7 (2.4–2.9)*	2.3 (1.9–2.6)	2.4 (2.2–2.7)	2.4 (1.9–2.7)	2.8 (2.5–3.3)	2.18 (2.0–2.3)
HB g/dl	16.3 (15.7–17.3)	14.8 (13.3–16.5)	12.9 (11.6–14.6)	13.8 (12.1–15.2)	16.2 (13.1–20.6)	16.7 (15.2–18.6)
Hct l/l	0.54 (0.51–0.58)	0.43 (0.37–0.46)	0.38 (0.34–0.42)	0.41 (0.35–0.47)	0.46 (0.38–0.59)	0.46 (0.42–0.50)
MCV fl	204 (194–224)	190 (183–206)	159 (151–171)	174 (160–184)	165 (149–173)	208 (201–216)
MCH pg	61.7 (58.6–65.0)	67.7 (65.2–72.9)	53.8 (48.8–57.5)	58.9 (56.3–62.7)	57.8 (51.6–62.4)	76.7 (73.4–80.8)
MCHC g/dl	30.2 (28.6–32.0)	35.2 (35.0–35.5)	33.9 (31.4–36.0)	34.0 (32.3–35.9)	35.2 (34.0–36.0)	36.9 (35.3–37.6)
WBC × 10⁹/l	20.1 (10.5–31.9)	7.6 (4.7–10.6)	9.1 (4.6–13.9)	13.1 (11.7–14.7)	6.8 (3.3–11.6)	8.1 (6.8–10.0)
Heterophils × 10⁹/l	11.8 (6.7–19.8)	4.0 (1.2–5.5)	5.5 (2.3–8.8)	10.4 (9.5–12.7)	4.2 (0.6–5.9)	5.3 (3.0–9.0)
Lymphocytes × 10⁹/l	3.3 (0.8–5.6)	2.5 (1.5–3.4)	1.7 (1.1–2.4)	2.2 (1.6–3.2)	2.4 (0.9–5.6)	2.4 (0.8–4.2)
Monocytes × 10⁹/l	(0.0–0.4)	(0.0–0.4)	0	0	(0.0–0.6)	(0.0–0.4)
Eosinophils × 10⁹/l	(1.5–7.5)	(0.3–1.4)	(0.1–3.1)	(0.2–0.6)	(0.0–0.3)	(0.0–0.2)
Basophils × 10⁹/l	(0.0–2.3)	0	(0.0–0.6)	(0.0–0.2)	(0.0–0.3)	(0.0–0.4)
Thrombocytes × 10⁹/l	14 (7–22)	13 (6–15)	27 (18–36)	14 (4–21)	27 (18–35)	9 (7–10)
Fibrinogen g/l	–	1.6 (1.0–1.9)	2.3 (1.3–3.3)	2.9 (2.0–4.1)	2.4 (1.2–3.8)	2.7 (2.0–3.3)

Mean ± standard error of mean (minimum–maximum)
* Range.
Source: Hawkey CM, Samour JH (1988) The value of clinical hematology in exotic birds. In: Jacobson ER, Kollias GV Jr (eds) *Exotic Animals: Contemporary Issues in Small Animal Practice*, pp. 109–141. Churchill Livingstone, New York.

Hematology values for selected Falconiformes (*continued*)

Species	Harris hawk n = 53	Ferruginous hawk n = 18	Red tailed hawk n = 15	Northern goshawk n = 43	Tawny eagle n = 29
Scientific name	Parabuteo unicinctus	Buteo regalis	Buteo jamaicensis	Accipiter gentilis	Aquila rapax
RBC × 10¹²/l	2.13–2.76*	2.41–3.59	2.2–3.35	2.6–3.48	2.32–2.83
HB g/dl	10.1–16.7	10.7–16.6	12.3–17.5	12.1–17.7	10.8–17.5
Hct l/l	0.32–0.44	0.37–0.48	0.35–0.53	0.43–0.53	0.37–0.47
MCV fl	147–163	150–178	157–168	141–156	163–188
MCH pg	45.4–51.1	46–57.4	43–50.4	44.5–51.6	54–62
MCHC g/dl	30.1–33.0	297–345	312–350	305–343	296–360
WBC × 10⁹/l	4.8–10	4.5–6.8	3.4–7.5	4–11	5–9.5
Heterophils × 10⁹/l	2.3–6.71	1.89–3.76	1.9–3.5	3.5–6.97	3.58–6.45
Lymphocytes × 10⁹/l	0.6–2.36	0.78–1.74	1.3–1.1	1.38–1.93	0.51–2.72
Monocytes × 10⁹/l	0.2–1.49	0.24–1.5	0.12–1.2	0–0.1	0.2–1.07
Eosinophils × 10⁹/l	0–0.75	0.3–0.7	0.1–0.9	0–0.65	0.3–2.1
Basophils × 10⁹/l	0–1.55	0.15–0.6	0–0.5	0–0.35	0–0.4
Thrombocytes × 10⁹/l	10–59	8–47	4–33	15–35	19–25
Fibrinogen g/l	< 4.3	< 3.5	< 3	< 3.5	< 3.5

* Range
Source: Jennings IB (1996) Haematology. In: Beynon PH, Forbes NA, Harcourt-Brown NH (1996) *Manual of Raptors, Pigeons and Waterfowl*, pp 68–78. British Small Animal Veterinary Association, Cheltenham.

Hematology values for selected Falconiformes (*continued*)

Species	Saker falcon* n = 25	Peregrine falcon† n = 48	Gyrfalcon‡ n = 187	Lanner falcon§ n = 42	Laggar falcon§ n = 13	Merlin§ n = 33
Scientific name	*Falco cherrug*	*Falco peregrinus*	*Falco rusticolus*	*Falco biarmicus*	*Falco jugger*	*Falco columbarius*
RBC × 10^{12}/l	2.65 ± 0.08 (2.05–3.90)	3.49 ± 0.21 (2.76–4.05)	3.23 ± 0.28	2.63–3.98	2.65–3.63	2.85–4.1
HB g/dl	15.93 ± 0.38 (13.3–21.2)	14.82 ± 1.32 (11.6–19.1)	15.00 ± 1.33	12.2–17.1	12.8–16.3	13.2–17.9
Hct l/l	0.47 ± 0.59 (0.42–0.53)	0.40 ± 0.38 (0.26–0.58)	0.45 ± 0.04	0.37–0.53	0.39–0.51	0.39–0.51
MCV fl	183.16 ± 3.84 (135.8–219.5)	117.51 ± 7.70 (100.8–176.0)	139.32 ± 5.44	127–150	123–145	105–130
MCH pg	60.74 ± 1.42 (50.62–78.94)	–	45.78 ± 1.84	42.3–48.8	38–47.7	36–45.9
MCHC g/dl	33.28 ± 0.63 (28.33–40)	–	–	317–353	312–350	340–360
WBC × 10^9/l	5.7 ± 0.31 (2.8–8.4)	12.56 ± 3.06 (7.6–21.2)	8.71 ± 3.80	3.5–11	5–9	4–9.5
Heterophils × 10^9/l	4.14 ± 0.24 (2.18–5.96)	4.52 ± 1.2 (1.38–7.53)	58.53 ± 12.90%	1.65–8.8	3.5–6.57	3.2–4.03
Lymphocytes × 10^9/l	1.33 ± 0.09 (0.52–2.29)	5.52 ± 1.36 (1.75–7.53)	37.54 ± 12.98%	1.1–5.13	1.7–4	1.2–1.56
Monocytes × 10^9/l	0.21 ± 0.03 (0.04–0.64)	0.25 ± 0.03 (0.12–0.62)	3.72 ± 2.50%	0–0.9	0–0.85	0–0.5
Eosinophils × 10^9/l	0	2.3 ± 0.9 (1–4.77)	0.20%	0–0.2	0–0.2	0–0.15
Basophils × 10^9/l	0.08 ± 0.01 (0–0.32)	–	0.0	0–0.45	0.17–0.83	0–0.15
Thrombocytes × 10^9/l	0.41 ± 0.03 (0.17–0.76)	2.97 ± 1.2 (1.25–7.15)	–	5–40	12–35	–
Fibrinogen g/l	2.82 ± 0.14 (1.78–4.7)	–	–	< 4	< 4	< 4

* Source: Samour JH, D'Aloia M-A, Howlett JC (1996) Normal haematology of captive saker falcons (*Falco cherrug*). *Comparative Haematology International* **6**: 50–52.

† Source: Dötlinger HS, Bird DM (1995) Haematological parameters in captive peregrine falcons (*Falco peregrinus*). In: *Falco Newsletter 4*, Middle East Falcon Research Group, National Avian Research Centre, United Arab Emirates.

‡ Mean ± SD. Source: Wernery *et al.* (2004) *Colour Atlas of Falcon Medicine*, pp. 12–36. Schlütersche, Hannover.

§ Range. Source: Jennings IB (1996) Haematology. In: Beynon PH, Forbes NA, Harcourt-Brown NH (1996) *Manual of Raptors, Pigeons and Waterfowl*, pp 68–78. British Small Animal Veterinary Association, Cheltenham.

Hematology values for selected Pelicaniformes

Species	American white pelican *n* = 10	Brown pelican *n* = 5
Scientific name	*Pelecanus erythrorhynchos*	*Pelecanus occidentalis*
RBC × 10^{12}/l	2.3 ± 0.3 (1.9–2.7)	2.7 (2.6–2.8)
HB g/dl	13.0 ± 1.8 (9.8–16.6)	14.5 (14.3–14.8)
Hct l/l	0.39 ± 0.04 (0.33–0.45)	0.46 (0.43–0.49)
MCV fl	166 ± 9 (152–182)	168 (166–173)
MCH pg	52.3 ± 2.9 (46.0–59.3)	53.4 (51.2–56.8)
MCHC g/dl	32.6 ± 2.0 (28.4–35.2)	31.7 (30.4–32.9)
WBC × 10^9/l	9.5 ± 3.4 (5.0–15.0)	11.9 (6.6–19.4)
Heterophils × 10^9/l	7.2 ± 3.0 (4.2–9.3)	6.7 (4.0–9.5)
Lymphocytes × 10^9/l	3.4 ± 0.7 (2.7–4.5)	4.0 (2.5–7.0)
Monocytes × 10^9/l	(0.0–0.2)	(0.0–0.20)
Eosinophils × 10^9/l	(0.0–0.3)	(0.0–0.2)
Basophils × 10^9/l	(0.1–1.6)	(0.0–0.2)
Thrombocytes × 10^9/l	29 ± 6 (21–38)	(17–38)
Fibrinogen g/l	0.9 ± 0.4 (0.3–1.5)	2.9 (2.6–3.1)

Mean ± standard error of mean (minimum–maximum)
Source: Hawkey CM, Samour JH (1988) The value of clinical hematology in exotic birds. In: Jacobson ER, Kollias GV Jr (eds) *Exotic Animals: Contemporary Issues in Small Animal Practice*, pp. 109–141. Churchill Livingstone, London.

Hematology values for selected Spheniciformes

Species	Gentoo penguin *n* = 9–20	King penguin *n* = 6–7	Rockhopper penguin *n* = 11–17	Black-footed penguin *n* = 12–42	Humboldt penguin *n* = 10–24
Scientific name	*Pygoscelis papua*	*Aptenodytes patagonica*	*Eudyptes crestatus*	*Spheniscus demersus*	*Spheniscus humboldti*
RBC × 10^{12}/l	1.61 ± 0.14 (1.39–1.76)	1.58 ± 0.30 (1.18–2.02)	1.94 ± 0.20 (1.69–2.30)	1.74 ± 0.20 (1.32–2.12)	2.05 ± 0.31 (1.46–2.46)
HB g/dl	15.7 ± 1.9 (12.7–19.2)	16.9 ± 4.2 (10.2–22.0)	17.9 ± 1.1 (16.1–19.2)	16.8 ± 1.6 (13.4–19.5)	17.6 ± 2.5 (14.5–21.3)
Hct l/l	0.45 ± 0.04 (0.37–0.51)	0.45 ± 0.08 (0.32–0.55)	0.46 ± 0.03 (0.41–0.50)	0.44 ± 0.04 (0.36–0.51)	0.48 ± 0.04 (0.41–0.54)
MCV fl	258 ± 31 (215–301)	288 ± 18 (270–301)	234 ± 18 (210–267)	254 ± 11 (232–273)	228 ± 17 (194–267)
MCH pg	95.0 ± 8.8 (81.4–110.5)	108.0 ± 12.5 (86.4–120.9)	91.7 ± 7.7 (80.3–104.0)	95.1 ± 4.5 (87.2–104.3)	85.3 ± 5.2 (76.0–94.3)
MCHC g/dl	37.7 ± 1.7 (34.8–40.0)	37.5 ± 3.8 (31.9–41.5)	39.1 ± 0.8 (37.5–40.0)	37.8 ± 1.4 (35.4–40.0)	38.0 ± 1.7 (35.0–40.6)
WBC × 10^9/l	8.2 ± 4.1 (3.2–16.1)	4.3 ± 1.4 (2.8–6.7)	4.7 ± 1.4 (3.0–7.7)	9.3 ± 3.5 (3.5–16.3)	15.9 ± 5.1 (5.6–25.8)
Heterophils × 10^9/l	3.9 ± 1.3 (2.2–6.0)	2.3 ± 1.0 (1.4–3.9)	3.6 ± 1.1 (1.5–5.2)	8.1 ± 2.3 (5.0–12.3)	11.9 ± 4.5 (4.1–17.9)
Lymphocytes × 10^9/l	2.2 ± 1.0 (0.6–4.8)	2.0 ± 0.6 (1.3–2.8)	1.6 ± 0.8 (0.3–2.5)	3.1 ± 1.4 0.8–5.2	2.7 ± 1.8 (1.0–5.0)
Monocytes × 10^9/l	0	0	< 0.1 (0.0–0.1)	0	< 0.5 (0.0–0.5)
Eosinophils × 10^9/l	0	0	< 0.3 (0.0–0.3)	< 0.1 (0.0–0.2)	< 0.2 (0.0–0.02)
Basophils × 10^9/l	0	0	< 0.1 (0.0–0.1)	< 0.1 (0.0–0.3)	< 0.5 (0.0–0.5)
Thrombocytes × 10^9/l	–	–	7.3 ± 4.2 (4–15)	11 ± 5 (5–19)	9.5 ± 4.9 (7–20)
Fibrinogen g/l	3.2 ± 0.8 (2.1–4.2)	2.4	2.9 ± 0.4 (2.2–2.7)	2.9 ± 0.4 (2.2–3.7)	3.5 ± 0.9 (2.0–5.3)

Mean ± standard error of mean (minimum–maximum)
Source: Hawkey CM, Samour JH (1988) The value of clinical hematology in exotic birds. In: Jacobson ER, Kollias GV Jr (eds) *Exotic Animals: Contemporary Issues in Small Animal Practice*, pp. 109–141. Churchill Livingstone, New York.

Hematology values for selected Ciconiiformes

Species	Rosy flamingo n = 36	Chilean flamingo n = 24	Lesser flamingo n = 10	Greater flamingo n = 9
Scientific name	*Phoenicopterus ruber ruber*	*Phoenicopterus chilensis*	*Phoeniconaias minor*	*Phoenicopterus rube*
RBC × 10^{12}/l	2.6 ± 0.2 (2.3–3.0)	2.7 ± 0.2 (2.4–3.0)	2.7 ± 0.1 (2.3–2.9)	2.6 (2.3–2.8)
HB g/dl	17.1 ± 1.4 (13.8–19.1)	16.2 ± 1.1 (14.1–18.1)	16.8 ± 1.6 (15.2–19.5)	17.3 (15.9–19.6)
Hct l/l	0.47 ± 0.04 (0.40–0.54)	0.46 ± 0.03 (0.41–0.51)	0.51 ± 0.03 (0.46–0.54)	0.50 (0.47–0.57)
MCV fl	184 ± 7 (168–196)	171 ± 6 (161–183)	188 ± 6 (179–195)	193 (170–207)
MCH pg	66.4 ± 4.0 (59.0–73.5)	60.6 ± 2.1 (57.3–64.8)	62.0 ± 5.4 (55.4–70.4)	66.2 (57.6–70.0)
MCHC g/dl	35.9 ± 2.3 (31.7–39.8)	35.6 ± 0.9 (33.3–37.9)	33.0 ± 2.5 (30.8–37.5)	34.4 (33.5–35.2)
WBC × 10^9/l	5.1 ± 1.7 (2.4–8.7)	4.9 ± 2.5 (1.6–9.0)	61 ± 2.0 (3.8–8.5)	2.4 (0.9–3.4)
Heterophils × 10^9/l	2.4 ± 0.9 (1.0–4.4)	2.4 ± 1.7 (0.4–4.8)	4.6 ± 1.8 (1.7–6.9)	1.2 (0.2–3.0)
Lymphocytes × 10^9/l	1.6 ± 0.6 (0.7–3.0)	1.8 ± 0.6 (0.8–2.7)	1.2 ± 0.6 (0.5–2.4)	0.9 (0.4–1.6)
Monocytes × 10^9/l	(0.0–0.5)	0	(0.0–0.4)	(0.0–0.2)
Eosinophils × 10^9/l	(0.0–0.6)	(0.0–0.7)	0	(0.0–0.4)
Basophils × 10^9/l		(0.0–0.4)	(0.0–0.3)	(0.0–0.4)
Thrombocytes × 10^9/l	14 ± 6 (4–29)	15 ± 6 (6–33)	16 ± 8 (3–23)	4 (2–7)
Fibrinogen g/l	2.7 ± 0.6 (1.7–3.7)	2.3 ± 0.6 (1.3–3.6)	2.3 ± 0.4 (1.4–2.9)	2.6 (1.5–3.3)

Mean ± standard error of mean (minimum–maximum)
Source: Hawkey CM, Samour JH (1988) The value of clinical hematology in exotic birds. In: Jacobson ER, Kollias GV Jr (eds) *Exotic Animals: Contemporary Issues in Small Animal Practice*, pp. 109–141. Churchill Livingstone, New York.

Hematology values for selected Ciconiiformes (*continued*)

Species	Night heron n = 22	Marabou stork n = 8	White stork n = 16	Maquari stork n = 5	Australian white ibis n = 8	Scarlet ibis n = 15
Scientific name	*Nycticorax nycticorax*	*Leptoptilos crumeniferus*	*Ciconia ciconi*	*Ciconia maguari*	*Threskiornis m. molucca*	*Eudocimus ruber*
RBC × 10^{12}/l	2.6 ± 0.2 (2.3–2.9)	2.3 ± 0.1 (2.2–2.5)	2.4 ± 0.1 (2.1–2.7)	2.3 (2.2–2.7)	3.0 ± 0.2 (2.6–3.3)	3.2 ± 0.3 (2.6–3.8)
HB g/dl	15.1 ± 1.4 (12.9–17.8)	15.8 ± 0.9 (14.8–17.1)	15.9 ± 1.1 (14.4–17.7)	16.1 (13.8–17.8)	18.2 ± 1.8 (14.6–19.5)	15.3 ± 1.0 (13.3–17.1)
Hct l/l	0.45 ± 0.03 (0.40–0.50)	0.47 ± 0.04 (0.42–0.52)	0.45 ± 0.03 (0.41–0.48)	0.46 (0.42–0.50)	0.48 ± 0.04 (0.39–0.51)	0.49 ± 0.05 (0.41–0.53)
MCV fl	178 ± 8 (162–194)	202 ± 12 (175–212)	189 ± 6 (172–195)	195 (186–210)	159 ± 7 (150–170)	153 ± 7 (142–164)
MCH pg	59.5 ± 3.4 (53.2–64.0)	67.3 ± 3.4 (62.1–70.9)	67.2 ± 2.9 (60.2–69.9)	69.0 (61.3–75.7)	60.5 ± 3.6 (55.5–67.2)	48.8 ± 2.9 (45.2–53.4)
MCHC g/dl	33.6 ± 1.7 (30.3–35.8)	33.5 ± 1.8 (31.1–35.9)	35.3 ± 1.5 (31.0–36.9)	35.3 (32.9–36.2)	38.1 ± 1.1 (36.8–39.4)	31.5 ± 1.3 (29.2–33.7)
WBC × 10^9/l	9.9 ± 2.8 (5.8–15.2)	19.5 ± 4.1 (14.4–23.3)	10.8 ± 3.1 (7.0–14.3)	9.8 (7.2–15.5)	6.7 ± 2.8 (2.1–10.0)	7.1 ± 3.2 (2.6–12.6)
Heterophils × 10^9/l	7.1 ± 2.4 (3.7–11.5)	12.7 ± 4.1 (7.6–18.7)	9.2 ± 3.2 (5.1–14.9)	5.9 (2.0–11.5)	5.7 ± 2.6 (1.4–8.8)	4.5 ± 2.5 (1.6–8.5)
Lymphocytes × 10^9/l	2.5 ± 0.9 (1.4–4.2)	4.1 ± 0.9 (2.5–5.3)	0.8 ± 0.4 (0.2–1.6)	2.6 (1.4–3.3)	1.0 ± 0.3 (0.5–1.5)	2.0 ± 0.7 (0.8–3.0)
Monocytes × 10^9/l	(0.0–0.9)	(0.0–2.3)	(0.0–0.3)	(0.0–0.7)	0	0
Eosinophils × 10^9/l	(0.0–1.1)	(0.2–4.1)	(0.0–0.7)	(0.7–2.2)	(0.0–0.3)	(0.0–0.8)
Basophils × 10^9/l	0	(0.0–0.7)	(0.0–0.5)	(0.0–0.8)	(0.0–0.3)	(0.0–0.7)
Thrombocytes × 10^9/l	16 ± 4 (8–5)	16 ± 3 (12–19)	19 ± 8 (8–32)	10 (8–11)	33 ± 12 (18–48)	22 ± 8 (11–35)
Fibrinogen g/l	1.8 ± 0.6 (1.1–3.1)	3.2 ± 0.6 (2.6–4.4)	2.3 ± 0.4 (1.7–3.2)	1.7 (1.3–2.1)	2.3 ± 0.3 (1.9–2.7)	2.6 ± 0.6 (1.9–3.7)

Mean ± standard error of mean (minimum–maximum)
Source: Hawkey CM, Samour JH (1988) The value of clinical hematology in exotic birds. In: Jacobson ER, Kollias GV Jr (eds) *Exotic Animals: Contemporary Issues in Small Animal Practice*, pp. 109–141. Churchill Livingstone, New York.

Hematology values for selected Gruiformes

Species	Manchurian crane n = 11	Sarus crane n = 9	Stanley crane n = 8	Crowned crane n = 11–22	Demoiselle crane n = 11
Scientific name	*Grus japonensis*	*Grus antigone*	*Anthropoides paradisea*	*Balearica regulorum*	*Anthropoides virgo*
RBC × 10¹²/l	2.2 ± 0.3 (1.9–2.7)	2.2 (2.0–2.5)	2.4 (2.2–2.7)	2.8 ± 0.3 (2.4–3.1)	2.7 ± 0.2 (2.3–3.0)
HB g/dl	14.3 ± 1.3 (12.6–16.8)	15.5 (13.8–17.7)	15.0 (13.4–16.8)	15.6 ± 1.9 (11.9–18.8)	14.9 ± 1.0 (13.1–16.2)
Hct l/l	0.42 ± 0.04 (0.38–0.50)	0.45 (0.42–0.49)	0.42 (0.39–0.46)	0.47 ± 0.03 (0.44–0.52)	0.43 ± 1.1 (0.39–0.47)
MCV fl	191 ± 9 (180–204)	203 (196–209)	174 (158–190)	171 ± 7 (156–182)	162 ± 7 (154–172)
MCH pg	64.8 ± 4.5 (56.0–68.8)	69.6 (60.0–77.0)	61.9 (57.3–65.1)	64.3 ± 3.0 (59.8–70.2)	55.6 ± 2.4 (51.5–60.0)
MCHC g/dl	34.3 ± 1.5 (32.7–37.2)	34.5 (30.6–37.0)	35.5 (33.1–39.5)	36.2 ± 2.3 (34.5–39.2)	34.3 ± 1.1 (32.6–36.2)
WBC × 10⁹/l	9.5 ± 1.9 (5.7–11.6)	9.4 (3.5–12.2)	9.1 (2.9–16.9)	11.1 ± 2.8 (6.3–15.6)	5.3 ± 1.7 (2.9–8.6)
Heterophils × 10⁹/l	6.7 ± 1.6 (4.5–9.3)	6.5 (1.4–9.5)	4.5 (1.0–10.0)	8.2 ± 3.0 (4.1–13.3)	3.8 ± 1.4 (1.7–6.6)
Lymphocytes × 10⁹/l	1.9 ± 0.8 (0.5–2.9)	2.1 (1.2–3.0)	2.5 (1.1–4.2)	1.6 ± 0.6 (0.6–2.7)	0.8 ± 0.4 (0.4–1.5)
Monocytes × 10⁹/l	0	(0.0–0.6)	(0.0–0.8)	(0.0–0.3)	(0.0–0.4)
Eosinophils × 10⁹/l	(0.0–1.2)	(0.1–0.7)	(0.4–2.1)	(0.0–1.3)	(0.0–0.9)
Basophils × 10⁹/l	(0.0–0.9)	(0.0–0.9)	(0.0–0.5)	(0.1–0.8)	(0.0–0.3)
Thrombocytes × 10⁹/l	13 ± 2 (11–15)	15 (11–21)	18 (11–27)	(5–18)	12 ± 10 (4–32)
Fibrinogen g/l	2.7 ± 0.4 (2.3–3.6)	2.7 (1.6–5.0)	3.5 (2.7–4.5)	–	2.5 ± 0.8 (1.4–3.7)

Mean ± standard error of mean (minimum–maximum)
Source: Hawkey CM, Samour JH (1988) The value of clinical hematology in exotic birds. In: Jacobson ER, Kollias GV Jr (eds) *Exotic Animals: Contemporary Issues in Small Animal Practice*, pp. 109–141. Churchill Livingstone, New York.

Hematology values for selected Strigiformes

Species	African eagle owl n = 6	European eagle n = 14	Spectacled owl n = 4	Tawny owl n = 14	Boobook owl n = 5	Barn owl n = 10
Scientific name	*Bubo africanus*	*Bubo bubo*	*Pulsatrix perspicillata*	*Strix aluco*	*Ninox novaeseelandiae*	*Tyto alba*
RBC × 10¹²/l	2.4 (2.1–2.8)	1.9 ± 0.2 (1.4–2.3)	1.6 (1.4–1.8)	2.5 ± 0.2 (2.0–2.9)	2.5 (2.4–2.9)	2.7 ± 0.3 (2.2–3.0)
HB g/dl	15.8 (13.9–19.9)	14.2 ± 1.5 (11.7–16.8)	14.2 (12.4–16.3)	14.6 ± 1.1 (12.9–16.4)	15.1 (14.4–15.9)	14.2 ± 1.5 (12.7–16.4)
Hct l/l	0.45 (0.41–0.53)	0.39 ± 0.04 (0.31–0.45)	0.42 (0.37–0.45)	0.40 ± 0.03 (0.36–0.47)	0.42 (0.40–0.45)	0.46 ± 0.03 (0.42–0.51)
MCV fl	189 (171–214)	207 ± 17 (178–239)	261 (245–267)	158 ± 9 (147–177)	172 (165–175)	176 ± 22 (145–216)
MCH pg	66.4 (58.9–76.2)	75.1 ± 8.1 (67.1–87.1)	87.8 (86.1–89.1)	56.8 ± 4.8 (49.8–66.6)	61.5 (60.8–61.6)	51.1 ± 5.7 (44.9–60.7)
MCHC g/dl	35.1 (33.9–36.6)	36.3 ± 2.0 (33.8–38.4)	33.7 (32.3–36.2)	36.3 ± 0.9 (34.9–38.0)	36.0 (34.8–37.3)	31.8 ± 2.2 (28.9–34.9)
WBC × 10⁹/l	6.2 (4.7–8.0)	10.8 ± 4.0 (5.3–18.6)	9.6 (6.9–11.1)	6.7 ± 3.3 (2.4–11.8)	6.4 (3.7–11.2)	16.6 ± 4.2 (11.5–22.3)
Heterophils × 10⁹/l	3.0 (1.3–5.2)	6.9 ± 3.2 (2.6–11.8)	4.9 (2.8–7.6)	3.4 ± 2.0 (1.1–7.2)	4.6 (2.3–9.1)	8.9 ± 3.0 (5.2–12.5)
Lymphocytes × 10⁹/l	2.3 (1.9–3.2)	3.8 ± 1.9 (1.9–6.7)	4.3 (2.7–7.3)	3.3 ± 1.4 (0.9–5.1)	1.4 (0.9–1.7)	5.0 ± 1.7 (2.5–7.5)
Monocytes × 10⁹/l	0	0	0	(0.0–0.3)	(0.0–0.5)	(0.0–1.0)
Eosinophils × 10⁹/l	(0.0–1.0)	(0.0–1.6)	(0.0–0.6)	(0.0–1.9)	(0.0–0.5)	(0.0–2.5)
Basophils × 10⁹/l	(0.0–0.6)	(0.0–0.6)	(0.0–0.4)	(0.0–0.9)	(0.0–0.2)	(0.0–0.9)
Thrombocytes × 10⁹/l	22 (14–29)	15 ± 3 (9–17)	18	17 ± 5 (10–24)	–	33 ± 15 (14–58)
Fibrinogen g/l	5.2 (3.6–7.7)	3.3 ± 0.9 (1.4–5.0)	7.0 (6.4–8.8)	3.6 ± 0.7 (2.6–5.3)	2.8 (1.6–3.8)	2.7 ± 0.5 (1.9–3.3)

Mean ± standard error of mean (minimum–maximum)
Source: Hawkey CM, Samour JH (1988) The value of clinical hematology in exotic birds. In: Jacobson ER, Kollias GV Jr (eds) *Exotic Animals: Contemporary Issues in Small Animal Practice*, pp. 109–141. Churchill Livingstone, New York.

Hematology values for selected Psittaciformes

Species	Bare-eyed cockatoo $n = 11$	Greater sulfur-crested cockatoo $n = 10–15$	Roseate cockatoo $n = 24–31$	African gray parrot $n = 11$	Amazon green parrot $n = 15$	Kea $n = 8$
Scientific name	Cacatua sanguinea	Cacatua galerita	Eolophus roseicapilus	Psittacus erithacus	Amazona sp.	Nestor notabilis
RBC × 10^{12}/l	2.9 ± 0.3 (2.5–3.4)	2.7 ± 0.2 (2.4–3.0)	3.6 ± 0.2 (3.1–3.9)	3.3 ± 0.2 (3.0–3.6)	2.9 ± 0.3 (2.6–3.5)	2.6 ± 0.3 (2.3–3.1)
HB g/dl	17.0 ± 1.2 (15.4–19.0)	15.7 ± 1.0 (13.8–17.1)	16.7 ± 1.3 (14.0–18.8)	15.5 ± 1.0 (14.2–17.0)	15.5 ± 1.3 (13.8–17.9)	13.4 ± 2.2 (10.6–16.9)
Hct l/l	0.53 ± 0.04 (0.47–0.60)	0.45 ± 0.03 (0.41–0.49)	0.54 ± 0.03 (0.49–0.60)	0.48 ± 0.03 (0.43–0.51)	0.51 ± 0.03 (0.44–0.56)	0.40 ± 0.04 (0.34–0.46)
MCV fl	188 ± 11 (181–200)	165 ± 9 (145–187)	149 ± 8 (136–164)	145 ± 6 (137–155)	173 ± 11 (156–194)	154 ± 17 (137–186)
MCH pg	60.5 ± 2.4 (56.6–63.1)	57.6 ± 2.1 (53.8–60.6)	45.9 ± 2.9 (43.5–51.3)	47.2 ± 3.0 (41.9–52.8)	52.6 ± 5.0 (44.7–58.6)	51.2 ± 9.0 (41.6–68.1)
MCHC g/dl	32.1 ± 2.4 (28.7–36.9)	34.9 ± 1.3 (33.3–37.6)	31.0 ± 1.7 (27.5–33.9)	32.5 ± 2.0 (28.9–34.0)	31.6 ± 2.8 (28.9–35.8)	33.2 ± 2.6 (30.4–37.0)
WBC × 10^9/l	7.3 ± 2.8 (4.2–11.8)	6.4 ± 2.9 (1.4–10.7)	6.3 ± 3.1 (1.6–11.9)	7.0 ± 2.3 (3.3–10.3)	4.6 ± 1.4 (2.3–6.5)	16.0 ± 3.8 (12.1–22.6)
Heterophils × 10^9/l	5.2 ± 2.7 (2.8–10.6)	3.7 ± 1.7 (1.0–6.6)	4.6 ± 2.5 (0.6–9.2)	4.9 ± 1.7 (1.8–7.3)	2.9 ± 0.7 (1.6–3.8)	13.8 ± 3.5 (9.4–20.1)
Lymphocytes × 10^9/l	1.5 ± 0.9 (0.5–3.9)	1.9 ± 0.8 (1.0–3.6)	1.2 ± 0.5 (0.5–2.0)	1.4 ± 0.4 (0.7–2.1)	1.7 ± 0.8 (0.6–2.8)	1.9 ± 0.6 (1.1–2.7)
Monocytes × 10^9/l	(0.0–0.5)	(0.0–0.2)	(0.0–0.1)	(0.0–0.3)	(0.0–0.1)	0
Eosinophils × 10^9/l	(0.0–0.7)	(0.0–0.2)	(0.0–0.2)	0	(0.0–0.1)	(0.0–0.5)
Basophils × 10^9/l	(0.0–0.8)	(0.0–0.9)	(0.0–0.8)	(0.0–0.8)	(0.0–0.2)	(0.0–0.6)
Thrombocytes × 10^9/l	12 ± 7 (5–24)	13 ± 7 (7–24)		22 ± 9 (11–42)	32 ± 12 (10–67)	16 ± 5 (11–24)
Fibrinogen g/l	2.0 ± 0.4 (1.5–2.8)	1.4 ± 0.3 (0.9–2.0)	1.8 ± 0.7 (0.8–3.5)	2.2 ± 0.5 (1.5–2.8)	2.2 ± 0.5 (1.4–3.0)	1.5 ± 0.2 (1.1–1.8)

Mean ± standard error of mean (minimum–maximum)

Hematology values for selected Psittaciformes (*continued*)

Species	Hyacinth macaw *n* = 6	Military macaw *n* = 5	Red-fronted macaw *n* = 7	Scarlet macaw *n* = 7	Severe macaw *n* = 4	Blue and gold macaw *n* = 12–15	Green-winged macaw *n* = 10–14	Yellow-naped macaw *n* = 7
Scientific name	*Anodor-hynchus hyacinthinus*	*Ara militaris*	*Ara rubrogenys*	*Ara macao*	*Ara severa*	*Ara ararauna*	*Ara chloroptera*	*Ara auricollis*
RBC × 10^{12}/l	3.2 (2.9–3.4)	2.9 (2.7–3.1)	3.3 (2.6–3.5)	3.0 (2.7–3.2)	3.3 (3.1–3.6)	3.2 ± 0.2 (2.7–3.5)	3.1 ± 0.2 (2.8–3.3)	3.5 (2.9–3.9)
HB g/dl	16.2 (15.4–18.0)	16.6 (14.4–19.6)	16.4 (14.4–19.6)	17.3 (15.8–18.4)	16.7 (16.0–17.1)	16.8 ± 1.2 (14.8–18.9)	16.2 ± 1.2 (14.7–18.8)	17.4 (15.0–19.2)
Hct l/l	0.48 (0.43–0.53)	0.47 (0.44–0.50)	0.46 (0.41–0.51)	0.48 (0.46–0.52)	0.49 (0.45–0.53)	0.46 ± 0.03 (0.41–0.51)	0.48 ± 0.05 (0.41–0.56)	0.50 (0.43–0.53)
MCV fl	150 (145–156)	159 (154–160)	142 (136–158)	160 (143–175)	149 (145–156)	146 ± 7 (132–157)	158 ± 9 (141–174)	144 (133–150)
MCH pg	50.0 (45.2–54.6)	55.9 (40.6–59.6)	50.8 (40.6–59.6)	57.6 (51.1–64.2)	51.4 (47.9–55.2)	52.3 ± 2.2 (49.4–56.4)	53.4 ± 2.4 (50.5–57.7)	50.6 (48.0–53.8)
MCHC g/dl	33.5 (30.2–37.3)	35.3 (34.2–37.0)	35.3 (29.3–38.4)	35.9 (32.6–38.5)	34.5 (32.1–35.6)	36.6 ± 1.7 (34.7–39.8)	33.9 ± 3.0 (29.1–38.3)	35.0 (32.9–36.9)
WBC × 10^9/l	7.3 (5.6–8.9)	14.8 (12.6–17.8)	5.9 (3.0–8.1)	10.2 (6.4–15.4)	7.8 (4.2–10.2)	8.5 ± 3.6 (4.5–15.4)	10.6 ± 4.7 (6.0–19.3)	10.4 (5.0–16.9)
Heterophils × 10^9/l	5.7 (3.3–6.8)	13.1 (10.0–15.3)	4.1 (1.8–6.2)	8.0 (4.9–12.8)	5.2 (3.0–6.7)	5.0 ± 1.5 (2.3–8.0)	4.1 ± 0.6 (3.7–5.8)	8.2 (4.0–15.2)
Lympho-cytes × 10^9/l	1.3 (0.8–2.0)	1.6 (0.7–2.5)	1.7 (1.0–2.6)	1.6 (1.2–2.2)	2.2 (0.5–3.6)	2.0 ± 0.6 (0.9–3.3)	3.9 ± 1.1 (2.3–5.5)	2.2 (0.9–4.8)
Monocytes × 10^9/l	0	(0.0–0.2)	0	(0.0–0.3)	(0.0–0.3)	(0.0–0.1)	(0.0–0.3)	
Eosinophils × 10^9/l	0	0	0	0	(0.0–0.5)	0	0	0
Basophils × 10^9/l	(0.0–0.3)	0	(0.0–0.2)	(0.0–0.8)	(0.0–0.1)	(0.0–0.2)	(0.0–0.2)	(0.0–0.4)
Thrombo-cytes × 10^9/l	19 (7–29)	24 (19–30)	13 (4–28)	22 (17–30)	12 (10–13)	21 ± 6 (11–34)	11 ± 3 (8–15)	18 (10–30)
Fibrinogen g/l	1.8 (1.3–2.4)	1.3 (1.0–2.0)	1.5 (1.3–2.8)	1.7 (1.0–2.2)	1.8 (1.6–2.1)	1.9 ± 0.6 (1.0–3.2)	2.0 ± 0.5 (1.1–2.7)	1.4 (1.0–1.9)

Mean ± standard error of mean (minimum–maximum)
Source: Hawkey CM, Samour JH (1988) The value of clinical hematology in exotic birds. In: Jacobson ER, Kollias GV Jr (eds) *Exotic Animals: Contemporary Issues in Small Animal Practice*, pp. 109–141. Churchill Livingstone, New York.

Hematology values for selected Psittaciformes (continued)

Species	White cockatoo n = 5	Black cockatoo n = 6	Palm cockatoo n = 12	Golden conure n = 7	Patagonian conure n = 6
Scientific name	Cacatua alba	Calyptorhynchus funereus	Probosciger aterrimus	Aratinga guarouba	Cyanoliseus patagonus
RBC × 10^{12}/l	2.98 ± 0.19 (2.75–3.20)	2.60 ± 0.10 (2.42–2.72)	2.62 ± 0.53 (1.96–3.59)	3.85 ± 0.19 (3.61–4.03)	3.54 ± 0.32 (3.16–4.09)
HB g/dl	15.7 ± 1.9 (13.9–18.4)	14.5 ± 1.6 (12.0–17.0)	14.6 ± 1.3 (12.8–16.7)	18.8 ± 1.0 (17.6–20.4)	15.0 ± 0.8 (14.3–16.2)
PCV%	44.8 ± 4.4 (37.0–48.0)	43.0 ± 2.5 (40.0–46.0)	44.0 ± 3.6 (36.3–47.3)	52.3 ± 1.3 (50.0–54.0)	47.6 ± 3.1 (45.0–52.0)
MCV fl	150.7 ± 14.3 (132.1–171.0)	165.6 ± 11.5 (154.2–183.6)	174.3 ± 32.9 (130.9–235.0)	136.1 ± 6.1 (125.9–143.7)	134.6 ± 7.1 (127.2–145.6)
MCH pg	52.4 ± 10.2 (43.4–67.1)	55.8 ± 5.7 (48.5–62.7)	57.4 ± 8.7 (46.1–74.1)	49.0 ± 3.1 (45.1–54.4)	42.5 ± 2.4 (39.7–46.8)
MCHC g/dl	33.5 ± 4.0 (30.0–39.2)	33.6 ± 1.9 (31.5–37.0)	33.1 ± 1.8 (31.1–35.5)	36.0 ± 2.5 (33.9–40.7)	31.6 ± 0.5 (30.9–32.3)
WBC × 10^9/l	6.7 ± 7.5 (1.3–18.7)	10.7 ± 6.5 (93.7–22.1)	6.5 ± 5.4 (1.4–17.60)	6.5 ± 1.6 (4.2–8.0)	5.8 ± 2.1 (2.5–8.7)
Heterophils %	45.1 ± 28.5 (17.6–83.0)	32.4 ± 20.9 (6.6–61.2)	53.9 ± 16.8 (23.6–75.0)	38.3 ± 8.7 (22.2–48.5)	40.7 ± 13.7 (23.5–62.7)
Lymphocytes %	52.7 ± 27.5 (15.0–80.3)	63.1 ± 22.1 (32.7–89.5)	42.5 ± 15.3 (24.0–69.4)	57.7 ± 6.8 (48.6–68.7)	54.3–10.7 (34.7–65.8)
Monocytes %	1.8 ± 1.6 (0.0–3.7)	4.1 ± 1.5 (2.7–6.7)	3.0 ± 2.2 (1.0–7.0)	2.5 ± 0.6 (1.4–3.1)	0.9 ± 1.1 (0.0–2.5)
Eosinophils %	0.2 ± 0.4 (0.0–1.0)	0.0	0.5- ± 0.6 (0.0–1.4)	0.5 ± 0.8 (0.0–2.0)	0.2 ± 0.4 (0.0–1.1)
Basophils %	0.2 ± 0.4 (0.0–1.0)	0.4 ± 0.9 (0.0–2.0)	0.2 ± 0.5 (0.0–1.4)	0.0	0.0

Mean ± SD (minimum–maximum)
Source: modified from: Polo FJ, Peinado VI, Viscor G, Palomeque J (1998) Hematologic and plasma chemistry in captive psittacine birds. *Avian Diseases* **42**: 523–535.

Hematology values for selected Psittaciformes (continued)

Species	Scarlet macaw n = 14	Green winged macaw n = 18	Military macaw n = 21	Hyacinthine macaw n = 16	Blue and yellow macaw n = 35	African gray parrot n = 15
Scientific name	Ara macao	Ara chloroptera	Ara militaris	Anodorhynchus hyacinthinus	Ara ararauna	Psittacus erithacus
RBC × 10^{12}/l	3.07 ± 0.43 (2.29–3.67)	3.20 ± 0.38 (2.65–4.05)	3.44 ± 0.59 (2.72–5.16)	3.19 ± 0.44 (2.45–4.260)	3.24 ± 0.50 (2.11–4.10)	3.47 ± 0.41 (2.96–4.03)
HB g/dl	16.4 ± 2.2 (13.1–19.90)	13.6 ± 2.8 (9.6–18.7)	15.6 ± 2.3 (11.1–19.6)	15.8 ± 0.9 (14.3–18.0)	14.4 ± 1.2 (11.7–17.0)	15.4 ± 3.4 (10.7–21.7)
Hct l/l	47.4 ± 4.4 (40.0–54.0)	46.1 ± 3.8 (39.0–54.0)	47.1 ± 4.3 (37.0–54.5)	46.9 ± 2.5 (43.0–51.0)	44.6 ± 4.6 (31.5–51.8)	46.4 ± 5.3 (32.0–54.0)
MCV fl	151.6 ± 10.7 (135.3–168.5)	145.0 ± 13.9 (116.1–176.5)	137.0 ± 16.0 (105.6–172.8)	149.0 ± 17.8 (119.1–180.6)	141.0 ± 21.4 (102.4–199.1)	134.7 ± 17.1 (105.6–165.8)
MCH pg	52.1 ± 3.8 (44.3–58.5)	42.2 ± 8.1 (31.3–61.1)	44.9 ± 4.7 (36.5–51.8)	50.3 ± 6.6 (38.7–62.8)	46.4 ± 6.5 (34.6–61.9)	43.9 ± 9.2 (29.0–59.3)
MCHC g/dl	34.4 ± 2.2 (29.7–37.3)	29.6 ± 4.6 (21.9–34.9)	33.5 ± 2.5 (33.9–40.7)	33.8 ± 1.4 (32.3–36.8)	32.7 ± 3.4 (28.1–43.5)	32.2 ± 5.4 (24.8–43.4)
WBC × 10^9/l	9.8 ± 4.5 (4.7–22.0)	16.9 ± 8.9 (3.8–30.0)	9.5 ± 4.5 (13.7–18.0)	9.7 ± 5.8 (1.5–19.2)	16.6 ± 9.0 (1.7–36.0)	9.0 ± 3.6 (4.0–20.0)
Heterophils %	39.9 ± 13.0 (26.0–67.0)	32.2 ± 13.4 (14.0–62.0)	41.5 ± 15.4 (12.0–62.5)	75.9 ± 12.1 (52.0–89.0)	37.2 ± 18.3 (12.8–60.0)	60.8 ± 20.6 (29.4–83.0)
Lymphocytes %	55.1 ± 11.4 (36.0–68.2)	34.0 ± 13.8 (35.0–84.2)	55.3 ± 14.5 (43.3–80.0)	30.3 ± 22.2 (10.0–77.3)	60.0 ± 17.6 (35.5–84.4)	35.5 ± 20.9 (15.5–67.7)
Monocytes %	3.4 ± 2.4 (0.0–8.1)	2.1 ± 2.2 (0.0–8.3)	2.4 ± 2.4 (0.0–8.0)	0.5 ± 0.6 (0.0–1.5)	1.3 ± 0.8 (0.0–2.0)	2.8 ± 2.0 (1.0–6.0)
Eosinophils %	1.2 ± 1.4 (0.0–4.0)	0.5 ± 0.9 (0.0–3.0)	0.3 ± 0.7 (0.0–2.1)	1.1 ± 1.4 (0.0–4.0)	0.7 ± 0.8 (0.0–2.0)	1.1 ± 1.4 (0.0–4.0)
Basophils %	0.4 ± 0.7 (0.0–2.0)	0.3 ± 0.5 (0.0–1.7)	0.2 ± 0.4 (0.0–1.2)	0.0	0.3 ± 0.6 (0.0–1.6)	0.0

Mean ± SD (minimum–maximum)
Source: modified from: Polo FJ. Peinado VI, Viscor G, Palomeque J (1998) Hematologic and plasma chemistry in captive psittacine birds. *Avian Diseases* **42**: 523–535.

Hematology values for selected Psittaciformes (*continued*)

Species	Blue-fronted Amazon *n* = 7	Orange winged Amazon *n* = 5	Yellow Amazon *n* = 8	Cuban Amazon *n* = 7	Festive Amazon *n* = 6	Red lory *n* = 18
Scientific name	*Amazona aestiva*	*Amazona amazonica*	*Amazona ochrocephala*	*Amazona leucocephala*	*Amazona festiva*	*Eos bornea*
RBC × 10^{12}/l	2.92 ± 0.55 (2.11–3.53)	3.08 ± 0.20 (2.81–3.32)	2.93 ± 0.16 (2.11–3.53)	3.30 ± 0.16 (3.09–3.49)	3.47 ± 0.29 (3.10–3.80)	3.17 ± 0.49 (2.62–4.72)
HB g/dl	17.3 ± 0.9 (16.0–18.4)	16.3 ± 0.8 (15.5–17.5)	15.3 ± 1.7 (12.1–17.4)	16.7 ± 0.9 (15.2–17.7)	16.7 ± 0.5 (16.1–17.4)	16.0 ± 1.4 (14.2–18.7)
PCV %	50.6 ± 6.2 (43.5–58.0)	48.4 ± 2.2 (46.0–51.0)	46.5 ± 4.4 (38.0–51.0)	49.6 ± 3.5 (44.0–54.0)	50.4 ± 2.6 (47.0–53.0)	48.8 ± 3.2 (44.0–54.0)
MCV fl	180.0 ± 19.7 (163.0–208.9)	157.6 ± 5.9 (150.6–165.8)	159.0 ± 12.4 (135.4–175.4)	150.4 ± 7.3 (141.9–162.4)	145.8 ± 11.8 (134.8–163.7)	155.9 ± 13.7 (111.2–171.6)
MCH pg	62.2 ± 9.9 (52.0–76.2)	53.1 ± 3.4 (48.3–57.3)	52.1 ± 4.9 (42.9–56.9)	50.8 ± 3.6 (44.8–55.2)	48.3 ± 4.5 (43.9–53.7)	51.7 ± 3.9 (39.6–55.7)
MCHC g/dl	34.3 ± 2.6 (31.7–37.8)	33.7 ± 1.5 (32.1–36.0)	32.5 ± 1.0 (31.0–34.1)	33.8 ± 2.2 (31.4–37.2)	33.2 ± 1.2 (31.5–34.5)	32.9 ± 1.0 (31.2–35.6)
WBC × 10^9/l	6.5 ± 2.4 (4.7–11.0)	6.1 ± 3.8 (91.2–10.1)	4.2 ± 1.9 (2.2–7.7)	8.3 ± 7.7 (1.9–24.7)	4.1 ± 1.8 (2.2–7.0)	3.3 ± 2.2 (0.8–9.0)
Heterophils %	30.7 ± 15.0 (12.4–46.6)	36.2 ± 7.2 (21.9–40.7)	30.6 ± 12.8 (12.3–51.9)	24.3 ± 3.3 (19.0–27.6)	25.1 ± 4.7 (21.9–32.2)	55.2 ± 17.4 (25.6–79.2)
Lymphocytes %	67.0 ± 14.2 (52.4–83.5)	63.4 ± 7.0 (55.8–73.2)	67.2 ± 10.9 (48.1–80.0)	77.3 ± 1.3 (71.4–75.0)	71.0 ± 4.3 (65.5–75.8)	41.7 ± 16.6 (18.7–70.1)
Monocytes %	1.7 ± 0.9 (1.0–3.1)	3.5 ± 1.5 (2.0–5.0)	1.9 ± 2.7 (0.0–7.7)	1.5 ± 2.1 (0.0–5.0)	2.4 ± 1.8 (0.0–4.2)	1.4 ± 1.2 (0.0–4.5)
Eosinophils %	0.3 ± 0.5 (0.0–1.0)	1.0 ± 2.2 (0.0–5.0)	0.2 ± 0.4 (0.0–1.2)	1.5 ± 2.1 (0.0–5.0)	1.3 ± 0.9 (0.0–2.3)	1.5 ± 1.5 (0.0–4.6)
Basophils %	0.2 ± 0.5 (0.0–1.0)	0.3 ± 0.7 (0.0–1.7)	0.2 ± 0.4 (0.0–1.2)	0.3 ± 0.4 (0.0–1.0)	0.0	0.2 ± 0.4 (0.0–1.2)

Mean ± SD (minimum–maximum)
Source: modified from: Polo FJ, Peinado VI, Viscor G, Palomeque J (1998) Hematologic and plasma chemistry in captive psittacine birds. *Avian Diseases* **42**: 523–535.

Hematology values for selected Psittaciformes (*continued*)

Species	African gray parrot *n* = 108	Amazon parrot *n* = 640	Blue-headed parrot *n* = 16	Budgerigar *n* = 251	Gray-cheeked parakeet *n* = 32
Scientific name	*Psittacus erithacus*	*Amazona* sp.	*Pionus menstruus*	*Melopsittacus undulatus*	*Brotogeris pyrrhopterus*
RBC × 10^6/mm^3	(2.4–4.5)	(2.5–4.5)	(2.4–4.1)	(2.5–4.5)	–
PCV %	(43–55)	(45–55)	(44–60)	(45–57)	(46–58)
WBC × 10^3/mm^3	(5–11)	(6–11)	(4–11)	(3–8)	(4.5–9.5)
Heterophils %	(45–75)	(30–75)	(40–70)	(45–70)	(40–75)
Lymphocytes %	(20–50)	(20–65)	(20–50)	(20–45)	(20–60)
Monocytes %	(0–3)	(0–3)	(0–2)	(0–5)	(0–3)
Eosinophils %	(0–2)	(0–1)	(0–1)	(0–1)	(0–1)
Basophils %	(0–5)	(0–5)	(0–5)	(0–5)	(0–5)

(Minimum–maximum)
Source: Woerpel RW, Rosskopf WJ (1984) Clinical experience with avian laboratory diagnostics. *Veterinary Clinics of North America* **14**: 254.

Hematology values for selected avian species

Species	Canary n = 62	Cockatiel n = 364	Cockatoo n = 242	Conure n = 85	Domestic duck n = 31
Scientific name	*Serinus canaria*	*Nymphicus hollandicus*	*Cacatua* spp.	*Aratinga* spp.	*Anas* spp.
RBC × 10^6/mm^3	(2.5–4.5)	(2.5–4.7)	(2.2–4.5)	(2.5–4.5)	(2.3–3.5)
PCV %	45–60)	(45–57)	(40–55)	(42–55)	(30–43)
WBC × 10^3/mm^3	(4–9)	(5–10)	(5–11)	(4–11)	(4.5–13.0)
Heterophils %	(20–50)	(40–70)	(45–75)	(40–75)	(30–70)
Lymphocytes %	(40–75)	(25–55)	(22–50)	(20–50)	(20–65)
Monocytes %	(0–1)	(0–2)	(0–4)	(0–3)	(0–3)
Eosinophils %	(0–1)	(0–2)	(0–2)	(0–3)	(0–4)
Basophils %	(0–5)	(0–6)	(0–5)	(0–5)	(0–5)

(Minimum–maximum)
Source: Woerpel RW, Rosskopf WJ (1984) Clinical experience with avian laboratory diagnostics. *Veterinary Clinics of North America* **14**: 254.

Hematology values for selected avian species (*continued*)

Species	Grand eclectus parrot n = 9	Finches n = 21	Lovebirds n = 78	Macaws n = 219	Greater Indian hill mynah n = 35	Philippines blue-naped parrot n = 7	Toucans n = 8
Scientific name	*Eclectus roratus riedeli*	*Atlapetes* spp.	*Agapornis* spp.	*Ara* spp.	*Gracula religiosa*	*Tanygnathus lucionensis*	*Ramphastos* spp.
RBC × 10^6/mm^3	(2.5–4.0)	(2.5–4.6)	(3.0–5.1)	(2.5–4.5)	(2.4–5.0)	(2.4–4.0)	(2.5–4.5)
PCV %	(45–55)	(45–62)	(44–57)	(45–55)	(44–55)	(45–55)	(45–60)
WBC × 10^3/mm^3	(6–11)	(3–8)	(3–8)	(6–13.5)	(6–11)	(4.5–11.5)	(4–10)
Heterophils %	(40–75)	(20–65)	(40–75)	(45–70)	(25–65)	(35–70)	(35–65)
Lymphocytes %	(20–50)	(20–65)	(20–55)	(20–50)	(20–60)	(20–60)	(25–50)
Monocytes %	(0–2)	(0–1)	(0–2)	(0–3)	(0–3)	(0–5)	(0–4)
Eosinophils %	(0–1)	(0–1)	(0–1)	(0–2)	(0–3)	(0–0)	(0–4)
Basophils %	(0–5)	(0–5)	(0–6)	(0–5)	(0–7)	(0–5)	(0–5)

(Minimum–maximum)
Source: modified from: Woerpel RW, Rosskopf PF, Monahan-Brennan M (1987) Clinical pathology and laboratory diagnostic tools. In: Burr EW (ed.) *Companion Bird Medicine*, pp. 180–196. Iowa State University Press, Ames, IA.

Hematology values for Quaker parrot

Species	Quaker parrot n = 6
Scientific name	*Myopsitta monachus*
RBC × 10^6/µl	3.35 ± 0.27 (2.81–3.89)
HB g/dl	14.7 ± 1.3 (12.1–17.3)
PCV %	50 ± 10 (30–70)
MCV fl	150 ± 32 (86–214)
MCH pg	44 ± 5 (34–54)
MCHC g/dl	30 ± 4 (22–38)
WBC µl	5958 ± 2367 (1224–10 692)
Heterophils %	11.5 ± 6.4 (0–24.3)
Lymphocytes %	82 ± 4 (74–90)
Monocytes %	2.5 ± 0.7 (1.0–4.0)
Eosinophils %	0.5 ± 0.7 (0–1.9)
Basophils %	1.5 ± 2.1 (0–5.7)
Azurophils %	2 ± 1 (0–4)

Mean ± SD (minimum–maximum)
Source: Goodwin JS, Jacobson ER, Gaskin JM (1982) Effects of Pacheco's parrot disease on hematologic and blood chemistry values of Quaker parrot (Myopsitta monachus). Journal of Zoo Animal Medicine **13**: 127–132.

Hematology values for selected Columbiformes

Species	Rock pigeon	Eastern turtle dove
Scientific name	*Columba livia*	*Streptopelia orientalis*
Erythrocytes 10^6/mm^3	3.7	(3.0–4.1)
PCV %	50.0	–
Hb g %	16.5	13.9
Leukocytes mm^3	–	11.1
Heterophils %	39.0	17.9
Lymphocytes %	53.0	70.8
Monocytes %	5.0	4.9
Eosinophils %	1.0	2.6
Basophils %	2.0	3.8
Thrombocytes mm^3	–	19.1

Source: Vogel C *et al.* (1983) *Taubenkrankheiten*. Schober Verlag, Hengersberg; Vogel C *et al.* (1992) *Tauben*. Deutscher Landwirtschaftsverlag, Berlin.

Hematology values for endangered Columbiformes

Species	Nicobar pigeon n = 16	Pheasant pigeon n = 3	Common crowned pigeon n = 9	Victoria crowned pigeon n = 6	Scheepmaker's crowned pigeon n = 1
Scientific name	Caloenas nicobarica	Otidiphas nobilis	Goura cristata	Goura victoria	Goura scheepmakeri
PCV %	50.7 ± 2.6 (45–56)	41.7 ± 9.0 (33–51)	34.3 ± 3.3 (30.0–39.5)	37.6 ± 3.8 (33.8–42)	42.0
HB g/dl	17.0 ± 1.5 (12.7–19.7)	13.9 ± 2.8 (11.4–17.0)	10.8 ± 1.5 (8.2–12.7)	12.3 ± 1.6 (10.6–14.7)	12.7
RBC 10^6/ml	3.40 ± 0.47 (2.67–4.33)	2.6 ± 0.4 (2.26–3.0)	2.23 ± 0.35 (1.80–2.80)	2.31 ± 0.23 (1.95–2.60)	2.30
MCV fl	149.8 ± 16.5 (127.6–168.5)	158.9 ± 12.1 (146–170)	158.7 ± 14.7 (142.9–175.0)	166.9 ± 18.2 (134.6–178.3)	182.6
MCH pg	50.0 ± 5.5 (41.3–57.6)	53.3 ± 3.1 (50.4–56.6)	50.8 ± 5.2 (44.2–57.3)	55.0 ± 7.3 (42.5–61.3)	55
MCHC g/dl	33.5 ± 1.8 (28.3–36.1)	33.6 ± 0.8 (33.1–34.5)	31.9 ± 4.3 (27.9–38.0)	32.6 ± 1.5 (31.1–35.0)	30.1
WBC 10^3/ml	4.23 ± 1.92 (2.0–8.25)	6.91 ± 2.43 (4.12–8.62)	17.71 ± 4.87 (11.75–25.12)	10.85 ± 6.54 (5.13–20.75)	19.38
Heterophils %	52.2 ± 15.7 (42–71)	54.1 ± 11.4 (46–67)	66.0 ± 9.0 (55–78)	52.8 ± 12.0 (40–70)	56
Lymphocytes %	37.4 ± 9.9 (27–51)	42.5 ± 13.6 (27–51)	30.3 ± 8.4 (18–40)	44.6 ± 12.1 (27–58)	37
Monocytes %	2.1 ± 1.6 (1–5)	1.6 ± 0.8 (0–2)	1.0 ± 0.5 (0–2)	0.7 ± 0.8 (0–2)	2
Eosinophils %	2.7 ± 2.3 (1–9)	0.6 ± 1.1 (0–2)	2.4 ± 1.4 (1–5)	2.5 ± 1.1 (1–4)	3
Basophils %	0	1.2 ± 1.2 (0–2.5)	0.25 ± 0.5 (0–1)	0.3 ± 0.5 (0–1)	2

Mean ± SD (minimum–maximum)
Source: Peinado VI, Polo FJ, Celdran JF, Viscor G, Palomeque J (1992) Hematology and plasma chemistry in endangered pigeons. *Journal of Zoo Wildlife Medicine* **23**: 65–71.

Hematology values for selected Galliformes

Species	Scientific name	RBC × 10^6/ml	PCV %	Hb g %	MCV µm^3	WBC × 10^3/ml
Domestic fowl	Gallus domesticus	(2.2–3.3)	(24–43)	(8.9–13.5)	(120–137)	(19.8–32.6)
Domestic turkey	Meleagris gallopavo	(2.3–2.8)	(36–41)	(10.3–15.2)	(129)	(23.5–26.8)
Pheasant	Phasianus colchicus	(2.2–3.6)	(28–42)	(8.0–18.9)	(104–150)	–
Guinea fowl	Numida meleagris	(1.7–2.8)	(39–48)	(11.4–14.9)	–	(15.5)
Peafowl	Pavo cristatus	(2.1)	(33–41)	(12.0)	–	–
Common partridge	Perdix perdix	(1.8–3.3)	(28–34)	(7.4–11.8)	(117–155)	–
Rock partridge	Alectoris graeca	(2.6)	(37)	(11.1)	–	–
Bobwhite quail	Colinus virginianus	(3.4–5.4)	(38)	(11.6–15.8)	–	–
Common quail	Coturnix coturnix	(3.8–5.4)	(40–53)	(12.9–15.8)	–	(16.2–24.0)
Japanese quail	Coturnix japonica	(3.3–4.1)	(37–46)	(10.7–15.8)	–	(19.7–25.0)
Chachalaca	Ortalis vetula	(2.7)	(35–45)	–	–	–

(Minimum–maximum)
Source: Gylstorff I (1983) Blut, Blutbildung und Blutkreislauf. In: Mehner A, Hartfiel W (eds) Handbuch der Geflügelphysiologie, vol 1. Gustav Fischer, Jena, pp. 280–393; Gylstorff I, Grimm F (1987) *Vogelkrankheiten*. Eugen Ulmer, Stuttgart; Vollmerhaus B, Sinowatz F (1992) Atmungsapparat der Vögel. In: Nickel, R, Schummer A, Seiferle E. (eds) *Lehrbuch der Anatomie der Haustiere, Band V: Anatomie der Vögel*, 2nd edn. pp. 159–175, Verlag Parey, Berlin,.

Hematology values for selected Anseriformes

Species	Black duck	Wood duck	Canvasback	Red head duck	Lesser scaup	Greater scaup	Ring-necked duck	Bufflehead
Scientific names	*Anas superciliosa*	*Chenonetta jubata*	*Aythya valisineria*	*Aythya americana*	*Aythya affinis*	*Aythya marila*	*Aythya colaris*	*Bucephala albeola*
RBC × 10^6/mm^3	2.78 ± 0.22	2.79 ± 0.28	2.5–2.6 2.61–3.51 2.61 ± 0.4	2.78 ± 0.3	2.4–2.5 2.45 ± 0.13 2.84	2.27 ± 0.7	2.50 2.54	2.6–2.7 2.64
Hb g/dl	12.96 ± 1.36	14.95 ± 1.22	13.8–18.1 15.2 ± 2.0	44.0 ± 7.1	56.5–58.0 57.1 ± 3.1 47.0	15.9 ± 2.0	14.3	–
PCV %	40.24 ± 4.21	45.54 ± 3.41	51.4–53.0 46.3–60.4 47 ± 6.2	13.5 ± 1.8	16.0	43.0 ± 1.4	49.1 47.0	53.9–54.7 54.3
MCV μg	144.68 ± 9.96	164.24 ± 14.43	165–209	–	–	–	–	–
MCH μg	46.60 ± 3.00	54.08 ± 6.74	47–63	–	–	–	–	–
MCHC %	32.23 ± 1.16	32.99 ± 3.7	28–31	–	–	–	–	–
RBC size μm	–	–	6.6 × 12.7	–	.5 × 13.0	–	–	–
WBC 10^3/mm^3	19.70 ± 6.60	23.58 ± 5.72	–	–	–	–	–	–
Heterophils × 10^3/mm^3	4.86 ± 1.37	8.45 ± 2.59	–	–	–	–	–	–
Lymphocytes × 10^3/mm^3	13.03 ± 1.53	13.28 ± 1.77	–	–	–	–	–	–
Monocytes × 10^3/mm^3	1.46 ± 0.99	1.05 ± 0.68	–	–	–	–	–	–
Basophils × 10^3/mm^3	0.16 ± 0.15	0.41 ± 0.23	–	–	–	–	–	–
Eosinophils × 10^3/mm^3	0.22 ± 0.16	0.51 ± 0.06	–	–	–	–	–	–
RBC × 10^6/mm^3	1.6–2.6 2.15–2.82	2.3 ± 0.4	2.25	2.6 ± 0.2	2.9 ± 0.2		2.30 ± 0.3	–
Hb g/dl	12.7–19.1	13.48 ± 2.01^m 12.8 ± 1.81^f	14.0	15.25 ± 0.74^m 15.72 ± 0.60^f	14.76 ± 1.54^m 15.43 ± 0.76^f		14.6 ± 1.7	41.6 ± 2.6
PCV %	38–58 41.7–56	42 ± 3	46	46 ± 2	43 ± 2		43.0 ± 3.4	–
MCV μ^3	145–174 168.1–229.5	–	–	–	34.6 ± 1.2^m 35.6 ± 0.6^f		–	–
MCH μg	53.7–70	32 ± 5.4^m 4.6 ± 0.7^f	–	32.5 ± 2.7^m 34.7 ± 1.7^f	4.9 ± 0.4^m 5.6 ± 0.4^f		–	32.6 ± 36.4
MCHC %	28–29 27.6–34.7	5.2 ± 0.8^m 4.6 ± 0.7^f	–	5.6 ± 0.3^m 6.3 ± 0.5^f	–		–	–
RBC size μ	6.9 × 13.2	–	–	–	–		–	–
WBC × 10^9/l	13.1–18.5	–	20.1 ± 4.71	–	–		–	–
Heterophils × 10^9/l	23.0–42.8	–	7	–	–		–	–
Lymphocytes × 10^9/l	47.8	–	12.3	–	–		–	–
Monocytes × 10^9/l	5.1	–	0.2	–	–		–	–
Eosinophils × 10^9/l	2.4	–	0.1	–	–		–	–
Basophils × 10^9/l	1.9	–	0.5	–	–		–	–

Mean ± SD (minimum–maximum)

m, male; f, female

Source: modified from: Kocan RM, Pitts SM (1976) Blood values of the canvasback duck by age, sex and season. *Journal of Wildlife Diseases* **12**: 341; Kocan RM (1972) Some physiologic blood values of wild diving ducks. *Journal of Wildlife Diseases* **8**: 115; Mulley RC (1980) Hematology of the wood duck (*Chenonetta jubata*). *Journal of Wildlife Diseases* **16**: 271; Mulley RC (1979) Hematology and blood chemistry of the black duck (*Anas superciliosa*). *Journal of Wildlife Diseases* **15**: 437; Shave HJ, Howard V (1976) A hematologic survey of captive waterfowl. *Journal of Wildlife Diseases* **12**: 195; William JI, Traines DO (1971) A hematological study of snow, blue and Canada geese. *Journal of Wildlife Diseases* **7**: 258.

Hematology values for selected ratites

Species	Ostrich	Cassowary
Scientific name	*Struthio camelus*	*Casuarius* spp.
RBC × 10⁶/μl	1.7 (0.4)	2.1 (0.3)
HB g/d	12.2 (2)	14.5 (0.5)
PCV	32.0 (3.0)	50.8 (3.7)
MCV fl	174 (42.0)	245.0 (41.0)
MCH pg	61.0 (16.0)	70.0 (11.5)
MCHC g/d	33.0 (5.0)	28.5 (1.6)
WBC 10³/μl	5.5 (1.9)	18.0 (4.5)
Heterophils %	62.6 (7.6)	77.7 (25.8)
Lymphocytes %	34.1 (7.0)	19.7 (10.4)
Monocytes %	2.8 (1.3)	2.4 (2.4)
Eosinophils %	0.3 (0.5)	–
Basophils %	0.2 (0.5)	–

Mean (SD)
Source: Stewart JS (1989) Husbandry, medical and surgical management of ratites, part 2. *Proceedings of the Association of Zoo Veterinarians*, Greensboro, pp. 119–122.

Hematology values for juvenile eclectus parrots (*Eclectus roratus*)

Parameter	30 day	90 day	All
RBC × 10⁶/μl	1.95 (0.28)	3.22 (0.51)	2.69 (0.67)
HB g/d	8.83 (1.15)	15.42 (2.38)	12.46 (3.01)
HCT %	33.7 (4.4)	53.8 (3.0)	43.8 (8.4)
MCV fl	174 (25)	169 (27)	166 (26)
MCH pg	43.9	49.1 (9.9)	45.5 (10.7)
MCHC g/dl	26.1 (2.5)	28.7 (4.1)	27.7 (5.0)
WBC #/μl	18 500 (6900)	10 900 (3700)	13 700 (6300)
WBC #/#(est.)/μl	17 000 (6000)	10 500 (4000)	13 500 (6000)
Bands %	0.2 (1.1)	0.4 (0.9)	0.5 (1.5)
Heterophils %	62.8 (7.7)	52.1 (10.2)	53.9 (11.4)
Lymphocytes %	30.4 (6.3)	40.8 (10.4)	39.5 (11.5)
Monocytes %	5.5 (3.0)	5.2 (2.7)	5.0 (2.7)
Eosinophils %	0.0 (0.0)	0.1 (0.4)	0.1 (0.3)
Basophils %	1.2 (1.0)	1.5 (1.0)	1.1 (1.0)
Bands #/μl	34 (188)	48 (111)	70 (221)
Heterophils #/μl	11 800 (5400)	5900 (2800)	7700 (4800)
Lymphocytes #/μl	5500 (2100)	4200 (1200)	5100 (2000)
Monocytes #/μl	930 (520)	532 (331)	639 (428)
Eosinophils #/μl	0	9 (43)	8 (44)
Basophils #/μl	209 (199)	175 (158)	152 (169)
Heterophils: lymphocytes (ratio)	2.2 (0.8)	1.4 (0.6)	1.6 (0.8)
PP (refrac) g/dl	2.8 (0.6)	3.9 (0.6)	3.5 (0.8)

Mean (SD)
Source: Clubb SL, Schubot RM, Joyner K *et al.* (1990) Hematologic and serum chemistry reference intervals in juvenile eclectus parrots. *Journal of the Association of Avian Veterinarians* **4**: 218–225.

Hematology values for juvenile cockatoos (*Cacatua* spp.)

Parameter	30 day	90 day	All
RBC × 10[6]/μl	196 (0.22)[a]	2.84 (0.49)[b]	2.53 (0.63)
HB g/d	8.12 (0.83)[a]	14.04 (1.23)[c]	11.43 (2.90)
HCT %	30.1 (2.8)[a]	47.6 (4.1)[c]	39.7 (9.0)
MCV fl	155 (17)[a]	172 (28)[b]	160 (23)
MCH pg	38.9 (11.7)[a]	49.0 (12.9)[b]	43.8 (10.8)
MCHC g/dl	24.6 (7.9)[a]	28.5 (6.2)[b,c]	27.2 (6.1)
WBC #/μl	13 700 (7400)[a]	10 000 (2800)[b]	12 900 (6300)
WBC #/#(est.)/μl	13 200 (6700)[a]	10 400 (2800)[b]	13 100 (5900)
Bands %	1.3 (2.3)[a,b]	1.3 (2.3)[a,b]	1.3 (2.3)
Heterophils%	54.8 (9.7)[a]	49.0 (8.1)[b]	50.8 (11.7)
Lymphocytes%	36.4 (8.1)[a]	43.6 (8.4)[b]	41.2 (11.9)
Monocytes%	6.9 (3.4)[a]	4.9 (3.4)[b,c]	5.8 (3.4)
Eosinophils%	0 (0)	0 (0.2)	0 (0.0)
Basophils%	0.6 (0.9)[a,c]	1.2 (1.1)[b]	0.9 (1.1)
Bands #/μl	150 (275)[a]	130 (290)[a]	160 (325)
Heterophils #/μl	7800 (5000[a])	4400 (2200)[b]	6500 (4500)
Lymphocytes #/μl	4900 (2600)[a]	3900 (2000)[a]	4900 (2500)
Monocytes #/μl	880 (530)[a]	440 (450)[a]	690 (525)
Eosinophils #/μl	0 (0)	0 (0)	0 (0)
Basophils #/μl	67 (130)[a]	115 (130)[a]	100 (140)
Heterophil: lymphocyte (ratio)	1.6 (0.6)[a]	1.2 (0.4)[b]	1.4 (0.8)
PP (refrac) g/dl	2.3 (0.5)[a]	4.0 (0.8)[b]	3.2 (0.9)

Mean (SD)
Source: Clubb SL, Schubot RM, Joyner K *et al.* (1991) Hematologic and serum biochemical reference intervals in juvenile cockatoos. *Journal of the Association of Avian Veterinarians* **5**: 16–26.

Hematology values for juvenile cockatoos (*Cacatua* spp.)

Parameter	30 day	90 day	All
RBC × 10[6]/μl	196 (0.22)[a]	2.84 (0.49)[b]	2.53 (0.63)
HB g/d	8.12 (0.83)[a]	14.04 (1.23)[c]	11.43 (2.90)
HCT %	30.1 (2.8)[a]	47.6 (4.1)[c]	39.7 (9.0)
MCV fl	155 (17)[a]	172 (28)[b]	160 (23)
MCH pg	38.9 (11.7)[a]	49.0 (12.9)[b]	43.8 (10.8)
MCHC g/dl	24.6 (7.9)[a]	28.5 (6.2)[b,c]	27.2 (6.1)
WBC #/μl	13 700 (7400)[a]	10 000 (2800)[b]	12 900 (6300)
WBC #/#(est.)/μl	13 200 (6700)[a]	10 400 (2800)[b]	13 100 (5900)
Bands %	1.3 (2.3)[a,b]	1.3 (2.3)[a,b]	1.3 (2.3)
Heterophils %	54.8 (9.7)[a]	49.0 (8.1)[b]	50.8 (11.7)
Lymphocytes %	36.4 (8.1)[a]	43.6 (8.4)[b]	41.2 (11.9)
Monocytes %	6.9 (3.4)[a]	4.9 (3.4)[b,c]	5.8 (3.4)
Eosinophils %	0 (0)	0 (0.2)	0 (0.0)
Basophils %	0.6 (0.9)[a,c]	1.2 (1.1)[b]	0.9 (1.1)
Bands #/μl	150 (275)[a]	130 (290)[a]	160 (325)
Heterophils #/μl	7800 (5000)[a]	4400 (2200)[b]	6500 (4500)
Lymphocytes #/μl	4900 (2600)[a]	3900 (2000)[a]	4900 (2500)
Monocytes #/μl	880 (530)[a]	440 (450)[a]	690 (525)
Eosinophils #/μl	0 (0)	0 (0)	0 (0)
Basophils #/μl	67 (130)[a]	115 (130)[a]	100 (140)
Heterophil: lymphocyte (ratio)	1.6 (0.6)[a]	1.2 (0.4)[b]	1.4 (0.8)
PP (refrac) g/dl	2.3 (0.5)[a]	4.0 (0.3)[b]	3.2 (0.9)

Mean (SD)
a,b,c,: Values for parameters are statistically different ($p < 0.05$) when letters are different.
Source: Clubb SL, Schubot RM, Joyner K *et al.* (1991) Hematologic and serum biochemical reference intervals in juvenile cockatoos. *Journal of the Association of Avian Veterinarians* **5**: 16–26.

Hematology values for juvenile umbrella cockatoos (*Cacatua alba*)

Parameter	30 day	90 day	All
RBC × 10^6/µl	1.98 (0.51)n	2.75 (0.49)n	2.54
HB g/d	7.9 (1.64)n	14 (0.92)n	11.6
HCT %	29.5 (5.65)n	46.9 (2.92)n	39.3
MCV fl	151 (25.6)n	175 (28.5)n	158.0
MCH pg	35.3 (10.03)n	51.9 (8.57)n	43.6
MCHC g/d	21.8 (10.5)n	29.9 (1.1)n	27.0
WBC #/µl	20 311 (5717)n	10 238 (3368)n	16 567.0
WBC #/#(est.)/µl	19 190 (5127)s	10 500 (3184)n	16 412.0
Bands %	1 (2.57)n	1.93 (2.76)n	1.31
Heterophils %	58.4 (11.4)s	50 (9.7)n	54.1
Lymphocytes %	34.4 (11.5)n	41.2 (9.9)n	38.1
Monocytes %	5.77 (3.1)	5.29 (3.27)n	5.35
Eosinophils %	0 (0.14)	0.07 (0.27)n	0.02
Basophils %	0.45 (1.05)n	1.43 (0.94)n	1.03
Bands #/µl	185 (331)n	192 (368)	202.0
Heterophils #/µl	12 041 (4993)s	4465 (2595)n	8917.0
Lymphocytes #/µl	6893 (2581)s	3663 (2076)n	5695.0
Monocytes #/µl	118 (624)s	492 (529)n	843.0
Eosinophils #/µl	0 (0)n	0 (0)n	0.00011
Basophils #/µl	83 (181)n	137 (135)n	143.0
Heterophils: lymphocytes (ratio)	1.83 (1.05)s	1.33 (0.54)n	1.64
PP (refrac) g/dl	2.69 (0.71)	4.26 (0.55)n	3.56

Mean (SD)
s, mean is statistically different (*p* < 0.05) from the same parameter in all juvenile cockatoos; n, mean is not statistically different (*p* > 0.05) from the same parameter in all juvenile cockatoos.
Source: Clubb SL, Schubot RM, Joyner K *et al.* (1991) Hematologic and serum biochemical reference intervals in juvenile cockatoos. *Journal of the Association of Avian Veterinarians* **5**: 16–26.

Hematology values for juvenile macaws (*Ara* sp.)

Parameter	30 day	90 day	All
RBC × 10^6/µl	1.9 (0.3)[a]	3.7 (0.5)[c]	2.9 (0.8)
HB g/d	7.7 (0.9)[a]	15.4 (1.0)[c]	12.3 (3.3)
HCT %	30.9 (3.3)[a]	49.5 (2.5)[c]	41.7 (8.4)
MCV f	165.5 (25.4)[a]	137 (19.2)[c]	149 (24.7)
MCH pg	41.7 (6.1)[a]	42.8 (5.8)[a]	42.3 (6.2)
MCHC g/d	25.1 (1.9)[a]	31.1 (1.3)[b]	28.7 (2.9)
WBC #/µl	19 300 (8300)[a,b]	17 700 (4900)[b]	19 200 (6900)
WBC #/#(est.)/µl	17 700 (5100)[a,b]	18 300 (4500)[a,b]	18 600 (5880)
Bands %	0.8 (1.6)[a]	0.3 (1.2)[a]	0.6 (1.7)
Heterophils %	58.9 (11.1)[a]	53.9 (9.4)[a,b]	55.3 (1.0)
Lymphocytes %	33.8 (9.7)[a]	41.6 (9.6)[b,c]	39.0 (10)
Monocytes %	5.9 (3.3)[a]	3.6 (2.0)[b]	4.4 (2.9)
Eosinophils %	0 (0)[a]	0.1 (0.2)[a]	0 (0.2)
Basophils %	0.7 (0.9)[a]	0.6 (1.2)[a,b]	0.5 (1.0)
BAND #/µl	134 (344)[a]	59 (230)[b,c]	110 (313)
Heterophils #/µl	10 200 (7600)[a,b]	9400 (4000)[b,c]	10 100 (5800)
Lymphocytes #/µl	5500 (3100)[a]	7000 (2500)[b]	6800 (3200)
Monocytes #/µl	910 (643)[a]	627 (418)[b]	750 (545)
Eosinophils #/µl	0 (0.0)[a]	9.3 (51)[a]	4.6 (35)
Basophils #/µl	115 (190)[a]	75 (165)[a,b]	91 (175)
Heterophil: lymphocyte (ratio)	2.0 (1.0)[a,b]	1.4 (0.6)[b,c]	1.6 (0.8)
PP (refrac) g/d	1.8 (0.40)[a]	3.5 (0.4)[c]	2.9 (0.8)

Mean (SD)
a,b,c: Values for parameters are statistically different (*p* < 0.05) when letters are different.
Source: Clubb SL, Schubot RM, Joyner K *et al.* (1991) Hematologic and serum biochemical reference intervals in juvenile macaws (*Ara* sp). *Journal of the Association of Avian Veterinarians* **5**: 154–162.

Hematology values for juvenile blue and gold macaws (*Ara ararauna*)

Parameter	30 day	90 day	All
RBC × 10^6/µl	1.9 (0.3)[a,n]	3.5 (0.4)[c,n]	2.7 (0.7)
HB g/d	7.9 (0.9)[a,n]	15 (0.9)[c,s]	11 (2.9)
HCT %	30 (2.7)[a,n]	48 (2.0)[c,s]	40 (7.7)
MCV f	163 (27)[a,n]	137 (14)[b,n]	149 (122)
MCH pg	43 (7.1)[a,n]	41 (3.7)[a,n]	38 (13)
MCHC g/d	26 (1.6)[a,n]	31 (1.4)[c,n]	25 (9.5)
WBC #/µl	19 200 (5600)[a,n]	16 600 (4300)[b,n]	18 928 (5561)
WBC #/#(est.)/µl	18 300 (5600)	16 800 (4300)	18 300 (5600)
Bands %	0.36 (1.3)[a,n]	0 (0)[a,n]	0.12 (0.7)
Heterophils %	57 (11.6)[a,n]	48 (11)[a,n]	52 (10)
Lymphocytes %	37 (10)[a,n]	47 (11)[c,n]	42 (10)
Monocytes %	5.3 (2.9)[a,n]	3.8 (2.2)[a,n]	4.3 (2.7)
Eosinophils %	0 (0)[a,n]	0 (0)[a,n]	0 (0)
Basophils %	0.9 (1.1)[a,n]	1.1 (1.7)[a,n]	0.9 (1.3)
Band #/µl	0.36 (1.3)[a,n]	0 (0)[a,n]	0.12 (0.7)
Heterophils #/µl	11 000 (4600)[a,n]	8100 (3000)[a,r]	10 000 (3800)
Lymphocytes #/µl	7000 (2600)[a,n]	7700 (2600)[b,n]	8000 (3100)
Monocytes #/µl	949 (498)[a,n]	639 (421)[a,n]	756 (446)
Eosinophils #/µl	0 (0)[a,n]	0 (0)[a,n]	0 (0)

Hematology values for juvenile blue and gold macaws (*Ara ararauna*) (continued)

Parameter	30 day	90 day	All
Basophils #/µl	194 (245)[a,n]	156 (256)[a,n]	154 (229)
Heterophils: lymphocytes (ratio)	1.75 (0.85)[a,n]	1.19 (0.77)[a,n]	1.38 (0.69)
PP (refrac) g/dl	1.87 (0.2)[a,n]	3.62 (0.5)[c,n]	2.86 (0.8)

Mean (SD)
a,b,c: Values for parameters are statistically different (*p* < 0.05) when letters are different; s, mean is statistically different (*p* < 0.05) from the same parameter in all juvenile macaws; n, mean is not statistically different (*p* > 0.05) from the same parameter in all juvenile macaws.
Source: Clubb SL, Schubot RM, Joyner K *et al.* (1991) Hematologic and serum biochemical reference intervals in juvenile macaws (*Ara* sp). *Journal of the Association of Avian Veterinarians* **5**: 154–162.

Age-related hematological changes in captive kori bustards (Ardeotis kori)

Parameter	1 month	2 months	3 months	4 months	5 months	6 months	7 months	8 months	9 months	15 months
RBC × 10^{12}/l	1.28 ± 0.06 (1.04–1.61)	1.57 ± 0.06 (1.22–2.01)	1.76 ± 0.08 (1.31–2.4)	2.06 ± 0.08 (1.39–2.63)	2.07 ± 0.08 (1.79–2.59)	2.14 ± 0.07 (1.84–2.46)	2.12 ± 0.07 (1.79–2.61)	2.0 ± 0.1 (1.72–2.6)	2.1 ± 0.04 (1.91–2.23)	2.08 ± 0.06 (1.81–2.47)
HB g/dl	7.5 ± 0.2 (6.8–8.3)	9.7 ± 0.3 (7.4–10.9)	10.9 ± 0.3 (9.6–13.1)	12.1 ± 0.3 (10.3–14.0)	12.1 ± 0.4 (9.1–14.0)	11.4 ± 0.4 (9.9–13.2)	11.7 ± 0.3 (10.5–13.1)	12.5 ± 0.4 (10.9–14.3)	12.8 ± 0.4 (10.9–14.2)	14.2 ± 0.4 (12.1–16.1)
Hct l/l	0.23 ± 0.7 (0.19–0.26)	0.30 ± 0.9 (0.24–0.34)	0.35 ± 0.7 (0.30–0.41)	0.37 ± 0.7 (0.32–0.41)	0.39 ± 0.9 (0.33–0.44)	0.38 ± 0.9 (0.34–0.42)	0.39 ± 0.9 (0.35–0.45)	0.39 ± 1.0 (0.36–0.45)	0.39 ± 0.9 (0.36–0.43)	0.47 ± 0.9 (0.41–0.51)
MCV #fl	178.4 ± 17.9 (152.2–219.6)	195.2 ± 6.6 (159.2–225.4)	204.3 ± 8.1 (168.8–262.8)	185.2 ± 7.9 (144.0–241.0)	194.2 ± 7.8 (152.5–225.4)	179.9 ± 5.0 (160.6–210.1)	188.2 ± 5.6 (165.1–220.7)	200.5 ± 7.4 (138.5–219.3)	186.5 ± 3.6 (168.2–200.5)	226.5 ± 7.3 (195.5–273.5)
MCH pg	59.3 ± 3.4 (42.2–77.6)	62.0 ± 1.5 (52.2–69.0)	63.5 ± 2.4 (49.2–79.4)	59.6 ± 2.3 (45.9–74.1)	59.5 ± 3.1 (42.1–73.7)	53.7 ± 2.1 (40.2–66.5)	55.8 ± 2.1 (43.7–66.5)	64.4 ± 2.5 (45.4–74.6)	60.5 ± 1.3 (57.1–68.6)	68.7 ± 2.4 (58.2–84.0)
MCHC g/dl	33.2 ± 1.0 (27.8–37.2)	32.0 ± 0.9 (28.2–40.4)	31.2 ± 0.8 (27.5–38.1)	32.3 ± 0.5 (29.2–35.3)	30.5 ± 0.7 (24.3–33.0)	29.8 ± 0.7 (25.1–32.4)	29.6 ± 0.6 (25.6–32.3)	32.2 ± 0.6 (29.5–36.3)	32.5 ± 0.7 (29.8–35.5)	30.3 ± 0.5 (27.6–33.2)
WBC × 10^9/l	8.78 ± 0.45 (6.65–10.85)	10.2 ± 0.6 (6.1–14.75)	10.7 ± 0.7 (7.05–16.2)	12.7 ± 0.7 (8–18.8)	12.5 ± 0.4 (10.35–15.15)	13.5 ± 0.7 (9.8–16.1)	15.6 ± 0.7 (9.2–18.5)	13.5 ± 0.9 (9.25–17.05)	14.5 ± 0.5 (12.8–16.9)	14.10 ± 0.61 (11.25–17.8)
Heterophils × 10^9/l	5.42 ± 0.38 (3.72–6.94)	4.28 ± 0.30 (2.62–6.34)	5.14 ± 0.65 (2.58–11.8)	6.2 ± 0.6 (2.9–10.2)	5.1 ± 0.5 (1.5–7.5)	5.1 ± 0.9 (1.9–11.4)	6.34 ± 0.58 (2.76–8.83)	5.41 ± 0.58 (2.59–8.35)	6.27 ± 0.76 (4.08–10.8)	5.84 ± 0.61 (2.70–10.63)
Lymphocytes × 10^9/l	2.63 ± 0.26 (1.37–3.70)	4.64 ± 0.33 (2.50–6.97)	4.19 ± 0.27 (3.08–6.35)	5.1 ± 0.4 (2.9–7.8)	5.49 ± 0.45 (3.6–9.05)	6.7 ± 0.6 (3.0–10.5)	7.32 ± 0.59 (4.5–11.84)	6.38 ± 0.52 (3.8–9.29)	6.49 ± 0.59 (2.85–8.45)	6.49 ± 0.43 (4.37–9.43)
Monocytes × 10^9/l	0.24 ± 0.06 (0.08–0.63)	0.66 ± 0.15 (0.24–1.92)	0.80 ± 0.12 (0.00–1.58)	0.81 ± 0.08 (0.35–1.50)	1.13 ± 0.16 (0.49–2.03)	0.93 ± 0.14 (0.14–1.64)	1.12 ± 0.13 (0.45–1.78)	1.18 ± 0.13 (0.63–1.70)	0.75 ± 0.17 (0.13–1.41)	1.13 ± 0.07 (0.80–1.53)
Eosinophils × 10^9/l	0.28 ± 0.08 (0.0–0.65)	0.32 ± 0.04 (0.1–0.5)	0.38 ± 0.08 (0.07–1.03)	0.35 ± 0.05 (0.0–0.78)	0.42 ± 0.08 (0.0–1.06)	0.36 ± 0.07 (0.14–0.76)	0.48 ± 0.08 (0.0–0.89)	0.21 ± 0.06 (0.0–0.63)	0.53 ± 0.09 (0.13–0.92)	0.35 ± 0.05 (0.13–0.68)
Basophils × 10^9/l	0.21 ± 0.06 (0.0–0.47)	0.12 ± 0.04 (0.0–0.43)	0.04 ± 0.01 (0.0–0.13)	0.11 ± 0.04 (0.0–0.48)	0.05 ± 0.01 (0.0–0.16)	0.23 ± 0.57 (0.0–0.57)	0.08 ± 0.01 (0.0–0.14)	0.03 ± 0.01 (0.0–0.08)	0.08 ± 0.01 (0.02–0.14)	0.29 ± 0.06 (0.0–0.69)
Thrombocytes × 10^9/l	7.03 ± 1.79 (3.1–15.0)	8.1 ± 0.8 (4.07–15.6)	6.7 ± 0.4 (4.6–9.2)	7.9 ± 0.7 (3.7–15.0)	7.35 ± 0.61 (3.7–10.8)	9.98 ± 1.09 (4.9–17)	11.61 ± 1.0 (5.5–16.7)	10.6 ± 0.9 (6.3–15)	7.0 ± 1.0 (4.8–9.5)	6.52 ± 0.54 (4.05–10.2)
Fibrinogen g/l	1.76 ± 0.18 (1.1–2.6)	2.0 ± 0.1 (1.2–2.8)	2.25 ± 0.2 (1.6–3.8)	2.57 ± 0.3 (1.6–4.0)	2.58 ± 0.49 (1.6–4.8)	2.83 ± 0.22 (1.7–4.0)	3.0 ± 0.2 (2.0–4.7)	2.7 ± 0.3 (1.1–5.4)	2.65 ± 0.27 (2.0–3.3)	3.0 ± 0.3 (1.3–5.3)

Mean ± standard error of mean (minimum–maximum)

RBC, red blood cells; HB, hemoglobin; Hct, hematocrit; MCV, mean cell volume; MCH, mean cell hemoglobin; MCHC, mean cell hemoglobin concentration; PCV, packed cell volume; WBC, white blood cells.

Extracted from: Howlett JC, Samour JH, Bailey TA, Naldo JL (1998) Age-related haematology changes in captive-reared kori bustards (Ardeotis kori). Comparative Haematology International, **8**: 26–30

Appendix 3

Blood chemistry reference values

Merle M. Apo, Tom Bailey

Blood chemistry values for endangered Columbiformes

Species	Nicobar pigeon $n = 16$	Pheasant pigeon $n = 3$	Common crowned pigeon $n = 9$	Victoria crowned pigeon $n = 6$	Scheepmaker's crowned pigeon $n = 1$
Scientific name	*Caloenas nicobarica*	*Otidiphaps nobilis*	*Goura cristata*	*Goura victoria*	*Goura scheepmakeri*
Glucose mmol/l	16.04 ± 1.9 (12.8–19.8)	19.6 ± 2.5 (17.0–22.1)	12.8 ± 0.92 (11.1–13.8)	14.2 ± 2.32 (11.6–17.7)	19.4
Urea mmol/l	0.97 ± 0.22 (0.66–1.38)	0.85 ± 0.08 (0.73–0.94)	1.41 ± 0.37 (0.87–2.09)	1.66 ± 0.38 (1.14–2.13)	1.63
Uric acid mmol/l	611.4 ± 158.8 (390.1–830.3)	779.1 ± 273 (465–967.7)	405.0 ± 274 (133.2–951)	412 ± 177 (215–717)	305.1
Creatinine mmol/dl	0.36 ± 0.15 (0.22–0.65)	0.38 ± 0.08 (0.30–0.45)	0.79 ± 0.15 (0.64–0.94)	0.77 ± 0.10 (0.66–0.90)	0.68
Total protein g/l	32.6 ± 4.1 (26.3–37.7)	32.7 ± 7.5 (28.4–41.4)	44.6 ± 3.7 (38.7–49.3)	35.8 ± 4.0 (30.1–40.3)	40.5
Prealbumin g/l	3.33 ± 0.46 (2.58–4.11)	2.86 ± 0.32 (2.50–3.10)	12.25 ± 2.34 (9.95–16.45)	9.33 ± 4.69 (3.03–13.92)	12.80
Albumin g/l	45.50 ± 6.05 (34.34–58.47)	47.20 ± 0.57 (46.80–47.60)	48.69 ± 2.82 (45.01–53.73)	56.10 ± 4.18 (51.33–62.17)	50.43
Globulin g/l	4.57 ± 1.78 (1.22–7.93)	8.70 ± 6.79 (3.90–13.50)	6.46 ± 1.43 (3.58–7.70)	6.06 ± 3.18 (3.58–7.70)	9.29 ± 3.18
α-globulin g/l	4.57 ± 1.78 (1.22–7.93)	8.70 ± 6.79 (3.90–13.50)	6.46 ± 1.43 (3.58–7.70)	6.06 ± 3.18 (3.04–8.28)	9.29
β-globulin g/l	10.93 ± 4.08 (4.79–21.48)	17.20 ± 14.9 (5.90–34.10)	20.29 ± 3.07 (17.81–25.62)	15.31 ± 3.20 (11.59–19.28)	16.63
γ-globulin g/l	5.71 ± 2.67 (1.54–9.20)	14.70 ± 9.81 (5.20–24.80)	12.31 ± 2.15 (8.68–15.01)	11.97 ± 3.40 (8.28–16.80)	10.85
Albumin/globulin ratio	3.80 ± 1.40 (2.41–7.23)	2.08 ± 1.53 (1.00–3.16)	1.57 ± 0.16 (1.36–1.80)	1.94 ± 0.25 (1.56–2.20)	1.72
ALT IU/l	9.72 ± 6.56 (2.38–19.4)	12.19 ± 4.91 (8.72–15.66)	7.16 ± 1.47 (6.06–10.31)	6.43 ± 2.42 (3.24–8.83)	6.78
AST IU/l	123.0 ± 82.6 (40.1–265.3)	65.6 ± 9.51 (58.9–72.35)	54.08 ± 8.42 (41.16–64.34)	42.80 ± 11.92 (23.5–54.2)	39.07
LDH IU/l	584.0 ± 496.3 (172.9–1808)	101.3 ± 72.2 (50.2–152.4)	257.6 ± 131.4 (134.6–518.5)	219.5 ± 94.3 (126.8–344.1)	ND
AP IU/l	225.2 ± 195.0 (22.6–684.9)	490.5 ± 195.0 (267.1–626.0)	44.3 ± 22.6 (27.9–79.3)	22.4 ± 11.9 (11.3–41.5)	15.37
CPK IU/l	251.3 ± 168.3 (43.3–510.4)	233.7 ± 213.1 (106.8–479.7)	117.2 ± 51.9 (65.8–220.5)	341.6 ± 235.2 (146.7–750.0)	63.3
γ-GT IU/l	2.21 ± 1.69 (0.5–4.5)	ND	0.30 ± 0.79 (0.00–2.08)	0.42 ± 0.41 (0.00–0.96)	2.88
Magnesium mmol/l	1.08 ± 0.20 (0.93–1.22)	1.20 ± 0.11 (1.12–1.27)	0.83 ± 0.16 (0.67–1.10)	0.94 ± 0.18 (0.74–1.17)	ND
Phosphorus mmol/l	13.6 ± 0.18 (13.5–13.7)	13.6 ± 9.5 (6.91–20.4)	6.89 ± 1.05 (5.94–8.46)	5.64 ± 1.71 (4.13–8.04)	ND
Calcium mmol/l	2.61 ± 0.55 (2.22–3.0)	4.04 ± 0.24 (3.87–4.22)	2.22 ± 0.11 (2.1–2.35)	2.42 ± 0.19 (2.25–2.7)	ND
Chloride mmol/l	100.5 ± 11.9 (86.2–126.8)	130.3 ± 12.6 (121.4–139.2)	101.1 ± 3.32 (96.4–106.8)	104.9 ± 4.34 (100.5–109.0)	100.0
Cholesterol mmol/l	11.08 ± 2.79 (7.65–15.16)	10.2 ± 4.44 (6.01–14.88)	6.79 ± 1.53 (5.37–9.46)	6.28 ± 3.50 (4.47–12.44)	6.98
Triglycerides mmol/l	2.02 ± 0.62 (0.01–3.16)	8.45 ± 3.54 (4.36–10.5)	1.72 ± 1.26 (0.49–4.41)	1.60 ± 2.22 (0.42–5.58)	0.74
Osmolality mosmol/kg	313.0 ± 18.7 (295.0–346.0)	311.3 ± 10.0 (301.0–321.0)	316.6 ± 8.5 (289.0–310.0)	315.4 ± 8.5 (305.0–328.0)	323.0

Mean ± SD (minimum–maximum)
ND, not determined
Source: modified from: Peinado VI, Polo FJ, Celdran JF, Viscor G, Palomeque J (1992) Hematology and plasma chemistry in endangered pigeons. *Journal of Zoo Wildlife Medicine* **23**: 65–71.

Plasma chemistry values for the kori and houbara bustard

Species	Kori bustard*	n	Houbara bustard[†]	n
Scientific name	*Ardeotis kori*	n	*Chlamydotis undulata*	n
Glucose mmol/l	13.2 ± 0.46 (9.21–1.98)	24	16.0 ± 0.38 (12.3–22.4)	38
Uric acid mmol/l	469 ± 29.7 (208–850.5)	26	585 ± 24.9 (344–904)	36
Creatinine µmol/l	57 ± 4 (20–110)	24	34 ± 2 (10–70)	35
Total bilirubin µmol/l	11.9 ± 0.51 (5.13–2.22)	25	8.55 ± 0.34 (1.71–13.6)	35
Total protein g/l	29.6 ± 1.6 (20.0–52.0)	25	35.8 ± 0.8 (26.0–50.0)	37
Albumin g/l	15.9 ± 0.8 (12.0–31.0)	25	14.3 ± 0.3 (11.0–19.0)	38
Globulin g/l	13.0 ± 0.8 (8.0–24.0)	22	21.2 ± 0.6 (13.0–34.0)	36
Albumin/globulin ratio	1.20 ± 0.47 (0.70–2.10)	23	0.70 ± 0.02 (0.50–1.10)	36
GGT IU/l	13.25 ± 0.47 (12.0–14.0)	4	372.91 ± 13.29 (200.0–508.0)	37
ALT IU/l	16.17 ± 2.24 (4.0–52.0)	23	36.03 ± 2.40 (8.0–76.0)	31
ALKP IU/l	–		137.28 ± 13.33 (24.0–333.0)	38
AST IU/l	226.50 ± 10.80 (200.0–251.0)	4	372.91 ± 13.29 (200.0–508)	37
LDH IU/l	3862.50 ± 307.0 (2637.0–4689.0)	6	–	
CK IU/l	135.60 ± 20.90 (47.0–510.0)	24	–	
Ammonia µmol/l	465.90 ± 47.40 (172.0–932.0)	21	309.93 ± 14.28 (174.0–486.0)	32
Carbon dioxide mmol/l	27.47 ± 4.41 (10.0–94)	19	26.24 ± 0.80 (19.0–38.0)	37
Magnesium mmol/l	0.35 ± 0.02 (0.12–0.78)	24	1.07 ± 0.03 (0.65–1.72)	38
Phosphorus mmol/l	1.32 ± 0.08 (0.83–2.36)	26	1.30 ± 0.10 (0.41–3.32)	38
Calcium mmol/l	3.11 ± 0.20 (1.52–5.27)	24	2.39 ± 0.08 (0.87–3.02)	38
Potassium mmol/l	2.94 ± 0.19 (1.80–6.10)	25	3.89 ± 0.14 (1.80–5.50)	35
Sodium mmol/l	154.48 ± 1.42 (145.0–174.0)	25	151.23 ± 2.30 (112.0–179.0)	38
Chloride mmol/l	403.69 ± 3.43 (381.5–444.5)	23	401.66 ± 4.9 (343.0–469.0)	34
Cholesterol mmol/l	3.11 ± 0.17 (1.70–4.99)	26	5.46 ± 0.21 (3.62–8.14)	33
Triglycerides mmol/l	1.21 ± 0.09 (0.68–2.54)	25	2.74 ± 0.21 (1.09–4.48)	24
VLDL mg/dl	21.18 ± 1.44 (12.0–37.0)	22	–	

Mean ± standard error of mean (minimum–maximum)
* Source: modified from: D'Aloia M-A, Samour JH, Bailey TA, Naldo J, Howlett JC (1996) Normal blood chemistry of the kori bustard (*Ardeotis kori*). *Avian Pathology*, **25**: 161–165. [†] Source: modified from: D'Aloia M-A, Samour JH, Howlett JC, Bailey TA, Naldo J (1996) Normal blood chemistry of the houbara bustard (*Chlamydotis undulata*). *Avian Pathology*, **25**: 167–173.

Plasma or serum chemistry values for racing pigeons

Species	Racing pigeon	
Scientific name	*Columba livia*	n
Sodium mmol/l	145 ± 0.3	68
Potassium mmol/l	4.4 ± 0.06	52
Calcium mmol/l	2.3 ± 0.03	52
Magnesium mmol/l	1.3 ± 0.03	50
Anorganic phosphorus mmol/l	0.83 ± 0.04	53
Chloride mmol/l	107 ± 0.5	55
Plasma iron µmol/l	23 ± 2.1	50
Iron binding capacity µmol/l	37.5 ± 0.8	50
Osmolality mosmol/kg	306 ± 0.9	55
Glucose mmol/l	16.6 ± 0.2	96
Creatinine µmol/l	28 ± 0.6	52
Uric acid µmol/l	375 ± 30	50
CK (EC 2.6.3.2) IU/l	203 ± 13.5	50
AP (EC 3.1.31.) IU/l	367 ± 25	65
LD (EC 1.1.1.27) IU/l	57 ± 3.2	50
ASAT (EC 2.6.1.1) IU/l	58.6 ± 2.5	50
ALAT (EC 2.6.1.2) IU/l	25 ± 1.6	50
Total serum protein g/l	27 ± 0.4	93
Pre-albumin g/l	2.8 ± 0.13	58
Albumin g/l	17.5 ± 0.36	58
α-globulin g/l	2.29 ± 0.08	58
β-globulin g/l	4.3 ± 0.14	58
γ-globulin g/l	1.9 ± 0.1	58

Mean ± standard error of mean
Source: modified from: Lumeij JT, de Bruijne JJ (1985) Blood chemistry reference values in racing pigeons (*Columba livia domestica*). *Avian Pathology* **14**: 401–408.

Blood chemistry values for blue and gold macaws

Species	Blue and gold macaw
Scientific name	*Ara ararauna*
Sodium mmol/l	145.7 (138–153)
Potassium mmol/l	7.4 (5.0–10.4)
Chloride mmol/l	106.5 (103–110)
Calcium mmol/l	2.77 (82.2–3.07)
Ionized Ca mmol/l	5.4 (4.6–6.2)
Phosphorus mmol/l	0.74 (0.61–0.83)
Total protein g/l	49.5 (43–56)
Albumin g/l	22.5 (19–26)
Globulin g/l	25.5 (21–30)
A/G	0.75 (0.6–0.9)
Iron µmol/l	19.16 (14.1–24.1)
Glucose mmol/l	17.1 (15.8–18.4)
BUN mmol/l	2.14 (0.74–3.57)
Creatinine µmol/l	35.3 (26.52–44.2)
BUN/Creatinine	8 (3–13)
Uric acid mmol/l	416.3 (237.9–600.7)
Cholesterol mmol/l	4.39 (3.59–5.22)
Triglycerides mmol/l	1.14 (33–170)
Total bilirubin µmol/l	2.56 (1.71–3.42)
Alkaline phosphatase IU/l	371 (162–580)
LDH IU/l	423.5 (183–664)
SGOT IU/l	247 (197–297)
SGPT IU/l	186 (99–263)

Mean (minimum–maximum)
Source: modified from: Raphael BL (1980) Hematology and blood chemistry of macaws. *Proceedings of the American Association of Zoo Veterinarians*, pp. 97–98. Washington.

Blood chemistry values for the Mauritius kestrel

Species	Mauritius kestrel
Scientific name	*Falco punctatus*
GGT IU/l 37°C	441 (30°C)
GOT IU/l 37°C	85.7–372.5 (30°C)
Creatinine mmol/l	3.9–11
Bilirubin mmol/l	923.4–4873.5
Total protein g/l	12–17

(Minimum–maximum)
Source: modified from: Cooper JE, Needham JR, Fox NC (1986) Bacteriological, haematological and clinical studies on the Mauritius kestrel (*Falco punctatus*). *Avian Pathology* **15**: 349–356.

Blood chemistry values for selected Falconiformes

Species	Golden eagle*	Bald eagle*	Tawny eagle[†] n = 29	Red-tailed hawk*,[‡]	Harris hawk*
Scientific name	*Aquila chrysaetos*	*Haliaëtus leucocephalus*	*Aquila rapax*	*Buteo jamaicensis*	*Parabuteo unicinctus*
Glucose mmol/l	13.8–22.6	15.8–22.2	10.19–14.4	17.3–22.8 16.9–22.2	16.2–21.6
Cholesterol mmol/l	–	3.87–6.25	7.90–10.70	2.58–3.87	2.58–3.87
Triglycerides mmol/l	–	–	–	–	1.69–3.16
GGT IU/l 37°C	–	–	1–2.7	–	–
GOT IU/l 37°C	95–210	153–370	124–226	113–180 136–307	–
GPT IU/l 37°C	–	–	–	–	–
Uric acid mmol/l	261–713.7	329.5–285.5	412–575	446.1–1058.7 481.7–999.2	523.4–1278.8
Creatinine mmol/l	0.5–1.2	0.4–1	0.3–0.59	0.5–1.2	0.7–1.5
Bilirubin µmol/l	5.13–8.55	3.42–8.55	–	8.55–10.26	8.55–20.5
Total protein g/l	25–39	30–41	29–41	33–45 4.8	39–52
Potassium mmol/l	–	–	1.5–3.1	2.6–4.3	–

Mean ± SD; minimum–maximum
* Source: modified from: Ivins GK, Weddle GD, Haliwell WH (1986) Hematology and serum chemistries in birds of prey. In: Fowler ME (ed.) *Zoo and Wildlife Medicine*, 2nd edn, pp. 286–290. WB Saunders, Philadelphia. † Modified from: Jennings IB (1996) Haematology. In: Beynon PH, Forbes NA, Harcourt-Brown NH (1996) *Manual of Raptors, Pigeons and Waterfowl*, pp. 68–78. British Small Animal Veterinary Association, Cheltenham. ‡ Modified from: Kollias GV, McLeish J (1978) Effects of ketamine hydrochloride in red-tailed hawks (*Buteo jamaicensis*), biochemical and hematology. *Comparative Biochemistry and Physiology* **60**: 211.

Blood chemistry values for selected Falconiformes

Species	Saker falcon*,† n = 30, 38	Peregrine falcon†,‡ n = 55, 14	Lanner falcon† n = 26	Gyrfalcon§ n = 53	Merlin† n = 39
Scientific name	*Falco cherrug*	*Falco peregrinus*	*Falco biarmicus*	*Falco rusticolus*	*Falco columbarius*
Glucose mmol/l	12–14	11–16	11–15	20.4 (1.7)	9–12 (1.7)
Cholesterol mmol/l	4.5–8.6	3.9–10.5	3–8.8	5.44 (1.03)	3–7.8 (1.03)
Triglycerides mmol/l	0.79–1.25	–	–	–	1.02 (0.27)
GGT IU/l 37°C	0.8–5.9	0–7	–	–	–
AST (GOT) IU/l 37°C	45–95	50–105	30–118	149 (110)	50–125
ALT (GPT) IU/l 37°C	36–55	15–51	–	135 (125)	
ALP IU/l	285–450	97–350	180–510	–	54–310
CK IU/l	355–651	357–850	350–650	–	521–807
LDH IU/l	551–765	625–1210	434–897	1917 (879)	329–630
Uric acid μmol/l	320–785	326–675	318–709	370 (170)	174–800
Urea mmol/l	0.5–2.6	0.9–2.8	1.3–2.7	3.6 (2.2)	–
Creatinine μmol/l	23–75	41–91	37–75	38 (14)	16–50
Bile acids μmol/l	20–90	20–118	–	–	–
Bilirubin μmol/l	146.2–470.7	1336.3	–	78.6 (29.07)	–
Total protein g/l	270–360	250–400	330–420	250 (87)	275–390
Albumin g/l	90–123	83–125	96–160	118 (17)	86–161
Globulin g/l	180–280	160–280	212–288	0.47–0.58	172–250
A:G ratio	0.45–0.57	0.4–0.55	0.44–0.57	0.47–0.58	0.47–0.58
Amylase IU/l	–	–	–	86 (116)	–
Potassium mmol/l	0.8–2.3	0.9–1.7	1–2.1	3.1 (0.9)	1–1.8
Chloride mmol/l	114–125	117–127	–	124 (8)	–
Sodium mmol/l	154–161	153–164	152–164	154 (12)	155–170
Calcium mmol/l	–	–	–	2.30 (0.27)	–
Phosphorus mmol/l	–	–	–	1.52 (0.40)	–

* Source: modified from: Samour JH, D'Aloia M-A (1996) Blood chemistry of the saker falcon (*Falco cherrug*). *Avian Pathology* **25**: 175–178; † Source: modified from: Jennings IB (1996) Haematology. In: Beynon PH, Forbes NA, Harcourt-Brown NH (1996) *Manual of Raptors, Pigeons and Waterfowl*, pp. 68–78. British Small Animal Veterinary Association, Cheltenham; ‡ Altman RB *et al.* (1997) Appendix 1, *Avian Medicine and Surgery*, pp. 1004–1024. WB Saunders, Philadelphia; § Lierz M (2003) Plasma chemistry reference values for gyrfalcons (*Falco rusticolus*). *Veterinary Record* **153**: 182–183.

Blood chemistry values for selected birds of prey

Species	Bald eagle	Peregrine falcon	Gyrfalcon	Red-tailed hawk	Great-horned owl
Scientific name	*Haliaëtus leucocephalus*	*Falco peregrinus*	*Falco rusticolus*	*Buteo jamaicensis*	*Bubo virginianus*
Acetylcholinesterase delta pH units/h	0.16 (0.06)	–	–	–	–
Alanine aminotransferase (ALT) IU/l	25 (13)	62 (56)	–	31 (5)	39 (14)
Albumin g/l	10.9 (1.8)	9.6 (1.3)	7.3 (0.9)	13.4 (4.1)	12.7 (3.5)
Alkaline phosphatase IU/l	57 (12)	99 (44)	257 (61)	53 (18)	31 (7)
Amylase IU/l	1158 (376)	–	–	–	–
Aspartate aminotransferase (AST) IU/l	218 (63)	78 (31)	97 (33)	303 (22)	287 (65)
Bilirubin, total µmol/l	5.30 (1.36)	78.1 (34.8)	–	2.73 (1.36)	1.19 (1.02)
Blood urea nitrogen (BUN) mmol/l	2.21 (1.76)	2.32 (0.09)	3.33 (0.58)	3.33 (0.33)	3.57 (2.09)
Calcium mmol/l	2.48 (0.11)	2.23 (0.11)	2.40 (0.06)	–	2.54
Chloride mmol/l	120 (3)	114.38 (43.36)	125 (2)	125 (3)	122
Creatine kinase IU/l	383 (300)	783 (503)	402 (163)	1124 (251)	977 (407)
Creatinine µmol/l	61.88 (22.9)	45.08 (19.4)	–	–	–
Glucose mmol/l	16.76 (1.38)	20.3 (1.60)	17.6 (2.16)	19.7 (0.88)	19.7
Osmolality mmol/kg	319 (6)	–	–	–	–
Phosphorus mmol/l	0.97 (0.16)	1.08 (0.22)	1.15 (0.36)	1.01 (0.16)	1.40
Potassium mmol/l	3.0 (0)	2.04 (0.81)	1.99 (0.56)	2.42 (0.73)	2.8
Protein, total g/l (biuret)	35.1 (7.5)	26.3 (4.8)	28.9 (3.1)	41.7 (6.9)	43.3
Sodium mmol/l	156 (4)	143 (54)	160 (3)	157 (1)	156
Uric acid mmol/l	301.5 (198.0)	267.6 (252.1)	828.5 (335.4)	644 (303.3)	814.8 (642.0)

Source: modified from: Altman RB, Clubb SL, Dorrestein GM, Quesenberry K (eds) (1997). *Avian Medicine and Surgery*. WB Saunders Co., Philadelphia. Information from Professor Patrick Redig, Raptor Center, University of Minnesota, Minneapolis.

Blood chemistry values for selected Psittaciformes

Species	Cockatiel n = 364	Cockatoo n = 242	African gray parrot n = 108	Conure n = 85	Grand eclectus parrot n = 9	Philippine blue-naped parrot n = 7
Scientific name	Nymphicus hollandicus	Cacatua spp.	Psittacus e. erithacus	Aratinga spp.	Eclectus roratus riedeli	Tanygnathus lucionensis
Total protein g/l	22–50	25–50	30–50	25–45	30–50	30–50
Glucose mmol/l	13.8–24.9	10.5–19.4	10.5–19.4	13.8–19.4	9.99–19.9	10.5–19.4
Calcium mmol/l	2.12–3.25	2.0–3.25	2.0–3.25	2.0–3.75	2.25–4.0	2.5–4.0
SGOT IU/l	100–350	150–350	100–350	125–350	130–350	130–350
LDH IU/l	125–450	225–650	150–450	125–420	100–200	130–425
Creatinine μmol/l	8.84–35.3	8.84–35.3	8.84–35.3	8.84–44.2	8.84–35.3	8.84–35.3
Uric acid mmol/l	208.1–654	208.4–654	237.0–594.8	148.7–624.5	178.4–594.8	237–594.8
Potassium mmol/l	2.5–4.5	2.5–4.5	2.6–4.2	3.4–5.0	–	–
Sodium mmol/l	132–150	131–157	134–152	134–148	–	–
Thyroxine mmol/l	9.0–30.8	10.2–56.6	38.6–25.7	3.21–11.5	6.43–12.8	3.86–12.87

(Minimum–maximum)

Source: modified from: Woerpel RW, Rosskopf WJ (1984) Clinical experience with avian laboratory diagnostics. *Veterinary Clinics of North America* **14**: 254.

Blood chemistry values for selected Psittaciformes (*continued*)

Species	Lovebird n = 78	Macaw n = 219	Amazon parrot n = 640	Blue-headed parrot n = 16	Budgerigar n = 251	Gray-cheeked parakeet n = 32
Scientific name	Agapornis spp.	Ara spp.	Amazona spp.	Pionus menstruus	Melopsittacus undulatus	Brotogeris pyrrhopterus
Total protein g/l	22–51	30–50	30–50	26–50	25–45	25–45
Glucose mmol/l	11.1–22.2	11.1–19.4	12.2–19.4	9.99–16.6	11.1–22.2	11.1–19.4
Calcium mmol/l	2.25–3.75	2.25–3.25	2.0–13.25	2.5–3.75	–	–
SGOT IU/l	100–350	100–280	130–350	150–350	150–350	150–400
LDH IU/l	100–350	75–425	160–420	200–550	150–450	150–450
Creatinine μmol/l	8.84–35.3	8.87–44.2	8.84–35.3	8.84–26.5	8.84–35.4	8.84–35.4
Uric acid mmol/l	178.0–654.0	148.7–684.0	118.9–594.8	237.9–713.7	237.9–832.7	237.9–713.0
Potassium mmol/l	2.5–3.5	2.5–4.5	3.0–4.5	3.0–4.5	–	–
Sodium mmol/l	137–150	136–155	136–152	130–150	–	–
Thyroxine mmol/l	2.57–24.4	12.87–51.4	0.64–12.87	2.57–14.1	32.1–56.6	2.57–30.8

(Minimum–maximum)

Source: modified from: Woerpel RW, Rosskopf WJ, Monahan–Brennan M (1987) Clinical pathology and laboratory diagnostic tools. In: Burr EW (ed.) *Companion Bird Medicine*, pp. 180–196. Iowa State University Press, Ames, IA.

Blood chemistry values for selected Psittaciformes (*continued*)

Species	African gray parrot	Amazon parrot	Cockatoo	Macaw
Scientific name	*Psittacus erithacus*	*Amazona* spp.	*Cacatua* spp.	*Ara* spp.
Urea mmol/l	0.7–2.4	0.9–4.6	0.8–2.1	0.3–3.3
Creatinine μmol/l	23–40	19–33	21–36	20–59
Uric acid μmol/l	93–414	72–312	190–327	109–231
Urea:uric acid ratio	2.4:15.6	4.4:33	2.7:8.9	5:28
Osmolality mosmol/kg	320–347	316–373	317–347	319–378
Sodium mmol/l	154–164	149–164	152–164	150–175
Potassium mmol/l	2.5–3.9	2.3–4.2	3.2–4.9	1.9–4.1
Ca mmol/l	2.1–2.6	2.0–2.8	2.2–2.7	2.2–2.8
Glucose mmol/l	11.4–16.1	12.6–16.9	12.8–17.6	12.0–17.9
AST U/l	54–155	57–194	52–203	58–206
ALT U/l	12–59	19–98	12–37	22–105
GGT U/l	1–3.8	1–10	2–5	<1–5
LDH U/l	147–348	46–208	203–442	66–166
CPK U/l	123–875	45–265	34–204	61–531
Bile acids μmol/l	18–71	19–144	23–70	25–71
TP g/l	32–44	33–50	35–44	33–53
Albumin:globulin ratio	1.4:4.7	2.6:7.0	1.5:4.3	1.4:3.9

Mean ± SD, (minimum–maximum)
Source: modified from: Lumeij JT, Overduin LM (1990) Plasma chemistry references values in Psittaciformes. *Avian Pathology* **19**: 235–244.

Blood chemistry values for selected Psittaciformes (*continued*)

Species	Budgerigar	African gray parrot	Amazon parrot	Cockatoo	Macaw
Scientific name	*Melopsittacus undulatus*	*Psittacus erithacus*	*Amazona* spp.	*Cacatua* spp.	*Ara* spp.
TP g/l	20–30	26–49	33–53	28–43	25–44
Ca mmol/l	1.6–2.8	1.75–2.3	1.87–2.42	1.9–2.22	1.7–2.47
P mmol/l	0.9–1.9	1.0–5.2	0.8–3.4	1.0–3.6	1.3–4.8
Uric acid mmol/l	178.4–511.5	184.3–416.3	77.3–333	208.1–553.1	172–505
Creatinine μmol/l	8.84–35.3	8.84–35.3	8.84–35.3	8.84–35.3	8.84–35.3
AST IU/l	55–154	28–200	35–200	32–180	45–125
ALT IU/l	5–20	2–21	4–13	5–12	5–15
LDH IU/l	154–271	105–420	65–420	130–353	65–400
CK IU/l	54–252	71–408	64–322	27–253	39–384
AP IU/l	54–326	24–94	93–311	32–171	25–152
Amylase IU/l	187–582	211–519	106–524	–	276–594
Glucose mmol/l	14.5–22.1	12.4–17.0	12.2–16.6	11.6–17.6	12.7–18.0
Cholesterol mmol/l	4.44–7.39	5.61–8.53	4.68–8.01	–	2.79–5.17
Triglycerides mmol/l	1.23–3.05	0.57–1.58	0.66–2.25	–	0.75–1.41
K mmol/l	2.2–3.7	2.2–3.5	2.1–3.3	–	2.1–4.5
Na mmol/l	139–159	146–167	127–158	–	133–160
Cl mmol/l	95–144	110–128	97–127	–	97–126

Kodak Ektachem ® –25°C
Source: modified from: Hochleithner M (1989) References values for selected psittacine species using a dry chemistry system. *Journal of the Association of Avian Veterinarians* **3**: 207–209.

Blood chemistry values for selected Psittaciformes (*continued*)

Species	Hyacinthine macaw	Blue and yellow macaw	Green-winged macaw	Scarlet macaw	Military macaw
Scientific name	*Anododorhynchus hyacinthinus*	*Ara ararauna*	*Ara chloroptera*	*Ara macao*	*Ara militaris*
	n = 13	*n* = 30	*n* = 16	*n* = 12	*n* = 16
Glucose mmol/l	14.5 ± 0.9 (13.2–15.9)	15.1 ± 2.1 (10.1–19.0)	16.0 ± 1.7 (13.2–18.9)	13.8 ± 0.9 (12.0–15.2)	15.4 ± 1.7 (12.0–18.3)
Urea mmol/l	1.3 ± 0.4 (0.6–22.2)	1.3 ± 0.5 (0.4–2.1)	1.3 ± 0.6 (0.5–2.2)	1.9 ± 0.7 (1.2–3.9)	1.2 ± 0.7 (0.2–2.5)
Uric acid µmol/l	347 ± 136 (127–641)	296 ± 147 (113–629)	401 ± 216 (151–829)	277 ± 161 (143–583)	466 ± 210 (144–842)
Cholesterol mmol/l	3.1 ± 0.6 (2.2–4.3)	4.2 + 0.9 (3.1–6.7)	4.2 ± 0.9 (2.1–5.3)	4.3 ± 1.1 (2.3–6.4)	4.2 ± 1.3 (1.7–6.6)
Triglycerides mmol/l	0.8 ± 0.3 (0.4–1.3)	1.2 + 0.7 (0.4–2.5)	1.3 ± 0.5 (0.7–2.1)	1.0 ± 0.3 (0.5–1.6)	1.0 ± 0.5 (0.3–1.8)
Creatinine µmol/l	45.7 ± 8.8 (33.7–62.8)	49.1 ± 15.1 (26.1–76.8)	62.5 ± 14.3 (33.5–78.6)	49.3 ± 9.6 (31.6–61.0)	47.4 ± 8.9 (24.2–60.3)
	n = 12	*n* = 29	*n* = 15	*n* = 7	*n* = 14
LDH IU/l	160 ± 90.7 (59.7–309)	140 + 81.3 (61.7–349)	226 ± 91.6 (113–422)	368 ± 176 (132–610)	307 ± 101 (121–485)
ASAT IU/l	56.7 ± 12.8 (38.4–90.6)	56.2 ± 19.1 (33.0–105)	68.1 ± 24.1 (44.0–139)	49.0 ± 11.2 (34.2–65.6)	97.0 ± 65.5 (37.3–228)
ALAT IU/l	7.5 ± 3.4 (2.5–14.4)	8.1 + 3.3 (3.5–15.7)	6.4 ± 3.5 (1.7–13.2)	8.8 ± 5.4 (1.3–16.8)	13.2 ± 7.0 (2.6–23.7)
CPK IU/l	142 ± 128 (16.7–351)	131 + 109 (35.4–428)	86.9 ± 45.4 (25.1–151)	64.0 ± 41.9 (20.3–132)	136 ± 167 (10.1–430)
AP IU/l	45.6 ± 21.9 (12.7–82.9)	194 + 81.9 (79.0–357)	132 ± 30.0 (86.1–177)	80.9 ± 23.1 (51.7–99.9)	75.9 ± 44.0 (27.6–156)
γ-GT IU/l	–	3.7 ± 5.8 (0.0–18.5)	0.5 ± 0.7 (0.0–2.0)	0.4 ± 0.5 (0.0–1.1)	3.0 ± 3.8 (0.0–11.8)
	n = 7	*n* = 17	*n* = 8	*n* = 14	*n* = 11
Osmolality mosmol/kg	298 ± 17.6 (263–319)	319 ± 6.2 (309–328)	315 ± 14.2 (251–339)	331 ± 24.0 (281–366)	29.6 ± 8.2 (17.2–44.4)
Sodium mmol/l	151 ± 20.7 (135–191)	150 + 28.6 (119–252)	145 ± 6.3 (141–159)	–	9.5 ± 6.2 (0.0–18.5)
Potassium mmol/l	4.9 ± 1.7 (3.3–7.9)	2.4 ± 0.8 (1.7–4.7)	2.7 ± 0.5 (1.9–3.2)	–	50.0 ± 12.0 (34.5–70.6)
Chloride mmol/l	102 ± 11.1 (83–120)	101 ± 9.1 (75–122)	103 ± 8.3 (91–120)	96 ± 4.8 (90–108)	10.5 ± 3.9 (5.8–18.3)
Calcium mmol/l	2.2 ± 0.4 (1.9–2.9)	2.3 ± 0.4 (1.7–3.2)	2.3 ± 0.3 (2.0–2.9)	–	17.8 ± 7.2 (8.1–32.5)
Phosphorus mmol/l	3.0 ± 0.4 (2.3–3.4)	4.5 ± 1.1 (3.0–6.2)	4.1 ± 1.2 (2.4–5.8)	–	12.1 ± 5.1 (1.8–19.6)
Magnesium mmol/l	1.2 ± 0.5 (0.9–2.0)	1.0 ± 0.2 (0.7–1.4)	1.3 ± 0.5 (0.9–2.2)	–	1.6 ± 0.5 (0.6–2.4)

Mean ± SD, (minimum–maximum)

Source: modified from: Polo FJ, Peinado VI, Viscor G, Palomeque J (1998) Hematologic and plasma chemistry in captive psittacine birds. *Avian Diseases* **42**: 523–535.

Normal blood chemistry values for selected avian species

Species	Greater Indian hill mynah n = 35	Toucan n = 8	Canary n = 62	Finches n = 21
Scientific name	*Gracula religiosa*	*Rhamphastos* spp.	*Serinus canaria*	
Total protein g/l	23–45	30–50	30–50	30–50
Glucose mmol/l	10.5–19.4	12.2–19.4	11.1–24.9	11.1–24.9
Calcium mmol/l	9.0–13.0	10.0–19.0	–	–
SGOT IU/l	130–350	130–330	150–350	150–350
LDH IU/l	600–1000	200–400	–	–
Creatinine μmol/l	8.84–53.0	8.84–35.3	–	–
Uric acid mmol/l	237.9–594.8	237.9–832.7	237.9–713.7	237.0–713.7
Potassium mmol/l	3.0–5.1	–	–	–
Sodium mmol/l	136–152	–	–	–
Thyroxine mmol/l	6.43–11.5	6.43–41.1	9.0–43.7	–

(Minimum–maximum)
Source: modified from: Woerpel RW, Rosskopf PF, Monahan-Brennan M (1987) Clinical pathology and laboratory diagnostic tools. In: Burr EW (ed.) *Companion Bird Medicine*, pp. 180–196. Iowa State University Press, Ames, IA.

Blood chemistry values for captive Masai ostrich (*Struthio camelus*)

Species	Ostrich n = 4
Total protein g/l	38.7 (5.8)
Glucose mmol/l	11.5 (1.86)
Blood urea nitrogen mmol/l	1.67 (0.19)
Uric acid mmol/l	664.3 (125.5)
Cholesterol mmol/l	3.0 (0.70)
Total bilirubin μmol/l	2.46 (0.68)
Creatinine μmol/l	56.6 (11.4)
Lactic dehydrogenase IU/l	514.9 (286.1)
Alkaline phosphatase IU/l	171.5 (45.9)
Aspartate aminotransferase IU/l	190.5 (39.4)
Alanine aminotransferase IU/l	20.62 (4.36)
Creatinine phosphokinase IU/l	933.0 (269.0)
Sodium g/l	3.69 (0.26)
Potassium mg/100 ml	6.64 (0.98)
Chloride mmol/l	8.51 (1.18)
Calcium mmol/l	4.51 (0.40)
Phosphorus mmol/l	4.42 (0.94)
Magnesium mmol/l	0.92 (0.07)

Mean (SD)
Source: modified from: Palomeque J, Pinto D, Viscor G (1991) Hematologic and blood chemistry values of the Masai ostrich (*Struthio camelus*). *Journal of Wildlife Diseases* **27**: 34–40.

Biochemistry values for mourning doves (*Zenaida macroura*)

Blood chemistry values	Male	n	Female	n
Glucose mmol/l	26.53 ± 0.47 (19.48–36.80)	94	25.91 ± 0.47 (18.87–39.85)	87
Sodium mmol/l	144.0 ± 033 (137.0–154.0)	97	143.43 ± 0.41 (125.0–156.0)	87
Potassium mmol/l	7.78 ± 0.19 (4.0–14.9)	96	7.81 ± 0.18 (4.5–12.0)	87
Chloride mmol/l	113.64 ± 0.33 (107.0–121.0)	94	112.6 ± 0.42 (96.0–123.0)	88
Total protein g/l	26.2 ± 0.4 (18–39)	97	26.6 ± 0.5 (17.0–39.0)	87
Albumin g/l	12.1 ± 0.2 (9–17)	97	12.2 ± 0.2 (10–17)	87
Globulin g/l	14.2 ± 0.3 (9–26)	97	14.4 ± 0.3 (07–26)	87
Calcium mmol/l	2.36 ± 0.02 (1.8- ± 2.87)	97	2.43 ± 0.02 (1.6–3)	87
Phosphorus mmol/l	1.22 + 0.03 (0.61–2.39)	97	1.25 ± 0.03 (0.67–2.61)	87
Cholesterol mmol/l	5.79 ± 0.14 (3.05–13.75)	94	5.97 ± 0.19 (2.1–12.12)	87
Magnesium mmol/l	1.17 ± 0.01 (0.86–1.59)	97	1.17 ± 0.01 (0.86–1.51)	87
Uric acid mmol/l	429.44 ± 13.68 (178.44–844.61)	96	429.44 ± 18.43 (154.64–1017)	87
AST IU/l	252.60 ± 1137 (94–709)	97	270.07 ± 11.10 (143–659)	86
GGT IU/l	11.16 ± 0.40 (9–37)	94	10.87 ± 0.31 (9–27)	86
LDH IU/l	905.35 ± 36.38 (312–1822)	95	1175 ± 108.11 (320–8528)	87

Mean ± standard error of the mean (range)
Source: modified from: Schulz JH *et al.* (2000) Blood plasma chemistries from wild mourning doves held in captivity. *Journal of Wildlife Diseases* **36**: 541–545.

Serum biochemistry values for juvenile umbrella cockatoos (*Cacatua alba*)

Blood chemistry values	30 day	90 day	All
Na mmol/l	139 (1.78)[s]	149 (2.33)[n]	145
K mmol/l	4.23 (0.57)[n]	3.13 (0.44)[n]	3.54
Cl mmol/l	107 (2.8)[s]	115 (3.2)[n]	111
Ca mmol/l	2.41 (0.09)[s]	2.35 (0.32)[n]	2.44
Phosphorus mmol/l	2.09 (0.14)[s]	1.51 (0.28)[n]	1.79
Urea mmol/l	0.16 (0.29)[n]	0.32 (0.40)[s]	0.26
Creatinine mmol/l	30.0 (6.1)[n]	29.1 (3.53)[s]	32.7
UA mmol/l	49.3 (21.4)[s]	294.4 (99.9)[n]	162.3
Cholesterol mmol/l	4.65 (0.95)[s]	11.0 (1.81)[s]	7.52
Glucose mmol/l	13.5 (1.0)[n]	13.1 (1.56)[s]	13.5
LDH IU/l	326 (394)[n]	341 (174)[n]	325
AST IU/l	84 (17.7)[n]	187 (39.2)[n]	136
ALT IU/l	1.8 (1.7)[n]	2.69 (1.58)[n]	2.11
ALP IU/l	426 (100)[s]	404 (104)[s]	440
GGT IU/l	1.95 (1.73)[n]	2.81 (1.33)[n]	2.66
CK IU/l	629 (193)[n]	395 (115)[n]	517
TP g/l	24.7 (4.1)[s]	32.5 (5.9)[n]	30.3
A:G ratio	0.6 (0.1)	0.62 (0.08)	0.64
PRE ALB g/l	4.3 (1.2)[n]	4.9 (1.3)[n]	4.5
ALB (Elect) g/l	12.7 (2.7)[s]	18.6 (3.5)[n]	16.9
α- GLOB g/l	1.7 (0.5)[n]	2.9 (1.9)[n]	2.6
β GLOB g/l	3.9 (1.6)[n]	3.4 (1.4)[n]	3.8
γ GLOB g/dl	2.3 (0.6)[n]	3.1 (1.1)[n]	2.9

Mean (SD)

s, mean statistically different ($p > 0.05$) from the same parameter in all juvenile cockatoos; n, mean is not statistically different ($p < 0.05$) from the same parameter in all juvenile cockatoos.

Source: modified from: Clubb SL, Schubot RM, Joyner K et al. (1991) Hematologic and serum biochemical reference intervals in juvenile cockatoos. *Journal of the Association of Avian Veterinarians* **5**: 16–26.

Serum biochemistry values for juvenile eclectus parrot (*Eclectus roratus*)

Blood chemistry values	30 day	90 day	All
Na mmol/l	141 (2)	154 (3)	148 (6)
K mmol/l	2.9 (1.0)	2.7 (0.6)	2.8 (0.7)
Cl mmol/l	105 (3)	115 (3)	111 (5)
Ca mmol/l	2.37 (0.12)	2.77 (0.1)	2.32 (0.1)
Phosphorus mmol/l	2.55 (0.25)	1.84 (0.29)	2.19 (0.38)
Urea mmol/l	0.25 (0.38)	0.33 (0.51)	0.28 (0.40)
Creatinine μmol/l	26.5 (8.84)	35.3 (8.84)	35.3 (8.84)
UA mmol/l	47.5 (53.5)	231.9 (89.2)	118.9 (95.1)
Cholesterol mg/dl	181 (43)	300 (69)	268 (80)
Glucose mmol/l	13.8 (0.88)	14.7 (1.05)	14.5 (0.99)
LDH IU/l	235 (145)	268 (70)	228 (101)
AST IU/l	85 (21)	216 (47)	140 (58)
ALT IU/l	4 (3)	7 (3)	4 (3)
ALP IU/l	421 (85)	565 (217)	489 (159)
GGT IU/l	5 (2)	2 (1)	4 (2)
CK IU/l	555 (164)	643 (262)	616 (472)
TP g/l	26 (4)	29 (04)	29 (5)
ALB g/l	12 (2)	13 (2)	13 (3)
GLOB g/dl	13 (3)	16 (3)	15 (3)
A:G ratio	0.9 (0.1)	0.8 (0.1)	0.9 (0.2)
ALB (Elect) g/l	18 (5)	21 (4)	22 (4)
GLOB (Elect) g/l	7 (2)	7 (2)	8 (2)

Mean (SD)

Source: modified from: Clubb SL, Schubot RM, Joyner K *et al.* (1990) Hematologic and serum chemistry reference intervals in juvenile eclectus parrots. *Journal of the Association of Avian Veterinarians* **4**: 218–225.

Serum biochemistry values for juvenile cockatoos (*Cacatua* spp.)

Blood chemistry values	30 day	90 day	All
Na mmol/l	139 (3)[a]	139 (3)[c]	145 (6)
K mmol/l	4.0 (0.8)[a]	3.10 (0.4)[b]	3.6 (0.7)
Cl mmol/l	105 (4)[a]	115 (4)[c]	110 (6)
Ca mmol/l	2.3 (0.15)[a]	2.3 (0.25)[a,b]	2.4 (0.17)
Phosphorus mmol/l	2.26 (0.19)[a]	1.64 (0.38)[c]	1.97 (0.35)
Urea mmol/l	0.26 (0.31)[a]	0.43 (0.41)[b]	0.33 (0.36)
Creatinine μmol/l	27.4 (5.30)[a]	37.1 (6.1)[a,b]	35.3 (8.84)
UA mmol/l	71.3 (53.5)[a]	303 (107)[c]	172.4 (136.8)
Cholesterol mmol/l	4.26 (0.82)[a]	9.05 (3.1)[b]	6.49 (2.71)
Glucose mmol/l	13.7 (1.11)[a]	13.8 (1.60)[a,b]	14.0 (1.33)
LDH IU/l	393 (348)[a]	367 (218)[a]	371 (285)
AST IU/l	98 (54)[a]	195 (73)[c]	143 (79)
ALT IU/l	2 (2)[a]	3 (3)[a,b]	2 (3)
ALP IU/l	593 (202)[a]	478 (167)[c]	579 (239)
GGT IU/l	2.35 (1.75)[a]	2.79 (1.54)[a,c]	2.55 (1.67)
CK IU/l	595 (205)[a]	368 (156)[b]	510 (235)
TP g/l	22 (4)[a]	31 (6)[b]	28 (7)
ALB g/l	8 (2)[a]	12 (3)[b]	11 (3)
GLOB g/l	13 (4)[a]	19 (4)[b]	17 (5)
A:G ratio	0.6 (0.2)[a,b]	0.6 (0.1)[b]	0.6 (0.2)
PRE ALB g/l	4 (1)[a]	5 (2)[b]	5 (2)
ALB (Elect) g/l	11 (3)[a]	7 (5)[b,c]	15 (5)
α- GLOB g/l	2 (1)[a]	3 (2)[c]	2 (1)
β GLOB g/l	3 (2)[a]	3 (1)[a]	3 (1)
γ GLOB g/l	2 (1)[a]	3 (1)[b]	3 (1)

Mean (SD)

a,b,c = Values for parameters are statistically different when letters are different.

Source: modified from: Clubb SL, Schubot RM, Joyner K *et al.* (1991) Hematologic and serum biochemical reference intervals in juvenile cockatoos. *Journal of the Association of Avian Veterinarians* **5**: 16–26.

Blood chemistry for canary finches (*Serinus canaria*)

Blood chemistry values	Mean	SD	$P_{2.5}$–$P_{97.5}$
Ca mmol/l	1.99	0.46	1.27–3.35
P mmol/l	1.05	0.39	0.51–1.80
Na mmol/l	139.2	8.18	125–154
Cl mmol/l	108.88	8.85	93–123
K mmol/l	3.58	0.69	2.7–4.8
Glucose mmol/l	19.19	1.68	16.1–21.7
Triglycerides mmol/l	2.08	0.62	1.35–3.52
Creatinine μmol/l	42.4	22.1	8.84–88.4
NH_3 mmol/l	221.18	110.42	87–467
ALT IU/l	11.58	7.92	2–30
AST IU/l	98.93	34.73	45–170
LDH IU/l	1582.63	325.72	1580–1816[m] 1300–1632[f]
AP IU/l	265.05	79.62	146–397
Cholesterol mmol/l	4.27	1.15	2.84–7.39
Amyl IU/l	481.78	141.84	277–787
CK IU/l	302.1	106.94	177–556
TP g/l	2.84	0.75	2.0–4.4
Uric acid mmol/l	531.1	196.8	255.7–880.3

Kodak Ektachem® –25°C.

m = male; f = female.

Source: modified from: Schöpf A, Vasicek L (1991) Blood chemistry in canary finches (*Serinus canaria*). *Proceedings of the European Association of Avian Veterinarians*, Vienna, pp. 437–439.

Blood chemistry for selected Galliformes

Species	Scientific name	TP g/l	Albumin g/l	Globulin g/l	Creatine µmol/l	Uric acid mmol/l	Glucose mmol/l	Cholesterol mmol/l	Ca mmol/l	P mmol/l	Na mmol/l	K mmol/l
Domestic fowl	Gallus domesticus	33–35	13–2.8	15–41	79.5–159.1	148.7–481.7	12.6–16.6	2.22–5.45	3.3–5.92	2.0–2.55	131–171	3.0–7.3
Domestic turkey	Meleagris gallopavo	49–76	30–59	17–19	70.7–79.5	202.2–309.2	15.2–23.5	2.09–3.33	2.92–9.67	1.74–2.29	149–155	6.0–6.4
Pheasant	Phasianus colchicus	69	52	17	–	136.8–220.0	18.5–22.0	4.24–4.44	–	–	–	–
Guinea fowl	Numida meleagris	35–44	–	–	–	172.4–303.3	–	–	–	–	149–157	–
Common quail	Coturnix coturnix	34–36	–	–	–	–	–	–	–	–	180	1.4
Bobwhite quail	Colinus virginianus	–	–	–	–	–	–	–	3.52–3.85	–	–	–
Japanese quail	Coturnix japonica	–	12–19	–	–	–	–	–	–	–	–	–
Peafowl	Pavo cristatus	–	–	–	–	107.0–220.0	15.1–19.8	–	–	–	154–162	–
Rock partridge	Alectoris graeca	–	–	–	–	148.7–249.8	14.9–17.3	145–163	–	–	–	–
Chachalaca	Ortalis vetula	–	–	–	–	220.0–469.8	13.04–19.1	158–164	–	–	–	–

Source: modified from: Gylstorff I (1983) *Handbuch der Geflügelphysiologie*, pp. 280–393; Gylstorff I, Grimm F (1987) *Vogelkrankheiten*; : Vollmerhaus B, Sinowatz F (1992) *Anatomie der Vögel*. pp. 159–175.

Serum chemistry values for selected Anseriformes

Species	American black duck	Canada goose*	Aleutian Canada goose†	White-fronted goose*	Nene goose†	Canvas duck	Lesser scoup	Ringneck duck	Bufflehead	Trumpeter swan
Scientific name	Anas superciliosa	Branta canadensis	Branta c. leucopareia	Anser albifrons	Branta sandvicensis	Aythya valisineria	Aythya affinis	Aythya colaris	Bucephala albeola	Cygnus buccinator
Total protein g/l	43.2 ± 4.2	53.6 ± 2.7 / 42.6 ± 1.3	48.0 ± 7	44 ± 4	44 ± 7	36–68 / 42–46	42–45	32–40	36–41	45 ± 4.9
Albumin g/l	31.0 ± 3.6 / 30.4 ± 3.0	21.8 ± 1.3 / 15.3 ± 0.5	21 ± 2 / 20 ± 2	17 ± 2 / 18 ± 2	17 ± 2 / 19 ± 2	20.8	18.9	16.8	17.2	–
Globulin g/l	12.1 ± 5.2	–	28 ± 6	27 ± 3	26 ± 5	–	–	–	–	–
A/G ratio	2.71 ± 0.77	–	0.76 ± 0.13	0.64 ± 0.08	0.71 ± 0.09	–	–	–	–	–
Glucose mmol/l	9.76 ± 1.47	12.18 ± 0.68 / 17.7 ± 1.57	11.65 ± 1.72 / 13.1 ± 2.27	12.2 ± 1.55 / 13.82 ± 1.6	10.2 ± 0.55 / 10.6 ± 0.66	9.99–30.4				
Calcium mmol/l	–	2.30 ± 0.31 / 2.64 ± 0.17	2.55 ± 0.17 / 2.6 ± 0.12	2.52 ± 0.15 / 2.57 ± 0.1	2.5 ± 0.15 / 2.62 ± 0.12	–				
Phosphorus mmol/l	1.04 ± 0.37	–	0.90 ± 0.29 / 0.93 ± 0.19	1.16 ± 0.19 / 1.09 ± 0.25	0.77 ± 0.22 / 0.77 ± 0.22	–				
Sodium mmol/l	–	–	142 ± 4	146 ± 5	146 ± 3	–				
Chloride mmol/l	–	–	105 ± 4	112 ± 23	99 ± 4	–				
Potassium mol/l	–	–	3.4 ± 0.6	3.3 ± 0.6	2.5 ± 0.4	–				
Uric acid mmol/l	–	359.8 ± 35.0 / 342.0 ± 23.1	493 ± 136.8	642.3 ± 59.48	475.8 ± 95.1	–				
Creatinine μmol/l	–	–	70.7 ± 26.5	79.5 ± 17.6	70.7 ± 17.6	–				
Blood urea nitrogen mmol/l	1.06 ± 0.25	–	2.14 ± 1.42	2.14 ± 0.71	1.42 ± 0.71	–				
AAT IU/l	55.9 ± 29.7 / 18.6 ± 8.2	–	75 ± 19	98 ± 18	45 ± 17	–				
ALP IU/l	20.9 ± 11.7 / 131.8 ± 36.7	–	72 ± 43	78 ± 44	33 ± 8	–				
LDH IU/l	312.8 ± 83.5 / 244.7 ± 81.8	–	301 ± 80	256 ± 68	659 ± 319	–				
GGT IU/l	–	–	2 ± 3	1 ± 1	2 ± 2	–				
SGPT IU/l	–	–	43 ± 11	50 ± 9	37 ± 7	–				
SGOT IU/l	–	–	75 ± 17 / 76 ± 21	104 ± 15 / 89 ± 19	40 ± 13 / 49 ± 18	–				
Amylase IU/l	–	–	570 ± 184	454 ± 201	824 ± 32	–				
Total bilirubin μmol/l	–	–	3.42 ± 11.9	8.72 ± 5.13	2.05 ± 0.68	–				

Serum chemistry values for selected Anseriformes (continued)

Species	American black duck	Canada goose*	Aleutian Canada goose†	White-fronted goose*	Nene goose†	Canvas duck	Lesser scoup	Ringneck duck	Bufflehead	Trumpeter swan
Iron μmol/l	–	–	41.9 ± 12.8	49.4 ± 16.1	–	–	–	–	–	–
Total lipids g/l	14.3 ± 1.8	–	13.8 ± 6.7	16.9 ± 6.4	14.5 ± 4.8	–	–	–	–	–
Triglyceride mmol/l	–	2.91 ± 0.68 / 1.63 ± 0.28	1.70 ± 0.31	2.42 ± 0.57	1.84 ± 0.47	–	–	–	–	–
Total cholesterol mmol/l	–	1.54 ± 0.25 / 7.9 ± 0.79	4.44 ± 0.72 / 4.44 ± 0.74	3.46 ± 0.36 / 3.36 ± 0.25	5.94 ± 0.85 / 6.02 ± 0.59	6.72 ± 9.46	–	–	–	–

* Line 1 = spring; line 2 = fall. † Line 1 = male; Line 2 = female

Source: modified from: Degernes LA et al. (1989) Lead poisoning in trumpeter swan. *Proceedings of the Association of Avian Veterinarians*, pp. 144–155. Seattle; Franson JC (1982) Enzyme activities on plasma, liver and kidneys of black ducks and mallards. *Journal of Wildlife Diseases* **18**: 481; Gee CG, Carpenter JW, Hensler GL (1982) Species differences in hematological values of captive cranes, geese, raptors and quails. *Journal of Wildlife Management* **45**: 463; Kocan RM (1972) Some physiologic blood values of wild diving ducks. *Journal of Wildlife Diseases* **8**: 115; Mori JG, George JC (1978) Seasonal changes in serum levels of certain metabolites, uric acid and calcium in the migratory Canada goose (*Branta canadensis interior*). *Comparative Biochemistry and Physiology* **59B**: 263; Mulley RC (1979) Hematology and blood chemistry of the black duck (*Anas superciliosa*). *Journal of Wildlife Diseases* **15**: 437; Wallach JD, Boever WJ (1983) Gamebirds, waterfowl and ratites. In: *Diseases of Exotic Animals: Medical and Surgical Management*, pp. 831–888. WB Saunders Co. Philadelphia.

Serum chemistry and enzyme values for non-reproductive adult mallards (Anas platyrhynchos)

Assay	Male	Female
TPR g/l	38 ± 7	42 ± 5
ALB g/l	15 ± 4	17 ± 2
GLU mg/dl	185.0 ± 47.0	215.0 ± 34.0
AMY IU/l	2631.0 ± 630.0	2766.0 ± 684.0
CHE IU/l	794.0 ± 249.0	812.0 ± 197.0
ALT IU/l	26.3 ± 8.0	29.9 ± 9.9
AST IU/l	16.2 ± 4.3	15.8 ± 4.7
GGT IU/l	7.7 ± 4.2	8.0 ± 4.8
ALP IU/l	26.3 ± 8.0	44.2 ± 22.7
LDH IU/l	199.0 ± 83.0	147.0 ± 80.0
Ca mmol/l	2.35 ± 0.47	2.45 ± 0.27
Mg mmol/l	1.8 ± 0.4	1.8 ± 0.3
PHOS mmol/l	0.93 ± 0.32	0.96 ± 0.32
UA mmol/l	237 ± 77.3	267.6 ± 107

Mean ± SD
Source: modified from: Fairbrother A (1990) Changes in mallard (*Anas platyrhynchos*) serum chemistry due to age, sex and reproductive condition. *Journal of Wildlife Diseases* **26**: 67–77.

Serum chemistry and enzyme values for adult female mallards (Anas platyrhynchos) of differing reproductive states

Assay	Pre-egg laying	Egg laying	Incubating	Molt
TPR g/l	56 ± 29	63 ± 12	44 ± 6	45 ± 12
ALB g/l	20 ± 3	23 ± 2	16 ± 2	17 ± 2
GLU mmol/l	13.21 ± 1.16	14.3 ± 2.83	11.71 ± 2.94	11.04 ± 1.66
AMY IU/l	3058.0 ± 527.0	3821.0 ± 741.0	2700.0 ± 626.0	2346.0 ± 1012.0
CHE IU/l	1337.0 ± 280.0	1563.0 ± 592.0	1002.0 ± 266.0	894.0 ± 219.0
ALT IU/l	31.0 ± 10.3	34.2 ± 19.4	30.6 ± 13.1	41.1 ± 17.1
AST IU/l	18.0 ± 3.4	23.7 ± 6.7	22.1 ± 7.4	22.6 ± 12.6
GGT IU/l	19.8 ± 19.8	199.6 ± 283.0	7.5 ± 4.7	20.8 ± 36.9
ALP IU/l	63.6 ± 56.8	124.9 ± 56.7	34.3 ± 15.8	36.0 ± 18.1
LDH IU/l	165.0 ± 50.0	177.0 ± 57.0	215.0 ± 107.0	268.0 ± 2.2
Ca mmol/l	3.5 ± 1.02	5.47 ± 1.4	2.57 ± 0.5	2.63 ± 1.05
Mg mmol/l	2.3 ± 0.5	3.6 ± 0.8	1.6 ± 0.3	1.6 ± 0.5
PHOS mmol/l	1.48 ± 0.54	2.61 ± 0.77	1.19 ± 0.32	1.32 ± 0.71
UA mmol/l	309 ± 65.4	541.2 ± 303	327 ± 101.1	291 ± 101.1

Mean ± SD
Source: modified from: Fairbrother A (1990) Changes in mallard (*Anas platyrhynchos*) serum chemistry due to age, sex and reproductive condition. *Journal of Wildlife Diseases* **26**: 67–77.

Serum chemistry and enzyme values for adult male mallards (Anas platyrhynchos) of differing reproductive states

Assay	Pre-egg laying	Egg laying	Incubating	Molt
TPR g/l	46 ± 6	45 ± 8	42 ± 5	39 ± 8
ALB g/l	18 ± 2	16 ± 2	17 ± 3	15 ± 3
GLU mmol/l	15.7 ± 1.83	12.9 ± 1.77	11.0 ± 1.44	10.2 ± 1.60
AMY IU/l	3123.0 ± 583.0	2869.0 ± 614.0	3203.0 ± 785.0	2991.0 ± 748.0
CHE IU/l	1326.0 ± 344.0	1380.0 ± 399.0	984.0 ± 470.0	983.0 ± 452.0
ALT IU/l	34.6 ± 9.4	35.8 ± 13.1	27.6 ± 12.1	28.4 ± 19.2
AST IU/l	17.3 ± 4.0	20.5 ± 8.0	20.8 ± 15.7	18.1 ± 8.1
GGT IU/l	8.5 ± 7.6	10.6 ± 12.6	9.3 ± 6.0	16.5 ± 36.0
ALP IU/l	40.2 ± 25.3	44.1 ± 44.8	38.4 ± 48.0	35.3 ± 44.2
LDH IU/l	168.0 ± 66.0	219.0 ± 107.0	263.0 ± 203.0	202.0 ± 152.0
Ca mmol/l	2.72 ± 0.25	2.75 ± 0.47	2.47 ± 0.25	2.32 ± 0.55
Mg mmol/l	2.0 ± 0.2	2.0 ± 0.4	1.8 ± 0.4	1.8 ± 0.9
PHOS mmol/l	1.19 ± 0.24	0.9 ± 0.22	0.7 ± 0.12	0.77 ± 0.35
UA mmol/l	309.2 ± 71.3	309.2 ± 8.92	339.0 ± 113.0	279.5 ± 136.8

Mean ± SD
Source: modified from: Fairbrother A (1990) Changes in mallard (*Anas platyrhynchos*) serum chemistry due to age, sex and reproductive condition. *Journal of Wildlife Diseases* **26**: 67–77.

Serum chemistry and enzyme values for juvenile mallards (Anas platyrhynchos)

Assay	Age 5 d	Age 18 d	Age 42 d	Age 58 d
TPR g/l	34 ± 6	43 ± 13	40 ± 8	32 ± 10
ALB g/l	14 ± 2	15 ± 3	16 ± 4	14 ± 4
GLU mmol/l	13.2 ± 2.99	11.9 ± 5.16	10.4 ± 1.49	10.3 ± 2.49
AMY IU/l	3230.0 ± 760.0	3984.0 ± 1297.0	3005.0 ± 302.0	2395.0 ± 699.0
CHE IU/l	1423.0 ± 696.0	984.0 ± 559.0	827.0 ± 253.0	818.0 ± 248.0
ALT IU/l	21.3 ± 9.1	30.5 ± 10.5	26.1 ± 7.0	23.9 ± 7.1
AST IU/l	22.3 ± 7.4	88.5 ± 54.1	9.4 ± 5.1	17.4 ± 5.7
GGT IU/l	1.2 ± 2.8	4.6 ± 3.6	5.3 ± 5.7	6.1 ± 3.6
ALP IU/l	411.0 ± 89.0	386.0 ± 194.0	217.0 ± 32.0	185.0 ± 47.0
LD-LH IU/l	425.0 ± 153.0	629.0 ± 251.0	169.0 ± 70.0	233.0 ± 83.0
Ca mmol/l	3.25 ± 2.57	2.4 ± 0.42	2.72 ± 0.4	2.1 ± 0.45
Mg mmol/l	2.8 ± 0.8	1.8 ± 0.7	2.0 ± 0.2	1.6 ± 0.5
PHOS mmol/l	2.55 ± 0.90	2.45 ± 0.41	2.0 ± 0.41	1.61 ± 0.54

Continued overleaf

Serum chemistry and enzyme values for juvenile mallards (*Anas platyrhynchos*) (continued)

Assay	Age 5 d	Age 18 d	Age 42 d	Age 58 d
UA mmol/l	725.6 ± 321.1	684.3 ± 226.0	237.9 ± 41.6	237.9 ± 107.0

Mean ± SD
Source: modified from: Fairbrother A (1990) Changes in mallard (*Anas platyrhynchos*) serum chemistry due to age, sex and reproductive condition. *Journal of Wildlife Diseases* **26**: 67–77.

Blood chemistry values for captive American flamingoes (*Phoenicopterus ruber*)

Assay	Value	n
Alkaline phosphatase IU/l	166.35 ± 128.78* (18.26–737.55)	17
Aspartate aminotransferase IU/l	273.07 ± 103.39 (70.42–475.72)	27
Calcium mmol/l	3.34 ± 1.07 (1.23–5.44)	24
CO_2 total mmol/l	16.77 ± 3.72 (9.47–24.07)	13
Creatinine kinase IU/l	1058.40 ± 1096.12* (157.15–3521.44)	27
Uric acid mmol/l	768.4 ± 278.9 (221.8–1314.5)	28
Total protein g/l	40.6 ± 4.5 (31.8–49.4)	27
Glucose mmol/l	10.97 ± 2.56 (5.95–16.0)	26
Potassium mmol/l	2.84 ± 0.50 (1.86–3.83)	18
Chloride mmol/l	116.92 ± 3.25 (110.55–123.30)	13
Sodium mmol/l	12.92 ± 4.69 (3.73–22.10)	18

Mean ± SD (95% reference range)
Data obtained from 16 males, 8 females and 1 bird of unknown sex. Samples from 5 birds were obtained twice and not all samples were evaluated for every test.
* Intervals obtained by calculation with logarithmic transformation of data.
Source: modified from: Merritt EL, Fritz CL, Ramsay EC (1996) Hematologic and serum biochemical values in captive American flamingos (*Phoenicopterus ruber ruber*). *Journal of Avian Medicine and Surgery* **10**: 163–167.

Blood chemistry values for selected ratites

Species	Ostrich	Emu	Cassowary
Scientific name	*Struthio camelus*	*Dromiceius novaehollandiae*	*Casuarius* sp.
Total protein g/l	37 ± 7	42 ± 05	61 ± 5
Osmolality mosmol/kg	286.0 ± 49.0	–	–
Glucose mmol/l	13.8 ± 3.88	8.7 ± 1.22	11.54 ± 2.63
Triglycerides mmol/l	1.01 ± 0.50	3.66 ± 6.67	2.03 ± 0.81
Cholesterol mmol/l	2.50 ± 1.16	2.68 ± 0.80	2.06 ± 0.41
BUN mmol/l	1.71 ± 0.42	1.78 ± 0.64	6.64 ± 0.42
Uric acid mmol/l	487.7 ± 160.5	279.5 ± 118.9	356 ± 35.6
Calcium mmol/l	2.3 ± 0.6	2.62 ± 0.32	2.85 ± 0.05
Phosphorus mmol/l	1.55 ± 0.38	1.74 ± 0.32	1.61 ± 0.03
Sodium mmol/l	147.0 ± 34.0	–	149.0 ± 2.1
Potassium mmol/l	3.0 ± 0.8	–	4.1 ± 1.0
Chloride mmol/l	100.0 ± 16.0	–	108.0 ± 0.0
Magnesium mmol/l	2.2 ± 0.8	–	2.3 ± 0.3
ALP IU/l	575.0 ± 248.0	84.0 ± 44.0	–
ALT IU/l	2.0 ± 1.7	15.4 ± 4.3	80.0 ± 21.0
AST IU/l	131.0 ± 31.0	104.0 ± 24.0	698.0 ± 532.0
GGT IU/l	1.5 ± 2.9	4.4 ± 3.4	–
LDH IU/l	1565.0 ± 660.0	240.0 ± 91.0	1060.0 ± 516.0
CK IU/l	688.0 ± 208.0	264.0 ± 170.0	–

Modified from: Stewart JS (1989) Husbandry, medical and surgical management of ratites, part 2. *Proceedings of the Association of Zoo Veterinarians*, Greensboro, pp. 119–122.

Blood chemistry values for the Eurasian buzzard (*Buteo buteo*)

Assay	*n* = 20
Albumin g/l	145
Total protein g/l	38.4
Glucose mmol/l	18.7
AST U/l	330.9
ALT U/l	40.6
LDH U/l	2008.4
CK U/l	1604.1
GGT U/l	0.3
ALKP U/l	89.8
Total bilirubin µmol/l	0.51
Cholesterol mmol/l	4.97
Triglycerides mmol/l	1.31
Lipase IU/l	26.37
Amylase IU/l	616.93
Uric acid mmol/l	218.0
Creatinine µmol/l	13.2
Urea mmol/l	2.12
Calcium mmol/l	2.16
Phosphorus mmol/l	0.71
Magnesium mmol/l	0.99
Prealbumin g/l	3.06
Albumin g/l	14.65
α-globulin g/l	4.89
β-globulin g/l	5.78
γ-globulin g/l	13.08

Source: modified from: Gelli D, Ferrari V, Franceschini F *et al.* (2005) Serum biochemical and electrophoretic patterns in the Eurasian buzzard (*Buteo buteo*) – reference values. *Proceedings of the European Association of Avian Veterinarians*, Arles, pp. 166–170.

Age-related blood chemistry changes in captive buff-crested bustards (*Eupodotis ruficrista gindiana*)

Assay	2–8 weeks	*n*	9–16 weeks	*n*	17–24 weeks	*n*	> 1 year	*n*
Glucose mmol/l	14.93 ± 0.45 (14.11–15.67)	3	18.17 ± 0.81 (15.83–22.17)	8	16.32 ± 0.68 (13.94–17.78)	5	20.36 ± 0.55 (15.28–28.83)	25
Uric acid µmol/l	392.86 ± 47.14 (172.61–589.28)	7	337.5 ± 39.58 (113.1–726.19)	14	573.21 ± 47.29 (238.1–779.76)	12	533.93 ± 38.97 (202.38–928.57)	26
Total protein g/l	18.14 ± 1.37 (11.0–22.0)	7	26.88 ± 1.76 (13.0–39.0)	17	30.67 ± 1.56 (23.0–42.0)	12	32.81 ± 0.83 (25.0–41.0)	26
Albumin g/l	nd		nd		nd		12.91 ± 0.37 (10.0–16.0)	23
Globulin g/l	nd		nd		nd		19.61 ± 0.64 (14.0–26.0)	23
Albumin:globulin ratio	nd		nd		nd		0.67 ± 0.02 (0.52–0.79)	23
ALKP IU/l	975.33 ± 367.33 (511–2926)	3	1080.81 ± 143.73 (392–2132)	11	561.5 ± 143.94 (155–790)	4	475.16 ± 45.71 (160–868)	26
ALT IU/l	26 ± 7 (19–40)	3	28.25 ± 6.93 (17–76)	8	23.2 ± 2.48 (18–32)	5	nd	
AST IU/l	248.2 ± 20.17 (184–310)	5	256.46 ± 20.33 (151–388)	13	269 ± 29.51 (154–469)	9	334.96 ± 11.91 (217–482)	26
LDH IU/l	381.5 ± 183.5 (198–565)	2	447.57 ± 79.65 (220–831)	7	415 ± 130.1 (278–675)	3	373.96 ± 29.72 (152–788)	26
CK IU/l	nd		nd		nd		361.65 ± 41.27 (115–797)	26

Continued overleaf

Age-related blood chemistry changes in captive buff-crested bustards (*Eupodotis ruficrista gindiana*) (continued)

Assay	2–8 weeks	n	9–16 weeks	n	17–24 weeks	n	> 1 year	n
Magnesium mmol/l	nd		nd		nd		1.05 ± 0.03 (0.83–1.36)	26
Calcium mmol/l	1.49 ± 0.11 (1.23–1.73)	5	1.61 ± 0.09 (1.1–1.95)	8	2.05 ± 0.19 (1.23–2.83)	7	2.55 ± 0.06 (2.02–3.51)	26
Cholesterol mmol/l	nd		nd		nd		3.64 ± 0.15 (2.19–5.37)	26

Mean ± standard error of the mean (minimum–maximum)
nd, not determined.
Source: Bailey TA, Wernery U, Howlett J *et al.* (1998) Age-related plasma chemistry findings in the buff-crested bustard (*Eupodotis ruficrista gindiana*). *Journal of Veterinary Medicine* **45**: 635–640.

Age-related blood chemistry changes in captive kori bustards (*Ardeotis kori*)

Assay	p value	4–8 weeks n = 24	9–16 weeks n = 6–8	17–24 weeks n = 7–14	25–32 weeks n = 6–13	33–40 weeks n = 8–10	41–52 weeks n = 6–7	1 year (adult) n = 28
Glucose mmol/l				17.74 ± 0.45 (15.43–19.87)				
Uric acid µmol/l	0.057							
Total protein g/l				35.86 ± 1.96 (24.0–51.0)		37.0 ± 1.64 (28.0–43.0)		30.0 ± 0.82 (23.0–40.0)
Albumin g/l	nd	nd	nd	nd	nd	nd	nd	11.0 ± 0.3
Globulin g/l	nd	nd	nd	nd	nd	nd	nd	1.9 ± 0.06
Albumin: globulin ratio	nd	nd	nd	nd	nd	nd	nd	0.58 ± 0.01 (0.29–0.73)
ALKP IU/l				147.5 ± 16.35 (55–219)				85.9 ± 2.6 (37–98)
ALT IU/l	0.566	27 (n = 1)		28 ± 2.27 (20–34)	33.7 ± 1.54 (20–39)		34.4 ± 3.43 (20–10)	
AST IU/l		221.5 ± 8.5 (213–230)						207 ± 7.1 (168–369)
LDH IU/l	0.001	1114 ± 17 (1024–1158)						
CK IU/l	nd	nd	nd	nd	nd	nd	nd	
Magnesium mmol/l	nd	nd	nd	nd	nd	nd	nd	1.05 ± 0.02
Calcium mmol/l		0.83 ± 0.1 (0.7–1.03)	1.41 ± 0.12 (1.0–1.8)	1.42 ± 0.07 (1.1–1.83)	1.67 ± 0.06 (1.25–2.2)	1.98 ± 0.1 (1.5–2.4)	1.94 ± 0.1 (1.5–2.28)	2.34 ± 0.07 (1.71–3.44)
Cholesterol mmol/l	nd	nd	nd	nd	nd	nd	nd	3.7 ± 0.13

Mean ± standard error of the mean (minimum–maximum).
nd, not determined.
Source: Bailey TA, Wernery U, Howlett J *et al.* (1998) Age-related plasma chemistry changes in houbara and kori bustards. *Journal of Wildlife Diseases 33*: 31–37.

Age-related blood chemistry changes in captive houbara bustards (*Chlamydotis undulata macqueenii*)

Assay	p value	4–8 weeks n = 10–11	9–16 weeks n = 24–26	1 year (adult) n = 28
Glucose mmol/l	0.016	20.70 ± 2.45 (14.93–39.63)	16.90 ± 0.56 (13.21–24.37)	16.89 ± 0.26 (14.04–19.59)
Uric acid µmol/l	0.186	393.76 ± 55.61 (190.34–713.76)	402.32 ± 42.75 (107.1–856.51)	432.42 ± 39.79 (202.23–1005.21)
Total protein g/l	0.006	32.0 ± 0.97 (27.0–36.0)	33.12 ± 1.07 (23.0–48.0)	37.93 ± 0.9 (30.0–48.0)
Albumin g/l	nd	nd	nd	14.5 ± 0.28 (11.0–18.0)
Globulin g/l	nd	nd	nd	2.38 ± 0.09 (1.7–3.7)
Albumin:globulin ratio	nd	nd	nd	0.64 ± 0.03 (0.32–0.84)
ALKP IU/l	0.044	622.8 ± 82.43 (257–1131)	278.72 ± 23.97 (122–622)	80.39 ± 7.24 (17–175)
ALT IU/l	0.018	21 ± 1.31 (11–26)	22.2 ± 1.33 (14–42)	45.14 ± 3.27 (22–97)
AST IU/l	0.007	376.36 ± 16.21 (293–466)	342.2 ± 15.08 (247–528)	467.9 ± 24.93 (246–774)
LDH IU/l	0.006	934.6 ± 69.54 (676–1284)	690.72 ± 46.31 (406–1467)	609.57 ± 43.42 (246–774)
CK IU/l	0.01	228.1 ± 42.76 (55–427)	141.04 ± 24.52 (14–479)	778.4 ± 122.2 (12–2309)
Magnesium mmol/l	0.015	0.75 ± 0.05 (0.41–1.03)	0.80 ± 0.02 (0.58–1.03)	1.01 ± 0.03 (0.81–1.27)
Calcium mmol/l	0.013	2.07 ± 0.13 (1.5–2.75)	1.81 ± 0.08 (1.1–2.73)	2.49 ± 0.08 (1.46–3.01)
Cholesterol mmol/l	0.273	6.29 ± 0.33 (4.65–7.76)	6.08 ± 0.28 (1.09–8.83)	6.78 ± 0.33 (4.06–10.65)

Mean ± standard error of the mean (minimum–maximum)
Values significantly different among the groups ($p < 0.05$).
nd, not determined.
Source: Bailey TA, Wernery U, Howlett J et al. (1998) Age-related plasma chemistry changes in houbara and kori bustards. *Journal of Wildlife Diseases* **33**: 31–37.

Age-related blood chemistry changes in captive white-bellied bustards (*Eupodotis senegalensis*)

Assay	4–8 weeks	n	9–16 weeks	n	17–24 weeks	n	1 year (adult)	n
Glucose mmol/l	15.21 ± 1.19 (13.1–18.09)	4	16.97 ± 0.29 (16.65–17.54)	3	16.54 ± 0.43 (14.99–17.59)	5	19.09 ± 1.05 (16.32–23.04)	6
Uric acid µmol/l	400.0 ± 30.81 (356.88–487.74)	4	303.35 ± 38.66 (261.71–380.67)	3	457.99 ± 88.63 (273.61–808.93)	6	408.63 ± 15.39 (356.88–481.79)	7
Total protein g/l	16.4 ± 2.42 (10.0–24.0)	5	24.25 ± 5.41 (13.0–37.0)	4	30.33 ± 1.36 (27.0–34.0)	6	30.0 ± 1.71 (25.0–35.0)	6
Albumin g/l	nd		nd		nd		12.0 ± 0.9 (9.0–15.0)	6
Globulin g/l	nd		nd		nd		18.0 ± 0.89 (15.0–20.0)	6
Albumin:globulin ratio	nd		nd		nd		0.66 ± 0.03 (0.56–0.75)	6
ALKP IU/l	187.75 ± 23.99 (137–244)	4	139 ± 4 (135–143)	2	70.75 ± 8.89 (53–91)	4	44.17 ± 10.53 (23–86)	6
ALT IU/l	21.25 ± 2.32 (17–27)	4	24 ± 3 (21–27)	2	26.33 ± 5.17 (16–32)	3	nd	
AST IU/l	293 ± 32.5 (225–375)	4	397.67 ± 100.1 (256–591)	3	372.33 ± 82.57 (206–718)	6	444.67 ± 42.34 (266–574)	6
LDH IU/l	1235.25 ± 152.95 (944–1620)	4	1452 ± 231 (1221–1683)	2	978.67 ± 174.33 (704–1302)	3	755.17 ± 80.18 (474–985)	6
CK IU/l	410.5 ± 32.56 (335–492)	4	180 ± 16 (164–196)	2	378 ± 142.49 (164–648)	3	377.14 ± 42.77 (170–521)	7
Magnesium mmol/l	0.65 ± 0.04 (0.53–0.74)	4	0.69 ± 0.04 (0.66–0.74)	2	0.78 ± 0.02 (0.74–0.82)	3	1.01 ± 0.07 (0.84–1.32)	

Age-related blood chemistry changes in captive white-bellied bustards (*Eupodotis senegalensis*) (*continued*)

Assay	4–8 weeks	n	9–16 weeks	n	17–24 weeks	n	1 year (adult)	n
Calcium mmol/l	1.41 ± 0.19 (1.03–1.93)	4	1.59 ± 0.45 (1.48–1.7)	2	1.99 ± 0.09 (1.73–2.3)	5	2.42 ± 0.05 (2.25–2.56)	6
Cholesterol mmol/l	nd		nd		nd		3.30 ± 0.35 (2.66–4.97)	6

Mean ± standard error of the mean (minimum–maximum)
nd, not determined.
Source: from: Bailey TA, Wernery U, Naldo J *et al.* (1998) Normal blood chemistry and age-related changes in the white-bellied bustards. *Comparative Haematology International* **8**: 61–65.

Reference urine chemistry values in clinically normal falcons

Assay	Mean (minimum-maximum)	Median(95% CI for the median)
Chloride mmol/l	41.85 (0.3–121.64)	37.75 (20.81–52.46)
GGT IU/l	42.65 (2.41–426.11)	26.07 (17.82–40.73)
Glucose mmol/l	1.34 (0.26–1.85)	0.91 (0.87–1.02)
Total protein g/l	27 (0–12)	2 (2–3)
ALKP IU/l	80.15 (0–889.3)	36.4 (26.02–52.88)

Source: modified from: Tschopp R, Bailey TA, Di Somma A, Silvanose C (2007) Urinalysis in Falconidae. *Journal of Avian Medicine and Surgery.* **21**(1):1–7.

Plasma α-tocopherol and cholesterol concentrations in captive bustards (*Chlamydotis undulata*)

Species	Age	α-tocopherol (μg/ml)	n	Cholesterol (mg/ml)	n	α-tocopherol: cholesterol (μg/mg)
Houbara bustards (*Chlamydotis undulata*)	Adult	11.07 ± 0.41	32	1.93 ± 0.10	12	6.09 ± 0.44
	Juvenile	6.33 ± 0.48	12	2.08 ± 0.09	11	2.94 ± 0.22
Kori bustards (*Ardeotis kori*)	Adult	4.43 ± 0.42	21	1.23 ± 0.25	20	3.67 ± 0.44
	Juvenile	4.46 ± 0.26	11	1.28 ± 0.11	11	3.71 ± 0.36
Buff-crested bustards (*Eupodotis ruficrista*)	Adult	6.64 ± 0.33	19	1.22 ± 0.05	18	5.56 ± 0.32
White-bellied bustards (*Eupodotis senegalensis*)	Adult	7.75 ± 0.81	8	1.35 ± 0.13	8	5.83 ± 0.43
Black bustards (*Eupodotis afra*)	Adult	10.08 ± 0.06	2	1.37 ± 0.04	2	7.36 ± 0.17
Heuglin's bustards (*Neotis heuglinii*)	Adult	6.08 ± 0.64	4	1.16 ± 0.09	4	5.39 ± 0.86

Mean ± standard error of the mean
Adult = ≥ 12 months; juvenile: 6–12 months.
Source: Anderson SJ, Dawodu A, Patel M *et al.* (2002) Plasma concentrations of vitamin E in six species of bustard (Gruiformes: Otididae). *Journal of Wildlife Diseases* **38**: 414–419.

Vitamin A, B₁, C and E levels in the blood of clinically normal captive houbara bustards (*Chlamydotis undulata*)

Vitamin B₁ μg/l	Vitamin E μmol/l	Vitamin C mg/l	Vitamin A μmol/l
45.83 ± 1.87 (33–60)	17.81 ± 1.03 (11.9–30.9)	4.06 ± 0.32 (1.3–5.9)	5.42 ± 0.23 (4.1–7.6)

Mean ± standard error of the mean (minimum–maximum)
Source: Bailey TA Diseases of and medical management of houbara bustards and other Otididae. Environment Agency Abu Dhabi, Abu Dhabi, United Arab Emirates, in press.

Blood gas values for eight clinically normal houbara bustards (*Chlamydotis undulata*)

Assay	Range
pH	7.44 ± 0.02 (7.39–7.53; 8)
P_{CO_2} mmHg	24.44 ± 0.91 (21.3–28.7; 8)
P_{O_2} mmHg	48.13 ± 1.39 (43.7–55.3; 8)
S_{O_2} %	61.21 ± 2.45 (54–73.2; 8)
Na mmol/l	151.95 ± 0.69 (150.2–156; 8)
Ca^{2+} mmol/l	1.49 ± 0.02 (1.39–1.6; 8)
Glucose mg/dl	243.5 ± 3.73 (225–256; 8)
BEecf mmol/l	−7.71 ± 0.79 (10.6–−3.2; 8)
HCO_3 mmol/l	16.69 ± 0.63 (14.1–19.7; 8)
T_{CO_2} mmol/l	17.438 ± 0.6497 (14.7–20.4; 7)
Beb mmol/l	−5.06 ± 0.736 (7.5–0.8; 7)
SBC mmol/l	19.55 ± 0.63 (17.6–23.3; 7)
A mmHg	118.89 ± 1.09 (113.8–122.7; 7)
$A–aD_{O_2}$ mmHg	71.343 ± 1.77 (65.1–78.1; 7)
a/A	0.41 ± 0.01 (0.4–0.5; 7)
RI	1.5 ± 0.08 (1.2–1.8; 7)
P_{50} mmHg	43.09 ± 0.47 (41.7–45; 7)
O_2 Cap ml/dl	19.37 ± 0.58 (17.7–22.4; 7)
O_2Ct ml/dl	12.09 ± 0.66 (10–15.2; 7)
nCa mmol/l	1.54 ± 0.03 (1.46–1.64; 7)

Mean ± standard error of the mean (minimum–maximum; *n*)
Samples were collected from a brachial vein of manually restrained birds. P_{CO_2}, partial pressure of carbon dioxide; P_{O_2}, partial pressure of oxygen; S_{O_2}, oxygen saturation; T_{CO_2}, total carbon dioxide content; Beb, base excess of blood; SBC, standard bicarbonate concentration; BEecf, base excess extracellular fluid; O_2Ct, oxygen content; A, alveolar saturation; $A–aD_{O_2}$, arterial alveolar oxygen tension gradient; a/A, arterial alveolar oxygen tension ratio; P_{50}, the P_{O_2} of a sample at which the hemoglobin is 50% saturated with oxygen at pH 7.4; nCa, ionized calcium normalized to pH 7.4.
Source: Bailey TA Diseases of and medical management of houbara bustards and other Otididae. Environment Agency Abu Dhabi, Abu Dhabi, United Arab Emirates, in press.

I-STAT blood values in clinically normal gyrfalcons (*Falco rusticolus*) and gyr hybrid falcons (*Falco rusticolus–Falco cherrug, Falco rusticolus–Falco peregrinus*)

Assay	Range (*n* = 70)
Glucose mmol/l	18.79 ± 1.43 (15.7–22.5)
BUN mmol/l	2.45 ± 0.06 (2.14–5.71)
Na mmol/l	150.33 ± 2.30 (146–157)
K mmol/l	2.90 ± 0.69 (2.0–4.1)
Cl mmol/l	119.86 ± 2.22 (15.0–125.0)
T_{CO_2} mmol/l	26.41 ± 2.24 (21.0–30.0)
AnGAP mmol/l	6.76 ± 2.70 (1.0–14.0)
Hct %	46.57 ± 4.48 (40.0–57.0)
Hb g/dl	15.79 ± 1.51 (14.0–19.0)
pH $\log_{10}$	7.47 ± 0.04 (7.4–7.6)
P_{CO_2} mmHg	34.96 ± 4.20 (27.0–49.9)
HCO_3 mmol/l	25.34 ± 2.19 (26.0–29.0)
BEecf mmol/l	1.77 ± 2.41 (−3.0–6.0)

Mean ± SD (minimum–maximum)
BUN, blood urea nitrogen; T_{CO_2}, total CO_2; AnGAP, anion gap; Hct, hematocrit; Hb: hemoglobin; P_{CO_2}, partial pressure of CO_2; BEecf: base deficit.
Source: McKinney P (2003) Clinical applications of the I-STAT blood analyzer in avian practice. *Proceedings of the European Association of Avian Veterinarians*, pp. 341–346, Tenerife.

I-STAT blood values in clinically normal red-tailed hawks (*Buteo jamaicensis*)

Assay	Range (*n* = 40)
Glucose mmol/l	20.5 ± 2.4
Na mmol/l	151.7 ± 2.1
K mmol/l	3.06 ± 0.47
Cl mmol/l	119.2 ± 3.0
T_{CO_2} mmol/l	18.65 ± 4.25
AnGAP mmol/l	17.63 ± 4.8
Hct %	36.8 ± 3.2
Hb g/dl	12.65 ± 0.98
pH $\log_{10}$	7.43 ± 0.07
P_{CO_2} mmHg	26.78 ± 4.6
HCO_3 mmol/l	18.1 ± 4.25
BEecf mmol/l	−6.36 ± 5.22

Mean ± SD
Source: Heatley JJ, Demirjian SE, Wright JC *et al.* (2005) Electrolytes of the critically ill raptor. *Proceedings of the Association of Avian Veterinarians*, Monterey, pp. 23–25.

Serum copper, magnesium and zinc levels in six species of captive bustards and stone curlew

Species	Houbara bustard *n* = 56	Kori bustard *n* = 45	White-bellied bustard *n* = 33	Buff-crested bustard *n* = 31	Black bustard *n* = 3	Heuglin's bustard *n* = 4	Stone curlew *n* = 3
Scientific name	*Chlamydotis undulata*	*Ardeotis kori*	*Eupodotis senegalensis*	*Eupodotis ruficrista*	*Eupodotis afra*	*Neotis heuglinii*	*Burhinus oedicnemus*
Copper µg/dl	86.05 ± 0.71 (76.7–98.1)	82.91 ± 0.88 (67.8–101.6)	84.20 ± 0.59 (77.4–93.3)	81.61 ± 0.82 (70.9–89.9)	83.7 ± 0.81 (82.4–85.2)	82.43 ± 4.14 (71.6–91)	81.5 ± 1.28 (76–88.6)
Magnesium mmol/l	1.2 ± 0.04 (0.63–1.95)	1.08 ± 0.05 (0.63–1.84)	1.12 ± 0.04 (0.83–1.72)	1.01 ± 0.03 (0.71–1.27)	1.03 ± 0.09 (0.93–1.21)	1.12 ± 0.05 (0.97–1.22)	0.88 ± 0.03 (0.75–1.0)
Zinc µg/dl	161.55 ± 2.53 (111.1–215)	159.38 ± 5.53 (104–293.4)	175.5 ± 4.33 (121.5–220.2)	174 ± 3.37 (129.7–205)	171.9 ± 8.84 (156.3–186.9)	201.33 ± 4.92 (192–215.2)	180.56 ± 7.89 (147.4–231.7)

Mean ± SD (minimum–maximum)
Source: Bailey TA, Silvanose C, Combreau O, Howlett JC (2004) Normal blood concentrations of copper, magnesium and zinc in stone curlews and five species of bustards in the United Arab Emirates. *Proceedings of the European Association of Zoo and Wildlife Veterinarians*, Ebeltoft, pp. 297–301.

Summary of the physiology and effects of changes in vitamin levels in avian species

Vitamin	Physiology in avian species	Causes and effects of changes in vitamin levels
A	Fat-soluble vitamin essential for growth and differentiation of epithelial tissues, mucopolysaccharide formation, stability of cell membranes, growth of bones and normal reproduction. Also improves the immune system. It is stored in the liver and has the potential to act as a cumulative toxicant. Deficiencies can result from insufficient dietary fat, insufficient antioxidant protection or disorders that interfere with fat digestion or absorption. Liver disease may reduce the bird's ability to store vitamin A	Deficiency – Embryo mortality and abnormalities, susceptibility to respiratory infections, visual disorders, squamous metaplasia of mucous membranes, hyperkeratosis, decreased testes size and testosterone levels, urate deposits in the kidneys and ureters, egg binding, poorly formed eggs Toxicity – bone abnormalities, spontaneous fractures, conjunctivitis, enteritis, suppressed keratinization, internal hemorrhages, fatty liver and kidneys and secondary deficiencies of other fat-soluble vitamins
D_3	Fat-soluble vitamin essential for the absorption of calcium and consequently normal bone and eggshell formation. It is destroyed by excess radiation with ultraviolet light and oxidation in the presence of rancidifying fatty acids. There are two forms of this vitamin, ergocalciferol (D_2), a plant derivative and cholecalciferol (D_3) produced in the bird's body. Vitamin D_3 is synthesized in avian skin exposed to ultraviolet light and is 30–40 times more potent than vitamin D_2. A dietary source of vitamin D_3 is needed by animals that do not have access to ultraviolet light	Deficiency – thin, soft-shelled eggs, embryonic abnormalities and mortality, metabolic bone disease, leg weakness, seizuring, pathological bone fractures, poor feathering. Can be induced by high dietary vitamin A or E levels Toxicity – reduced fertility, decreased eggshell quality, soft tissue calcification, renal and artery calcification, bone demineralization and muscular atrophy
E	Fat-soluble vitamin that provides natural antioxidation protection for cells, fatty acids and other fat-soluble vitamins. Working in conjunction with vitamin E are several metalloenzymes that incorporate manganese, zinc, copper, iron and selenium. The selenium-containing glutathione peroxidase is the most important of these enzymes. Because of their similar activity, selenium and vitamin E tend to have a sparing effect on each other. Vitamin E is active in several metabolic systems including cellular respiration, normal phosphorylation reactions, ascorbic acid synthesis, sulfur amino acid synthesis. It also has effects on immunity by increasing phagocytosis and antibody production as well as stimulating macrophage and lymphocyte activity	Deficiency – low fertility, embryonic mortality, low hatchability, immunosuppression, testicular degeneration and specific clinical abnormalities such as encephalomalacia, exudative diathesis and muscular myopathies. May be predisposed by giardiasis Toxicity – enlarged fatty liver, waxy feathers. High levels can cause secondary deficiency signs of bone demineralization or blood clotting failure if vitamins D_3 and K are marginal
K	Fat-soluble vitamin essential for normal blood clotting. It comes from three sources: green plants, bacteria and synthetic forms. The microbial synthesis in the intestinal tract is significant in most species. The requirements of this vitamin vary according to the extent to which different species use the synthesized vitamin K and to which they practice coprophagy. It is destroyed by oxidation, alkaline conditions, strong acids, ultraviolet light and some sulfa drugs. Vitamin K also requires the presence of dietary fats and bile salts for absorption from the gut, so decreased pancreatic and biliary function can impair normal absorption	Deficiency – embryonic mortality, hemorrhaging, anemia, altered bone metabolism. Can be induced by high dietary levels of vitamins A or E or by prolonged antibiotic treatment Toxicity – high levels can cause chick mortality and anemia
B_1 Thiamine	Water-soluble vitamin essential for enzyme activity and cellular respiratory control as well as being involved in nerve activity. It is common in plant and animal food sources but generally at low concentration. Several compounds in nature possess antithiamine activity. These include amprolium, which inhibits thiamine absorption from the intestine, thiaminases, which are found in raw fish, and thiamine antagonists such as tannic acid. Thiamine is not stored in the body for long	Deficiency – embryonic mortality, muscular paralysis, ataxia, convulsions, neurological signs, organ atrophy Toxicity – not studied in birds. High levels in mammals can cause depression of the respiratory center and blockage of nerve transmission
B_2 Riboflavin	Water-soluble vitamin essential for enzyme activity, carbohydrate utilization, cellular metabolism and respiration, uric acid formation, amino acid breakdown and drug metabolism. It is destroyed by ultraviolet light and alkaline solutions. Very little riboflavin is stored in the body and it is rapidly excreted	Deficiency – embryonic abnormalities and mortality, chick mortality, curled toe paralysis and other neuromuscular disorders, dermatitis, poor feather pigmentation, splayed legs, fatty liver and dermatitis Toxicity – not reported in birds. Toxicity not thought to be a risk because it is not well absorbed from the gut
B_6 Pyridoxine	Water-soluble vitamin involved in a number of enzyme systems as a coenzyme. It is required in all areas of amino acid utilization, the synthesis of niacin and the formation of antibodies. It is destroyed by oxidation	Deficiency – reduced hatchability, ataxia, neuromuscular disorders, perosis, hemorrhaging and gizzard erosion Toxicity – not reported in birds
B_{12} Cyanoco-balamin	A product of bacterial biosynthesis and therefore must be obtained by consuming a bacterial source or animal tissues that accumulate the vitamin. It is a critical component of many metabolic pathways and is involved in the synthesis of nucleic acids and protein as well as carbohydrates and fats. Most vitamin B_{12} in the body is found in the liver, with secondary stores in the muscles. Vitamin B_{12} is stored efficiently with a long biological half-life of 1 year in humans	Deficiency – embryo abnormalities and mortality, chick mortality, gizzard erosion and poor feathering Toxicity – not reported in birds

Source: Bailey TA Diseases of and medical management of houbara bustards and other Otididae. Environment Agency Abu Dhabi, Abu Dhabi, United Arab Emirates, in press.

Continued

Summary of the physiology and effects of changes in vitamin levels in avian species *(continued)*

Vitamin	Physiology in avian species	Causes and effects of changes in vitamin levels
Biotin	Water-soluble vitamin that is an active part of four different carboxylase enzymes in the body in the metabolism of energy, glucose, lipids and some amino acids. It is destroyed by strong acids and bases, oxidizing agents and the protein avidin in raw egg albumin. Biotin is widely distributed in foods at low concentrations. The synthesis of biotin by intestinal microflora may be important	Deficiency – embryo abnormalities and mortality, poor growth, dermatitis, perosis and leg abnormalities, fatty liver–kidney syndrome Toxicity – not reported in birds
Choline	Water-soluble vitamin with four important metabolic functions: 1) as a component of phospholipids and therefore in maintaining cell integrity, 2) maturation of the cartilage matrix of bone, 3) fat metabolism in the liver, and 4) acetylated to form the neurotransmitter acetylcholine. While most animals synthesize choline, young animals cannot synthesize enough to meet the demands of growth	Deficiency – reduced hatchability, perosis and enlarged hocks, hepatic steatitis, fatty liver syndrome Toxicity – not reported in birds
Folic acid	Water-soluble vitamin involved in amino acid metabolism and bioconversion and in the synthesis of nucleotides. It is involved in red blood cell maturation, white cell production, functioning of the immune system, and uric acid formation. It is also essential for normal growth. Some sulfa drugs increase folic acid requirements. Zinc deficiency can decrease the absorption of folic acid by reducing activity of the mucosal enzyme that creates an absorbable form of folic acid. Enzyme inhibitors are present in some foods such as cabbage, oranges, beans and peas	Deficiency – embryo abnormalities and mortality, perosis, macrocytic anemia, poor feathering and loss of feather pigmentation Toxicity – not reported in birds
Niacin	Water-soluble vitamin that is an important component of coenzymes NAD and NADP, which are involved in carbohydrate, fat and protein metabolism	Deficiency – dermatitis, perosis, stomatitis, perosis and enlarged hocks, anemia, digestive disorders, general muscular weakness Toxicity – coarse dense feathering and anteriorly directed short legs in chickens
C Ascorbic acid	Has not been demonstrated to be a required nutrient for most avian species. It is easily manufactured in the liver and kidneys of birds, but biosynthesis can be inhibited by deficiencies of vitamins A, E and biotin. Ascorbic acid is involved in the synthesis of collagen, is an excellent antioxidant and can regenerate vitamin E	Deficiency – Signs of vitamin C deficiency have not documented in birds
Pantothenic acid	Water-soluble vitamin that is a structural component of coenzyme A, one of the most critical coenzymes in tissue metabolism. As such it is involved in fatty acid biosynthesis and degradation, and the formation of cholesterol, triglycerides, phospholipids and steroid hormones. It is destroyed by heat, acids and bases	Deficiency – embryonic mortality, dermatitis, perosis, poor feathering, poor growth, fatty liver–kidney syndrome, ataxia and reduced semen volume and fertility Toxicity – not reported in birds

Source: adapted from: Anderson S (1995) Bustard micronutrient review. National Avian Research Centre External Report No. 4, Abu Dhabi; Brue RN (1994) Nutrition. In: Ritchie BW, Harrison GJ, Harrison LR (eds) *Avian Medicine and Surgery: Principles and Applications*, pp. 63–95. Wingers Publishing, Lake Worth, FL; McWhirter P (1994) Malnutrition. In: Ritchie BW, Harrison GJ, Harrison LR (eds) *Avian Medicine and Surgery: Principles and Applications*, pp. 842–861. Wingers Publishing, Lake Worth, FL. Bailey TA Diseases of and medical management of houbara bustards and other Otididae. Environment Agency Abu Dhabi, Abu Dhabi, United Arab Emirates, in press.

Plasma protein electrophoresis in clinically normal birds of prey

Species	Bonelli's eagle n = 18	Golden eagle n = 33	Peregrine falcon n = 29	Imperial eagle n = 20	Griffon vulture n = 17	Booted eagle n = 12	Eagle owl n = 13	Barred owl n = 11
Scientific name	Hieraaetus fasciatus	Aquila chryaetos	Falco peregrinus	Aquila heliaca	Gyps fulvus	Hieraaetus pennatus	Bubo bubo	Strix varia
Total protein	3.61 ± 0.41 (2.79–4.17)	3.76 ± 0.39 (3.19–4.4)	3.19 ± 0.68 (2.13–5.32)	3.56 ± 0.39 (3.12–4.36)	4.36 ± 0.94 (2.73–5.6)	5.13 ± 0.45 (4.6–5.6)	4.14 ± 0.65 (3.38–5.25)	3.35 ± 0.87 (2.16–2.49)
Prealbumin	0.12 ± 0.04 (0.06–0.23)	0.12 ± 0.03 (0.09–0.19)	0.09 ± 0.03 (0.05–0.2)	0.11 ± 0.02 (0.06–0.15)	0.16 ± 0.05 (0.24–1.14)	0.22 ± 0.04 (0.17–0.27)	0.10 ± 0.03 (0.05–0.14)	0.10 ± 0.04 (0.06–0.7)
Albumin	1.55 ± 0.20 (1.26–1.92)	1.48 ± 0.17 (1.22–1.85)	1.09 ± 0.25 (0.65–1.6)	1.43 ± 0.19 (1.17–1.85)	2.06 ± 0.37 (1.35–2.35)	2.10 ± 0.33 (1.63–2.52)	1.53 ± 0.31 (1.13–2.05)	1.31 ± 0.36 (0.87–1.79)
Alpha 1	0.22 ± 0.04 (0.15–0.29)	0.22 ± 0.02 (0.17–0.27)	0.10 ± 0.03 (0.04–0.17)	0.22 ± 0.04 (0.15–0.28)	0.38 ± 0.09 (0.22–0.52)	0.34 ± 0.04 (0.3–0.4)	0.15 ± 0.04 (0.09–0.14)	0.19 ± 0.06 (0.13–0.27)
Alpha 2	0.82 ± 0.09 (0.61–0.98)	0.93 ± 0.15 (0.63–1.25)	1.01 ± 0.28 (0.59–1.92)	0.90 ± 0.13 (0.65–1.23)	0.77 ± 0.22 (0.49–1.16)	1.40 ± 0.17 (1.21–1.67)	1.07 ± 0.12 (0.89–1.24)	0.78 ± 0.17 (0.57–1.01)
Beta	0.66 ± 0.12 (0.5–0.86)	0.73 ± 0.15 (0.48–1.04)	0.53 ± 0.19 (0.34–1.05)	0.66 ± 0.11 (0.49–0.9)	0.51 ± 0.19 (0.29–0.83)	0.73 ± 0.09 (0.59–0.82)	1.02 ± 0.18 (0.78–1.32)	0.71 ± 0.28 (0.39–1.13)
Gamma	0.25 ± 0.04 (0.16–0.33)	0.28 ± 0.05 (0.19–0.4)	0.38 ± 0.12 (0.23–0.78)	0.26 ± 0.05 (0.17–0.34)	0.47 ± 0.15 (0.28–0.72)	0.35 ± 0.10 (0.25–0.39)	0.26 ± 0.06 (0.19–0.33)	0.26 ± 0.06 (0.16–0.32)
A:G ratio	0.72 ± 0.19 (0.0–0.92)	0.66 ± 0.09 (0.5–0.82)	0.52 ± 0.10 (0.3–0.67)	0.67 ± 0.08 (0.59–0.86)	0.92 ± 0.12 (0.72–1.03)	0.69 ± 0.10 (0.55–0.82)	0.59 ± 0.06 (0.5–0.67)	0.64 ± 0.09 (0.54–0.79)

Mean ± SD (minimum–maximum); values expressed in g/dl

Extracted from: Blanco JM, Hofle U (2003) Plasma protein electrophoresis as diagnostic and prognostic tool in raptors. *Proceedings of the European Association of Avian Veterinarians*, Tenerife, pp. 256–262.

Plasma protein electrophoresis in selected psittacine species

Species	Hyacinthine macaw n = 8	Blue and yellow macaw n = 11	Green winged macaw n = 10	Scarlet macaw n = 12	Military macaw n = 11
Scientific name	Anodorhynchus hyacinthinus	Ara ararauna	Ara chloroptera	Ara macaw	Ara militaris
Total protein	30.3 ± 3.9 (23.8–38.5)	29.2 ± 7.0 (17.9–46.5)	36.7 ± 9.8 (18.0–59.9)	38.3 ± 6.4 (28.6–47.5)	29.6 ± 8.2 (17.2–44.4)
Prealbumin	5.9 ± 5.7 (0.0–14.9)	10.1 ± 6.3 (3.0–21.8)	9.3 ± 7.2 (0.0–17.2)	10.2 ± 4.8 (0.0–14.3)	9.5 ± 6.2 (0.0–18.5)
Albumin	58.0 ± 9.9 (45.9–69.2)	54.6 ± 3.0 (51.4–59.2)	64.1 ± 5.1 (55.3–70.5)	55.6 ± 11.8 (34.6–66.6)	50.0 ± 12.0 (34.5–70.6)
Alpha	7.5 ± 3.2 (3.3–12.2)	7.8 ± 5.1 (1.7–15.9)	6.7 ± 3.6 (2.1–11.9)	8.8 ± 8.2 (2.0–28.5)	10.5 ± 3.9 (5.8–18.3)
Beta	14.4 ± 5.3 (5.6–20.3)	17.0 ± 7.0 (11.3–31.6)	12.3 ± 6.0 (4.9–24.3)	14.9 ± 9.1 (5.2–37.7)	17.8 ± 7.2 (8.1–32.5)
Gamma	14.3 ± 8.5 (2.2–25.6)	10.5 ± 4.7 (2.6–16.4)	7.5 ± 4.6 (1.7–16.5)	10.4 ± 5.6 (1.5–20.1)	12.1 ± 5.1 (1.8–19.6)
A:G ratio	1.9 ± 0.6 (1.3–3.0)	1.9 ± 0.5 (1.3–2.8)	2.9 ± 0.8 (1.6–4.1)	2.3 ± 1.1 (0.6–4.1)	1.6 ± 0.5 (0.6–2.4)

Mean ± SD (minimum–maximum)
Source: modified from: Polo FJ, Peinado VI, Viscor G, Palomeque J (1998) Hematologic and plasma chemistry in captive psittacine birds. *Avian Diseases* **42**: 523–535.

Plasma protein electrophoresis in selected psittacine species (continued)

Species	Yellow shouldered amazon n = 29	Red-browed amazon n = 18
Scientific name	Amazona barbadensis	Amazona rhodocorytha
Total protein	4.8 ± 6.1	45.06 ± 3.26
Prealbumin	11.42 ± 3.67 (24.99 ± 6.87)	7.74 ± 1.21 (17.28 ± 3.16)
Albumin	23.79 ± 3.86 (53.31 ± 5.60)	27.30 ± 3.27 (60.35 ± 3.61)
Alpha	2.88 ± 0.66 (6.37 ± 1.24)	2.68 ± 0.73 (5.97 ± 1.60)
Beta	3.19 ± 0.96 (7.11 ± 2.20)	3.39 ± 0.46 (7.4 ± 1.07)
Gamma	3.74 ± 1.22 (8.23 ± 2.33)	4.0 ± 1.1 (8.83 ± 2.21)
A:G ratio	3.80 ± 1.04	3.56 ± 0.69

Mean ± SD (minimum–maximum); values expressed in g/dl, percentage in parentheses
Source: Bürkle M, Silveira Viera L, Dreisörner CJ et al. (2003) Electrophoresis in Psittaciformes normal values and selected cases. *Proceedings of the European Association of Avian Veterinarians*, Tenerife, pp. 253–255.

Plasma protein electrophoresis in selected birds

Species	Bar-headed goose n = 62	White storkn n = 42	Domestic pigeon n = 36	Jackdaw n = 44	Black kite n = 34	Indian peafowl n = 40	African gray parrot n = 13	Blacksmith plover n = 18
Scientific name	Anser indicus	Ciconia ciconia	Columba livia	Corvus monedula	Milvus migrans	Pavo cristatus	Psittacus erithacus	Vanellus armatus
Total protein	4.11 ± 0.51	4.10 ± 0.34	3.68 ± 0.49	3.60 ± 0.55	4.01 ± 0.32	4.43 ± 0.24	3.71 ± 0.40	3.61 ± 0.40
Albumin	2.53 ± 0.26	1.60 ± 0.17	1.06 ± 0.15	1.41 ± 0.22	1.76 ± 0.24	2.48 ± 0.25	1.99 ± 0.24	1.55 ± 0.26
Alpha 1	0.23 ± 0.05	0.84 ± 0.17	0.08 ± 0.01	0.09 ± 0.27	0.29 ± 0.13	0.20 ± 0.03	0.06 ± 0.01	0.19 ± 0.04
Alpha 2	0.75 ± 0.17	0.60 ± 0.11	0.13 ± 0.17	0.81 ± 0.15	1.03 ± 0.23	0.75 ± 0.06	0.90 ± 0.19	0.93 ± 0.19
Beta	0.57 ± 0.16	0.43 ± 0.09	0.97 ± 0.27	1.05 ± 0.27	0.61 ± 0.16	0.55 ± 0.06	0.57 ± 0.09	0.63 ± 0.20
Gamma	0.20 ± 0.07	0.53 ± 0.11	0.33 ± 0.10	0.20 ± 0.08	0.31 ± 0.08	0.44 ± 0.10	0.23 ± 0.04	0.29 ± 0.05
A:G ratio	0.13 ± 0.02	0.06 ± 0.00	0.04 ± 0.01	0.06 ± 0.01	0.07 ± 0.01	0.12 ± 0.01	0.11 ± 0.02	0.07 ± 0.01

Mean ± SD (minimum–maximum); values expressed in g/dl
Source: modified from: Ordonneau D, Roman Y, Chaste-Duvernoy D, Bomsel MC (2005) Plasma electrophoresis reference ranges in various bird species. *Proceedings of the European Association of Avian Veterinarians*, Arles, pp. 283–287.
ALKP, alkaline phosphatase; ALT, alanine aminotransferase; ALB, albumin; GLO, globulin; AST, aspartate aminotransferase; LDH, lactate dehydrogenase; CK, creatine kinase; CPK, creatine phosphokinase; γ-GT, gamma glutamyltranspeptidase; GGT, X-glutamyl transferase; Mg, magnesium; PHOS, phosphorus; TP, total protein; BUN, blood urea nitrogen.

Appendix 4

Incubation periods for selected avian species

Merle M. Apo

Hatching

Calculation of hatch date

- The hatch date is calculated from the laying date or the date that incubation started if eggs were stored for any length of time
- As the hatch date approaches, the egg is candled daily to monitor air cell and embryo position
- The egg is transferred from the incubator to the hatcher after pipping.

Anatomical and physiological changes during hatching

- As the embryo grows and develops, the head moves from the narrow end of the egg up toward the air cell in the wide end of the egg, eventually becoming positioned just under the right wing
- Allantoic circulation gradually fails to meet the embryo's gaseous gas exchange needs
- The elevated level of carbon dioxide leads to twitching of the neck muscles
- During twitching the beak penetrates the air cell and the embryo begins to breathe
- As the embryo begins breathing, the lungs begin to function for the first time in air exchange, and the right-to-left cardiovascular shunt closes

- In some species, vocalizations (peeping) can be heard for the first time
- The elevated carbon dioxide level also causes abdominal muscle contractions, which pull the yolk sac into the abdomen
- As the embryo continues to breathe air from the air cell, the carbon dioxide level again rises, to as high as 10%
- The elevated carbon dioxide level leads to further muscle contractions
- During one of the contractions, the beak breaks through the shell, forming a pip hole
- Species vary considerably in the length of the interval between entry into the air cell and pipping (the range is 3 h to 3 d, generally longer in larger species)
- Alternating between contractions of the head and neck and of the neck, back, and abdominal muscles, the embryo first chips at the shell, then shifts position slightly before the next head and neck contraction results in further chipping; this process is called cutting out
- Finally, the top of the shell is pushed away, and the chick kicks free
- The interval from pipping to kicking free ranges from 30 min to 3 d and is also species-specific
- The newly hatched chicks are usually wet and exhausted and will rest and dry off.

Description and prognosis of malpositioned embryos		
Malposition number	**Embryo position**	**Prognosis**
1	Head between the thighs	Initially a good prognosis, because this is the early normal position; as time progresses the prognosis becomes poor and the embryo may die
2	Head in the small end of the egg	Guarded prognosis: the position is lethal in about 50% of cases; Assistance with hatching improves the chances of survival
3	Head under the left wing	Poor prognosis: this position is generally lethal to the embryo
4	Body rotated with the head under the right wing but not pointing at the air cell	Guarded to poor prognosis, because the head will not enter the air cell; may be possible to assist hatching
5	Feet over the head	Guarded to poor prognosis, because embryo cannot kick to rotate its body during cutting out; assistance with hatching improves survival
6	Head over instead of under the right wing	Good prognosis; embryo usually hatches with minimal complications or help
7	Embryo crosswise in the egg	Poor prognosis; this position is often fatal. It is seen with small embryos and spherical eggs, and other defects are commonly present

Source: modified from Olsen GH, Orosz SE (2000) Embryologic considerations. *Manual of Avian Medicine*, pp. 189–212. Mosby, St Louis.

Incubation requirements for some commonly reared birds

Common name	Scientific name	Incubation temperature, °C (°F)	Relative humidity, %	Incubation, d
Budgerigar	Melopsittacus undulatus	37.1 (98.7)	18	
Cockatiel	Nymphicus hollandicus	37.5 (99.5)	56	21
Moluccan cockatoo	Cacatua moluccensis	37.2–37.4 (99–99.3)	58–61	29.3
Eclectus parrot	Eclectus roratus	37.2–37.4 (99–99.3)	50–53	28
African gray parrot	Psittacus erithacus erithacus	99–99.4 (37.2–37.5)	50–53	29.8
Macaw	Ara spp.	37.3–37.4 (99.1–99.3)	50–53	25.1–26.5
Hyacinth macaw	Anodorhynchus hyacinthinus	37.2–37.4 (99–99.3)	50–53	26.5
Rose-breasted cockatoo	Eolophus roseicapillus	37.4–37.6 (99.3–99.7)	50–53	21.9
Yellow-naped Amazon parrot	Amazona ochrocephala	37.3–37.5 (99.1–99.5)	50–53	27.3

Source: modified from Olsen GH, Orosz SE (2000) Embryologic considerations. *Manual of Avian Medicine,* pp. 189–212. Mosby, St. Louis.

Incubation requirements for some commonly reared birds

Common name	Scientific name	Incubation temperature, °C (°F)	Relative humidity, %	Incubation, d
Ostrich	Struthio camelus	36–36.4 (96.8–97.5)	20–25	42–45
Cassowary	Casuarius spp.	36.1 (97)	68	46–49
Rhea	Rhea americana	36.5 (97.7)	62–65	36–44
Emu	Dromaius novaehollandiae	(97–97.5)	25–30	51

Source: modified from Shane SM (1996) Hatchery management in emu production. In: Tully TN Jr, Shane SM (eds) *Ratite Management, Medicine, and Surgery,* pp. 69–73. Krieger, Malabar, FL.

Incubation requirements for some commonly reared birds

Common name	Scientific name	Incubation (d)
Conures	Pyrrhura spp. and Aratinga spp.	23–24
Monk parakeets	Myiopsitta monachus	24–48
Senegal parrots	Poicephalus senegalus	24–48
Lories	Eos spp., Lorius spp., Chalcopsitta spp.	24–36
Lovebirds	Agapornis spp.	24–48
Caiques	Poinites spp.	24–48
Pionus parrots	Pionus spp.	24–48

Source: modified from Olsen GH, Clubb SL (1997) Embryology, incubation and hatching. In: Altman RB, Clubb SL, Dorrestein GM, Quesenberry K (eds) *Avian Medicine and Surgery,* pp. 54–71. WB Saunders, Philadelphia.

Incubation requirements for some commonly reared birds

Common name	Scientific name	Incubation (d)
Amboina king parrot	Alisterus amboiensis	20
Blue-fronted Amazon parrot	Amazona aestiva	26
Goldie's lorikeet	Psitteuteles iris	24–48
Grass parakeet	Neophema chrysostoma	24–48
Quaker parakeets	Myiopsitta monachus	24–48
Palm cockatoo	Probosciger aterimus	24–72

Source: modified from Clubb S, Flammer K, Kim JL (1994) Theriogenology. In: Ritchie BW, Harrison GJ, Harrison LR (eds) *Avian Medicine: Principles and Application,* pp. 749–804. Wingers Publishing, Lake Worth, FL.

Incubation requirements for some commonly reared birds

Common name	Scientific name	Incubation (d)
Mute swan	*Cygnus olor*	35–40
Pink-footed goose	*Anser brachyrhynchus*	26–27
Bar-headed goose	*Anser indicus*	27
Hawaiian goose	*Branta sandvicensis*	29
Red-breasted goose	*Branta ruficollis*	23–25
European widgeon	*Anas penelope*	23–25
Mallard	*Anas platyrhynchos*	23–29
Common eider	*Somateria mollissima*	25–30
Tufted duck	*Aythya fuligula*	23–25
Mandarin duck	*Aix galericulata*	28–30
Muscovy duck	*Cairina moschata*	35
European goldeneye	*Bucephala clangula*	27–32

Source: modified from Parsons DG (1996) Breeding problems and neonate diseases. In: Beynon PH, Forbes NA, Harcourt-Brown NH (eds) *Manual of Raptors, Pigeons and Waterfowl*, pp. 284–298. British Small Animal Veterinary Association, Cheltenham.

Incubation requirements for some commonly reared birds

Common name	Scientific name	Incubation (d)
Bearded vulture	*Gypaetus barbatus*	53–58
European black vulture	*Aegypius monachus*	50–55
Griffon vulture	*Gyps fulvus*	48–54
Egyptian vulture	*Neophron perenopterus*	42
White-tailed sea eagle	*Haliaeetus albicilla*	38–40
Pallas sea eagle	*Haliaeetus leucoryphus*	38
Osprey	*Pandion haliaeetus*	35–38
Peregrine falcon	*Falco peregrinus*	31–33
Gyrfalcon	*Falco rusticolus*	30–34
Saker falcon	*Falco cherrug*	31–33
Lanner falcon	*Falco biarmicus*	32
European hobby	*Falco subbuteo*	(28) 31–33
Common kestrel	*Falco tinnunculus*	28–30
Merlin	*Falco columbarius*	28–30
Eleonora's falcon	*Falcon eleonorae*	28–30
Northern goshawk	*Accipiter gentilis*	32–34 (39)
European sparrowhawk	*Accipiter nisus*	32–34
Common buzzard	*Buteo buteo*	31–33
Rough-legged buzzard	*Buteo lagopus*	31–34
Long-legged buzzard	*Buteo rufinus*	33–35
Golden eagle	*Aquila chrysaetus*	43–45
Imperial eagle	*Aquila heliaca*	43
Tawny or steppe eagle	*Aquila rapax*	35
Lesser spotted eagle	*Aquila pomarina*	38–41
Greater spotted eagle	*Aquila clanga*	42–44
Bonelli's eagle	*Hieraaetus fasciatus*	37–39
Booted eagle	*Hieraaetus penatus*	35–38
Red and black kites	*Milvus milvus and Milvus migrans*	30–32
Marsh harrier	*Circus aeruginosus*	33–35
Montagu's harrier	*Circus pygargus*	28–30

Source: modified from Heidenreich M (1997) *Birds of Prey, Medicine and Management*, pp. 45–61. Blackwell Science, Oxford.

Incubation requirements for some commonly reared birds

Common name	Scientific name	Incubation (d)
Northern sparrowhawk	*Accipiter nisus*	35
Eurasian buzzard	*Buteo buteo*	36–38
Harris hawk	*Parabuteo unicinctus*	32
Barn owl	*Tyto alba*	30–31
Northern eagle owl	*Bubo bubo*	34–36
Snowy owl	*Nyctea scandiacea*	30–33

Source: modified from Parsons DG (1996) Breeding problems and neonate diseases. In: Beynon PH, Forbes NA, Harcourt-Brown NH (eds) *Manual of Raptors, Pigeons and Waterfowl*, pp. 20–215. British Small Animal Veterinary Association, Cheltenham.

Incubation requirements for some commonly reared birds

Common name	Scientific name	Incubation period (d)
ORDER PROCELLARIIFORMES		
Albatross		
Royal	*Diomeda epomophora*	79
ORDER PSITTACIFORMES		
Amazon		
Blue-fronted	*Amazona aestiva*	26–27
Cuban	*Amazona leucocephala*	26–28
Green-cheeked	*Amazona viridigenalis*	24
Hispaniolan	*Amazona ventralis*	25
Lilac-crowned	*Amazona finschi*	26
Puerto Rican	*Amazona vittata*	25–27
Red-lored	*Amazona autumnalis*	25–26
Cockatoo		
Bare-eyed	*Cacatua sanguinea*	23–24
Blue-eyed	*Cacatua ophthalmica*	30
Citron-crested	*Cacatua sulphurea citrinocristata*	25–26
Galah	*Eolophus roseicapillus*	22–24
Gang-gang	*Callocephalon fimbriatum*	30
Glossy	*Calyptorhynchus lattami*	29
Goffin's	*Cacatua goffini*	25
Greater sulfur-crested	*Cacatua galeria*	27–28
Leadbeater's	*Cacatua leadbeateri*	26
Lesser sulfur-crested	*Cacatua sulphurea*	24–25
Moluccan	*Cacatua moluccensis*	28–29
Philippine red-vented	*Cacatua haematuropygia*	24
Red-tailed black	*Calyptorhynchus banksii*	30
Slender-billed	*Calyptorhynchus latirostris*	23–24
Umbrella	*Cacatua alba*	28
Conure		
Blue-crowned	*Aratinga acuticaudata*	23
Blue-throated	*Pyrrhura cruentata*	24–26
Brown-throated	*Aratinga pertinax*	23
Dusky-headed	*Aratinga weddellii*	23
Green-cheeked	*Pyrrhura molinae*	22–24
Nanday	*Nandayus nenday*	21–23
Orange-fronted	*Aratinga canicularis*	30
Patagonian	*Cyanoliseus patagonus*	24–25
Pearly	*Pyrrhura lepida*	25
Sun	*Aratinga solstitialis*	28

Continued

Incubation requirements for some commonly reared birds (continued)

Common name	Scientific name	Incubation period (d)
White-eared	Pyrrhura leucotis	27
Kea	Nestor notabilis	28–29
Lorikeet		
Fairy	Charmosyna pulchella	25
Goldie's	Psitteuteles goldiei	24
Johnstone's	Trichoglossus johnstoniae	21–23
Little	Glossopsitta pusilla	22
Meyer's	Trichoglossus flavoviridis	23–24
Musk	Glossopsitta concinna	25
Ornate	Trichoglossus ornatus	26–28
Purple-crowned	Glossopsitta porphyrocephala	22
Red-flanked	Charmosyna placentas	25
Scaly-breasted	Trichoglossus chlorolepidotus	23
Stella's	Charmosyna papou	26–27
Varied	Psitteuteles versicolor	22
Lory		
Black	Chalcopsitta atra	25
Blue-crowned	Vini australis	23
Chattering	Lorius garrulous	26
Collared	Phigys solitarius	30
Dusky	Pseudeos fuscata	24
Duyvenbode's	Chalcopsitta duivenbodei	24
Papuan	Charmosyna papou	21
Purple-naped	Lorius domicella	24–26
Rainbow	Trichoglossus haematodus	25–26
Red (Moluccan)	Eos squamata	24
Tahitian	Vini peruviana	25
Violet-necked	Eos squamata	27
Yellow-backed chattering	Lorius garrulus	26
Yellow-streaked	Chalcopsitta scintillata	24
Lovebird		
Black-cheeked	Agapornis nigregenis	24
Black-winged	Agapornis taranta	25
Fischer's	Agapornis fischeri	23
Gray-headed	Agapornis canus	23
Masked	Agapornis personatus	23
Nyasa	Agapornis lilianae	22
Peach-faced	Agapornis roseicollis	23
Red-faced	Agapornis pullarius	22
Macaw		
Blue and gold	Ara ararauna	26
Buffon's	Ara ambigua	26–27
Caninde	Ara glaucogularis	26
Chestnut-fronted	Ara severa	28
Green-winged	Ara chloroptera	26
Hyacinth	Anodorhynchus hyacinthinus	26–28
Illiger's	Propyrrhura maracana	26–27
Military	Ara militaris	26
Red-bellied	Orthopsittaca manilata	25
Red-fronted	Ara rubrogenys	26
Red-shouldered	Diopsittaca nobilis	24
Scarlet	Ara macao	26
Yellow-collared	Propyrrhura auricollis	26

Continued overleaf

Incubation requirements for some commonly reared birds (continued)

Common name	Scientific name	Incubation period (d)
Rosella		
Eastern	*Platycercus eximius*	21
Western	*Platycercus icterotis*	20
ORDER CICONIIFORMES		
Bittern		
American	*Botaurus lentiginosus*	28–29
Eurasian	*Botaurus stellaris*	25
Least	*Ixobrychus exilis*	19–20
Little	*Ixobrychus minutus*	16–17
Yellow	*Ixobrychus sinensis*	22
Heron		
Black-headed	*Ardea melanocephala*	25
Goliath	*Ardea goliath*	28
Gray	*Ardea cinerea*	25–26
Squacco	*Ardeola ralloides*	21
Ibis		
Bald	*Geronticus calvus*	24–25
Glossy	*Plegadis falcinellus*	26
Hadada	*Bostrychia hagedash*	26
Northern bald	*Geronticus eremita*	27–28
Oriental	*Threskiornis melanocephalus*	23–25
Sacred	*Threskiornis aethiopicus*	28–29
Scarlet	*Eudocimus rubber*	21–23
Spoonbill		
African	*Platalea alba*	23–24
European	*Platalea leucorodia*	25
Stork		
Asian open-billed	*Anastomus oscitans*	24–25
Black	*Ciconia nigra*	30–35
Marabou	*Leptoptilos crumeniferus*	30
White	*Ciconia ciconia*	30
ORDER GRUIFORMES		
Bustard		
Great	*Otis tarda*	25–28
Crane		
Australian	*Grus rubicunda*	35–36
Black-necked	*Grus nigricollis*	31–33
Canadian sandhill	*Grus canadensis*	27
Common (Eurasian)	*Grus grus*	28–31
Demoiselle	*Anthropoides virgo*	27–30
Florida sandhill	*Grus canadensis pratensis*	31–32
Greater sandhill	*Grus canadensis tabida*	31–32
Japanese	*Grus japonensis*	30–34
Sarus	*Grus antigone*	28
Siberian white	*Grus leucogeranus*	29
Stanley	*Anthropoides paradisea*	29–30
Wattled	*Bugeranus carunculatus*	35–40
White-naped	*Grus vipio*	28–32
Whooping	*Grus americana*	30
Moorhen		
Common	*Gallinula chloropus*	19–22

Continued

Incubation requirements for some commonly reared birds *(continued)*

Common name	Scientific name	Incubation period (d)
ORDER FALCONIFORMES		
Buzzard		
Common	*Buteo buteo*	33–38
Honey	*Henicopernis longicauda*	30–35
Caracara		
Crested	*Polyborus plancus*	28
Condor		
Andean	*Vulture gryphus*	54–58
Falcon		
Eleonora's	*Falco eleonorae*	28
Red-footed	*Falco vespertinus*	28
Saker	*Falco cherrug*	30
Goshawk		
Common	*Accipiter gentilis*	35–38
Harrier		
Hen	*Circus cyaneus*	29–31
Marsh	*Circus aeruginosus*	31–38
Montagu's	*Circus pygargus*	27–30
Pallid	*Circus macrourus*	29–30
Hawk		
Red-tailed	*Buteo jamaicensis*	28–32
Kestrel		
Common	*Falco tinnunculus*	27–29
Lesser	*Falco raumanni*	29
Kite		
Brahminy	*Haliastur indus*	26–27
Red	*Milvus milvus*	31–32
Osprey	*Pandion haliaetus*	38
Merlin	*Falco columbarius*	28–32
Sparrowhawk		
Common	*Accipiter nisus*	33–35
Levant	*Accipiter brevipes*	30–35
Vulture		
Bearded	*Gypaetus barbatus*	55–60
Egyptian	*Neophron pecnopterus*	42
King	*Sarcoramphus papa*	56–58
ORDER STRUTHIONIFORMES		
Cassowary		
Twin-wattled	*Casuarius casuarius*	49–56
Ostrich	*Struthio camelus*	40–42
Rhea		
Greater	*Rhea americana*	36–40
ORDER GALLIFORMES		
Curassow		
Nocturnal	*Nothocrax urumutum*	26–30
Grouse		
Blue	*Dendragapus obscurus*	24–25
Hazel	*Bonasa bonasia*	25
Ruffed	*Bonasa umbellus*	24

Continued overleaf

Incubation requirements for some commonly reared birds (continued)

Common name	Scientific name	Incubation period (d)
Sage	*Centrocercus urophasianus*	24–25
Spruce	*Falcipennis falcipennis*	21
Willow/red	*Lagopus lagopus*	21–22
Guinea fowl		
Helmeted	*Numida meleagris*	24–25
Vulturine	*Acryllium vulturinum*	25–26
Junglefowl		
Ceylon	*Gallus lafayetti*	18–20
Green	*Gallus varius*	21
Pheasant		
Blood	*Ithaginis cruentus*	28
Blue eared	*Crossoptilon auritum*	26–28
Blyth's tragopan	*Tragopan blythii*	28
Brown eared	*Crossoptilon mantchuricum*	26–27
Bulwer's wattled	*Lophura bulweri*	25
Cabot's tragopan	*Tragopan caboti*	28
Cheer	*Catreus wallichii*	26
Common ring-necked	*Phasianus colchicus*	24–25
Copper	*Syrmaticus soemmerringii*	24–25
Crested argus	*Rheinaraia ocellata*	25
Crested fireback	*Lophura ignita*	24
Crestless fireback	*Lophura erythrophthalma*	21–24
Edwards's	*Lophura edwardsi*	21–24
Elliot's	*Syrmaticus ellioti*	25
Golden	*Chrysolophus pictus*	23
Great argus	*Argusianus argus*	24–25
Green	*Phasianus versicolor*	24–25
Himalayan monal	*Lophophorus impejanus*	28
Hume's bar-tailed	*Syrmaticus humige*	27–28
Imperial	*Lophura imperialis*	25
Kalij	*Lophura leucomelanus*	23–25
Koklass	*Pucrasia macrolopha*	26–27
Lady Amherst's	*Chrysolophus amherstiae*	22
Mikado	*Syrmaticus mikado*	26–28
Reeve's	*Symaticus reevesii*	24–25
Salvadori's	*Lophura inornata*	25
Satyr tragopan	*Tragopan satyra*	28
Siamese fireback	*Lophura diardi*	24–25
Silver	*Lophura nycthemera*	25
Swinhoe's	*Lophura swinhoii*	25
Temminck's tragopan	*Tragopan temminckii*	28
Western tragopan	*Tragopan melanocephalus*	28
White eared	*Crossoptilon crossoptilon*	24
Quail		
Bobwhite	*Colinus virginianus*	22
California	*Callipepla californica*	22–23
Harlequin	*Coturnix delegor guei*	14–18
Partridge		
Chukar	*Alectoris chukar*	23
Gray	*Arborophila orientalis*	23–25
Red-legged	*Alectoris rufa*	23–25
Rock	*Alectoris graeca*	24–26

Continued

Incubation requirements for some commonly reared birds (continued)

Common name	Scientific name	Incubation period (d)
Peafowl/peacock		
Congo	Afropavo congensis	26–28
Bronze-tailed	Polyplectron chalcurum	22
Germain's	Polyplectron germaini	22
Gray	Polyplectron bicalcaratum	22
Green	Pavo muticus	28
Indian	Pavo cristatus	27–28
Malayan	Polyplectron malacense	22
Palawan	Polyplectron emphanum	18–19
Rothschild's	Polyplectron inopinatum	22
ORDER CHARADRIIFORMES		
Curlew		
Eurasian	Numenius arguata	29
Stone	Burhinus oedicnemus	21–23
Gull		
Herring	Larus argentatus	27–31
Lapwing		
Spur-winged	Vanellus spinosus	22–24
Oystercatcher		
European	Haematopus ostralegus	24–27
Snipe		
Common	Gallinago gallinago	20
Tern		
Artic	Sterna paradisaca	20–22
Caspian	Hydroprogne caspia	20–22
Thick-knee		
Water	Burhinus vermiculatus	24
Woodcock		
Eurasian	Scolopax rusticola	20–22
Avocet		
American	Recurvirostra americana	22–24
Common	Recurvirostra avosetta	22–24
ORDER PHOENICOPTERIFORMES		
Flamingo		
Lesser	Phoeniconaias minor	28
Greater	Phoenicopterus ruber	30–32
ORDER CAPRIMULGIFORMES		
Frogmouth		
Tawny	Podargus strigoides	30
ORDER ANSERIFORMES		
Goose		
Abyssinian blue-winged	Cyanochen cyanopterus	31
Andean	Chloephaga melanoptera	30
Ashy-headed	Chloephaga poliocephala	30
Atlantic brant	Branta bernicla	23
Atlantic Canada	Branta canadensis	28
Bar-headed	Anser indicus	28
Barnacle	Branta leucopsis	28
Black brant	Branta nigricans	23
Cereopsis	Cereopsis novaehollandiae	35
Cackling Canada	Branta canadensis minima	28

Continued overleaf

Incubation requirements for some commonly reared birds (continued)

Common name	Scientific name	Incubation period (d)
Dusky Canada	Branta canadensis occidentalis	28
Eastern graylag	Anser anser rubrirostris	28
Egyptian	Alopochen aegyptiacus	30
Emperor	Anser canagisus	25
European white-fronted	Anser albifrons	26
Giant Canada (maxima)	Branta canadensis maxima	28
Hawaiian	Branta sandvicensis	29
Kelp	Chloephaga hybrida	32
Lesser white-fronted	Anser erythropus	25
Magellan	Chloephaga picta	30
Magpie	Anseranas semipalmata	30
Moffitt's Canada	Branta canadensis mofitti	28
Orinoco	Neochen jubata	30
Pink-footed	Anser brachyrhynchus	28
Red-breasted	Branta ruficollis	25
Ross's	Anser rossii	23
Ruddy-headed	Chloephaga rubidiceps	30
Snow	Anser caerulescens	25
Spur-winged	Plectropterus gambensis	32
Swan	Anser cygnoides	28
Teverner's Canada	Branta canadensis traverneri	28
Western graylag	Anser anser	28
Vancouver	Branta canadensis fulva	28

Swan

Bewick's	Cygnus columbianus bewickii	30
Black	Cygnus atratus	36
Black-necked	Cygnus melanocorypha	36
Coscoroba	Coscoroba coscoroba	35
Mute	Cygnus olor	37
Trumpeter	Cygnus buccinator	33
Whistling	Cygnus columbianus	36
Whooper	Cygnus cygnus	33

ORDER PODICIPEDIFORMES
Grebe

Great crested	Podiceps cristatus	25–29
Little	Tachybaptus ruficollis	20–24

ORDER CORACIIFORMES
Hornbill

Red-billed	Tockus erythrorhynchus	30

Kookaburra

Laughing	Dacelo novaeguineae	25

ORDER PASSERIFORMES
Oriole

Golden	Oriolus oriolus	14–15

Raven

Common	Corvus corax	20–21

ORDER STRIGIFORMES

Owl

Barn	Tyto alba	32–34
Great-horned	Bubo virginianus	35
Hawk	Surnia ulula	26–30
Little scops	Otus sunia	24–25

Continued

Incubation requirements for some commonly reared birds *(continued)*

Common name	Scientific name	Incubation period (d)
Snowy	*Nyctea scandiaca*	33–36
Tawny	*Strix aluco*	28–30
ORDER PELICANIFORMES		
Pelican		
Brown	*Pelecanus occidentalis*	28–29
White	*Pelecanus onocrotalus*	28
Shag		
European	*Phalacrocorax aristotelis*	30
ORDER SPHENISCIFORMES		
Penguin		
Adelie	*Pygoscelis adeliae*	33–38
Emperor	*Aptenodytes forsteri*	62–64
Humboldt	*Spheniscus humboldti*	36–42
King	*Aptenodytes patagonicus*	51–57
ORDER COLUMBIFORMES		
Pigeon		
Rock dove	*Columba livia*	17–19
Wood	*Columba palumbus*	17
ORDER TRAGONIFORMES		
Quetzal	*Pharomachrus mocinno*	17–18
ORDER CORACIIFORMES		
Roller		
Eurasian (European)	*Coracias garrulas*	18–19
ORDER TINAMIFORMES		
Tinamou		
Elegant crested	*Eudromio elegans*	17–21
ORDER PICIFORMES		
Woodpecker		
Greater spotted	*Dendrocopos major*	16
ORDER OPISTHOCOMIFORMES		
Hoatzin	*Opisthocomus hoazin*	28
ORDER UPUPIFORMES		
Hoopoe		
European	*Upupa epops*	16–19

Source: modified from Harvey R (1990) Incubation periods. In: *Practical Incubation*, pp. 122–133. Hancock House, Blaine, WA.

Appendix 5

Selected avian literature

Merle M. Apo

Al Timimi F (1987) *Falcons and Falconry in Qatar*. Ali bin Ali Printing Press, Doha, Qatar.

Altman RB, Forbes NA (1998) *Self Assessment Color Review of Avian Medicine*. Iowa State University Press, Ames, IA. ISBN 0-8138-2339-0.

Altman RB, Clubb SL, Dorrestein GM, Quesenberry K (1997) *Avian Medicine and Surgery*. WB Saunders, Philadelphia. ISBN 0-7216-5446-0.

Arnall L, Keymer IF (1975) *Bird Diseases: An Introduction to the Study of Birds in Health and Disease*. THF Publications, Neptune City, NJ. ISBN 0-87666-950-X.

Beer JV (1988) *The Game Conservancy Diseases of Gamebirds and Wildfowl*. Game Conservancy, Fordingbridge, Hampshire.

Beynon PH, Forbes NA, Lawton MPC (1995) *Manual of Psittacine Birds*. British Small Animal Veterinary Association, Cheltenham, Gloucestershire. ISBN 0-905214-30-7.

Beynon PH, Forbes NA, Harcourt-Brown NH (1996) *Manual of Raptors, Pigeons and Waterfowl*. British Small Animal Veterinary Association, Cheltenham, Gloucestershire. ISBN 0-905214-29-3.

Brearley MJ, Cooper JE, Sullivan M (1991) *A Colour Atlas of Small Animal Endoscopy*. Wolfe Publishing, London. ISBN 0-7234-1559-5.

Campbell TW (1988) *Avian Hematology and Cytology*, 2nd edn. Iowa State University Press, Ames, IA. ISBN 0-8138-2970-4.

Coles BH (1997) *Avian Medicine and Surgery*, 2nd edn. Blackwell Science, Oxford ISBN. 0-632-03356-8.

Coles BH, Krautwald-Junghanns ME (1998) *Avian Medicine: Self Assessment Picture Test in Veterinary Medicine*. Mosby, St Louis. ISBN 0-7234-30008-X.

Cooper JE (1978) *Veterinary Aspects of Captive Birds of Prey*. Standfast Press, Saul, Gloucestershire. ISBN 0-904602-04-4.

Cooper JE (1989) *Disease and Threatened Birds*. Anagram Editorial Service, Guildford, Surrey. ISBN 0-946888-18-3.

Cooper JE (2002) *Birds of Prey: Health and Disease*, 3rd edn. Blackwell Science, Oxford, UK. ISBN 0-632-05115-9.

Cooper J, Cooper M (2003) *Captive Birds in Health and Disease*. World Pheasant Association/Hancock House Publishers, Fordingbridge, Hampshire. ISBN 0-906864-80-1.

Cooper JE, Greenwood AG (1981) *Recent Advances in the Study of Raptor Diseases*. Chiron Publications, Keighley, West Yorkshire. ISBN 0-9507716-00.

Cooper JE, Hutchison MF, Jackson OF, Maurice RJ (1985) *Manual of Exotic Pets*. British Small Animal Veterinary Association, Cheltenham, Gloucestershire. ISBN 0-905214-04-8.

Drenowatz C (1995) *Ratite Encyclopedia: Ostrich, Emu and Rhea*. Ratite Record, San Antonio, CA.

Fowler ME (1978) *Zoo and Wildlife Animal Medicine*. WB Saunders, Philadelphia. ISBN 0-7216-6559-4.

Fowler ME (1986) *Zoo and Wild Animal Medicine*, 2nd edn. WB Saunders, Philadelphia.

Fowler ME (1993) *Zoo and Wild Animal Medicine: Current Therapy 3*. WB Saunders, Philadelphia. ISBN 0-7216-3667-5.

Fowler ME (1999) *Wild Animal Medicine: Current Therapy 4*. WB Saunders, Philadelphia. ISBN 0-7216-8664-8.

Friend M (1987) *Field Guide to Wildlife Diseases: General Field Procedures and Diseases of Migratory Birds*. United States Government Printing, Washington, DC.

Fudge AM (2000) *Laboratory Medicine: Avian and Exotic Pets*. WB Saunders, Philadelphia. ISBN 0-7216-7679-0.

Ginn HB, Melville DS (2000) *Moult in Birds*. British Trust for Ornithology, Thetford, Norfolk. ISBN 0-903793-02-4.

Harrison GJ, Harrison LR (1986) *Clinical Avian Medicine and Surgery*. WB Saunders, Philadelphia. ISBN 0-7216-1241-5.

Harrison GJ, Lightfoot TL (2006) *Clinical Avian Medicine*. Spix Publishing, Palm Beach, FL. ISBN 00-9754994-0-8.

Heidenreich M (1982) *Diseases of Parrots*. THF Publications, Neptune City, NJ.

Heidenreich M (1997) *Birds of Prey: Medicine and Management*. Blackwell Science, Oxford. ISBN 0-632-04186-2.

Jacobson ER, Kollias GV Jr (1988) *Exotic Animals: Contemporary Issues in Small Animal Practice*. Churchill Livingstone, New York. ISBN 0-443-08408-4.

Johnson-Delaney C (1996) *Exotic Companion Medicine Handbook for Veterinarians* (2 vols). Wingers Publishing, Lake Worth, FL.

King AS, McLelland J (1984) *Birds: Their Structure and Function*, 2nd edn. Baillière Tindall, Eastbourne, East Sussex. ISBN 0-7020-0872-9.

Klasing RC (2000) *Comparative Avian Nutrition*. CAB International, Wallingford, Oxfordshire. ISBN 0-85199-219-6.

Lumeij JT (1987) *Clinical Investigative Methods for Birds*. Vakgroep Geneeskunde van het Kleine Huisdier Faculteit der Diergeneeskunde, Rijksuniversiteit Utrecht, Netherlands. ISBN 90-9001845-X.

Lumeij JT, Remple JD, Redig PT, Lierz M, Cooper JE (2000) *Raptor Biomedicine III, Including Bibliography of Diseases of Birds of Prey*. Zoological Education Network, Lake Worth, FL. ISBN 0-9636996-1-X.

McLelland J (1990) *Avian Anatomy*. Wolfe Publishing, London. ISBN 0-7234-1575-7.

Olsen GH, Orosz SE (2000) *Manual of Avian Medicine*. Mosby, St Louis. ISBN 0-8151-8466-2.

Olsen J (1990) *Caring for Birds of Prey*. Wild Ones Animal Books, Springville, CA.

Orosz SE, Ensley PK, Jaynes CJ (1992) *Avian Surgical Anatomy. Thoracic and Pelvic Limbs*. WB Saunders, Philadelphia. ISBN 0-7216-3654-3.

Petrak ML (1982) *Diseases of Cage and Aviary Birds*, 2nd edn. Lea & Febiger, Philadelphia.

Petrie A, Watson P (2003) *Statistics for Veterinary and Animal Science*. Blackwell Science, Oxford. ISBN 0-632-03742-3.

Randall C, Reece RL (1996) *Color Atlas of Avian Pathology*. Mosby–Wolfe, London. ISBN 0-7234-20874.

Randall CJ (1991) *A Colour Atlas of Diseases and Disorders of the Domestic Fowl and Turkey*, 2nd edn. Wolfe Publishing, London. ISBN 0-7234-16281.

Randall CJ (1997) *Diseases and Disorders of the Domestic Fowl and Turkey*, 2nd edn. Mosby–Wolfe, London. ISBN 0-7234-1628-1.

Randall CJ, Reece RL (1996) *Color Atlas of Avian Histopathology*. Mosby–Wolfe, New York. ISBN 0-7234-20874.

Redig PT, Cooper JE, Remple DJ, Hunter DB (1993) *Raptor Biomedicine*. University of Minnesota Press, Minneapolis. ISBN 0-8166-2219-1.

Remple D, Gross C (1993) *Falconry and Birds of Prey in the Gulf*. Motivate Publishing, Dubai, United Arab Emirates. ISBN 1-873544391.

Riddell C (1996) *Avian Histopathology*, 2nd edn. American Association of Avian Pathologists, Saskatoon, Saskatchewan. ISBN 0-915538-04-0.

Ritchie BW (1995) *Avian Viruses: Function and Control*. Wingers Publishing, Lake Worth, FL. ISBN 0-9636996-3-6.

Ritchie BW, Harrison GJ, Harrison LR (1994) *Avian Medicine: Principles and Application*. Wingers Publishing, Lake Worth, FL. ISBN 0-9636996-0-1.

Rosskopf W, Woerpel R (1996) *Diseases of Cage and Aviary Birds*, 3rd edn. Williams & Wilkins, Philadelphia. ISBN 0 683 07382.

Rupley AE (1997) *Manual of Avian Practice*. WB Saunders, Philadelphia. ISBN 0-7216-4083-4.

Saif YM, Barnes HJ, Glisson JR et al. (2003) *Diseases of Poultry*, 11th edn. Iowa State University Press, Ames, IA. ISBN 0-8138-0423-X.

Schmidt RE, Reavill DR, Phalen DN (2003) *Pathology of Pet and Aviary Birds*. Iowa State Press, Iowa, USA. ISBN 0-8138-0502-3.

Stark JM, Ricklefs RE (1998) *Avian Growth and Development*. Oxford University Press, Oxford, UK. ISBN 0-19-510608-3.

Tudor DC (1991) *Pigeon Health and Disease*. Iowa State University Press, Ames, IA.

Tully TN, Lawton MPC, Dorrestein GM (2000) *Avian Medicine*. Butterworth-Heinemann, Oxford. ISBN 0-7506-3598-3.

Tully TN, Shane SM (1996) *Ratites: Management, Medicine and Surgery*. Krieger Publishing, Malabar, FL. ISBN 0-89464-874-8.

Wernery R, Wernery U, Kinne J, Samour J (2004) *Colour Atlas of Falcon Medicine*. Schlütersche, Hannover, Germany. ISBN 3-89993-007-X.

Whiteman CE, Bickford AA (1989) *Avian Diseases Manual*, 3rd edn. American Association of Avian Pathologists, Saskatoon, Saskatchewan. ISBN 0-8403-5795-8.

Whittow GC (2000) *Sturkie's Avian Physiology*, 3rd edn. Academic Press, London. ISBN 0-12-747605-9.

Appendix 6

Legislation and codes of practice relevant to avian medicine

Margaret E. Cooper

It is useful and, indeed, important for those who work in avian medicine to be aware of the legislation relevant to their work, their clients and their patients.

Legislation is very largely produced by individual countries and is therefore subject to variation on any particular topic from nation to nation. Moreover within a country that has a federal constitution, law-making powers may be given to provincial authorities, creating further variety. Consequently, in an international publication such as this, it may be more helpful to indicate the types and fields of legislation that are most commonly encountered and of significance to the avian practitioner than to discuss specific pieces of national legislation. Individuals may use this summary to identify the sorts of law that are appropriate and then seek in their own jurisdiction for specific legal provisions.

Legislation

Legislation is made at several levels.

Level	Source	Example
International	Global treaties	CITES
Regional	Several countries	EU regulations, directives
National	Single countries	Primary and secondary legislation, e.g. statutes, orders
Provincial	Within a country, i.e. state, province, canton, land, etc.	Regulations, decrees, etc.
Local	District, city	Bye-laws

Note: For abbreviations, see below.

Legislation on particular topics may be found at several levels; for instance, trade in endangered species is subject to global, regional and national legislation although, in practice, the effective administration and enforcement of the laws is usually implemented at national or provincial level.

In some countries the keeping and use of birds is highly regulated, yet in others the legislation is not well developed or little control is exercised and/or laws are not effectively enforced.

In some situations there are voluntary, non-legal provisions, often in the form of guidelines, codes of practice or rules. These are followed on a voluntary basis as a matter of self-regulation or because no legislation is in place.

It should always be remembered that legislation can change from time to time and it is important that the reader should ensure that s/he has up-to-date information on the law.

Fields of law relevant to avian medicine

The veterinarian and veterinary practice

- Professional – qualification and the right to practice: registration, professional ethics
- Malpractice/negligence
- Medicines, prescription and controlled (dangerous) drugs
- Employment
- Health and safety
- Health certification and quarantine supervision under animal health legislation, disease surveillance
- Law enforcement and forensic skills.

Birds

Several areas of law are applicable to captive or free-living birds.

- *In captivity*, birds may be kept as pets, for show, sport, breeding, trade, research, treatment or rehabilitation. Authorization (e.g. permit/license) may be required: to keep a bird privately; for commercial or sporting purpose; to take a wild bird into captivity; or to study them in the wild. Responsibility must be taken for the welfare of a bird in captivity: in its day-to-day life, when being transported, and if used for experimental research. Special authorization is often required.
- *Many species of free-living bird* are protected against: hunting, killing, injury or capture, and the use of certain methods of killing or capture. Eggs, young and nests may also be protected. Habitat protection (e.g. national parks, forests, etc.) restricts access to, and protects, free-living birds. Authorization (permit, license) may allow certain activities for purposes such as possession, breeding, research, zoological collections, the rehabilitation of sick or injured birds, and commerce. Legal attitudes to falconry can vary from total prohibition (e.g. Norway) to not being regulated by law as a sport (as in the UK), although possession of the birds, taking the quarry and the sale of quarry, which count as game, are regulated. In the USA, falconry training and permits are required, in most cases under state law. Falconry clubs may impose rules and standards. In the UK they are responsible for a measure of self-regulation in respect of bird licensing.
- *Trade in birds*: at a national level trade in protected species may be controlled as part of wildlife legislation – permits to sell may be restricted to captive-bred specimens.
- *International trade and movement of birds*: the movement of endangered species between countries is regulated by CITES (see below) legislation implemented by individual countries. Permits are required to import and export species listed on Appendices I, II and III of CITES. Permits are not given for primarily commercial purposes for Appendix I species. Import and export for commercial and non-commercial purposes of Appendix II species is allowed under permit. This applies to whole birds, parts or derivatives (e.g. diagnostic samples) of a bird. Some countries apply stricter controls or list more species than does CITES itself. CITES management authorities (usually the government department responsible for the environment, but sometimes for agriculture) may issue guidance notes for permit applicants. In the EU, CITES is operated under EU Regulations that apply uniformly amongst all 27 member states whereas national laws deal only with enforcement. Once a CITES bird is legally present in a member state, it may be moved freely within the EU. A wide range of birds is listed in the Convention Appendices, including most birds of prey. The EU CITES Regulation lists and upgrades many additional birds in its Annexes A–D.
- *Animal health*: birds moving from one country to another are likely to need a veterinary health check and certificate and, in some countries, to go into quarantine (around 35 d) on arrival. This is normally regulated by the government department responsible for agriculture. Special restrictions may operate when there is a risk of a pandemic as in the case of Highly Pathogenic Avian Influenza (H5N1).
- *Customs control and charges* apply to imported birds.

Abbreviations

CITES: Convention on International Trade in Endangered Species of Wild Fauna and Flora.
EU: European Union: The EU has 27 member states. It has legislation (regulations or directives) on a number of subjects relevant to avian medicine. Regulations (e.g. on CITES) need no further legislation and one refers to the provisions of the actual regulations. Directives (e.g. on veterinary laws, medicinal products, animal health, health and safety, wild birds, habitat conservation) take the form of directives and require national legislation to implement their provisions. Enforcement (including powers, offenses and penalties), even for regulations, is normally a matter for national law.

Useful contacts

UK

Department for Environment, Food and Rural Affairs (DEFRA)

For DEFRA contacts see:
http://www.defra.gov.uk/corporate/contacts/contact.asp

DEFRA is responsible for both the environment and agriculture.

Wildlife

The Wildlife Licensing and Registration Section provides information sheets on the law relating to wild birds in the UK, including the legal aspects of falconry and the special controls on birds of prey.
http://www.defra.gov.uk/wildlife-countryside/gwd/birdreg/index.htm

For a summary and explanation of the UK wildlife law at various levels see:
http://www.jncc.gov.uk/page-1359

CITES (and bird registration)

The Global Wildlife Division issues guidance notes on import and export, particularly CITES controls, and on other international wildlife treaties:
http://www.defra.gov.uk/wildlife-countryside/gwd/cites/contact.htm

UK CITES website

http://www.defra.gov.uk/wildlife-countryside/gwd/cites/index.htm

http://www.ukcites.gov.uk/default.asp

http://www.ukcites.gov.uk/intro/leg_frame.htm

CITES global website of the Convention

http://www.cites.org/

http://www.cites.org/eng/app/appendices.shtml

DEFRA

http://www.defra.gov.uk/corporate/contacts/index.htm

DEFRA Agriculture

http://www.defra.gov.uk/animalh/index.htm

International trade: http://www.defra.gov.uk/animalh/int-trde/default.htm

http://www.defra.gov.uk/animalh/int-trde/imports/iins/birds/index.htm

Avian influenza: http://www.defra.gov.uk/animalh/diseases/notifiable/disease/ai/keptbirds/index.htm

EU

Main website: EU portal: http://europa.eu.int/

Links to government websites of the 27 member states of the EU: http://europa.eu/abc/european_countries/eu_members/index_en.htm

Legislation website: http://europa.eu.int/eur-lex/

EU CITES website: http://ec.europa.eu/environment/cites/legis_wildlife_en.htm

Species lists: http://www.ukcites.gov.uk/intro/13322005.pdf

USA

The US Fish and Wildlife Service (USFWS)

Legislation and regulation: http://www.fws.gov/birds/Laws.htm

US federal laws on wildlife in general: http://www.llrx.com/columns/environment.htm

http://www.llrx.com/features/esa.htm

http://training.fws.gov/library/Pubs9/wildlife_laws.pdf

USFWS Division of Migratory Bird Management

Migratory species legislation:

http://www.fws.gov/migratorybirds/

http://www.fws.gov/migratorybirds/intrnltr/treatlaw.html

USFWS Endangered Species Program

http://www.fws.gov/endangered/policies/index.html

USFWS International (CITES)

http://www.fws.gov/international/cites/cites.html

http://www.fws.gov/permits/importExport/ImportExport.shtml

The United States Department of Agriculture (USDA)

Veterinary Service Import/Export/National Center for Import and Export

http://www.aphis.usda.gov/vs/ncie/

Animal Regulations Library: http://www.aphis.usda.gov/vs/import_export.htm

Online application for USDA, APHIS, VS, NACIE permit: https://www.aphis.usda.gov/permits/learn_epermits.shtml

Export: http://www.aphis.usda.gov/import_export/animals/animal_exports.shtml

Approval of animal health status of countries/regions: http://www.aphis.usda.gov/import_export/animals/animal_disease_status.shtml

US Geological Service (USGS) / National Wildlife Health Center (NWHC)

http://www.nwhc.usgs.gov/

Wildlife Health Bulletins: Highly Pathogenic Avian Influenza H5N1

http://www.nwhc.usgs.gov/disease_information/ avian_influenza/index.jsp

http://www.nmhc.usgc.gov/publications/wildlife_ health_bulletins/

http://www.nwhc.usgs.gov/publications/wildlife_ health_bulletins/WHB_04_01.jsp

Field research

http://www.nwhc.usgs.gov/publications/wildlife_ health_bulletins/WHB_05_03.jsp

http://www.nmhc.usgs.gov/publications/field_ manual/index.jsp

Guidelines for proper care and use of wildlife in field research

The USGS-National Wildlife Health Center Field Manual of Wildlife Diseases: General Field Procedures and Diseases of Birds: http://www.nwhc.usgs.gov /publications/ field_manual/chapter_22.pdf

Field Research Animal Welfare Act USA: http://www.nal. usda.gov/awic/legislat/awabrief.htm#Q11

Other countries

Contacts and information can be obtained from diplomatic missions and from the internet.

FURTHER READING

Wildlife, bird and animal welfare organizations are often useful sources of information on the law. The veterinary literature and professional bodies provide information on professional matters.

British Field Sports Society Falconry Committee and the Hawk Board (undated) *Code of Welfare and Husbandry of Birds of Prey and Owls.* British Field Sports Society, London.

British Wildlife Rehabilitation Council (1989) *Ethics and Legal Aspects of Treatment and Rehabilitation of Wild Animal Casualties.* British Wildlife Rehabilitation Council, London.

Cooper ME (2003) Legislation for bird-keepers. In: Cooper JE (ed.) *Captive Birds in Health and Disease.* World Pheasant Association, Fordingbridge, Millsap BA, Cooper ME and Holroyd G (2007). Legal Considerations. In: DM Bird and Bildstein KL (eds) Raptor Research and Management Techniques. Hancock House Publishers, Blaine, WA UK.

Cooper ME (2000). Legislation and codes of practice relevant to working with raptors. In: Cooper JE (ed.) *Birds of Prey: Health and Disease,* 3rd edn. Blackwell Publishing, Oxford.

Gaunt AS and Oring LA (1999). Guidelines for the use of wild birds in research. The Ornithological Council. Washington DC

Van Heijnsbergen, P (1997) *International Legal Protection of Wild Fauna and Flora.* IOS Press, Amsterdam.

Wilson JF (1989) *Law and Ethics of the Veterinary Profession.* Priority Press, Yardley, PA.

Appendix 7

Organizations and electronic resources relating to avian medicine

F. Joshua Dein, Peter Thorsen

Introduction

This appendix is a compilation of organizations and resources that may be helpful to those interested in avian medicine. As with the text, the focus here is on non-psittacine species. These resources have been identified primarily from what is available on the World Wide Web (WWW) and should not be considered complete or exhaustive. In many situations, information is available from one source, which may lead to many non-WWW-based organizations.

The listings are offered in four major groups: General, Veterinary, Aviculture and Conservation. Within these, they are divided into organizations and WWW resources. Keep in mind that there is considerable overlap in all these groups and divisions, such as a WWW Universal Resource Locator (URL) listing under organizations, and organizations cited only by their URL. A short note with many of the entries tries to provide the organizational mission, or content, as taken from the resource.

General

WWW

Arctic Bird Library

A list of 124 species of water-bird that breed in the Arctic, as defined by Conservation of Arctic Flora and Fauna (CAFF). For 16 species we have provided information on the habitat, conservation status and population size; a distribution map and links to conservation information; and images for four other species.
E-mail: chrisz@wcmc.org.uk
URL: http://www.wcmc.org.uk/arctic/data/birds/birds.htm

Bird Links to the World

Comprehensive site with links to bird discussion groups, journals, organizations, materials and images.
URL: http://www.ntic.qc.ca/lnellus/links4.html

Birdnet Image Gallery

Bird photographs and artwork.
URL: http://www.interaktv.com/BIRDNET/CArt.html

Birds Databases

A compilation of searchable databases related to birds.
URL: http://www.internets.com/sbirds.htm

Ducks of the World

Pictures and information on many species.
E-mail: mfield@utm.edu
URL: http://www.utm.edu/departments/ed/cece/ducks.shtml

Eurobirdnet

A site dedicated to European birds and birding.
URL: http://ebn.unige.ch/ebn/ugebn_e.html

Hot Spot for Birds

Site designed for the pet bird owner with links and bird health and nutrition.
E-mail: hotspot@multiscope.com
URL: http://www.multiscope.com/hotspot/

Internet Flyway

Site with numerous links.
URL: http://www.netlink.co.uk/users/aw/index.html

Northern Prairie Wildlife Research Center

A site with many on-line biological resources.
E-mail: npscinfo@usgs.gov
URL: http://www.npwrc.usgs.gov/resource/resource.htm

The Aviary

Comprehensive site on birding, aviculture, bird care, etc.
URL: http://theaviary.com/

Veterinary/wildlife health

Veterinary/wildlife health organizations

American Association of Wildlife Veterinarians

A US organization of individuals interested in all areas of wildlife health.
Address: Dr. Victor Nettles, Secretary/Treasurer, Vet. Med., University of Georgia, Athens, GA 30602, USA
Phone: +1 706 542 1741; Fax: +1 706 542 5865
E-mail: vnettles@calc.vet.uga.edu
URL: http://www.emtc.nbs.gov/http_data/whip/aawvnet.html

American Association of Zoo Veterinarians

An international organization, with the mission to improve the health care and promote conservation of captive and free-ranging wildlife.
Address: Dr. Wilbur B. Amand, Executive Director, 6 North Pennell Road, Media, PA 19063, USA
Phone: +1 610 892 4812; Fax: +1 608 892 4813
E-mail: 75634.235@compuserve.com
URL: http://www.worldzoo.org/aazv/aazv.htm

Association of Avian Veterinarians

The purpose of the AAV is to educate its members and the general public as to all aspects of avian medicine and surgery, through conferences, practical labs, avicultural programs, client education brochures and a veterinary journal devoted to all aspects of avian medicine.
Address: AAV Central Office, PO Box 811720, Boca Raton, FL 33481, USA
Phone: +1 561–393–8901; Fax: +1 561–393–8902
E-mail: AAVCTRLOFC@aol.com
URL: http://www2.upatsix.com/aav/

Canadian Cooperative Wildlife Health Centre/Centre Canadian de la Santé de la Faune

The Centre was established as a vehicle to apply veterinary medical science to management and conservation of wild animals in Canada. The focus of the Centre is disease as a factor in wildlife biology. The central activity of the CCWHC/CCCSF is surveillance of wild animal diseases. This is achieved through programs to enhance the detection of disease by field personnel, diagnostic services provided by each Regional Centre, a national database of wildlife disease occurrences and regular reporting of relevant information to government and non-government wildlife agencies and to the public.

Address: c/o Veterinary Pathology, Western College of Veterinary Medicine, 52 Campus Drive, University of Saskatchewan, Saskatoon, Saskatchewan S7N 5B4, Canada

Phone: 800–567–2033 (Canada); +1 306–966–5099; Fax: 306–966–7439

E-mail: ccwhc@sask.usask.ca

URL: http://www.emtc.nbs.gov/http_data/whip/ccwhc.html

http://www.fas.org/ahead/news.ccwhc/index.html

IUCN Species Survival Commission – Veterinary Specialist Group

Address: Michael Woodford, 2440 Virginia Avenue N.W., Apt. D-1105, Washington, DC 20037, USA

Phone: +1 202 331–9448; Fax: +1 202 331–9448

URL: http://www.emtc.nbs.gov/http_data/whip/iucn-org.html

Newsletter: http://www.fas.org/ahead/news/iucn/index.html

E-mail: Dinton@aol.com

National Wildlife Health Center

The National Wildlife Health Center (NWHC) is a Science Center of the Biological Resources Division of the US Geological Survey located in Madison, WI. The NWHC was established in 1975 as a biomedical laboratory dedicated to assessing the impact of disease on wildlife and to identifying the role of various pathogens in contributing to wildlife losses.

Address: 6006 Schroeder Road, Madison, WI 53711, USA

Phone: +1 608 270 2400; Fax: +1 608 270 2415

E-mail: nwhc.do@usgs.gov

URL: http://www.emtc.nbs.gov/nwhchome.html

The Raptor Center

The Raptor Center is an international medical facility for birds of prey. Our mission is to preserve biological diversity among raptors and other avian species through medical treatment, scientific investigation, education and management of wild populations.

Address: University of Minnesota, Gabbert Raptor Building, 1920 Fitch Ave, St Paul, MN 55108, USA

Phone: +1 612 624–4745; Fax: +1 612 624–8740

E-mail: raptor@umn.edu

URL: http://www.raptor.cvm.umn.edu

Southeastern Cooperative Wildlife Disease Study

The Southeastern Cooperative Wildlife Disease Study is recognized internationally as a leader in wildlife health research, service and teaching. This special unit is supported jointly by multiple federal and state agencies. This cooperative support has provided wildlife conservationists and animal health authorities with far greater capabilities for wildlife health investigations than they can afford individually. (Quarterly newsletter, see URL.)

Address: College of Veterinary Medicine (Building 6), Athens, GA 30602–7393, USA

Phone: +1 706 542 1741; Fax: +1 706 542 5865

URL: http://www.vet.uga.edu/scwds.html

Veterinarian Association for the Care of Exotic and Savage (Wild) Animals

AVAFES is an association of students and veterinarians. It was born in the Veterinary College of the Universidad Autonoma de Barcelona, through the interest in veterinary medicine applied to wild animals.

Address: Facultad de Veterinaria, Universidad Autonoma de Barcelona, 08193 Bellaterra, Spain

Phone: +34 3 581.21.07; Fax: +34 3 581.20.06

E-mail: avafes@blues.uab.es

URL: http://tau.uab.es/associacions/avafes/

Wildlife Disease Association

The Wildlife Disease Association is an international, nonprofit organization dedicated to wildlife conservation through the study and understanding of diseases in wildlife. The WDA has more than 1300 members from 45 countries who are engaged in research, teaching and service activities related to wildlife.

Address: Department of Veterinary Pathology, College of Veterinary Medicine, University of Georgia, Athens, GA 30602, USA

Phone: +1 706 542–5833; Fax: +1 706 542–5828

E-mail: ehowerth@calc.vet.uga.edu

URL: http://www.vet.uga.edu/wda/

World Association of Wildlife Veterinarians

Address: Secretary, WAWV, Department of the Marine Fish Health Unit, Teagasc, Malahide Road, Kinsealy, Dublin 17, Ireland

Phone: +353 1 8460644; Fax: +353 1 8460524

URL: http://www.emtc.nbs.gov/http_data/whip/wawv-org.html

Veterinary/wildlife health

WWW

Association of Avian Veterinarians – Australian Committee

Links to Birdmed discussion group and other sites.
E-mail: gcross@extro.ucc.su.oz.au
URL: http://www.vet.murdoch.edu.au:80/birds/aav-aus2.htm

Avian Hematology

A site offering basic information on techniques in avian hematology.
URL: http://agweb.clemson.edu/Poultry/bld/Avian_hematology.html

Avian Pathology

Searchable database of tables of contents and abstracts for articles about avian pathology.
URL: http://www.bdt.org.br/bioline/ap

Bird Medicine Related Links

Site from Murdoch University with links to veterinary related sites, as well as others.
URL: http://numbat.murdoch.edu.au/birds/avi_links.htm

Medical formulary

(Pigeon-focused) Compiled and recommended for use by the Association of Avian Veterinarians.
URL: http://members.aol.com/duiven/vet.htm

The Oklahoma State Ostrich Book

A complete online resource on ratite management and medicine, by Dr. Alan Kocan.
E-mail: aak4453@okstate.edu
URL: http://www.cvm.okstate.edu/instruction/kocan/ostrich/ostbk2.htm

Wildlife Health Information Partnership

WHIP is a collaborative project that gathers and disseminates information in the broad context of wildlife health, including the areas of disease and health management in freeranging and captive wildlife, environmental toxicology, conservation biology, and zoonoses and public health. Link to WildlifeHealth discussion group.
E-mail: whadmin@usgs.gov

URL: http://www.emtc.nbs.gov/http_data/whip/whiphmpg.html

Aviculture

Aviculture organizations

American Emu Association

Address: PO Box 740814, Dallas, TX 75374–0814, USA

Phone: +1 214 559–2321; Fax: +1 214 528–2359

E-mail: info@aea-emu.org

URL: http://www.aea-emu.org/

American Federation of Aviculture

The AFA is a nonprofit educational organization for individual members nationwide and worldwide and also a federation, composed of over 200 affiliated bird clubs and organizations representing over 50 000 aviculturists.
Address: PO Box 56218, Phoenix, AZ 85017, USA

Phone: +1 602–484–0931; Fax: +1 602–484–0109

E-mail: nwrvp@byway.com

URL: http://www.afa.birds.org/afa/

American Ostrich Association

Organizational site with information and links to ostrich organizations worldwide.
Address: 3950 Fossil Creek Blvd., Suite 200, Fort Worth, TX 76137, USA

Phone: +1 817 232–1200; URL: http://www.ostriches.org

American Pheasant and Waterfowl Society

An organization devoted to education, aviculture and conservation of pheasants, waterfowl, and other upland aquatic and ornamental birds.
Address: W2270 US HWY 10, Granton, WI 54436, USA

American Racing Pigeon Union

The American Racing Pigeon Union is an association of some 11 000 members, from all areas of the USA. Our objectives include the promotion of registered homing pigeons as a recreational alternative.
Also: Vet Tip of the Month

Address: PO Box 18465, Oklahoma City, OK 73154–0465, USA

Phone: +1 405–478–2240; Fax: +1 405–670–4748

E-mail: arpu@pigeon.org

URL: http://www.pigeon.org/

International Aviculturists Society

IAS is a group of aviculturists from around the world striving to protect, preserve and enhance the keeping and breeding of all exotic birds through educational programs, cooperative breeding programs and the funding of avian research and avian conservation programs.
Address: PO Box 2232, LaBelle, FL 33975, USA

Phone: +1 941 674–0321; Fax: +1 941 675–8824

E-mail: Richard@funnyfarmexotics.com

URL: http://www.funnyfarmexotics.com/IAS/

International Wild Waterfowl Association

Conservation of endangered and threatened species through captive breeding.
Address: 5614 River Styx Road, Medina, OH 44256, USA

Phone: +1 216 725 8782

National Pigeon Association

America's foremost all breed pigeon club, the NPA has served the pigeon fancy for over 75 years and provides leadership and service throughout the country. Also: Association of Pigeon Veterinarians; Pigeon Health Questions and Answers.
Address: PO Box 439, Newalla, OK 74857–0439, USA

E-mail: James4bird@aol.com

URL: http://www.angelfire.com/md/
nationalpigeonassn/

World Bird Sanctuary (Raptor Rehabilitation and Propagation Project)

Mission is biodiversity conservation through education, propagation and rehabilitation.
Address: Box 270270, St. Louis, MO 63127, USA

Phone: +1 314 938–6193; Fax: +1 314 938–9464

WWW

Care and Incubation of Hatching Eggs

On-line incubation resource, primarily for galliformes, by Dr. Tom W. Smith.
URL: http://www.msstate.edu/dept/poultry/hatch.
htm

Dr. Robert Cook's Home Page

Site with information on pigeon behavior, learning, and visual perception.
Address: Tufts University Department of Psychology, Research Building, 490 Boston Avenue, Medford, MA 02155, USA

E-mail: rcook1@emerald.tufts.edu

URL: http://www.pigeon.psy.tufts.edu/

International Pigeon Page

Site focused on show pigeons with information on organizations around the world.
URL: http://members.aol.com/PigeonNet/pigeon/
docl.htm

Ostrich–Emu Infonet

Commercial site with information about ratites, associations and publications.
URL: http://channel.isle.net/lkapala/

Pet Bird

Site devoted to pet bird care and aviculture with links to many avicultural organizations.
URL: http://www.afa.birds.org/

Pigeon Links All Over the World

Expansive list of pigeon sites.
E-mail: Freddy. Thienpont@cevi.be

URL: http://www.cevi.be/pp/freddy/

Conservation

Conservation organizations

American Zoo and Aquarium Association

AZA supports membership excellence in conservation, education, science and research. Conserving our natural world is AZA's central mission. On behalf of its 182 accredited zoos and aquariums throughout North America, AZA promotes education and habitat

protection programs and manages cooperative Species Survival Plans (SSP) for over 135 endangered species.
Address: 7970–D Old Georgetown Road, Bethesda, MD 20814, USA

Phone: +1 301 907–7777; Fax: +1 301 907–2980

URL: http://www.aza.org

Birds Australia

Site of Birds Australia (formerly Royal Australasian Ornithological Society).
Address: 415 Riversdale Road, Hawthorn, East Victoria, Australia 3123

Phone: +61 3 9882 2622; Fax: +61 3 9882 2677

E-mail: raou@raou.com.au

URL: http://avoca.vicnet.net.au/lbirdsaus/

British Ornithologists Union

The British Ornithologists' Union aims to encourage the study of birds in Britain, Europe and throughout the world, in order to understand their biology and to aid their conservation.
Address: c/o The Natural History Museum, Tring, Hertfordshire HP23 6AP, UK

Phone: +44 1442 890080; Fax: +44 1442 890693

E-mail: bou@bou.org.uk

URL: http://www.bou.org.uk/

Cornell Laboratory of Ornithology

A membership institute dedicated to the study, appreciation, and conservation of birds. The Lab fosters understanding about nature and contributes to efforts to protect biologic diversity through programs of research, education, and citizen science. The Lab of Ornithology and Cornell University together form a global center for amateur and professional training in the ecology, evolutionary biology, and conservation of birds.
Address: 159 Sapsucker Woods Road, Ithaca, NY 14850, USA

Phone: +1 607 254–2473

http://birdsource2.ornith.cornell.edu/Feedback.html

URL: http://www.ornith.cornell.edu/

Delta Waterfowl Foundation

Central mission is to train resource managers, conduct ecological and policy research related to waterfowl and wetlands, and ensure that the results of its research are applied. We are dedicated to ensuring a sustainable North American waterfowl population for the hunting enjoyment of future generations.

Address: 102 Wilmot Road, Suite 410, Deerfield, IL 60015, USA

Phone: +1 708 940–7776 +1–888–987–3695; Fax: +1 708 940–3739

E-mail: dw4ducks@portage.net

URL: http://www.deltawaterfowl.com

Ducks Unlimited, Inc.

The world's largest nonprofit wetlands, waterfowl and wildlife conservation organization. Projects nurture waterfowl and 900 species of other wildlife throughout the USA, Canada and Mexico.
Address: One Waterfowl Way, Memphis, TN 38120–2351, USA

Phone: +1 901 758–3825; Fax: +1 901 758–3850

E-mail: webmaster@ducks.org

URL: http://www.ducks.org/

George Miksch Sutton Avian Research Center, Inc.

The George Miksch Sutton Avian Research Center is dedicated to finding cooperative conservation solutions for birds and the natural world through science and education. The scope of our projects ranges from the reintroduction of Southern Bald Eagles to the use of NASA thermoimaging cameras to study incubation temperatures, to captive breeding of endangered species, raptor surveys worldwide and to intensive field research on declining grassland birds. The Sutton Research Center is a private, nonprofit organization affiliated with the University of Oklahoma's Oklahoma Biological Survey.
Address: PO Box 2007, Bartlesville, OK 74005, USA

Phone: +1 918 336–7778; Fax: +1 918 336–7783

E-mail: GMSARC@aol.com

URL: http://www.suttoncenter.org/

Hawk and Owl Trust

The Hawk and Owl Trust is the only UK charity dedicated solely to the conservation of wild birds of prey and their habitats.
Address: c/o Birds of Prey Section, London NW1 4RY, UK

Phone: +44 1494 876262; E-mail: webmaster@mycenae.demon.co.uk

URL: http://www.mycenae.demon.co.uk/HawkAndOwl/HOTHome.htm

Hawkwatch International, Inc.

Dedicated to monitoring and promoting the conservation of eagles, hawks and other birds of prey.

Striving to increase public awareness and instill a commitment to protect these magnificent birds and the ecosystems in which they live.
Address: PO Box 660, Salt Lake City, UT 84110–0660, USA

Phone: +1 800 726–4295/801; Fax: +1 801 524–8520

E-mail: hawkwatch@juno.com

URL: http://www.info-xpress.com/hawkwatch/

International Crane Foundation

The International Crane Foundation (ICF) works world-wide to conserve cranes and the wetland and grassland communities on which they depend. ICF is dedicated to providing experience, knowledge and inspiration to involve people in resolving threats to these ecosystems. Information on all crane species.
Address: E-11376 Shady Lane Road, PO Box 447, Baraboo, WI 53913–0447, USA

Phone: +1 608 356–9462; Fax: +1 608 356–9465

E-mail: gordon.icf@baraboo.com

URL: http://www.baraboo.com/bus/icf/whowhat.htm

IUCN – The World Conservation Union

A union of governments, government agencies and non-governmental organizations working at the field and policy levels, together with scientists and experts, to protect nature.
Address: Rue Mauverney, 28, 1196 Gland Vaud, Switzerland

E-mail: mail@hq.iucn.org

URL: http://iucn.org/index.html

Middle East Falcon Research Group

The MEFRG intends to bring together experts in falcons and falconry, veterinary surgeons, falcon biologists and conservationists working in the Middle East and other professionals interested in falcons and falconry from around the world.
Address: PO Box 45553, Abu Dhabi, United Arab Emirates

Phone: +971 (2) 414441; Fax: +971 (2) 414131

URL: http://www.ead.ae

National Avian Research Center

The National Avian Research Center (NARC) is a research organization dedicated to the ecologically sustainable use of avian wildlife. NARC's flagship species are the houbara bustard and the saker falcon.
Address: PO Box 45553, Abu Dhabi, United Arab Emirates

URL: http://www.ead.ae

Ornithological Council

A combine of 8 North American ornithological societies. WWW site has links to each member plus many other bird links.
Address: 3713 Chevy Chase Lake Dr, Apt. 3, Chevy Chase, MD 20815, USA

Phone: +1 301 986–8568; E-mail: epaul@dclink.com

URL: http://www.nmnh.si.edu/BIRDNET/

Patuxent Wildlife Research Center

Patuxent Wildlife Research Center is an international research institute for wildlife and applied environmental research, for transmitting research findings to those responsible for managing our nation's natural resources and for providing technical assistance in implementing research findings so as to improve natural resource management.
Address: 12100 Beech Forest Road, Laurel, MD 20708–4039, USA

Phone: +1 301–497–5500; Fax: +1 301–497–5505

E-mail: director@patuxent.nbs.gov

URL: http://www.pwrc.usgs.gov/

The Peregrine Fund

The Peregrine Fund works nationally and internationally, focusing on birds to conserve nature.
Address: 5666 W. Flying Hawk Lane, Boise, ID 83709, USA

Phone: +1 208 362–3716; Fax: +1 208 362–2376

E-mail: tpf@peregrinefund.org

URL: http://www.peregrinefund.org/

Raptor Research Foundation, Inc.

The Raptor Research Foundation (RRF) is a nonprofit scientific society whose primary goal is the accumulation and dissemination of scientific information about raptors (hawks, eagles, falcons and owls).
Address: OSNA, PO Box 1897, 810 E. 10th Street, Lawrence, KS 66044–8897, USA

URL: http://catsis.weber.edu/rrf/

Wild Bird Society of Japan

Bird conservation in Japan and region.
Address: Bird and Greenery Information Centre, NEXT21 Bldg, 6–16 Simizudani-cho, Tennouji-ku, Osaka 543, Japan

Phone: +81 6–766–2307; Fax: +81 6–766–2308

E-mail: marutani@st.rim.or.jp

URL: http://www.kt.rim.or.jp/lbirdinfo/japan/index.html

WWW

Birdlife International– Asia Council

Site organized by Asian bird conservation groups, with other international links.
URL: http://www.kt.rim.or.jp/lbirdinfo/

Birdlinks

One of several mirrored sites with multiple birding/conservation links.
URL: http://www.phys.rug.nl/mk/people/wpv/birdlink.html

Raptor Information Clearinghouse

An extensive collection of raptor information sources.
URL: http://www.charweb.org/organizations/science/raptorcenter/ClearingHouse.html#nsrehabilitation

The Wildlife Rehabilitation Information Directory

Information on what to do with injured wildlife and who to contact in North America. Information is provided for the public and for the professional wildlife rehabilitator. Many links are provided to sites of interest relating to the field.
URL: http://www.cc.ndsu.nodak.edu/instruct/devold/twrid/html/hp.htm

World Conservation Monitoring Centre

'Threatened Animals of the World' Searchable database with basic info about a number of birds as well as more detail for birds threatened with extinction.
URL: http://www.wcmc.org.uk/species/data/birdlife/index.html

Appendix 8

Pharmaceutics commonly used in avian medicine

Thomas A. Bailey, Merle M. Apo

Antibiotics					
Generic name	Trade name	Species	Route	Dosage	Remarks
Amikacin sulfate	Amiglyde 50 mg/ml, 240 mg/ml, (Aveco); Amikin (Bristol Labs)	Most species	IV, IM	10–15 mg/kg b.i.d.	Indicated against acute infections. Active in vitro Gram-negative bacteria including *Pseudomonas* spp., *E coli*, *Proteus* spp., *Klebsiella* spp., *Enterobacter* spp. and Gram-positive bacteria including *Staphylococcus* spp. and *Streptococcus* spp. The risk of nephrotoxicity increased with dehydrated patients. Synergistic effect when used with third generation penicillins and cefalosporins. Risk factors predisposing to aminoglycoside nephrotoxicosis: prior renal insufficiency, advanced age, increased dose or frequency, hepatic disease, hypovolemia, dehydration, metabolic acidosis, exposure to other nephrotoxins, severe sepsis, endotoxemia

Continued overleaf

Antibiotics (continued)

Generic name	Trade name	Species	Route	Dosage	Remarks
Amoxicillin trihydrate	Amoxinsol 150 Injection (Univet) Amoxinsol LA (Univet) Amoxinsol 50 Soluble Powder (Univet)	Pigeons / Waterfowl	IM or SC / PO	150 mg/kg daily for 5 d; every other day if using long-acting preparation 1 g per 3 l of drinking water. Provide on alternate days for 3 d	Broad-spectrum antibiotic active against a wide range of Gram-positive and Gram-negative microorganisms. However, many bacterial organisms affecting birds are resistant to amoxicillin and antibiotic sensitivity tests should be conducted before treatment is embarked upon. Injections of large volumes should be given SC in valuable athletic birds such as falcons to avoid any possible complications associated with muscle necrosis
	Clamoxyl Ready to Use Injection (SmithKline Beecham) 150 mg/ml Clamoxyl LA (SmithKline Beecham) 150 mg/ml	Bustards / Bustards	IM or SC / IM or SC	100 mg/kg b.i.d. / 100–250 mg/kg	Pharmacological studies on houbara bustards indicate that therapeutic levels may be maintained for 5–7 d after a dose of 250 mg/kg IM. If doses of 100 mg/kg IM are used, therapeutic levels greater than 2 µg/ml are maintained for 72 h
	Betamox 40 mg Tablets (Norbrook) Amoxypen 40 mg Tablets (Mycofarm)	Pigeons	PO	40 mg/kg b.i.d. for 5 d	
	Vetremox Powder for Poultry/Pigeons (Vetrepharm)	Pigeons	In drinking water	1–1.5 g/l of drinking water for 5–7 d	
Amoxicillin/ clavulanic acid	Synulox Ready to Use Injection (Pfizer); Synulox Palatable Drops (Pfizer); Clavamox (SmithKline Beecham) Synulox (Pfizer); Clavamox (SmithKline Beecham)	Psittacines / Raptors	IM or PO	100 mg amoxicillin/ 30 mg clavulanic acid per kg b.i.d. / 150 mg/kg b.i.d. for 5–7 d	Broad-spectrum antibiotic active against a wide range of Gram-positive and negative organisms. Effective against beta-lactamase-producing bacteria, among them Staphylococcus aureus, Escherichia coli and Proteus spp. Fewer cases of resistance than amoxicillin alone. Injection can cause renal failure in dehydrated birds
Sodium amoxicillin	Amoxil (sodium amoxicillin) (SmithKline Beecham)	Bustards	SC/IM/IV	100 mg/kg	Pharmacokinetic studies in houbara bustards using 100 mg/kg have shown that administrations every 8 h (IV) or 4 h (IM) will maintain levels above 2 µg/ml
Ampicillin	Polyflex 100 mg/ml (Fort Dodge)	Psittacines / Galliformes	PO / IM / PO	100–200 mg/kg q.i.d. / 100 mg/kg q.4 h / 250 mg/8 oz of drinking water	Broad-spectrum antibiotic active against a wide range of Gram-positive and Gram-negative organisms. However, minimum activity for the common Gram-negative infections of birds. Poor gastrointestinal absorption. May be useful for treating sensitive pathogens restricted to gastrointestinal tract
Carbenicillin	Pyopen (Link); Geopen (Roerig) Pyopen (SmithKline Beecham)	Raptors / Psittacines	IM / IM or IV	100–200 mg/kg t.i.d. for 3–5 d / 200 mg/kg b.i.d.	Effective against Gram-negative organisms, especially Pseudomonas spp. and Proteus spp. resistant to other antibiotics. Synergistic with aminoglycosides. May also be given as IT injection 100 mg/kg s.i.d.
Cefotaxime	Claforan Injectable Solution, variable concentrations (Hoechst–Roussel)	Most species	IM, IV	75–100 mg/kg	Broad-spectrum activity for many avian Gram-positive and Gram-negative pathogens. Penetrates blood-brain barrier. For best result q.i.d. therapy is recommended. Reconstituted vial stable for 13 weeks if frozen
Ceftiofur	Naxcel Injectable Solution, variable concentrations (Upjohn)	Most species	IM	50–100 mg/kg q.i.d.	Similar treatment regimen to other third-generation cefalosporins
Ceftriaxone	Rocephin Injectable Solution, variable concentration (Roche)	Most species	IM, IV	75–100 mg/kg q.i.d. or every 4 h	Can be reconstituted into 10–250 mg/ml concentrations. When reconstituted into lower concentrations the Rocephin should be administered IV. Reconstituted

Continued

Antibiotics (continued)

Generic name	Trade name	Species	Route	Dosage	Remarks
					solution is stable for 10 d refrigerated. Useful for Gram-positive and Gram-negative bacteria, including some activity against *Pseudomonas* spp.
Cefuroxime	Zinacef 250 mg vials (Glaxo)	Most species	IM, IV	100 mg/kg	Bactericidal cephalosporin antibiotic resistant to beta-lactamases active against Gram-positive and Gram-negative organisms. Highly effective against *Staphyloccus aureus*. 100 mg/kg t.i.d. is the dose rate of other cephalosporins
Cephalexin	Ceporex (Mallinckrodt) Keflex (Dista)	Raptors, bustards, other species	IM or PO	40–100 mg/kg for 3–5 d t.i.d. or q.i.d.	Active against many Gram-positive and Gram-negative bacteria. Active against *E. coli* and *Proteus* spp., but not *Pseudomonas* spp. Useful for *Staphylococcus* spp. dermatitis. Reconstituted suspension stable for 14 d if refrigerated
Chloramphenicol *Salmonella*	Chloramphenicol	Raptors	IM	50 mg/kg t.i.d.	Effective in flock treatment for
	Injection (Willows Francis, Fort Dodge, Parke-Davis)			for 3–5 d	spp. infections. May be useful for cases of enteritis in young birds. Use with caution on patients with renal or kidney disease. Causes bone marrow suppression in humans. Associated with temporary infertility in male pigeons
	Chloramphenicol Injection (Willows Francis, Fort Dodge, Parke-Davis); Intramycetin (Upjohn)	Budgerigar	IM	200 mg/kg, b.i.d. for 5 d	
			PO	50 mg/kg t.i.d. or q.i.d.	
Chlortetracycline Gram-	Aureomycin Soluble Powder (Cyanamid)	Pigeons	PO	130 mg activity per liter drinking water for 5–8 d (2.4 g powder/l)	Broad-spectrum antibiotic active against a wide range of Gram-positive and negative bacteria
			PO	400 mg activity per liter drinking water for 5–8 d (7.25 g powder/l)	
			PO	400 mg activity per liter drinking water for 21 d (7.25 g powder/l)	
		Waterfowl	PO	1000 ppm (18.2 g/kg) in feed for 45 d	
	Aureomycin Ophthalmic Ointment (Cyanamid)	Pigeons	Topical	Apply to affected eye b.i.d. for 7 d	
Clindamycin	Antirobe Capsules (Upjohn)	Raptors	PO	50 mg/kg b.i.d. for 7–10 d	Indicated for osteomyelitis and tendon sheath infections. Has been used for up to 12 weeks without deleterious effects
		Psittacines Pigeons	PO PO	100 mg/kg s.i.d. 100 mg/kg s.i.d.	Recommended for osteomyelitis. Monitor renal and hepatic function during long-term use for secondary yeast infections (has been noted in mammals). Recommended for bone and joint infection
Clofazimine	Lamprene (Ciba)	Psittacines	PO	1.5 mg/kg s.i.d.	Recommended for the treatment of mycobacteriosis
Cloxacillin	Amplicox Syrup/ Capsules (SmithKline Beecham); Cloxapen (SmithKline Beecham); Tegopen (Bristol)	Raptors	PO	250 mg/kg b.i.d. for 7–10 d	Recommended in the treatment of infected bumblefoot
Doxycycline	Ronaxan Tablets (Rhône Mérieux, Henry Schein, Roerig) Vibravenos (Pfizer);	Raptors Waterfowl	PO PO	50 mg/kg b.i.d. for 3–5 d (45 d for chlamydophilosis)	Drug of choice for the treatment of chlamydophilosis. The agent has greater activity, less immunosuppression and fewer side effects including fungal

Continued overleaf

Antibiotics (continued)

Generic name	Trade name	Species	Route	Dosage	Remarks
	ßRonaxan Tablets (Rhône Mérieux, Henry Schein, Roerig)			50 mg/kg b.i.d. for 3–5 d (45 d for chlamydophilosis)	overgrowth and disturbance to the normal bacteria of the gastrointestinal tract than other tetracycline preparations. Monitor feces for *Candida* spp. infections
				240 ppm in feed for 45 d	
		Pigeons	PO	1 tablet daily for 5–7 d (40 mg/kg)	Respiratory infections
		Psittacines	IM IM PO	10 mg/kg s.i.d. 75–100 mg/kg every 5–7 d 25–50 mg/kg b.i.d.	Treat for 45 d for chlamydophilosis. Some injectable doxycycline preparations can cause myositis. Vomiting has been reported in macaws
		Bustards	IM	100 mg/kg once every week	Pharmacokinetic studies in houbara bustards have shown that therapeutic levels are maintained in birds given a dose of 100 mg/kg IM every 7 d. Doxycycline hydrate may be given IV once at a dose of 22–44 mg/kg for initial severe cases of chlamydophilosis followed by PO or IM treatment
Enrofloxacin	Baytril 2.5% or 5% Injection, Baytril 2.5% Oral Suspension, Baytril 10% Solution (Bayer)	Raptors Waterfowl	IM or PO Baytril 10% Solution can be used either in water or PO undiluted in food	10–15 mg/kg b.i.d. for 5–7 d	Broad-spectrum antimicrobial, bactericidal in action and effective against a wide range of Gram-positive and Gram-negative bacteria including *Pseudomonas* spp. and *Klebsiella* spp. as well as *Mycoplasma* spp. Higher doses (15 mg/kg b.i.d.) are more effective for less susceptible organisms such as *Pseudomonas* spp. IM or PO route can cause emesis in some species (e.g. falcons) if the bird has eaten in previous six hours. The injectable solution may be administered orally. Useful for bacterial hepatitis or septicemia in neonates. Used widely in growing chickens and poultry of all ages without incidence of articular cartilage problems: at normal therapeutic levels (10–15 mg/kg b.i.d.) it is unlikely to produce joint deformity in neonatal birds (or in pigeons or waterfowl). Baytril 10% Solution can be used either in water or PO undiluted in food; the water dose should be based on the water drinking habits of the species
	Baytril Tablets (Bayer)		Nasal flushing	4 mg in 20 ml saline for a 1 kg bird daily for 10 d	
	Baytril 2.7% (Haver/Diamond)			500 ppp in feed for 45 d (for chlamydophilosis)	
	Baytril 10% Oral Solution (Bayer) Baytril 2.7% (Haver/Diamond)	Pigeons	PO	150 mg/l drinking water for up to 10 d; may need 300 mg/l to prevent reappearance of infection	
		Bustards	PO	10–15 mg/kg b.i.d. for 5–7 d	
	Baytril 10% Injection (Bayer)	Pigeons	IM or SC	20 mg/kg initially, followed by oral treatment	
	Baytril 2.5% or 5% Injection, Baytril 2.5% or 10% Oral Solution (Bayer)	Psittacines	IM	5–15 mg/kg b.i.d.	Treat for 21 d for chlamydophilosis, use 15 mg/kg or 2 ml/l
			PO	1–2 ml 10% solution/l drinking water	
	Baytril 2.7% (Haver/Diamond)	Bustards	IV or IM	15 mg/kg	
Erythromycin	Erythrocin Soluble (11.56 g erythromycin activity/70 g sachet) (Sanofi, Lextron)	Pigeons	PO	13–26 mg erythromycin activity per liter drinking water for 3 d (1.5 g powder/l)	Gram-negative bacteria affecting birds are resistant to this antibiotic. May be effective in sinusitis and air sacculitis caused by *Mycoplasma* spp.
		Psittacines	PO	10–20 mg/kg b.i.d. 500 mg/4.5 l drinking water	

Continued

Antibiotics (continued)

Generic name	Trade name	Species	Route	Dosage	Remarks
Ethambutol	Myambutol (Lederle)	Psittacines	PO	15–20 mg/kg b.i.d.	Treatment of mycobacteriosis
Gentamicin	Gentacin (Nicholas, Butler, Schering-Plough)	Psittacines	IM	5–10 mg/kg t.i.d. for 5 d	Bactericidal antibiotic that is most effective against Gram-negative pathogens, especially *Pseudomonas* spp. Effective in respiratory tract. Inject between tracheal rings in the neck region. The drug is nephrotoxic and can cause a transient polyuria. It is better to use amikacin if available. May be given IV and nebulized for treatment of upper respiratory tract infections
Lincomycin	Lincocin Injection/ Tablets (Upjohn)	Raptors	IM or PO Intra-articular injection	50–75 mg/kg b.i.d. for 7–10 d 0.25–0.5 ml daily for 7–10 d	This drug has a poor activity against most Gram-negative bacteria, but it has a good activity for many Gram-positive bacteria. Useful for bumblefoot, chronic dermatitis and respiratory infections caused by mycoplasmas. Has been used in raptors for up to 12 weeks without ill effect. Patients should be monitored for secondary yeast infections
		Psittacines	IM PO	100 mg/kg b.i.d. 75 mg/kg b.i.d.	
	Lincocin Soluble Powder (Upjohn)	Waterfowl	PO	10 g/5 l drinking water for 5–7 d	
Lincomycin/ spectinomycin Lincomycin HCl 33.3% spectinomycin 66.7%	Linco-Spectin 100 Soluble Powder (Upjohn)	Pigeons	PO	50 mg (16.7 mg lincomycin/33.3 mg spectinomycin)/kg for 3–7 d, e.g. 1 g powder/l drinking water	Susceptible infections, mycoplasmal infections
		Waterfowl	PO	3 g/4 l drinking water for 3–7 d	Mycoplasmal tenosynovitis, sinusitis
	Linco-Spectin Soluble Powder (Upjohn)	Psittacines	PO	0.125–0.25 teaspoonfuls per 568 ml drinking water	Water-soluble treatment for enteritis and mycoplasmal sinusitis
Marbofloxacin	Marbocyl 2% and 10% Injection (Univet) Marbocyl 5 mg and 20 mg Tablets (Univet)	Raptors	IV, IM, PO	5–10 mg/kg b.i.d. for 5–7 d 15 mg/kg s.i.d.	As for enrofloxacin but less likely to cause emesis. Pharmacokinetic studies in buzzards have indicated that doses of 2 mg/kg IV b.i.d. can maintain therapeutic plasma levels
Metronidazole	Flagyl Tablets (Rhône Poulenc Rorer); Flagyl (Searle)	Raptors	PO	50 mg/kg s.i.d. 5 d	Anaerobic infections (and giardiasis and trichomonosis)
Oxytetracycline	Various standard preparations and tablets	Raptors	IM or PO	25–50 mg/kg t.i.d. for 5–7 d	A broad-spectrum bacteriostatic antibiotic, although high prevalence of resistant bacteria
	Long-acting Injection	Raptors	IM	50–200 mg/kg every 3–5 d	IM injection may cause significant muscle necrosis
	Terramycin Soluble Powder (Pfizer)	Waterfowl	PO	37 g/15 l drinking water 5–7 d	Pasteurellosis and other sensitive bacterial infections
Oxytetracycline dihydrate	Oxycare 50 mg Tablets (Animalcare)	Waterfowl	PO	One tablet daily for 5–7 d	*Chlamydophila psittaci* infections
	Terramycin (Pfizer) Terramycin Injection (Pfizer)	Psittacines Pigeons	IM	50 mg/kg s.i.d. 0.1–0.5 ml/kg on alternate days for 21 d in conjunction with oral tetracycline	For birds over 700 g use 20 mg/kg. For birds under 400 g use 80 mg/kg. Birds under treatment with long-acting oxytetracycline need to be monitored for secondary yeast infections
Piperacillin	Pipril (Lederle); Pipracil (Lederle)	Raptors	IV or IM	100 mg/kg b.i.d. for 5–7 d	Broad-spectrum bactericidal penicillin. Recommended for the treatment of systemic and local infections caused by susceptible Gram-negative and Gram-positive aerobic and anaerobic organisms, particularly *Pseudomonas* spp., *Proteus* spp., *Klebsiella* spp., *Enterobacter* spp., *Serratia* spp., *E. coli* and *Haemophilus* spp.
		Psittacines	IV or IM	100–200 mg/kg b.i.d. or t.i.d.	
Rifampin (rifampicin)	Rimactane (Ciba); Rifadin (Marion Merrell Dow)	Psittacines	PO	15 mg/kg b.i.d.	Used for the treatment of avian tuberculosis. It has been associated with hepatitis, central nervous system signs, depression and vomiting

Continued overleaf

Antibiotics (continued)

Generic name	Trade name	Species	Route	Dosage	Remarks
Spectinomycin	Spectam (Sanofi, Syntex)	Psittacines	IM	10–30 mg/kg b.i.d., t.i.d.	Has been used to treat enteritis in Galliformes caused by Gram-negative bacteria. It can be also given into sinuses at 35 mg/kg: one third into each sinus and the rest IM
Sulfachlorpyridazine	Vetisulid Water Soluble Powder (Solvay)	Most species	PO	0.25–tsp/gallon 5–10 d	Excellent flock treatment for *E. coli* infections. Check sensitivity
Tetracycline HCl 80%	Tetsol 800 (C-Vet, Generic)	Pigeons	PO	1 g/1.5 l drinking water for 5–7 d (60 mg/kg)	*Chlamydophila psittaci* infections
Tiamulin	Tiamutin 12.5% Solution (Leo Laboratories, Denaquard)	Pigeons	PO	225 mg (2 ml)/l drinking water for 6 d	Mycoplasmal infections
Tobramycin	Nebcin Injection (Lilly)	Raptors	IM	5–10 mg/kg b.i.d. for 5–7 d	Least nephrotoxic of all current aminoglycosides; should be used only for severe infections caused by resistant *Pseudomonas* spp. Also useful to treat joint injections by direct irrigation of toe joints in raptors. Use with caution in neonatal and geriatric birds, birds with neuromuscular disorders, and pre-existing renal disease
		Pheasants	Intra-articular flush	0.25–0.5 ml daily for 7–10 d	
		Cranes	IM	2.5–5 mg/kg b.i.d.	
	Nebcin (Lilly), Tobralax (Alcan)	Psittacines	IM or topical	2.5–10 mg/kg t.i.d.	Septic arthritis
Trimethoprim/ sulfonamide	Borgal (Hoechst); Duphatrim (Solvay Duphar); Cosumix Plus (Ciba); Bactrin (Roche)	Psittacines	IM PO	8 mg/kg b.i.d. 20 mg/kg b.i.d. or t.i.d. Cosumix Plus should be given at a rate of 1 g/l drinking water daily for 5 d	Good lipid solubility and well distributed in tissues. Bacteriocidal for Gram-positive and Gram-negative pathogens including *E. coli*, *Pasteurella* spp., *Proteus* spp., *Salmonella* spp. and *Listeria* spp. Recommended for the treatment of nephritis, bacterial hepatitis and septicemia in neonates. May also be effective for treating some forms of coccidiosis. Regurgitation is reported to occur in some species. Do not use in dehydrated birds or patients with liver disease or bone marrow suppression. Cosumix is a water-soluble powder and is useful for providing sulfachlorpyradizine in the drinking water.
	Cosumix Plus Soluble Powder (Ciba); Duphatrim Poultry Suspension (Solvay Animal Health); Tribrissen Piglet Suspension (Mallinckrodt); Bactrin (Roche)	Most species	PO	12–60 mg/kg b.i.d. (combined constituents for 5–7 d)	
	Cosumix Plus Soluble Powder (Ciba); Duphatrim Poultry Suspension (Solvay Animal Health); Bactrin (Roche)	Waterfowl	PO	1 ml/5 l drinking water for 5–7 d	
		Raptors	SC	30 mg/kg b.i.d. for 5–7 d	
	Duphatrim 24% Injection (Solvay Duphar)	Bustards	IM	8–30 mg/kg b.i.d. for 5–7 d	
Tylosin	Tylan Injection (Elanco) (Butler)	Raptors	IM	30 mg/kg b.i.d. for 3 d	60 mg/kg t.i.d. for birds of 50–250 g 25 mg/kg t.i.d. for birds 250–1000 g 15 mg/kg t.i.d. for birds > 1000 g
	Tylan (Elanco) (Butler)	Psittacines	IM PO	20–40 mg/kg t.i.d. 2 teaspoonfuls/4.5 l drinking water	Well distributed in tissues. Upper respiratory tract infections. *Mycoplasma* spp., *Pasteurella* spp., *Chlamydophila psittaci* Most Gram-negative organisms are resistant to this drug
	Tylan 50 or 200 Injection (Elanco, Butler)	Waterfowl	IM	20–30 mg/kg t.i.d. for 3–7 d; or 100 mg in 10 ml saline daily nasal flush for 10 d	
	Tylan Soluble Powder (100g tylosin activity per bottle) (Elanco, Butler)	Pigeons	PO	550 mg tylosin activity/l drinking water for 3 d (activity approx. 100%)	
		Waterfowl	PO	2.5 g/5 l drinking water for 3 d	

Antimycotic agents

Generic name	Trade name	Species	Route	Dosage	Remarks
Amphotericin B	Fungizone (Squibb, Bristol-Meyers)	Raptors	IV	1.5 mg/kg t.i.d. for 7 d	Organisms with an MIC < 1 μ/ml are considered susceptible. There is good correlation between MIC values and clinical response. Treatment failure due to fungal resistance is rare in humans but *Aspergillus* spp. are the most frequently reported resistant fungi. Give by slow intravenous administration with 10–15 ml/kg fluids for 7 d. Absorption from the lungs following aerosol administration is poor and this route is used to treat pulmonary aspergillosis. Improved clinical efficacy when used in combination with flucytosine or azole antifungal agent. Poorly absorbed from the gastrointestinal tract so must be given IV, IO or IT. Most important clinical toxicosis is nephrotoxicity, which is dose-related and seen clinically as increases in BUN and creatinine in mammals. Dosing every other day, electrolyte loading and slow infusion of amphotericin B decrease severity and rate of development of renal toxicity. Other adverse effects include phlebitis, fever, nausea, vomiting and hypokalemia with resulting cardiac arrhythmia. Measures to prevent vomiting include giving antiemetic drugs before infusion. In dogs doses > 5 mg/kg resulted in death due to cardiac abnormalities; doses of 2–5 mg/kg occasionally caused cardiac problems but doses < 1 mg/kg were without effect on the heart. Treatment protocols should include pretreatment with sodium chloride and it should be infused at a slow rate. It can be mixed with 5% dextrose solution during infusion. Administration of amphotericin B in 0.45% saline with 0.5% dextrose SC in dogs/cats is a way of administering large quantities of amphotericin B without producing the marked azotemia associated with IV injection
		Psittacines	IT	1 mg/kg b.i.d. for 12 d, reduce to every other day for 5 weeks	
			Nebulized	1 mg/ml saline solution b.i.d. × 20 min	
			IV	1.5 mg/kg t.i.d. together with 1 mg/kg, IT b.i.d. for 3–5 d 0.25–1 ml daily for 4–5 d	
	Fungilin Suspension (Squibb)	Psittacines	PO	1 ml/kg b.i.d. for 3–5 d	Candidiasis. Especially in young neonates as not absorbed from the alimentary tract
Amphotericin B lipid complex	Abelcet Amphotericin B Lipid Complex (Squibb)	Raptors	IV	1.5 mg/kg s.i.d.	New, less toxic lipid-based formulation, has been used in humans. Can be given at higher doses with less toxicity. In humans daily dose is 3–5 mg/kg daily, whereas the dose of the conventional form is 0.5–1 mg/kg every 48 h. Indicated for aspergillosis. The pharmacokinetics of Abelcet and conventional amphotericin B are different. In dogs peak blood levels and kidney levels are lower after Abelcet administration. Appears well tolerated in raptors and can be given SC
Caprillic acid	Kaprycidin A Capsules 325 mg, (Ecological Formulas)	Most species	PO	1/4 capsules/300 g	Adjunct treatment of antifungal therapy using imidazole
Chlorhedixine	Nolvasan Solution 20 mg/ml (Fort Dodge)	Most species	PO	10–30 ml/gallon drinking water	Disinfectant. For flock or individual treatment of mild gastrointestinal candidiasis. Toxic to finches. Use properly. This drug may also slow the spread of viral diseases. Give for 2–4 weeks duration in drinking water. Not absorbed from the gut. May irritate eyes or mucous membranes
			Topical	0.5% as a wound cleanser	
Enilconazole	Imaverol (Janssen) Clinafarm (Sterwin)	Raptors	IT	Dilute 1:10, administer 0.5 ml/kg daily for 7–14 d	Excellent antifungal activity. Residual effect after topical application and used to treat topical dermatophyte infections. Indicated for dermatomycoses such as *Trichophyton* spp. and *Microsporum* spp. Treatment of choice for nasal aspergillosis in dogs and local infusion is used in the treatment of guttural pouch mycosis in the horse. Can be given topically or nebulized and the Clinafarm-EC formulation is used in the environmental decontamination of poultry facilities and equipment to prevent aspergillosis. Indicated for dermatomycoses such as
			Topical	Dilute 1:10, apply topically b.i.d. for 3–4 weeks	
			Nebulized	1 ml in 9 ml saline solution	
		Psittacines	IT or topical	1:10–1:100 dilution	

Continued overleaf

Antimycotic agents (continued)

Generic name	Trade name	Species	Route	Dosage	Remarks
					Trichophyton spp. and *Microsporum* spp. Dilute solution in 50 parts of water and apply topically 3–4 × d. Also used intratracheally for aspergillosis treatment – dilute 1:20 and give 0.5–1.0 ml/kg IT q.8 h. Used as a nebulizing agent at 0.5 ml in 25 ml saline for systemic and topical fungal infections. Corrosive and may cause damage to the eyes
Flucytosine 5-Fluorocytosine	Alcobon (Roche), Ancobon (Roche)	Raptors	PO	20–30 mg q.i.d. for 20–90 d 40–50 mg /kg t.i.d.	Flucytosine has a narrow spectrum of activity and few *Aspergillus* sp. strains are susceptible. Strains with MIC < 16 µg/ml are susceptible. Two-thirds of fungal isolates change from susceptible to resistant during treatment, so flucytosine should only be used in combination with other antifungal agents. Combination with amphotericin B is synergistic because amphotericin B increases fungal permeability to flucytosine. Total dose of 120 mg/kg/d divided into 18–30 mg/kg q.6 h. Used as a preventative agent for aspergillosis. May be indicated for the long term treatment of aspergillosis infections or severe candidiasis infections that are resistant to nystatin. Toxic to the bone marrow
		Psittacines	PO	20–75 mg/kg b.i.d. for 21 d	Generalized yeast or fungal infections
F10	F10 (Health & Hygiene)	Most species	Nebulized	1:250 dilution 1–3 × d	Complete-spectrum virucidal, bactericidal, fungicidal and sporicidal but aldehyde-free compound of six synergistic active ingredients. Has been tested against every significant animal/human pathogen and has outperformed other disinfectants during efficacy testing, over a range of temperatures, in the presence of organic material, at low concentrations, short contact times, without any corrosive effects on infrastructure, metal nozzles or any tissue irritation on workers and animals. Can be used to disinfect animal environments in their presence, lowering the environmental pathogen challenge significantly, with no side effects. Using either a nebulizer or a 'smogger' unit, has been used to treat both individuals and groups of falcons with aspergillosis. Nebulized at a concentration of 1:250 and can also be added at the same concentration to drinking water, where it may limit the spread of bacterial or viral diseases
Gentian violet	Gentian Violet Powder or Solution 16 mg/ml	Psittacines	Topical	Apply affected area with cotton swabs	Topical application as drying agent. Excellent for crop candidiasis and skinfold candidiasis in hyacinth macaw chicks
Itraconazole aspergillosis infections.	Sporanox	Raptors	PO		Prophylactic dose: Drug of choice to treat
	Capsules (Janssen)			10 mg/kg s.i.d. for 7–10 d Therapeutic dose: 10–15 mg/kg b.i.d. for 4–6 weeks	Organisms with MIC < 0.12 µ/ml are susceptible; those with MIC 0.25–0.5 µ/ml are susceptible depending on dose and those with MIC > 1 µ/ml are considered resistant. Absorbtion is increased in an acidic environment
		Waterfowl	PO	Prophylactic dose: 10 mg/kg s.i.d. for 7–10 d Therapeutic dose: 10 mg/kg b.i.d. for 4–6 weeks	and when taken with meals. Bioavailability increases from 40% after fasting to 99.8% when given with food. Extensively distributed throughout the body. Hepatometabolized and eliminated mainly in the bile. Therapeutically active concentrations maintained longer in tissues than in plasma. Used to treat superficial and systemic infections and to treat and prevent aspergillosis in birds. As oral absorbtion is pH-dependent, dosage adjustments are necessary if gastric pH is increased. Oral capsules should be given with food but the oral suspension is better absorbed on an empty stomach. Higher tissue concentrations are reported when itraconazole is dissolved in acid

Continued

Antimycotic agents (continued)

Generic name	Trade name	Species	Route	Dosage	Remarks
					and gavaged with orange juice in pigeons. Treatment of serious infections should be prolonged (> 3 months) and relapses occur. Better tolerated than ketoconazole. Fewer side effects are seen than with other antifungal agents. Beads dissolve best in 5% acetic acid (cola-based fizzy drinks or orange juice may also be used) left to stand overnight. Diarrhea and inappetance has been associated with the use of this drug in juvenile kori bustards. Dose of 10 mg/kg for 1 month considered prophylactic. Sporanox liquid (10 mg/ml) is often more convenient
		Psittacines	PO	5–10 mg/kg for 3 weeks to 3 months	Adverse reaction observed in certain species, in particular African gray parrots
Ketoconazole	Nizoral (Janssen)	Raptors	IM	25 mg/kg b.i.d. for 7 d	Used for treatment of candidiasis when other therapies have been ineffective.
	Nizoral Suspension (Janssen)	Raptors Pigeons	PO Crop tube	60 mg/kg b.i.d. 3 mg/kg daily for 7–21 d	Treatment for 14 d. Effective against *Candida* spp. *Mucor* spp. and *Penicilium* spp. Can also use ketoconazole tablets,
		Psittacines	PO	10 mg/kg b.i.d.	dissolving a 200 mg tablet in 1.2 liters of water. Reported to be nephro- and hepatotoxic after long-term application in mammals
Miconazole	Daktarin (Janssen-Cilag)	Raptors Psittacines	Topical	b.i.d. for 3–5 d	Highly effective against candidiasis infections in the oro-pharynx and crop of falcons
Nystatin	Nystatin Oral Suspension (Lagap)	Raptors	PO	300 000 u (3 ml/kg) b.i.d. for 7 d	Antifungal agent active against yeast infections localized to the alimentary tract, including *Candida albicans*. For oral and intestinal
		Waterfowl	PO	300 000 u (3 ml) b.i.d. for 7 d	*Candida* spp. infections. Give 1–3 × d for 7–14 d. Not absorbed after oral application, so very safe. Not effective against *Aspergillus*
		Pigeons Psittacines	Crop tube PO	20 000 u daily for 7 d	spp. May be used in conjunction with antibiotic therapy to prevent yeast overgrowth
	Nystatin Feed Premix Myco 20 Mycozo (Squibb)	Most species	With feed	300 000 u/kg b.i.d. for 10 d	
Griseofulvin	Grisovin 125 mg Tablets (Mallinckrodt)	Pigeons	Crop tube	10 mg/kg for 21 d	Dermatophytosis
	Grisol-V Powder (Univet)	Pigeon	PO	10 mg/kg for 7 d	Dermatophytosis
STA Solution	Salicyclic acid (3 g), tannic acid 3 g and ethyl alcohol to 100 ml	Most species	Topical	As needed	For fungal dermatitis
Terbinafine	Lamisil, Terbinafine 125 mg Tablet (Novartis)	Raptors	Nebulized PO	1 mg/ml solution q.8–12 h 10–15 mg/kg b.i.d.	Synthetic allylamine drug, highly fungicidal. Allylamines decrease the fungal synthesis of ergestrol and cause fungal death by disrupting the cell membrane. Active against *Aspergillus* spp. but to date clinical use has been limited in veterinary medicine, although preliminary nebulization results are promising. Oral and topical antifugal primarily used for dermatophytic infections. Use with caution if liver or kidney disease present
Voriconazole	Vfend 50 mg Tablets (Pfizer)	Raptors	Nebulized PO	10–15 mg/kg b.i.d.	New triazole with *in vitro* activity against a wide range of fungi and potential for use in the treatment of avian aspergillosis. Human studies have shown that the MIC of voriconazole at which 90% of *Aspergillus fumigatus* isolates is inhibited is lower (1 mg/l, range 0.25–2.0 mg/l) than those of amphotericin B and itraconazole. Highly efficacious experimentally in prevention and treatment of *Aspergillus* endocarditis in guinea pigs and superior to itraconazole. Appears to be well tolerated in falcons

Antiprotozoal agents

Generic name	Trade name	Species	Route	Dosage	Remarks
Albendazole	Valbazen 113–116 mg/ml Suspension (SmithKline Beecham)	Ratites	PO	1 ml/50 lb body-weight b.i.d. for 3 d. Repeat in 2 weeks	For protozoal infections in ratites
Amprolium	Corid, Amprol plus (MSD, Ag Vet)	Raptors	PO	30 mg/kg daily for 5 d	Indicated for coccidiosis. Some coccidial strains of mynahs and toucans may be particularly resistant. Ideal for flock treatment
		Most species	PO	2–4 ml/gallon (5–100 mg/l) for 5–7 d	
Amprol	Coccoid 3.4% Solution (Harkers); Corid (MSD, Agvet)	Pigeons	PO	28 ml/4.5 l drinking water for 7 d, i.e. 25 mg/kg. Use half strength for extended regimen	Coccidiosis
Aminothiazole	Tricoxine (Fabry)	Pigeons	PO	5 ml/l drinking water for 7 d	Susceptible trichomonads, avoid overdosing
Carnidazole	Spartrix 10 mg tablets (Harkers, Wildlife Laboratories, Janssen)	Raptors Pigeons Psittacines	PO PO PO	20–25 mg/kg once 0.5–1 tablet once, e.g. 12.5–25 mg/kg 20–30 mg/kg once	Treatment for trichomonosis, hexamitiasis and histomoniasis. Highly effective as a single dose but use lower dose for juvenile birds. Use together with dimetridazole in rest of the loft, susceptible trichomonads. Has been used in other species, although single doses have not always been effective in falcons and in bustards with advanced infections in the Middle East; use with caution
Clazuril	Appertex (Harkers, Janssen)	Raptors Waterfowl	PO PO	5–10 mg/kg every 3rd day; give three times	Indicated for coccidiosis
		Pigeons	PO	1 tablet/bird single dose, e.g. 6.25 mg/kg	
		Psittacines	PO	7 mg/kg 3 d, 2 d off, 3 d on	
Co-trimazine (trimethoprim +sulfadiazine)	Cosumix Plus Soluble Powder (Ciba); Duphatrim Poultry Suspension (Solvay Animal Health); Bactrin (Roche)	Raptors	PO	60 mg/kg (combined constituents) b.i.d. 3 d on, 2 d off, 3 d on	Indicated for coccidiosis; do not use with dehydrated birds
		Waterfowl	PO	60 mg/kg (combined constituents) b.i.d. 3 d on, 2 d off, 3 d on	
	Duphatrim 24% Injection (Solvay Duphar)	Raptors	SC	30 mg/kg b.i.d. 3 d on, 2 d off, 3 d on	
		Waterfowl	SC	30 mg/kg b.i.d. 3 d on, 2 d off, 3 d on	
Chloroquine	Reschin R Tablet 500 mg (Bayer); Arlen (Winthrop)	Penguins	PO	10 mg/kg once then 5 mg/kg at 6, 18, 24 h	Primarily used to treat *Plasmodium* spp. usually in combination with primaquine. Overdose may result in death
Dimetridazole	Harkanka 40% Powder (Harkers); Emtryl Prescription (40%) Soluble Powder (Rhône-Mérieux)	Pigeons	PO	666 mg powder/l drinking water for 7–12 d	Soluble powder indicated for water treatment against gardiasis, trichomonosis and hexamitiasis. Also used at a dose of 2.5 g/kg food in bustards. Drug of choice for flock treatment of trichomonosis in bustards housed in naturalistic aviaries. Dimetridazole also has some activity against some anaerobic bacteria. Low therapeutic index. Toxic to Peking robin and some other Passeriformes. Very toxic if overdosed in parrots.
		Bustards	PO	3 g/10 l water for 10 d; prevention 9 g/10 l for 5 d followed by 7 g/10 l for 10 d	

Continued

Antiprotozoal agents (continued)

Generic name	Trade name	Species	Route	Dosage	Remarks
					Acute hepatitis reported in fledging birds. Recommended not to be given in the breeding season. No problems associated with use of this drug in bustards
Metronidazole	Flagyl Tablets (Rhône-Poulenc Rorer); Flagyl (Searle)	Raptors	PO	50 mg/kg daily for 3–5 d	Treatment of choice for trichomonosis in raptors. In severe cases repeat after 7 d upon completion of treatment
	Metronidazole 200 mg Tablets (Centaur); Flagyl (Searle)	Pigeons	PO	10 g powder/l drinking water for 5 d	Susceptible trichomonads; provides moderate control of hexamitiasis
	Metronidazole 25% Powder (Vetrepharm)	Pigeons	PO	100–150 mg in total for 5 d	
	Torgyl (Rhône Mérieux), Flagyl S Suspension (Rhône Poulenc Rorer); Flagyl (Searle)	Psittacines	PO IM	10–30 mg/kg b.i.d. for 10 d 10 mg/kg s.i.d.	Antiprotozoal
Pyrimethamine	Daraprim (Glaxo-Wellcome)	Raptors	PO	0.25–0.5 mg/kg b.i.d. for 30 d	Indicated for *Sarcocystis* spp., toxoplasmosis
		Waterfowl	PO	0.25–0.5 mg/kg b.i.d. for 30 d	
Pyrimethamine/ sulfaquinoxaline	Microquinox (C-Vet Livestock Products)	Waterfowl	PO	60 mg/l drinking water, 3 d on, 2 d off, 3 d on	Indicated for coccidiosis
Ronidazole	Ronidazole 10% Powder (BP)	Pigeons	PO	1 g powder/l drinking water for 6 d, e.g. 12.5 mg/kg/d	Indicated in the treatment of trichomonosis. Recommended flock treatment dose 60 g/100 l water for 5–7 d. Preventive dose 40 g/100 l water for 5–7 d
Sulfaquinoxaline/ pyrimethamine	Microquinox (Microbiologicals)	Psittacines	PO	15 ml/10 liters drinking water, 3 d on, 2 d off, 3 d on, 2 d off	Coccidiostatic
Sulfadimidine sodium 33.3%	Vesadin (Rhône Mérieux); Intradine (Norbrook); Bimadine (Bimeda)	Pigeons	PO	10–20 ml/l drinking water for 5 d (or 3 d on, 2 d off, 3 d on, 2 d off, 3 d on)	Coccidiosis. May be effective against toxoplasmosis
Tetracycline plus furaltadone		Pigeons	PO	400 mg tetracycline + 400 mg furaltadone/l drinking water for 7 d	Avoid in adults feeding young less than 10 d of age; indicated for trichomonosis and hexamitiasis
Toltrazuril	Baycox (Bayer, Bayvet)	Raptors	PO	10 mg/kg 3 times on alternate days or 15–25 mg/kg daily for 2 consecutive days	Treatment of choice for coccidiosis in falcons. Bitter taste. Mixing in equal parts (e.g. 1 ml to 1 l) with a soft drink (e.g. cola-based) prevents spitting of medication
Baycox 2.5%	Waterfowl Solution (Bayer, Baycox, Bayvet)	PO		1 ml of 2.5% solution/2 l drinking water for 48 h	
		Pigeons	PO	5 ml/l drinking water for 5 d, e.g. 10 mg/kg	

Anthelmintics

Generic name	Trade name	Species	Route	Dosage	Remarks
Chlorsulon	Curatrem (MSD, Agvet)	Raptors	PO	20 mg/kg 3 times at 2 week intervals	Control trematodes and cestodes
		Waterfowl	PO	20 mg/kg 3 times at 2 week intervals	
Cambendazole	Ascapilla 30 mg Capsules (Chevita); Equiben (MSD, Agvet)	Pigeons	PO	75 mg/kg on 2 consecutive days	Ascariasis and capillariasis
Doramectin	Dectomax 10 mg/ml injection (Pfizer)	Raptors Bustards	SC, IM	1 mg/kg	Used to treat alimentary tract nematodes, lungworms, eyeworms and mites
Febantel	Avicas 15 mg Tablets (Orthopharma) Rintal Suspension (Miles)	Pigeons	PO	37.5 mg/kg single dose	Ascariasis and capillariasis
Fenbendazole	Panacur 2.5% or 10% Liquid, 8 mg Capsules (Hoechst)	Raptors	PO PO PO	100 mg/kg once 20 mg/kg daily for 14 d 20 mg/kg daily for 5 d	Ascarids, some microfilariae, capillariasis, other nematodes, trematodes. May be effective against *Syngamus* spp.; not effective against the gizzard worms that infect finches. Can cause feather abnormalities during molt and also have adverse effect if used during the breeding season
	Panacur 2.5% or 10% Liquid, 8 mg Capsules (Hoechst)	Waterfowl	PO	20 mg/kg once	
	Panacur 8 mg Capsules (Hoechst)	Pigeons	PO	One capsule/pigeon > 8 weeks old, single dose	20–50 mg/kg daily for 5 d for capillariasis. Do not use during molt
	Panacur (Hoechst)	Psittacines	PO	15 mg/kg daily for 5 d; or 20–50 mg/kg once and repeat after 10 d	Medicate feed for 7 consecutive days. Broad-spectrum anthelmintic. Dosed according to bodyweight has produced no side effects in bustards
		Bustards	PO	30 mg/kg	Used, in addition to ivermectin treatment, to treat *Serratospiculum* spp. in falcons at a dose of approximately 20 mg/kg/d for 14 d. Dose of 60 mg/kg PO used in pheasants. Use all benzimidazole anthelmintics with care in molting birds – feather stunting has been reported in other species. Appears to be well tolerated by bustards
Levamisole	Levacide (Norbrook), Ripercol-L (American Cyanamid)	Raptors	SC PO PO	10–20 mg/kg once 20 mg/kg once 40 mg/kg once	Control nematodes, including *Capillaria* spp.
	Levacide 7.5% Injection (Norbrook)	Waterfowl	SC	25–50 mg/kg once	Low therapeutic index. Do not use in debilitated birds. Toxic if given parentally to finches Immunostimulant 2 mg/kg IM or SC every 14 d three times
		Pigeons	IM	0.1 ml once. Can repeat after 7 d	
			PO	5 m/l drinking water as sole source of water over 24 h. Repeat 7 d later	Loft treatment of capillariasis and ascariasis. Follow up to parenteral treatment
	Nilverm (Mallinckrodt); Lavasole (Pitman-Moore)	Psittacines	PO	Use 1:40 dilution of 7.5% solutions: 20–50 mg/kg (5–15 ml/4.5 l) for 1–3 d	Has a low therapeutic index, therefore beware use as a wormer
			IM or SC	2–5 mg/kg, repeated 10–14 d on 3 occasions as an immunostimulant	

Continued

Anthelmintics (continued)

Generic name	Trade name	Species	Route	Dosage	Remarks
Mebendazole	Mebenvet (Janssen); Telmin (Pitman–Moore)	Raptors	PO	20 mg/kg daily for 14 d	Broad-spectrum ovicidal anthelmintic but primarily use for capillaria. May be given by oral gavage but most commonly administered in the food of Galliformes and waterfowl. Toxic in pigeons, cormorants, finches and raptors. Has been associated with hepatitis in some mammals and raptors. Appears to be well tolerated by bustards
		Waterfowl	PO	5–15 mg/kg daily for 2 d	
			PO	120 ppm (1.2 g/tonne) in feed for 14 d	
Moxidectin	Imox Tablets 1000 μg/tablet (Vetafarm)	Raptors	PO	500 μg/kg	For the treatment of internal and external parasites by oral dosing. Drug recommended by J. Samour for the control of *Serratospiculum seurati*, *Capillaria* spp., *Acanthocephalan* spp., *Paraspiralatus sakeri* and *Psysaloptera alata* in falcons
Piperazine	Espelix Piperazine Citrate Elixir (BP) (750 mg/ml); Wazine 34 (Salisbury)	Pigeons	PO	1g/l drinking water (12.5 mg/kg)	Has been used for ascarids in gallinaceous birds. Not effective in psittacines and finches. Repeat the dose every 10–14 d
Praziquantel	Droncit 50 mg Tablets (Bayer, Bayvet), Droncit Injectable 56.8 mg/ml	Raptors	SC or PO / SC or PO	5–10 mg/kg once / 5–10 mg/kg for 14 d	Active against cestodes and trematodes. May need to repeat treatment 14 d after first dose
		Bustards Waterfowl	/ SC or PO / SC or PO	1 mg/kg / 10–20 mg/kg. Repeat after 10 d / 10 mg/kg daily for 14 d	Has been used in bustards. Cestodes are expelled within 24 h. Injectable form may be toxic in finches and has been associated with depression and death in some species. Appears to be well tolerated by bustards
		Psittacines	IM / PO / IM or SC	9 mg/kg / 10–20 mg/kg / 10 mg/kg daily for 3 d, then 10 mg/kg daily for 11 d PO	For tapeworms repeat after 10 d
		Pigeons	PO	20 mg/kg single dose	For flukes
Pyrantel	Strongid (Pfizer); Nemex (Pfizer)	Raptors Psittacines	PO / PO	20 mg/kg once / 4.5 mg/kg. For nematodes repeat after 10 d	Control of nematodes
Thiabendazole	Equizole 4 mg/30 ml Suspension, (MSD agent)	Most species	PO	250–500 mg/kg repeat 10–14 d / 100 mg/kg s.i.d for 7–10 d	Treatment for ascarids. For treatment of helminth parasites especially *Syngamus trachea*. Maybe toxic to cranes, ratites and diving ducks
Carbaryl	Sevin 5% Powder, (Southern Agricultural Insecticides, Inc.)	Most species	Topical	Light dusting on feathers	Recommended for ectoparasite control when lightly dusted on to feathers. Add 1–2 teaspoons, depending on size of box, to nesting material to control insects
Crotamiton	Eurax Cream 10% and Lotion 10%, (Westwood Squibb)	Psittacines	Topical	Apply to affected areas	Cnemidocoptic mite infestation
Cypermethrin	Dy-Sect (Deoson)	Raptors Psittacines	Spray	Dilute to 2% (avoid contact with bare skin)	Treatment of premises infested with *Dermanyssus* spp.
Cypermethrin 5% concentrated	Barricade (Lever)	Pigeons	Spray or dip	1:100 dilution	Lice, mites
Fipronyl	Frontline (Rhône Mérieux)	Raptors	Topical	Spray direct on to skin. One treatment usually sufficient. Repeat after 1 month if required	All ectoparasites. Beware drying action of alcohol on feather structure – may reduce durability of feathers

Ectoparasiticides

Generic name	Trade name	Species	Route	Dosage	Remarks
High-cis permethrin	Harker's Louse Powder (Harker, Generic)	Raptors	Topical application		Ectoparasite control
		Psittacines	Topical dusting		
Ivermectin	Ivomec 1% Cattle Injection (MSD, Agvet)	Raptors	SC	1–2 mg/kg. Repeat after 14 d	Some nematodes, feather mites, lice, *Cnemidocoptes* spp. May be effective also for some coccidia, microfilariae, *Syngamus* spp., *Capillaria* spp. and *Sternostoma* spp. Has been used undiluted in raptors by IM injection for the control of *Serratospiculum* spp. May be toxic when given by injection in some small birds, some finches and budgerigars. Appears to be well tolerated by bustards. Percutaneously used in canaries, finches and budgerigars. Control nematodes and nasal or duck leeches. Dilute 1.9 with sterile water and use 0.2 ml/kg. Active against nematodes, feather mites, lice and *Cnemidocoptes* spp. Repeat 7–10 d after first dose. Can also be administered topically or orally
		Psittacines	IM, SC, PO	200 µg/kg	Lice, mites
		Pigeons	IM	Dilute 1:9 in sterile water just before use. Give 200 µg (0.2 ml)/kg	
	Ivermectin 0.8% w/v in propylene glycol (Vetrepharm)	Pigeons	Topical	Apply one drop to the skin once a week for 3 weeks	
Malathion	Duramitex (Harkers, Generic)	Raptors	Paint or spray on to perches	Dilute to 0.93%	Treatment of premises infested with *Dermanyssus* spp.
Piperonyl butoxide/ pyrethrin	Ridmite Powder (Johnson)	Raptors	Topical dusting	Repeat after 3 weeks	Control lice, hippoboscids
		Psittacines	Topical	Apply to plumage. Repeat after 10 d	
Permethrin	Companion Flea Powder (Battle, Haywood & Bower, Generic)	Pigeons	Dusting powder		Fleas, lice
Permethrin/ piperonyl butoxide/ methoprene	Avian Insect Liquidator (Vetafarm)	Most species	Ready to use spray, concentrate	Apply to plumage, spray cages, aviaries, bird rooms and surroundings	Fleas, lice, mites, flies, mosquitoes, moths

Sedatives/tranquilizers/anesthetics

Generic name	Trade name	Species	Route	Dosage	Remarks
Alphaxalone/ Alphadalone	Saffan (Mallinckrodt)	Psittacines	IV–IM/IP	5–10 mg/kg /36 mg/kg	May cause a transient apnea
		Cranes, flamingoes, bustards	IV	4–8 mg/kg	Surgical anesthesia lasts for 8–10 min Practical and effective for short surgical procedures e.g. surgical sexing
Atipamezole	Antisedan (Pfizer)	Psittacines	IM	250–380 µg/kg	Used to reverse xylazine or medetomidine
Diazepam	Valium (Roche)	Raptors	IV or IM	0.5–1 mg/kg b.i.d. or t.i.d. as required	Control of fits
		Waterfowl	IV or IM	0.5–1 mg/kg b.i.d. or t.i.d., as required	
Halothane	Halothane (Rhône Mérieux), Flouthane (Mallinckrodt; Fort Dodge)	Psittacines	Inhalation agent		Slower recovery than with isoflurane, marked respiratory depression, moderate myocardial depression. Metabolism is impaired with liver disease, in particular fatty liver in obese captive birds
Isoflurane	Isoflo (Mallinckrodt) Isoflurane (Abbots Laboratories); Aerrane (Anaquest)	Raptors Psittacines	Inhalation anesthetic Inhalation agent		Anesthetic of choice in avian species
Sevoflurane	Ultane (Abbot)	Psittacines Raptors	Inhalation anesthetic		Expensive, requires specific vaporizer. Induction and recovery faster than isoflurane
Ketamine	Ketaset (Willows Francis); Vetalar (Upjohn); Ketaset (Fort Dodge/Aveco); Ketalar (Parke-Davies)	Raptors	PO	100 mg/kg in a 30 g piece of meat	Sedation to capture an escaped bird
			IM	5–30 mg/kg	Reversible anesthetic in combination with medetomldine
		Psittacines	IV, IM or SC	20–50 mg/kg	Ketamine on its own does not produce good muscle relaxation nor adequate analgesia
Medetomidine	Domitor (Pfizer)	Raptors Psittacines	IM IM	150–350 µg/kg 60–85 µg/kg	Reversible anesthetic (by equal volume of Antisedan) in combination with ketamine. Use atipamezole to reverse
Midazolam	Hypnovel (Roche); Versed (Roche)	Raptors	IV or IM	0.5–1 mg/kg t.i.d.	Control of fits; shorter duration than diazepam
		Psittacines	IM or SC	0.2 mg/kg	For use in combination with ketamine
Propofol	Rapinovet (Mallinckrodt); Diprivan (Stuart)	Psittacines	IV	1.33 mg/kg	Useful to induce anesthesia
Tiletamine/ zolazepam	Telazol (Robins; Fort Dodge)	Psittacines	IM	5–10 mg/kg	Provides good immobilization
Xylazine	Rompun (Bayer, Miles); Virbaxyl, (Virbac)	Raptors Psittacines	IM or IV IV or IM	1–2.2 mg/kg 1–2.2 mg/kg	Xylazine in combination with ketamine (1:3 or 1:5) is still widely used in raptors by many veterinarians in developing countries. Its effect can be reverse using yohimbine hydrochloride 0.1–0.2 mg/kg IV

Topical preparations

Generic name	Trade name	Species	Route	Dosage	Remarks
Oil of proflavine	Proflavine Cream (Loveridge)	Most species	Topical	Apply to wounds s.i.d. or b.i.d. to effect	Very safe. Stimulates granulation. May cause yellow coloration of urates
Povidone-iodine	Pevidine Surgical Scrub (BK); Vetasept (Animalcare)	Most species	Topical	Apply and wash off after 3 min	Very safe cleansing agent for open wounds
Propylene glycol, malic acid, benzoic acid, salicylic acid	Dermisol (Pfizer)	Most species	Topical	Apply s.i.d. or b.i.d. to effect	Removes skin debris, scabs and crusts. Antiseptic properties. Very safe
Sodium fusidate	Fucidin	Most species	Topical	Apply sparingly b.i.d. to effect	Antibacterial, particularly against Staphylococcus spp. infections Useful for mild/early bumblefoot and other skin lesions. Reported to penetrate intact skin
Sodium fusidate /hydrocortisone	Fucidin H (Leo)	Raptors	Topical	Apply sparingly b.i.d. to effect	Antibacterial, particularly against Staphylococcus spp. infections plus anti-inflammatory action. Reported to penetrate intact skin. Excess application will cause polydipsia

Miscellaneous

Generic name	Trade name	Species	Route	Dosage	Remarks
Aciclovir	IV Solution Powder, 200 mg Capsule, 50 mg/ml, 40 mg/ml Suspension, Gel (Zovirax, Burroughs, Wellcome)	Most species	PO, IM, IV Topical	80 mg/kg t.i.d. up to 240 mg/kg of food	Muscle necrosis if given IM. Phlebitis and neurologic signs if given IV. Has been shown to affect sperm development and fetal development in mammals. Herpesvirus DNA polymerase inhibitor. Use to control Pacheco's disease virus. Most effective when administered before clinical signs occur. Also suggested that it can be used topically in pox virus infections
Activated charcoal	Forgastrin (Arnolds); Toxiban (Vet-A-Mix)	Psittacines	PO	2–8 g/kg as required	Used to absorb ingested toxins, including insecticides, heavy metals and chemotherapeutic agents from the alimentary tract. Can be mixed with hemicellulose to act as a bulk laxative and aid in the passage of ingested toxins
Aloe vera, sodium lauryl sulfate, sodium dodecyl and benzene sulfonate	Bird Rain (Avian Care Products)	Cage and aviary birds	Topical	Spray on to feathers	Revitalize skin and feathers
Aloe vera, ammonia solution	Soother Ointment (Avian Care Products)	Cage and aviary birds	Topical	Apply on to affected areas	Promote healing of skin irritation and superficial lesions. Do not use in birds with kidney disorders
Allopurinol	Zyloric (Glaxo-Wellcome)	Psittacines	PO	Dissolve one 100 mg tablet in 10 ml water – 1 ml of diluted solution/ 30 ml drinking water	Used to treat gout. Well absorbed from the gut. Functions to inhibit purine catabolism, which prevents the formation of uric acid. Provide fresh drinking water and ensure that birds are well hydrated
Aminoloid	Aminoloid (Schering)	Raptors	IM	0.25–0.75 mg/kg repeat 10–14 d	Induction of molt in raptors
Aminopentamide hydrogen sulfate	Centrine Injectable Solution (Aveco)	Most species	IM, SC	0.05 mg/kg b.i.d. 5 doses maximum	Antiemetic. Antidiarrheal, slows gastrointestinal motility
Amitryptyline	Lentizol (Upjohn); Elavil (Stuart)	Psittacines	PO	1–5 mg/kg s.i.d. or b.i.d.	Behavior modifier. Useful with some feather pluckers
Apple cider vinegar	Apple Cider Vinegar (organic) (Avian Care Products)	Cage and aviary birds	PO	1 teaspoonful per pint of water as the sole drinking water for 10–14 d	Helps restore normal intestinal flora. Control of many Gram-negative bacterial and yeast problems
Atropine	Atropine Injection (C-Vet)	Raptors	IV or IM	0.1 mg /kg every 3–4 h	Acetylcholinesterase poisoning, e.g carbamates. Not recommended as preanesthetic in avian species. Thicker respiratory secretions, which may block endotracheal tube. Used in organophosphate poisoning in avian species. Does not dilate pupils in avian species
		Waterfowl	IV or IM	0.1 mg/kg every 3–4 h	
		Psittacines	IM or SC	0.05 mg/kg repeat hourly	
Avipro	Contains *Lactobacillus*, *Streptococcus*, *Saccharomyces*, electrolytes, trace minerals and vitamins, amylase, cellulase and proteases (Vetark)	Psittacines, raptors, bustards	PO	1 scoop/200 ml water; for stressed birds use 1 scoop/100 ml	Probiotic combination of bacteria, enzymes, electrolytes and vitamins. Highly palatable. Can be added to drinking water
Avipro Paediatric	Contains *Lactobacillus*, *Streptococcus*, *Saccharomyces*, amylase, cellulase and proteases	Psittacines, raptors, bustards	PO	1/4 teaspoon per 60 g food	An enzyme and probiotic blend for hand-rearing or feeding convalescent birds. Use Avipro starter packs at 6 h of age to start the chick off

Continued

Miscellaneous (continued)

Generic name	Trade name	Species	Route	Dosage	Remarks
Biotin	Biotin Tablets (Arnolds); (Generic)	Raptors	PO	50 μg/kg daily for 30–60 d	Aid in beak or claw regrowth
Bismuth subsalicylate	Bismuth Subsalicylate Oral Suspension 1.75% subsalicylate	Most species	Oral	2 ml/kg b.i.d.	For gastrointestinal irritation. May help to remove ingested toxins
Brewer's yeast	Dried Yeast Tablets BP 300 mg (Lloyds Chemists)	Pigeons	PO	1 tablet crushed over feed/10 birds/d during the molt	For the treatment of brittle feathers if suspected to be nutritional in origin
Buprenorphine	Vetergesic (Animalcare); Buprenex (Norwich Eaton)	Psittacines	IV or IM	0.1 mg/kg b.i.d.	Anti-inflammatory and analgesic
Butorphanol	Torbugesic (Willows Francis); Torbutrol (Bristol Laboratories)	Psittacines	IV or PO	3–4 mg/kg t.i.d.	Anti-inflammatory and analgesic. Use with caution in liver-compromised patients
Calcium gluconate or borogluconate 10%	Various Calcium Sandoz Injection (10 ml Ampoules) (Sandoz, SmithKline Beecham, Fort Dodge)	Raptors Pigeons	IV or SC SC or slow IV	1–5 ml/kg slowly, once 0.1–0.2 ml (25–50 mg)/kg injection	Initial treatment of hypocalcemia, hypocalcemic fits and egg binding. Also useful for bone healing
	Calcium borogluconate 20%, Calcibor CBG20 (Arnolds)	Psittacines	IV or IM	0.5–1 ml/kg	
	Calcium gluconate 20% (Sandocal, Sandoz, SmithKline Beecham, Fort Dodge)	Psittacines	IV IM or SC	50–100 mg/kg slowly to effect 5–10 mg/kg b.i.d. as required	
Carprofen	Zenecarp (C- Vet)	Psittacines	IV, IM or SC	2–10 mg/kg s.i.d.	Nonsteroidal anti-inflammatory drug with analgesic and antipyretic properties. Used in mammals for the control of postoperative pain and inflammation following orthopedic and tissue surgery (including intraocular surgery). Second dose can be administered 24 h after the first
Cisapride	Propulsid (Janssen)	Psittacines	PO	0.5–1.5 mg/kg t.i.d.	Used to stimulate gastrointestinal motility
Clofazimine	Lamprene Tablets (Geigy)	Raptors	PO	1–5 mg/kg s.i.d. for 3 months to 1 year	Tuberculosis in combination with enrofloxacin, cycloserine and ethambutol. Beware zoonotic risk of M. avium infection
Clomipramine	Anafranil (Geigy, Baker Cummings)	Psittacines	IM	0.5–1 mg/kg s.i.d. or b.i.d.	Behavior modifier
Copper sulfate	Caustic Powder 51% (Phoenix Butler)	Most species	Topical	Apply to affected area as needed	Treatment of cases of ulcerative dermatitis
Cycloserine	Seromycin Pulvules (Lilly)	Raptors	PO	5 mg/kg b.i.d. for 3 months to 1 year	Tuberculosis in combination with enrofloxacin, cyclofazamine and ethambutol. Beware zoonotic risk of M. avium infection
Dandelion	Dandelion root (Avian Care Products)	Cage and aviary birds	PO	Mix 5 drops in 1/2 oz lactulose and use 1 drop/ 100 g bodyweight b.i.d.	Liver stimulant
D-penicillamine	Distamine (Dista); Cuprimine (Merk); Depen (Wallace); Titratabs (Wallace)	Raptors Waterfowl	PO PO	55 mg/kg b.i.d. for 7–14 d 55 mg/kg b.i.d. for 7–14 d	Heavy metal poisoning, e.g. copper, lead, zinc
Diclophenac	Voltarol 25 mg Tablets (Geigy)	Pigeons	PO	12.5 mg as a single dose	Arthritis
Dimercaprol	Bal Injectable Solution 100 mg/ml (Becton Dickinson)	Most species	PO	25–35 mg/kg b.i.d. 5 d per week for 3–5 weeks	Painful injections IM. Less toxic and better at reducing blood lead levels than calcium EDTA

Continued overleaf

Miscellaneous (continued)

Generic name	Trade name	Species	Route	Dosage	Remarks
Doxepin	Sinequan (Pfizer,	Psittacines	PO	0.5–1 mg/kg	Behavior modifier. Useful in some feather pluckers
D-tubocurarine	D-tubocurarine Solution 3 mg/ml	Raptors	Ophthalmic drops	Every 5 min × 3 times	Mydriatic
Dimethylsulfoxide	Fluvet DMSO (Univet); DOMOSO (Syntex)	Pigeons, raptors	Topical application		A method of reducing swelling and a vehicle for carrying some antibiotics and anti-inflammatories into difficult-to-reach sites of infection, particularly in the hock and foot region. Avoid contact with human skin
Dinoprost	Lutalyse (Upjohn)	Raptors	Topical	0.02–0.1 mg/kg on to cloacal mucosa, once	Egg binding
		Waterfowl	IM or topical	0.02–0.1 mg/kg on to cloacal mucosa, once	
		Psittacines	IM or per cloacum	0.02–0.1 mg/kg once	
Doxapram	Dopram Injection (Willows Francis, Fort Dodge)	Raptors	IV	10 mg/kg once	Respiratory stimulant. Reversal of respiratory depression associated with overdose of general anesthetic, hypnotic and sedative drugs. Speed up recovery from ketamine/xylazine anesthesia. Be aware with excessive doses hyperventilation may lead to cerebral vasoconstriction and cerebral hypoxia
	Dopram Injection (Willows Francis, Robins)	Waterfowl	IV	10 mg/kg once	
	Dopram–V (Willows Francis, Fort Dodge)	Psittacines	IV or IM	5–10 mg/kg once	
Echinacea	Echinacea Solution (Biobotanica) Echinacea (Avian Care Products)	Cage and aviary birds	PO	2.5 drops/kg 5 d/cup of water Mix 5 drops in 1/2 oz lactulose and use 1 drop/100 g bodyweight b.i.d.	Immunostimulant especially in viral infections. Holistic use
EDTA-TRIS	Lysozyme Solution Mix 3.07 g Trizma HCl, 3.17 g Trizmabase, 1.12 g disodium EDTA in 100 ml water	Most species	Topical	Used intratracheally, intranasally or for wound lavage	Helps antibiotics penetrate bacterial wall
Electrolytes, vitamins, amino acids, dextrose	Duphalyte (Solvay Duphar)	Psittacines, raptors, bustards	IV, SC, PO	10 ml/kg	Indicated for the prevention and treatment of dehydration, electrolyte imbalance and hypoproteinemia. Administer SC in the groin or administer PO by stomach tube. Use very slow IV
Electrolyte solution	Tyrode's Solution (Avian Care Products)	Cage and aviary birds	PO	Add envelope to 1 quart drinking water. Use as sole source of drinking water	Electrolyte imbalance, cases of polyuria and polydipsia.
Epinephrine	Epinephrine injection 1:1000 epinephrine (Elkins-Sinn)	Most species	IV, IO, IT, IC	Emergency drug. Dilute with 10 parts Lactated Ringers Solution and use 0.5–1.0 ml/kg.	Clinical indications for attempts to restore cardiac function in cases of peracute death from anesthesia. Use drug with caution in birds. The therapeutic index for this drug is low
Ethambutol	Myambutol Tablets (Lederle)	Raptors	PO	20 mg/kg b.i.d. for 3 months to 1 year	Tuberculosis in combination with enrofloxacin, cyclofazamine and cycloserine. Beware zoonotic risk of *M. avium* infection.
Essential fatty acid	Dermplus Liquid (C-Vet)	Raptors	PO	0.5 ml/kg daily for 50 d or indefinitely	Pruritic dermatitis (atopy)
	Vetreplume (Vetrepharm)	Pigeons	PO	5 ml per 1 kg feed once weekly	Improve feather quality

Continued

Miscellaneous (continued)

Generic name	Trade name	Species	Route	Dosage	Remarks
Ferric subsulfate	Monsel's Solution, liquid or powder	Most species	Topical	As needed to stop bleeding, especially after nail trim	May cause feather cysts if applied into damaged follicles
Fluoxetine	Prozac (Dista)	Psittacines	PO	0.4 mg/kg s.i.d.	Antidepressant. Useful in some feather pluckers
Flunixin	Finadyne (Schering-Plough); Bonamine (Schering-Plough)	Raptors	IM	1–10 mg/kg s.i.d. for 1–5 d only	Potent nonsteroidal non-narcotic analgesic agent with anti-inflammatory, anti-endotoxic and antipyretic properties. Not recommended to treat for more than 5 consecutive days in mammals. Reported to cause vomiting
		Psittacines	IM	1–10 mg/kg	
Furosemide	Lasix Injection (Hoechst)	Raptors	IM	1.5 mg/kg q.i.d. as required	Diuretic. Beware of overdose, which causes dehydration and electrolyte abnormalities. Toxic reactions characterized by neurological signs and death
		Psittacines	IM, SC	0.15–2 mg/kg, s.i.d. or b.i.d.	
Goldenseal	Goldenseal (Avian Care Products)	Cage and aviary birds	PO	Mix 5 drops in 1/2 oz lactulose and use 1 drop/100 g bodyweight b.i.d.	Immune stimulation. Short term use only, i.e. < 5 d
Glucose polymer	Energix (Vetrepharm)	Pigeons	PO	15 g/l drinking water for 4 d	Racing pigeon tonic
Glucose 5%	Aquapharm No. 6 (Animalcare)	Most species	IV, SC or PO	50 mg/kg (1 ml/kg)	Isotonic solution. Useful in the treatment of hypoglycemia and dehydration. IV slowly
Haloperidol 2 mg/ml solution	Dozic (RP Drugs); Haldol (Henry Schein)	Psittacines	PO	0.4 mg/kg s.i.d.	For feather plucking
Heparin	Heparin sodium 25 000 IU/ml (Leo Labs)	Most species	IV		Use for flushing IV locks and IV catheters. Use diluted at 100 IU/ml in saline for flushing. Heparin therapy should be given with caution to patients about to undergo surgery and those with impaired renal or hepatic function
Hyaluronidase	Hyalase, 150 IU/ml (CP Pharmaceuticals)	Most species		150 IU/l fluids	Increases the rate of absorption of subcutaneous fluids
Iodine and trace minerals	Budgie Builder (Avian Care Products)	Cage and aviary birds	PO	Dilute content to 1 gallon of water. Use as only source of drinking water	Nutritional supplement
Iodine	Lugols	Psittacines	PO	2 parts iodine + 28 parts water – add 3 drops to 100 ml drinking water	For treatment of goiter in budgerigars
Iron dextran	Vet Iron Injection (Animalcare, Butler, Lextron, Vedco)	Raptors	IM	10 mg/kg. Repeat after 1 week if required	Hemopoiesis
		Waterfowl	IM	10 mg/kg. Repeat after 1 week	
		Psittacines	IM	10 mg/kg, repeat in 7–10 d as required	
Isoxsuprine	Navicox (Univet)	Raptors	PO	5–10 mg/kg s.i.d. for 20–40 d	Wing-tip edema, dry gangrene syndrome
Kaolin	Kaogel (Upjohn); Koalin (Vet-A-Mix, Evsco)	Psittacines	PO	2 ml/kg b.i.d. or t.i.d	For treatment of nonspecific diarrhea
Ketoprofen	Ketofen (Rhône Mérieux) (Fort Dodge/Aveco)	Raptors	IM	1 mg/kg s.i.d. for 1–10 d	Pain relief, arthritis. Anti-inflammatory and analgesic
		Waterfowl	IM	1 mg/kg s.i.d. for 1–10 d	
	Ketofen 1% Injection (Rhône Mérieux, Fort Dodge/Aveco)	Pigeons	IM or SC	0.1 ml s.i.d. or b.i.d. on two consecutive days	
		Psittacines	IM	2 mg/kg	

Continued overleaf

Miscellaneous *(continued)*

Generic name	Trade name	Species	Route	Dosage	Remarks
Lactated Ringer's solution	Hartmann's Solution, Aquapharm No. 11 (Animalcare)	Most species	IV, IO or SC	10 ml/kg/min	Calculate fluid deficit from PCV. Give over 2–d period plus 50 ml/kg/d. Give the calculated daily requirement in 4 equal volumes during the day
Lactulose	Duphalac (Solvay Duphar); Cephulac (Marion Merrell Dow)	Psittacines	PO	0.2–0.4 mg/kg t.i.d.	Can be administered for a period of many weeks. To decrease toxin absorption from the alimentary tract and/or CNS symptoms from liver damage, stimulate appetite and improve intestinal flora
Leuprolide acetate	Lupron (TAP Pharmaceutical)	Cockatiels	IM	0.375 mg/kg once	Prevention of ovulation
Lipoform Tabs	Lipoform Chewable Tablet (Vet-A-Mix)	Most species	PO	500 mg s.i.d.	Prevent liver damage in face of viral infection
Liquid iron	Ferripar (Vetrepharm)	Pigeons	PO	2 ml per 2 kg feed daily for 3 d, then once weekly	Racing pigeon tonic
Magnesium sulfate crystals	Magnesium Sulfate (various)	Raptors	PO	0.5–1 g/kg s.i.d. for 1–3 d	Increase gut motility to aid passage of lead if present in intestine
		Waterfowl	PO	0.5–1 g/kg s.i.d. for 1–3 d	
Medroxy-progesterone	Promone–E (Upjohn)	Psittacines	IM or SC	5–50 mg/kg every 4–6 weeks: 150 g bird – 0.05 mg/g; 300–700 g bird – 0.03 mg/g; > 700 g bird – 0.025 mg/g	Used for excessive egg production, especially in cockatiels. Can cause lethargy, inappetence, polydipsia and fatty liver syndrome
Meloxicam	Metacam 1.5 mg/ml Suspension (Boehringer Ingelheim)	Most species	PO	0.2 mg/kg s.i.d.	Nonsteroidal anti-inflammatory drug with analgesic and antipyretic properties. Used in mammals for the control of postoperative pain and inflammation following orthopedic and tissue surgery (including intraocular surgery)
	Metacam 5 mg/ml Injection (Boehringer Ingelheim)		IM, SC		
Metoclopramide	Emequell (Pfizer);	Raptors	IV or IM	2 mg/kg t.i.d. as required	Anti-emetic. Control of gastrointestinal stasis, e.g. sour crop
	Reglan (Robins)	Waterfowl	IV or IM	2 mg/kg t.i.d. as required	
		Psittacines	IM, IV or PO	0.5 mg/kg, repeat q.8 h as required	
Milk thistle	Milk Thistle (Avian Care Products)	Cage and aviary birds	PO	Mix 5 drops in 1/2 oz lactulose and give 1 drop/ 100 g bodyweight b.i.d.	Supports and protects the liver and helps restore liver function. Antioxidant
Minerals/ vitamin B$_1$	Vetreplex (Vetrepharm)	Pigeons	PO	10 g per 3.5 l drinking water once weekly	Nutritional supplement
Monoglycerides of edible fatty acids in organic denude oil	Booster (Avian Care Products)	Cage and aviary birds	PO	1 drop of the liquefied product/ 100 g bodyweight	Stimulant of immune system
Naltrexone	Nalorex (Du Pont); Trexan (Du Pont)	Psittacines	PO	1.5 mg/kg b.i.d.	An opioid antagonist used to prevent self-mutilation
Nandrolene laurate	Laurabolin 50 mg/ ml (Intervet)	Psittacines, raptors, bustards	IM or SC	0.4 mg/kg once	Testosterone derivative recommended as part of treatment after chronic and debilitating diseases. Give every 3 weeks. Can cause liver disease
N-butyl-cyanoacrylate	Vet-Seal Tissue Adhesive (Braun)	Topical			Surgical glue. Indicated for the closure of skin wounds, surgical incisions, mucosa in oral surgery and skin punctures. Useful for closing incision following surgical pinioning of young birds

Continued

Miscellaneous *(continued)*

Generic name	Trade name	Species	Route	Dosage	Remarks
Nutrobal	Per gram, 200 mg Ca, 150 IU Vitamin D$_3$ and other vitamins and minerals (Vetark)	Psittacines, raptors, bustards	PO	Sprinkle on food at a rate of 1 pinch/kg of animal being supplemented	Calcium balancer and multivitamin supplement to help during growth and breeding in all birds. High potency: do not exceed normal levels
Oseltamivir phosphate	Tamiflu (Roche)	Bustards	PO	8–10 mg/kg b.i.d.	Antiviral agent active against influenza virus in humans. Has been used in white-bellied bustards by one of us (T.A.B.) with confirmed avian influenza. Clinical signs resolved and no side effects were observed
Organic denude oil	Sunshine Factor (Avian Care Products)	Cage and aviary birds	PO	1 teaspoon of the liquefied product with 1 lb of food	Indicated for dry flaky skin, balding feet, lack of sheen and improper feather color, especially in older birds
Oxyglobin	Hemoglobin glutamer-200 (Oxyglobin, Biopure)	Raptors	IV	10 ml/kg once	Provides oxygen-carrying support to dogs, improving clinical signs of anemia for at least 24 h, independent of the underlying conditions. Has been used as a one-off treatment in anemic falcons
Oxytocin	Oxytocin S (Intervet); Oxytocin (Leo, Butler, Lextron, Vedco)	Raptors Waterfowl Psittacines	IM IM IM	3–5 IU/kg 3–5 IU/kg 0.01–0.1 ml/kg once	For egg expulsion for cases of uncomplicated uterine stasis. Should be administered in conjunction with injectable calcium gluconate. Should not be used in cases where there is mechanical obstruction or damage to the reproductive tract
Pedialyte	Pedialyte (Abbott Laboratories): water, dextrose, sodium chloride, potassium citrate and sodium citrate	Most species	PO		Pedialyte is used in the maintenance of body water and electrolytes in neonatal birds with mild or moderate diarrhea and dehydration
Penicillamine	Distamin (Dista); Cuprimine (Merk)	Psittacines	PO	50–55 mg/kg b.i.d.	Chelating agent that binds copper, zinc, mercury and lead
Phenobarbital	Phenobarbital Poythress	Psittacines	PO	0.003 mg/g (e.g. 3 mg/kg) b.i.d.	Used in cases of feather plucking. May cause deep sedation and inability to perch
Plasma substitute	Haemaccel 3.5% Colloid Infusion (Hoechst)	Most species	IV	10 ml/kg	Indicated as a plasma volume substitute in cases of hypovolemic shock caused by hemorrhage, burns, water and electrolyte loss from persistent vomiting or diarrhea. Should be administered IV in a volume approximately equal to the estimated blood loss to restore circulatory volume
Poly-Aid	Poly-Aid Nutrient Supplement (Vetafarm)	Psittacines, raptors, bustards	PO	10 g/100 g bodyweight/d in 2 divided doses	A sustained release of carbohydrate and protein supplement with vitamins and electrolytes for debilitated birds. Add 5 ml water to 10 g Poly-Aid and make into a slurry
Pralidoxime chloride	Protopam (Wyeth-Ayerst)	Raptors	IM	100 mg/kg. Repeat once after 6 h	Organophosphate and acetylcholinesterase poisoning, e.g. carbamates. Contact National Poisons Bureau regarding availability
Pralidoxime mesylate	Mesylate (Ayerst); Protopam (Wyeth-Ayerst)	Waterfowl Psittacines	IM IM	100 mg/kg. Repeat once after 6 h 100 mg/kg, repeat once after 6 h	Organophosphate and acetylcholinesterase poisoning, e.g. carbamates
Prednisolone	Prednicare (Animalcare); Solu-Delta-Cortef (Upjohn)	Psittacines	PO	2 mg/kg b.i.d.	Anti-inflammatory and analgesic
Pyrimethamine	Daraprim (Glaxo-Wellcome)	Psittacines	PO	0.5 mg/kg b.i.d.	For treating *Plasmodium* spp., *Sarcocystis* spp. and *Toxoplasma* spp.
Propentofylline	Vivitonin (Hoechst)	Raptors	PO	5 mg/kg b.i.d. for 20–40 d	Wing-tip edema, dry gangrene syndrome
Sodium bicarbonate	8.4% Sodium Bicarbonate 1 mEq/ml (Abbott Laboratories)	Most species	IV	1 mEq/kg q.15–30 min to a maximum of 4 mEq/kg total dose	Emergency drug. Used to treat severe metabolic acidosis. Contraindicated in respiratory and metabolic alkalosis

Continued overleaf

Miscellaneous (continued)

Generic name	Trade name	Species	Route	Dosage	Remarks
Sodium chloride	Aquapharm No.1 (Animalcare) 0.9% sodium chloride	Psittacines, raptors, bustards	SC, PO or IV	50 ml/kg/d for maintenance	To correct water and electrolyte depletion. Indicated in severe vomiting of acute onset, or where lodgement of foreign bodies interferes with ingestion, e.g. where there is vomiting and/or endotoxic shock. Sodium overload may occur in cases with myocardial or renal damage
Sodium chloride and glucose	Aquapharm No.3 (Animalcare) sodium chloride 9 g and anhydrous glucose 50 g	Psittacines, raptors, bustards	IV, SC or PO	50 ml/kg/d for maintenance	For the treatment of dehydration to correct water and electrolyte depletion where the patient's carbohydrate store is considered to be depleted
Sodium lactate solution	Aquapharm 11 (Animalcare) sodium chloride 6.0 g, potassium chloride 0.4 g, calcium chloride dihydrate 0.27 g and molar sodium lactate 28.9 g	Psittacines, raptors, bustards	IV, SC or PO	50 ml/kg/d for maintenance	Give to severely diseased patients with diarrhea, dehydration and vomiting to combat metabolic acidosis. Sodium overload may occur in cases with myocardial and renal damage
Sodium calciumedetate	Strong (Animalcare); Calcium Disodium Versenate (3M Pharmaceuticals)	Raptors	IV or IM	10–40 mg/kg b.i.d. for 5–10 d	Lead and other heavy metal poisoning such as copper, lead and zinc. Dilution not required Up to 100 mg/kg b.i.d. IM has been used in falcons without any deleterious effect
		Waterfowl	IV or IM	10–40 mg/kg b.i.d. for 5–10 d	
		Psittacines	IV or IM	20–40 mg/kg b.i.d. for 5 d	
Soluble multivitamins	Duphasol (Solvay Duphar)	Pigeons	PO	1 g/l drinking water for 5–7 d or 1 day per week	Support in infectious disease. Nutritional dermatitis
Soluble multivitamins	Soluvet (Vetafarm)	Psittacines, raptors, bustards	PO	4 g in 400 ml water 1 g in 100 ml food	Support in infectious diseases, stress
Spark	Spark Carbohydrate and Oral Electrolyte Supplement (Vetafarm)	Psittacines, raptors, bustards	PO (water)	3 g/150 ml water	High-calorie electrolyte for use in birds that need extra energy and body salts. Use before birds are to be translocated and give for 3 d before and 2 d after any move
Stanozolol	Winstrol V Tablet, Injectable Solution 50 mg/ml	Most species	IM	25–50 mg/kg	Increases weight gain in anorectic cases. Monitor patients with hepatic or renal problems. May not achieve desired results
Thiamine	Thiamine Compound Tablets (Rhône Poulenc Rorer, Generic)	Raptors	PO	1–50 mg/kg s.i.d. for 7 d or indefinitely	For control of thiamine-responsive fits
Tolfenamic acid	Tolfedine 4% injectable (Vetoquinol)	Raptors	IM, SC	2–4 mg/kg	Nonsteroid anti-inflammatory drug with analgesic and antipyretic properties
Triamcinolone/ neomycin/ thiostrepton/ nystatin	Panalog Ointment (Ciba)	Pigeons	Topical	1 drop into the eye b.i.d. for 3–5 d	Conjunctivitis, 'one eyed cold'
Thyroxine	Soloxine Tablets (Vet-2-Vet, Butler)	Raptors	PO	Birds weighing 750–1000 g, e.g. female red-tailed hawk: 25 µg s.i.d. for 7 d 50 µg s.i.d. for 7 d 75 µg s.i.d. for 7 d 50 µg s.i.d. for 7 d 25 µg s.i.d. for 7 d	Stimulate molt. Scale dose up or down by up to 50% for larger or smaller birds
		Psittacines	PO	0–100 µg/kg b.i.d., (ie. 0.025 mg/100 ml water) for 4 weeks	Used to induce molt and treat hypothyroidism

Miscellaneous (continued)

Generic name	Trade name	Species	Route	Dosage	Remarks
Testosterone	Androject (Intervet, Henry Schein, Upjohn)	Psittacines	IM	8 mg/kg weekly as required	Use with great care. Usually contraindicated. May affect spermatogenesis
Vitamin A avian	Various injectable preparations	Raptors	IM	Maximum 20 000 IU/kg weekly as required	Hypovitaminosis A. To increase skin healing, e.g. in bumblefoot. Supplemental therapy for pox infections, sinusitis and ophthalmic disorders
Vitamin A, D, E	Various injectable preparations	Psittacines	IM	0.1–0.2 ml (10 000–20 000 IU)/300 g, weekly as required	Useful in the treatment of vitamin A + D deficiencies, reproductive disorders and bone healing
Vitamin B complex	Various injectable preparations	Raptors	IM	Sufficient to give 10–30 mg/kg of thiamine. Repeat weekly as required	Stimulate appetite. General health, neuromuscular disease, hepatic disorders. Control of thiamine responsive fits
		Psittacines	IM	To give 1–3 mg thiamine/kg every other day	
Vitamin B$_{12}$	Cyano (Bimeda); Cyanocobalamin (Butler)	Psittacines	IM	250–500 µg/kg weekly	Indicated in anemias and convalescence. Has been reported to produce pink droppings in other species but this has not been observed in bustards
Vitamin E/selenium	Dystosel (Upjohn); Seletoc (Schering–Plough)	Raptors	SC	0.05 mg selenium + 3.4 IU vitamin E. Repeat once after 72 h	Vitamin E/selenium deficiency. For prevention and treatment of muscular weakness, capture myopathy. Given to birds before transportation during translocation procedures
Vitamin E	Dystosel (Intervet); Seletoc (Schering–Plough)	Psittacines	IM	0.06 mg/kg weekly	
Vitamin K	Konakion (Roche, Butler, Phoenix, Vet-A-Mix)	Most species	IM	0.2–2.5 mg/kg daily as required	For hemorrhagic disorders and to prevent such problems when amprolium and sulfa drugs are administered or after long-term tetracycline treatment
Yeast Cell Derivatives	Preparation H Ointment (Whitehall Laboratories)	Most species	Topical	As needed	Stimulate epithelial healing, especially abrasions and lacerations

Vaccines

Generic name	Trade name	Species	Route	Dosage	Remarks
Canary pox virus strain Herzberg vaccine	Poulvac P Canary (Duphar, Holland)	Houbara bustards	Topical (wing-web)		Recommended for use in houbara bustards following research at the National Wildlife Research Center, Taif, Saudi Arabia
Newcastle Disease Vaccine–Living	NDV Hitchner B1 (Living)	Bustard chicks	Intraocular or intranasal	1–2 drops	For the primary vaccination of young growing bustards at 4, 8 and 20 weeks. Does not result in detectable serum hemagglutinating antibodies in bustards
Newcastle Disease Vaccine–Inactivated	Newcavac Nobilis (Inactivated)	Bustards	SC	1.0 ml/kg	For the secondary vaccination of bustards. Administered at 32 weeks of age. Must be used only when birds have been primarily vaccinated with NDV Hitchner B1 living vaccine. Annual vaccination will result in detectable serum HI antibodies. Response after 14 d
Paratyphoid vaccine	Bespoke– (Specialist Laboratories)	Pigeons	IM	Usually 0.25 ml	Persistent loft problem with paratyphoid
Pigeon pox vaccine	Pigeon Pox Vaccine (Living) Nobilis (Intervet, Vetrepharm)	Pigeons, falcons	Topical	Topical application on to 6–8 exposed feather follicles	Pigeon pox. Vaccinate on lower legs. Pluck 6–8 feathers and stretch skin to open feather follicles. Brush vaccine on to open follicles. For routine prophylaxis, vaccinate young birds before racing: vaccinate old birds at least 6 weeks before pairing. Vaccinated birds are infectious until the vaccine lesions have healed. Vaccinate every year in early autumn.
PMV-1 Vaccine	Colombovac PMV (Solvay Duphar)	Pigeons	SC	0.2 ml	PMV-1. Choose vaccination site carefully. Avoid vascular trauma
	Hartavac (Harkers) Nobi-Vac Paramyxo (Intervet, Vetrepharm)		SC SC	0.2 ml 0.25 ml	
Reovirus vaccine	Nobilis Reo inac Intervet International, France)	Bustards	SC		Inactivated reovirus vaccine used in some bustard collections
Psittimune PDV (Pacheco's disease vaccine, killed virus)	Biomune Co	Psittacines	SC, IM		Susceptible psittacine birds prior the breeding season, before fledging, during quarantine or prior to exposure to other psittacines
Psittimune APV (Avian polyomavirus vaccine, killed virus)	Biomune Co	Psittacines	SC	Dose rate for larger birds 200 g is 0.5 ml. Dose for birds < 200 g is 0.25 ml	Susceptible psittacine birds prior the breeding season, during quarantine or prior to exposure to other psittacines. Young birds are vaccinated at 5 weeks of age
Poximune C (Canary pox vaccine, modified live virus)	Biomune Co	Canaries	Wing web method	0.01 ml per bird	Susceptible canaries at least 4 weeks old

Sources:
Anonymous (1995) Compendium of Data Sheets for Veterinary Products 1995–1996. National Office of Animal Health, Enfield, Middlesex.
Bailey TA (1999) A contribution to preventive medicine and therapeutics of avian captive breeding programmes with special reference to the houbara bustard (Chlamydotis undulata macqueenii). PhD Thesis, Durrell Institute of Conservation and Ecology, University of Kent, Canterbury.
Bailey TA (2002) Aspergillosis: therapy and prevention in zoo animals with emphasis on birds. Falco 20: 18–22.
Bailey TA, Sullivan T (2001) Aerosol therapy using a novel disinfectant to treat upper and lower respiratory tract infections in birds. Exotic DVM Magazine 3: 17.
Bailey TA, Samour JH, Sheen RS, Garner AG (1996) Analysis of amoxicillin in houbara bustard plasma by HPLC after administration of a long-acting formulation. Journal of Veterinary Pharmacology and Therapeutics 19: 313–315.
Bailey TA, Sheen RS, Silvanose C et al. (1998) Clinical pharmacology and pharmacokinetics of enrofloxacin after intravenous, intramuscular and oral administration in houbara bustard (Chlamydotis undulata macqueenii). Journal of Veterinary Pharmacology and Therapeutics 21: 288–297.
Bailey TA, Manvell R, Gough RE et al. (2001) A review of Newcastle disease in bustards: presentation, diagnosis and control; results of vaccination trials. Proceedings of the European Association of Avian Veterinarians, Munich, pp. 202–207.
Bonn, Flammer K, Aucoin DP, Whitt DA (1991) Intramuscular and oral disposition of enrofloxacin in African grey parrots following single and multiple doses. Journal of Veterinary Pharmacology and Therapeutics 14: 359–366.
Carpenter JW, Mashima TY, Rupiper DJ (2001) Exotic Animal Formulary. WB Saunders, Philadelphia.
Clubb SL (1986) Therapeutics. In: Harrison GJ, Harrison LR (eds) Clinical Avian Medicine and Surgery, pp. 327–355. WB Saunders, Philadelphia.
Coles BH (1997) Avian Medicine and Surgery, 2nd edn, pp. 240–279. Blackwell Science, Oxford.
Debuf Y (1991) Veterinary Formulary. Pharmaceutical Press, London.
Di Somma A, Bailey TA (2003) Aspergillosi: la malattie che sfida i veterinari aviari [Aspergillosis: the challenging disease]. Proceedings of SIVAE, Rome.
Dorrestein GM (1991) The pharmacokinetics of avian therapeutics. Veterinary Clinics of North America: Small Animal Practice 21: 1241–1263.
Dorrestein GM (1993) Antimicrobial drug use in pet birds. In: Prescott JF, Baggot JD (eds) Antimicrobial Therapy in Veterinary Medicine, pp. 490–506. Iowa

Continued

Vaccines (continued)

Generic name	Trade name	Species	Route	Dosage	Remarks

State University Press, Ames, IA.

Dorrestein GM, Van Miert ASJAM (1988) Pharmacotherapeutic aspects of medication of birds. *Journal of Veterinary Pharmacology and Therapeutics* **11**: 33–44.

Dorrestein GM, Verburg E (1988) Pharmacokinetics of enrofloxacin (Baytril) in homing pigeons after different administration routes. *Proceedings of the Fourth Congress of the European Association for Veterinary Pharmacology and Toxicology*, Budapest, p. 172.

Flammer K (1993) An overview of antifungal therapy in birds. *Proceedings of the Association of Avian Veterinarians*, Nashville, pp. 1–4.

Forbes NA, Harcourt-Brown NH (1996) Formularies. In: Forbes NA, Harcourt-Brown N (eds) *Manual of Raptors, Pigeons and Waterfowl*, pp. 334–352. British Small Animal Veterinary Association, Cheltenham.

Greth A, Gerlach H, Gerbermann H, Vassart M, Richez P (1993) Pharmacokinetics of doxycycline after parenteral administration in the houbara bustard (*Chlamydotis undulata*). Avian Diseases **37**: 31–36.

Heidenreich M (1997) Clinical therapy. In: *Birds of Prey Medicine and Management*, pp. 91–101. Blackwell Science, Oxford.

Krautwald-Junghanns ME (1991) Avian therapeutics. In: *Proceedings of the European Association of Avian Veterinarians*, Vienna, pp. 30–39.

Lawrence K (1988) Therapeutics. In: Price CJ (ed.) *Manual of Parrots, Budgerigars and other Psittacine Birds*, pp. 175–176. British Small Animal Veterinary Association, Cheltenham.

McDonald SE (1989) Summary of medications for use in psittacine birds. *Journal of the Association of Avian Veterinarians* **3**: 124–127.

Martínez MR, Diaz MJ, Fernández-Cruz ML et al. (1997) Pharmacokinetics of marbofloxacin in broiler chickens after intravenous administration. *Journal of Veterinary Pharmacology and Therapeutics* **20**(Suppl 1): 197.

Michell AR (1994) Small animal fluid therapy 1. Practice principles. *Journal of Small Animal Practice* **35**: 559–565.

Michell AR (1994) Small animal fluid therapy 2. Solutions and monitoring. *Journal of Small Animal Practice* **35**: 613–619.

Michell AR (1998) Oral rehydration for diarrhoea: symptomatic treatment or fundamental therapy. *Journal of Comparative Pathology* **118**: 175–193.

Naldo JL, Bailey TA, Samour JH, (2000) Trichomonosis: a review of clinical pathology and control in bustard collection. In: *Proceedings of the European Association of Zoo and Wildlife Veterinarians*, Paris, pp. 347–352.

Ostrowski S, Dorrestein G, Burger L et al. (1996) Cross-protection of an avian poxvirus isolated from houbara bustards. *Avian Diseases* **40**: 762–769.

Plumb DC (2002) *Veterinary Drug Handbook*, 4th edn. Iowa State University Press, Ames, IA.

Pokras MA, Karas AM, Kirkwood JK, Sedgwick CJ (1993) An introduction to allometric scaling and its uses in raptor medicine. In: Redig PT, Cooper JE, Remple JD, Hunter DB (eds) *Raptor Biomedicine*, pp. 211–224. University of Minnesota Press, Minneapolis.

Pugh DM (1991) Blood formation, coagulation and volume. In: Brander GC, Pugh DM, Bywater RJ, Jenkins WL (eds) *Veterinary Applied Pharmacology and Therapeutics*, pp. 166–186. Baillière Tindall, London.

Redig P (1984) Fluid therapy and acid-base balance in the critically ill avian patient. In: *Proceedings of the Association of Avian Veterinarians*, Boulder, pp. 59–74.

Ritchie BW, Harrison GJ (1994) Formulary. In: Ritchie BW, Harrison GJ, Harrison LR (eds) *Avian Medicine: Principles and Application*, pp. 457–478. Wingers Publishing, Lake Worth, FL.

Robertson EL (1991) Farmaci antinematodici. In: Booth NH, McDonald LE (eds) *Farmacologia e Terapeutica Veterinaria Italia*, 6th edn. Iowa State University Press, Ames, IA.

Rosskopf WJ, Woerpel RW (1991) Practical avian therapeutics with dosages of commonly used medications. *Veterinary Clinics of North America: Small Animal Practice*, **21**: 1265–1271.

Rupiper DJ, Carpenter JW, Mashima TY (2000) Formulary. In: Olsen GH, Orosz SE (eds) *Manual of Avian Medicine*, pp. 553–589. Mosby, St Louis.

Rupley AE (1997) Formulary. *Manual of Avian Practice*, pp. 502–518. WB Saunders, Philadelphia.

Sedgwick CJ (1993) Allometric scaling and emergency care: the importance of body size. In: Fowler ME (ed.) *Zoo and Wildlife Medicine: Current Therapy 3*, pp. 34–37. WB Saunders, Philadelphia.

Tully TN (1997) Formulary. In: Altman RB, Clubb SL, Dorrestein GM, Quesenberry K (eds) *Avian Medicine and Surgery*, pp. 671–688. WB Saunders, Philadelphia.

ACKNOWLEDGMENTS

We are grateful to Dr. Paolo Zucca from the Laboratory of Animal Cognition and Comparative Neuroscience, Department of Psychology, University of Trieste, Italy for providing most of the information on antiparasitic drugs.

Index

ultimobranchial glands 302, 304
ultrasonography 103–12, *104*
    approaches 104–6, *105, 106*
    equipment 104
    examination procedure 104–6
    organs and organ systems 107–12
    patient preparation 104–6
Unopette™ 365851 system 43
Unopette™ 365877 system 46
upper gastrointestinal tract biopsy *71*
upper respiratory tract swabs 65
Upupa epops 473
Upupiformes 473
urates 31, *76*
urea 53, 54, *56, 175*
uric acid *53,* 54, *56,* 112, 269
urinalysis 60, *61*
urinary system, post-mortem 406, *406*
urine
    collection of 60
    color and consistency *61*
urogenital system, ultrasonography 106,
        110–12, *111*
urography 84
uropygial gland *23,* 156, 397, *397*
uterine torsion 160
uveitis 205, *205*

vaccination
    avian infectious laryngotracheitis 372
    avian pox 368
    Marek's disease 371
    metabolic drug scaling 180–2, *181*
    Newcastle disease 363
    vaccines *508*
vacuolation *40*
Vacutainer 62–3
vaginoscopes 123
Vanellus
    armatus 462
    spinosus 471
vapor-permeable adhesive film (MVP)
        dressings *198*
vaporizers 140, *140*
vasectomy, endoscopic 126–7
vasotocin 305
vecuronium bromide 205–6
vent gleet 296

ventilation 29
ventilation triggers 139
ventriculitis, traumatic 291
ventriculotomy 161
ventriculus *see* gizzard
Vernier measuring device *22*
villous atrophy 294
Vini
    australis 467
    peruviana 467
viral infections 358–60, *374*
    hepatic 298
    intestinal 293–4
    see also specific infection
virological examination *65,* 409
visceral gout 299, *299*
vitamin A *58, 278, 458, 507*
vitamin B$_1$ *58, 458, 505, 507*
vitamin B$_2$ *58, 458*
vitamin B$_6$ *58, 458*
vitamin B$_{12}$ *58–9, 458, 507*
vitamin B complex *507*
vitamin C *59, 459*
vitamin D 256, *507*
vitamin D$_3$ *58, 278, 458*
vitamin E *58, 458, 507*
vitamin K *58, 458, 507*
vitamins 54–7, *58–9, 502*
    summary of changes in levels of *458–9*
    toxic effects *278*
vitreous hemorrhage 205, 206
volatile anaesthesia 139–45
volvulus 294
vomitoxin 277, *277*
voriconazole 386, 387, *493*
vulture
    Egyptian *421, 465, 469*
    European black *465*
    griffon *460, 465*
    king *469*
    turkey *421*
Vulture gryphus 469

waders, handling and restraint *12*
water intake 174, *174*
waterfowl
    handling and restraint *12*
    transport of 14

weighing *21,* 21–2, *22*
wet pox 285, *366, 367*
wet vent 296
white blood cells (WBC) *32,* 35, *43*
    count 46, *46*
        absolute 47–9
        differential 47–9
        morphological and staining
            characteristics of 47, *47*
widgeon, European *see Anas* spp.
wing twitch 145
wings
    angel wing 258, 261
    bandaging *193, 194*
    clipping 191–2, *191–2*
    deformities 258
    examination 23
    feather classification *188*
    fracture *208,* 208–9, *209*
        physical therapy 246, *246–7*
    luxation *208,* 208–9
    tip injuries *208,* 208–9, *209,* 253
woodcock, Eurasian *471*
woodpecker, greater spotted *473*
wounds 249–54, *250–1*
    assessment of 195
    closed 249, 252
    healing of 252
    open 249, 252
    treatment of 156, 195–9, 252–4
    wing tip 208

X-ray unit 79
xanthoma 157
xylazine 145, *146, 147, 499*
xylazine hydrochloride 4

Yeast Cell Derivatives *507*
Yersinia pseudotuberculosis 350, 350
yersiniosis 293, *350,* 350–1
yolk sacculectomy 162

Zenaidura macroura 3, *3, 445*
zinc *53, 57,* 274–5, *275*
zinc gluconate 127
zolazepam 4, *147, 499*
Zoletil 4
zygomycosis 285